PRINCIPLES AND PRACTICE OF PHARMACOLOGY FOR ANAESTHETISTS

This book is dedicated to our wives

Principles and Practice of Pharmacology for Anaesthetists

T. N. CALVEY BSc, MD, PhD (Liverpool), FRCA
Honorary Senior Research Fellow, Department of Anaesthesia,
University of Liverpool;
Honorary Consultant, Whiston Hospital

N. E. WILLIAMS MB, ChB (Liverpool),
FFARCS (England) Consultant Anaesthetist, Whiston Hospital;
Part-time Lecturer in Clinical Pharmacology
University of Liverpool

FOREWORD BY

JACKSON REES MB, ChB, FFARCS
Formerly Honorary Director of Studies (Paediatric Anaesthesia)
and Clinical Lecturer, Department of Anaesthesia
University of Liverpool

THIRD EDITION

Blackwell
Science

Editorial Offices:
Osney Mead, Oxford OX2 0EL
25 John Street, London WC1N 2BL
23 Ainslie Place, Edinburgh EH3 6AJ
350 Main Street, Malden
MA 02148 5018, USA
54 University Street, Carlton
Victoria 3053, Australia
10, rue Casimir Delavigne
75006 Paris, France

Other Editorial Offices:
Blackwell Wissenschafts-Verlag GmbH
Kurfürstendamm 57
10707 Berlin, Germany

Blackwell Science KK
MG Kodenmacho Building
7–10 Kodenmacho Nihombashi
Chuo-ku, Tokyo 104, Japan

First published 1982
Second edition 1991
Reprinted 1995
Third edition 1997
Reprinted 1998, 2000

Set by Setrite Typesetters, Hong Kong
Printed and bound in the United Kingdom at the University Press, Cambridge

For further information on Blackwell Science, visit our website:
www.blackwell-science.com

DISTRIBUTORS

Marston Book Services Ltd
PO Box 269
Abingdon Oxon OX14 4YN
(*Orders*: Tel: 01235 465500
Fax: 01235 465555)

USA
Blackwell Science, Inc.
Commerce Place
350 Main Street
Malden, MA 02148 5018
(*Orders*: Tel: 800 759 6102
781 388 8250
Fax: 781 388 8255)

Canada
Login Brothers Book Company
324 Saulteaux Crescent
Winnipeg, Manitoba R3J 3T2
(*Orders*: Tel: 204 837-2987)

Australia
Blackwell Science Pty Ltd
54 University Street
Carlton, Victoria 3053
(*Orders*: Tel: 3 9347 0300
Fax: 3 9347 5001)

A catalogue record for this title is available from the British Library

ISBN 0–632–04156–0

Library of Congress
Cataloging-in-Publication Data

Calvey, T.N.
Principles and practice of pharmacology for anaesthetists/T.N. Clavey, N.E. Williams; foreword by Jackson Rees. — 3rd ed.
p. cm.
Includes bibliographical references and index.
ISBN 0-632-04156-0
1. Anesthetics. 2. Pharmacology.
I. Williams, N. E. (Norton Elwy) II. Title.
[DNLM: 1. Anesthetics — pharmacology.
QV81 C167p 1997]
RD82.C34 1997
615′.1′024617 — dc20 96-20973

Contents

Foreword to the First Edition

A book with a title such as this might be thought merely to present an account of the drugs used in anaesthesia. In this case, the authors have achieved much more. They have presented their subject in such a way as to give their reader an insight which will make him not only a more competent anaesthetist, but one who will derive more satisfaction from his work by a more acute perception of the nuances of drug administration.

The authors demonstrate their awareness of the unique nature of anaesthesia amongst the disciplines of medicine. This uniqueness arises from the necessity of the anaesthetist to induce in his patient a much more dramatic attenuation of a wide range of physiological mechanisms than colleagues in other disciplines seek to achieve. He must also produce these effects in such a way that their duration can be controlled and their termination may be acute. The anaesthetist may be called upon to do this on subjects already affected by diseases and drugs which may modify the effects of the drugs which he uses. To be well-equipped to meet these challenges he needs a knowledge of the factors influencing the response to and elimination of drugs, and of the mechanisms of drug interaction. Such knowledge is much more relevant to anaesthesia than to most other fields of medicine. The authors of this book have striven successfully to meet the need of anaesthetists for a better understanding of these basic mechanisms of pharmacology. This is illustrated by the fact that one-third of the work is devoted to these principles. This should relieve the teacher of the frustration of having students who seem always to produce answers on the effects of drugs, but respond to the question 'Why?' with a stony silence.

Those sections of the book which deal with specific drugs show the same emphasis on mechanisms of action, thus giving life to a subject whose presentation is so often dull. The trainee who reads this book early in his career will acquire not only a great deal of invaluable information, but also an attitude and approach to the problems of his daily activity which will enhance the well-being of his patients and his own satisfaction in his work.

Jackson Rees

Preface

In the 5 years since the publication of the second edition, a number of new drugs have been introduced into anaesthesia. In many instances accepted explanations for the mode of action of some drugs have been modified or revised. In the present edition, the authors have attempted to reflect these developments and present a topical, readable and practical account of drugs which have an important role in current practice.

All the existing chapters have been extensively revised and updated, although the general layout of the book remains unchanged. A new chapter on the important topic of drug isomerism has been introduced. We hope that the book will be of value to candidates preparing for the FRCA examination and also provide a useful reference for all anaesthetists. We are pleased to acknowledge the help and advice of Dr John O'Shea in the preparation of Chapter 16. The artistic help of Mrs Pamela Williams is also much appreciated. We are grateful to Dr Brenda Phillips for the electromyogram reproduced in Fig. 10.5.

Chapter 1
Drug Absorption, Distribution and Elimination

Drugs can be defined as agents that modify biological responses, and thus produce pharmacological effects. These effects are usually determined by their transfer across one or more cellular membranes. The rate and extent of this process are dependent on the structure and the physicochemical properties of the cell membrane. Most cell membranes are approximately 10 nm wide, and consist of a bimolecular layer of phospholipids and cholesterol with intercalated molecules of protein (Fig. 1.1). The bimolecular layer of lipid is generally regarded as fluid, and its components are free to move in the lateral plane of the membrane by the exchange of one molecule for another. Some protein molecules are permanently incorporated within the phospholipid membrane (intrinsic or integral proteins); others are situated on the internal or external aspects of the membrane, and can be removed by changes in pH or ionic strength (extrinsic or peripheral proteins). Intrinsic proteins often cross the entire width of the plasma membrane (i.e. from the internal to the external aspect), and may consist of an annulus surrounding small pores or ion channels approximately 0.5 nm in diameter (Fig. 1.1). In capillary endothelial cells the diameter of these pores or ion channels is considerably greater (i.e. 4–5 nm), and intercellular spaces are usually present. Both intrinsic and extrinsic proteins can act as enzymes or receptors, or mediate the active transport of drugs.

Approximately 5–10% of the cell membrane consists of carbohydrates, which are mainly present on the external aspect as glycolipids or glycoproteins. They are believed to be responsible for the immunological characteristics of cells, and play an important part in molecular recognition. In addition, there are inorganic constituents in many cellular membranes (e.g. calcium ions), which are associated with negatively charged groups on phospholipids and cholesterol.

The lipid plasma membrane is an excellent electrical insulator. Consequently, there may be differences in electrical potential across cellular membranes, which can facilitate or impede the transport of charged molecules through ion channels.

Transfer of drugs across cell membranes

In general, drugs cross cell membranes by three main methods:

1 Simple diffusion.

2 Non-ionic diffusion.

3 Carrier transport.

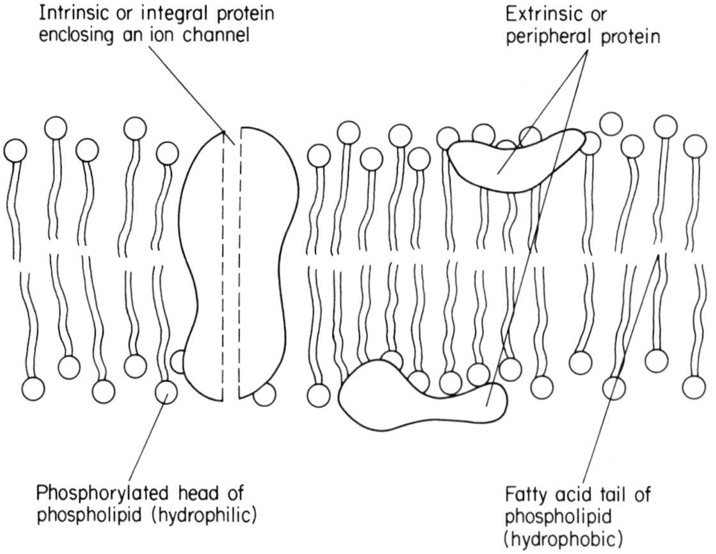

Fig. 1.1 A typical cell membrane.

Simple diffusion

Simple diffusion can be defined as the movement of molecules from a higher concentration to a lower concentration, due to the random molecular movement that results from thermal energy. Consequently, any drug that can dissolve in the membrane can cross the cell by diffusion. Simple diffusion is an entirely passive process that depends on differences in the concentration of drugs across cellular membranes; for any given drug, the rate of diffusion is directly proportional to the concentration gradient across the membrane (Fick's law of diffusion).

The diffusion of drugs also depends on the permeability of cellular membranes (i.e. the ability to dissolve in the membrane). Since cell membranes consist of a biomolecular layer of lipid, differences between the diffusion of drugs are usually related to their lipid solubility; molecular size is a factor of lesser importance.

Most lipid-soluble drugs (e.g. diazepam, fentanyl) readily dissolve in membrane phospholipids and rapidly diffuse into cells. Drugs with a lower lipid solubility (e.g. morphine) diffuse less readily. The diffusion of poorly lipid-soluble drugs (e.g. quaternary amines) across cells is usually restricted by the permeability barrier imposed by the phospholipid cell membrane. Some polar, small molecular weight drugs may diffuse through ion channels or pores, which are generally considered to be associated with intrinsic membrane proteins. Alternatively, they may penetrate small intercellular or paracellular channels (particularly in 'leaky' epithelial membranes). The permeability of vascular endothelium is greater than other tissues, and most ionized compounds can readily cross capillary membranes.

Non-ionic diffusion

Drugs that are weak acids (e.g. salicylates, probenecid, barbiturates) or weak bases (e.g. many opioid analgesics, local anaesthetics, antihistamines) are present in aqueous solutions (and in physiological conditions) in both an ionized and a non-ionized form. The ionization or dissociation can be expressed as the equations:

$AH \rightleftharpoons A^- + H^+$ (for acids)

and

$BH^+ \rightleftharpoons B + H^+$ (for bases)

and is obviously influenced by pH; weak acids and bases are predominantly present as the species AH and BH^+ in acidic conditions, but as A^- and B in alkaline conditions. Only the non-ionized forms AH and B have high lipid solubility, and can readily diffuse across cell membranes. The ionized forms A^- and BH^+ are effectively impermeable, and cannot readily cross the membrane. Since the proportion of the drug that is present in the non-ionized form is dependent on pH, differences in H^+ concentration across cellular membranes can provide a diffusion gradient for the passive transfer of the non-ionic fraction.

Consider a weakly acidic drug that dissociates in the manner:

$AH \rightleftharpoons A^- + H^+$

From the Henderson–Hasselbalch equation, it can be shown that:

$$pK_a - pH = \log\frac{[AH]}{[A^-]},$$

where [AH] and $[A^-]$ are the concentrations of the non-ionized and the ionized forms, and the constant pK_a (the negative logarithm of the dissociation constant) is the pH value at which $[AH] = [A^-]$. If the pK_a of the drug is 6, at pH 2 (e.g. in gastric fluid), almost 100% is present in the form AH (Fig. 1.2). This non-ionized form will rapidly diffuse into plasma (pH 7.4) where approximately 96% will be converted to A^-, providing a concentration gradient for the continued diffusion of AH. Subsequent transfer of the drug to other sites will also be dependent on the relative pH gradient. At pH 8 (e.g. in interstitial fluid or alkaline urine), the concentration of AH is less than at pH 7.4. In this manner, a gradient is created for the passive diffusion of AH across renal tubular epithelium, followed by its subsequent ionization to A^- and elimination from the body (Fig. 1.2). By contrast, at a urine pH of 7 or less, the concentration of AH is greater in urine than in plasma, and the excreted drug will tend to back-diffuse from urine to plasma.

In a similar manner, pH gradients govern the non-ionic diffusion of weak bases which associate with hydrogen ions in the manner:

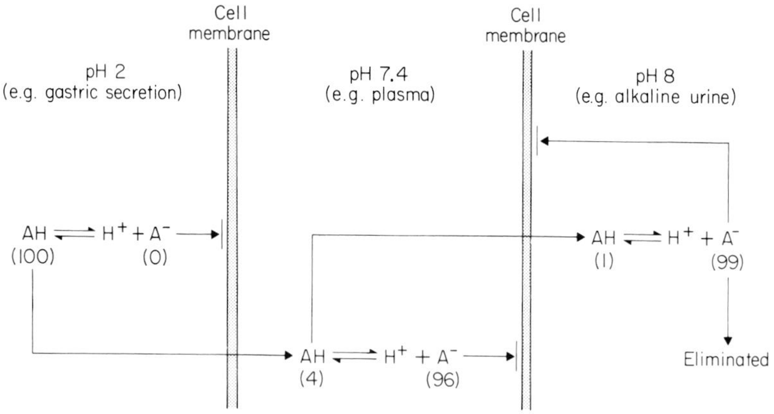

Fig. 1.2 Non-ionic diffusion of the weak acid AH ($pK_a = 6$). Only the non-ionized form AH can diffuse across cell membranes; the diffusion gradient is dependent on pH differences in compartments or tissues. Numbers in parentheses correspond to the percentage of the drug present as AH and A^- at pH 2, 7.4 and 8.

$$B + H^+ \rightleftharpoons BH^+$$

From the Henderson–Hasselbalch equation, it can be shown that:

$$pK_a - pH = \log\frac{[BH^+]}{[B]},$$

where $[BH^+]$ and [B] are the concentrations of the ionized and the non-ionized forms, and pK_a is the pH value at which $[BH^+] = [B]$. If the pK_a of the basic drug is 7, at pH 2 (e.g. in the stomach), almost 100% is present as the ionized, poorly lipid-soluble form BH^+ (Fig. 1.3); even at pH 5.5 (e.g. in the small intestine) only 3% is present as the non-ionized species B, and is available to diffuse across the cell membrane. Although the effective pH gradient does not facilitate the non-ionic diffusion of weak bases from the small intestine (pH 5.5) to plasma (pH 7.4), the continuous perfusion of intestinal capillaries provides a small concentration gradient for their absorption.

By contrast, weak bases at pH 7.4 (e.g. in plasma) are mainly present as the non-ionized species B. In these conditions, there is a large concentration gradient that facilitates their diffusion into the stomach (pH 2) and into acid urine (pH 5). After intravenous injection of the opioid analgesics fentanyl and phenoperidine, the initial decline in plasma concentration is followed by a secondary peak 30–40 min later. Both these weak bases are initially eliminated from plasma to the stomach, due to the large concentration gradient in favour of diffusion; their subsequent reabsorption from the small intestine is responsible for the secondary rise in the plasma concentration. Similarly, weak bases rapidly diffuse from plasma (pH 7.4) to urine (pH 5) as the non-ionized species B, where they are converted to the ionic form BH^+ and rapidly eliminated (Fig. 1.3).

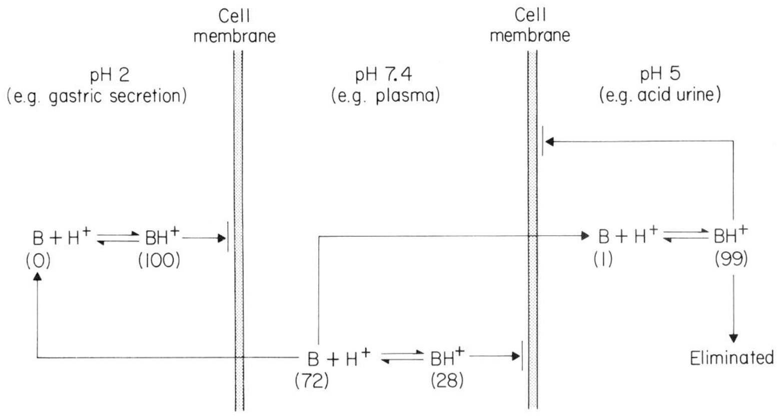

Fig. 1.3 Non-ionic diffusion of the weak base B ($pK_a = 7$). Only the non-ionized form B can diffuse across cell membranes; the diffusion gradient is dependent on pH differences in compartments or tissues. Numbers in parentheses correspond to the percentage of the drug present as B and BH^+ at pH 2, 7.4 and 5.

In theory, modification of urine pH can increase the proportion of weak acids ($pK_a = 3.0$–7.5) and weak bases ($pK_a = 7.5$–10.5) that are present in an ionized form in urine, and thus enhance their elimination in drug-induced poisoning. In practice, forced alkaline or acid diuresis has a limited applicability; it is only of value when toxic drugs are: (i) non-protein-bound; (ii) confined to extracellular fluid; and (iii) mainly eliminated unchanged in urine. Unfortunately, many acid and basic drugs are extensively metabolized, and have a large volume of distribution that is consistent with their significant sequestration in tissues. In these conditions, only small amounts of the unchanged drug are eliminated in acid or alkaline urine, and the amount of drug available for diffusion from plasma is relatively limited. In addition, forced diuresis is a potentially hazardous procedure, since it requires the infusion of relatively large amounts of fluid and the use of loop diuretics or mannitol to maintain a significant urinary output. Pulmonary and cerebral oedema are possible complications (particularly in elderly subjects). Nevertheless, forced alkaline diuresis is sometimes used in the management of salicylate and phenobarbitone overdosage, and in poisoning with the pesticides 2,4-D (2,4-dichlorophenoxyacetic acid) and mecoprop. Acid diuresis is only rarely of value, but may be used in amphetamine, fenfluramine and phencyclidine poisoning.

Carrier transport

Drugs may also cross cellular membranes by carrier transport, which is generally assumed to be mediated by intrinsic membrane proteins. In general, carrier transport is unidirectional, saturable, relatively specific, and can be inhibited (competitively or non-competitively) by other drugs. Carrier transport may occur through membrane channels in intrinsic proteins; alternatively, it may involve temporary combination with specific membrane components in the cell membrane. There are two main types of carrier transport: facilitated diffusion and active transport.

Facilitated diffusion is a type of carrier transport that does not require the expenditure of cellular energy, either as adenosine triphosphate (ATP) or as an electrochemical gradient. Many molecules of physiological importance enter cells down a concentration gradient, but at a faster rate than anticipated from their lipid solubility or molecular size (i.e. more rapidly than expected by simple diffusion). Facilitated diffusion is responsible for the absorption of some simple sugars, steroids, amino acids and pyrimidines from the small intestine, and for their subsequent transfer across cell membranes (e.g. in muscle and red blood cells). It is probably related to the combination of these substrates with specific sites on intrinsic proteins, followed by conformational (allosteric) changes which facilitate their transport to the opposite side of the membrane.

In contrast, active transport requires cellular or metabolic energy, and can transfer drugs against a concentration gradient. In some instances, metabolic energy is directly produced from the hydrolysis of ATP (primary active transport). More commonly, metabolic energy is provided by the active transport of Na^+ ions, or is dependent on the electrochemical gradient produced by the sodium pump, Na^+/K^+ ATPase (secondary active transport). It is generally considered that the drug or substrate initially combines with an intrinsic carrier protein (which may be an ion channel or Na^+/K^+ ATPase); the drug–protein complex is then transferred across the cell membrane, where the drug is released and the carrier protein returns to the opposite side of the membrane.

Active transport systems are widespread and ubiquitous, and play an important part in the transport of drugs across cell membranes at many sites (e.g. the small intestine, the proximal renal tubule, the biliary canaliculus and the choroid plexus). They are often concerned with the transfer of endogenous substances (e.g. neurotransmitters) across cellular membranes; for example, the uptake of noradrenaline by Uptake_1 at sympathetic nerve endings is coupled to the active transport of Na^+.

Active transport also plays an important role in the elimination of acids and bases from the body. In the proximal renal tubule many acidic and basic drugs are eliminated from plasma by active transport; in consequence, their renal clearance is greater than glomerular filtration rate. Competition between weak acids for proximal tubular secretion may be responsible for drug interactions; for example, the inhibition of urate secretion by diuretic drugs can induce acute gout, and probenecid affects the elimination and the plasma concentration of benzylpenicillin. Basic drugs, including some quaternary amines that are used in anaesthesia (Table 1.1), are eliminated by a separate active transport system in the proximal renal tubule. Both systems can be competitively or non-competitively inhibited by different drugs.

Acidic and basic drugs or conjugates may also be eliminated by active transport from the liver cell to the biliary canaliculus (Table 1.2). In general, drugs or conjugates

Table 1.1 Common acidic and basic drugs eliminated from plasma by active transport in the proximal renal tubule.

Acidic drugs	Basic drugs
Cephalosporins	Choline
Chlorpropamide	Dopamine
Ethacrynic acid	Histamine
Frusemide	Lignocaine
Glucuronide conjugates	Morphine
Indomethacin	Neostigmine
Methotrexate	Pyridostigmine
Oxyphenbutazone	Quinidine
Penicillins	Quinine
Probenecid	Thiamine
Salicylates	
Sulphate conjugates	
Sulphinpyrazone	
Spironolactone	
Sulphonamides	
Thiazide diuretics	

Table 1.2 Common acidic and basic drugs secreted from liver cells into biliary canaliculi.

Acidic drugs	Basic drugs
Amoxycillin	Alcuronium
Ampicillin	Dimethyltubocurarine
Bromosulphonphthalein	Glycopyrrolate
Cephaloridine	Mepenzolate
Glucuronide conjugates of many drugs	Pancuronium
Phenol red	Pipenzolate
Probenecid	Tubocurarine
Radiographic contrast media	Vecuronium
Rifampicin	
Sulphate conjugates of many drugs	

with a molecular weight of above 400 are eliminated in bile by a process of active secretion that is probably dependent on membrane Na^+/K^+ ATPase. The biliary excretion of some muscle relaxants (i.e. alcuronium, tubocurarine, vecuronium) probably accounts for their relative safety in patients with poor renal function.

Plasma concentration of drugs and its relation to their pharmacological effects

In humans, it is often impossible to determine the effective tissue concentration of drugs, although their plasma concentrations can usually be measured. Factors that

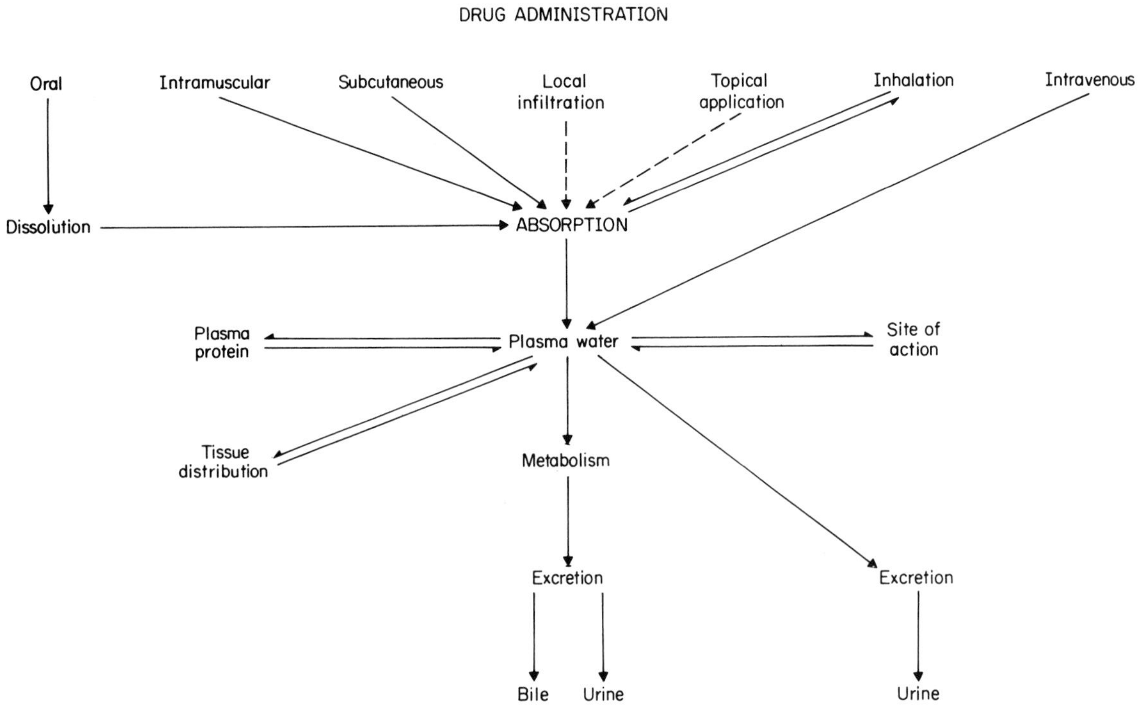

Fig. 1.4 The relation between drug absorption, distribution, metabolism and excretion, and the concentration of drugs at their site of action.

modify the plasma concentration of drugs (e.g. absorption, distribution, metabolism and excretion) may also affect the concentration of drugs at their site of action, and can thus modify the magnitude and duration of their effects. A diagrammatic representation of the relation between drug absorption, distribution, metabolism and excretion, and the effect of these processes on the tissue concentration of drugs, is shown in Fig. 1.4.

Drug administration

In general, drugs may be administered orally, by subcutaneous, intramuscular or intravenous injection, by topical application or local infiltration or by inhalation.

Oral administration

Oral administration is obviously most convenient and acceptable for the patient. Nevertheless, non-compliance with prescribed drug therapy is relatively common. Some drugs are unstable in the presence of gastric acid (e.g. benzylpenicillin and erythromycin); others may irritate the stomach and cause nausea, vomiting or gastrointestinal haemorrhage (e.g. salicylates, phenylbutazone and concentrated solutions of most salts). These problems can sometimes be circumvented by the use of enteric-coated tablets or slow-release preparations, which dissolve only in the small intestine.

When drugs are taken orally, there is usually a latent period of 30–120 min before they reach their maximum concentration in plasma or produce pharmacological effects. The presence of adequate drug concentrations in plasma is dependent on:

1 Drug dissolution;
2 Drug absorption;
3 The absence of significant first-pass effects in the gut wall or the liver.

Drug dissolution

Since drugs are only absorbed in solution, the dissolution of agents administered as tablets or capsules is essential before drug absorption can take place. Drug dissolution usually occurs in the stomach, and may be dependent on gastric acidity. Variations in the dissolution of tablets and capsules, and the rate and extent of gastric emptying, can thus affect the amount of drug in solution in the upper part of the small intestine (where absorption mainly occurs).

Many pharmaceutical factors may influence the dissolution of tablets and capsules (for instance, particle size, chemical formulation, the presence of inert fillers and the outer coating applied to the tablet core). In these circumstances, proprietary or generic preparations of the same drug may have different dissolution characteristics and thus produce a range of plasma concentrations after oral administration. Variations in drug dissolution mainly occur with relatively insoluble drugs that are administered orally. The subsequent differences in the proportion of the dose present in the systemic circulation (bioavailability) may be clinically significant. Approximately 20 years ago, differences in the potency of digoxin tablets suspected from clinical observations were eventually traced to variations in the dissolution of different preparations of the drug. Similarly, toxic effects were produced by tablets of diphenylhydantoin (phenytoin) when an excipient (calcium sulphate) was replaced by lactose. In these conditions, dissolution was more rapid, resulting in faster and more extensive absorption, and higher blood levels of the drug. Although other examples of differences in dissolution rate resulting in altered bioavailability are common, their clinical significance is a matter of conjecture.

Drug absorption

The absorption of drugs in the stomach and the small intestine is usually dependent on their ability to penetrate lipid cell membranes. Consequently, physicochemical properties of drugs (particularly lipid solubility, ionization and molecular weight) mainly determine the rate and extent of drug absorption. Non-ionized compounds (e.g. ethyl alcohol) and low molecular weight drugs (e.g. urea) readily cross cell membranes by passive diffusion, and are easily and rapidly absorbed from the gut. Drugs that are weak acids (e.g. aspirin) are predominantly non-ionized and lipid-soluble in acidic conditions, and therefore should diffuse into plasma more readily from the stomach than from the small intestine. By contrast, basic drugs (e.g. propranolol, amitriptyline, most benzodiazepines) are less ionized and more lipid-soluble in alkaline conditions, and should be preferentially absorbed from the duodenum (pH = 5–6). Strong bases (e.g. quaternary amines) are always ionized in solution and are not readily absorbed from the gut.

In practice, other factors influence the site of drug absorption. Mucosal surface area is more extensive in the upper small intestine than in the stomach, and most drugs, whether acids or bases, are predominantly absorbed from the duodenum. Nevertheless, significant amounts of non-ionized compounds and acidic drugs may be absorbed from the stomach, and can produce a relatively rapid increase in plasma concentration after oral administration.

Compounds that affect gastric motility can modify drug dissolution, and influence the rate (but not the extent) of drug absorption. In particular, drugs that slow gastric emptying (e.g. anticholinergic drugs, antihistamines, tricyclic antidepressants and opioid analgesics) decrease the rate of drug absorption. Other drug interactions (e.g. between tetracyclines and iron preparations, and between cholestyramine and digoxin) may affect the extent of drug absorption, and thus modify systemic bioavailability. Drug absorption may be reduced in pathological conditions affecting the gastrointestinal tract (e.g. coeliac disease, Crohn's disease, obstructive jaundice or after extensive resection of the small intestine).

Although most drugs are absorbed from the stomach and small intestine by passive transport (i.e. simple diffusion or non-ionic diffusion), occasionally their absorption is dependent on carrier-mediated processes. Thus, levodopa is absorbed by a carrier that normally transports amino acids, and fluorouracil is absorbed by the carrier that transports pyrimidine bases.

First-pass effects

After oral administration and absorption, drugs must pass through the intestinal mucosa and the liver in order to produce their pharmacological effects. Some drugs are absorbed from the small intestine but metabolized by the gut wall (e.g. chlorpromazine, dopamine, isoprenaline) or by the liver (e.g. lignocaine, pethidine, propranolol) before they gain access to the systemic circulation (first-pass metabolism). In these conditions, oral administration may not produce adequate plasma concentrations or reproducible pharmacological effects. First-pass metabolism by the liver is relatively common with drugs that have a high hepatic extraction ratio (i.e. when the concentration in the hepatic vein is less than 50% of the concentration in the portal vein). In these conditions, the hepatic clearance of drugs is primarily limited by liver blood flow rather than the activity of drug-metabolizing enzymes. Thus, drugs that modify hepatic blood flow (e.g. propranolol) may affect drug clearance, and influence the magnitude and effect of the first-pass effect after oral administration. Most drugs that are given orally have a low hepatic extraction ratio and a limited first-pass effect, and their clearance by the liver is dependent on intrinsic enzyme activity rather than hepatic blood flow. Drugs are sometimes given by sublingual or rectal administration in order to avoid first-pass effects in the liver.

Subcutaneous and intramuscular administration

Some drugs do not produce adequate plasma concentrations or pharmacological effects after oral administration and are usually given subcutaneously or intramuscularly. In particular, drugs that are broken down in the gut (e.g. benzylpenicillin, polypeptide hormones) are poorly or unpredictably absorbed (e.g. aminoglycoside antibiotics, many quaternary amines), or that have significant first-pass effects (e.g. opioid analgesics), are often given by these routes. Drugs are sometimes given intramuscularly when patients are intolerant of oral preparations (e.g. iron salts) or when patient compliance is known to be poor (e.g. in schizophrenia).

The absorption of drugs after subcutaneous or intramuscular administration is not usually dependent on the dissociation constant of the drug or its pH, but is often determined by regional blood flow. Thus, after intramuscular administration, the onset of drug action is usually more rapid (i.e. as fast as or faster than after oral administration) and the duration of action is usually shorter, due to differences in the perfusion of muscle and subcutaneous tissues. The subcutaneous administration of relatively insoluble drugs or drug complexes is sometimes used to slow the rate of drug absorption and prolong the duration of action (e.g. with preparations of insulin or penicillin). In these conditions, the dissolution of the drug from the complex and its subsequent absorption governs the duration of drug action.

Intravenous administration

Drugs are usually given intravenously when a rapid or immediate onset of action is necessary. When given by this route, their effects are usually dependable and reproducible. Intravenous administration often permits the dose of a drug to be accurately related to its effects, and thus eliminates some of the problems associated with interindividual variability in drug response. Most drugs can be safely given as a rapid intravenous bolus; in some instances (e.g. aminophylline) drugs must be given slowly to avoid the cardiac complications associated with the extremely high plasma concentrations. Irritant drugs must be given intravenously in order to avoid local tissue or vascular complications. Some drugs (e.g. diazepam) can cause local complications (e.g. superficial thrombophlebitis) after intravascular administration; it is uncertain if this is due to the pH of the injected solution or to other factors.

When drugs that release histamine from mast cells are given intravenously (e.g. tubocurarine, pethidine), local vasodilatation and oedema (flare and wheal) in the surrounding tissues may be observed.

Topical application and local infiltration

Most drugs are poorly absorbed through intact skin owing to their relatively high molecular weight and low lipid solubility. The stratum corneum is the main barrier to the diffusion of drugs; in particular, its lipid lamellar bilayers prevent the penetration of polar compounds. Nevertheless, some extremely potent drugs with a high lipid solubility (e.g. glyceryl trinitrate, hyoscine, ethinyloestradiol, fentanyl) are absorbed transcutaneously and can produce systemic effects when applied to the skin. In these conditions, the stratum corneum may act as a reservoir for lipid-soluble drugs for several days after administration is stopped. The absorption of drugs from the skin can be influenced by the carrier or vehicle used for administration, and can be increased by the use of various penetration enhancers (e.g. dimethylsulphoxide, dimethylacetamide, *N*-methyl-pyrrolidone).

In practice, drugs are usually given locally or topically (e.g. to skin or mucous membranes) when it is important to confine their action to a region or an area of the body. Local anaesthetics are most commonly given by this method; they are often combined with vasoconstrictors in order to restrict their absorption and prolong the duration of drug action. Local anaesthetics and other drugs that are used to relieve pain (e.g. opioid analgesics) are sometimes given by intrathecal and extradural routes (Chapters 9 and 11).

Inhalation

Drugs given by inhalation usually have a rapid onset of action, since there is an extremely extensive epithelial surface available for absorption. Corticosteroids and some bronchodilators are given to produce a local action on respiratory bronchioles and to avoid systemic effects. Particle size may influence the distribution to their site of action. In general, particles with a diameter greater than 10 μm are deposited in the upper respiratory tract; particles with a diameter of 2–10 μm are deposited in bronchioles, while those with a diameter less than 2 μm reach the alveoli. The factors that govern the absorption of general anaesthetics from pulmonary epithelium into capillary blood are considered in detail in Chapter 8.

Other methods of drug administration

During the past decade there has been considerable progress in the development of other methods of drug delivery, and some of these may have significant therapeutic advantages. In some instances the development of sustained and programmed-release preparations allows the use of novel methods of administration. This results in greater convenience and safety, improved bioavailability and less variability in plasma concentrations. Other advantages include a reduction in side-effects, drug dosage, frequency of administration and cost.

Timed-release oral preparations usually consist of multi-lamellated erodable polymers, and allow fixed doses of a drug to be released at regular intervals. Some formulations are designed for the slow continuous release of drugs; they may be osmotically active, or incorporate an ion-exchange resin (so that the drug is released in an aqueous medium at an appropriate ionic concentration and pH). A number of therapeutic agents may be administered in this manner (e.g. some opioid analgesics, non-steroidal anti-inflammatory drugs (NSAIDs), bronchodilators, antihypertensive drugs, antiarrhythmic agents and potassium salts).

Several drugs have been administered by non-invasive routes that avoid pre-systemic metabolism. The buccal route (i.e. the positioning of tablets between the teeth and the gum) may be used for the administration of glyceryl trinitrate, hyoscine and prochlorperazine. Similarly, oral transmucosal administration of opioid analgesics using drug-impregnated 'lollipops' has been employed in the management of postoperative pain.

Certain hypothalamic and pituitary polypeptides that are destroyed in the gut are given by nasal administration. A number of other drugs (e.g. opioid analgesics, steroids, histamine antagonists, propranolol and vitamin B_{12}) can also be given by this route. This method of drug delivery may allow the rapid and complete absorption of drugs from the nasal mucosa to the cerebrospinal fluid (CSF) and the cerebral circulation, since the submucous space of the nose is in direct contact with the subarachnoid space of the olfactory lobes. After nasal administration, the concentration of some drugs in the CSF may be significantly higher than in plasma.

In recent years, several drugs have been given by transdermal administration. In general, only extremely potent drugs with a high lipid solubility can be successfully given by this route. Glyceryl trinitrate was the first drug given by transdermal administration; the development of rate-controlled release devices with self-adhesive layers has greatly enhanced its applicability and use. Similar transdermal systems are available for the administration of ethinyloestradiol, fentanyl and hyoscine. There have also been advances in the delivery of drugs by parenteral administration. Implantable subcutaneous pellets are frequently used in hormone replacement therapy, and further improvements in this method of drug administration are anticipated (e.g. with insulin and similar polypeptides). Regulated controlled-release systems capable of providing increased release rates on demand (e.g. by the external application of magnetic or ultrasonic fields, or the use of enzymes) have also been investigated. The development of mini-infusion pumps for intermittent intravenous drug delivery is particularly valuable in pain relief; some of these devices incorporate electronic pumps to provide on-demand bolus release of the drug according to the patient's needs. Alternatively, the use of gravity methods and balloon reservoir devices provides accurate mechanical control of drug administration. Battery-operated syringe drivers for the continuous administration of opioid analgesics are particularly valuable in the domiciliary management of patients with intractable pain associated with malignant disease.

Delivery systems have been designed to target selectively drugs to their desired site of action, thus avoiding regions where their effects are too toxic or where rapid inactivation may occur. In the future, microparticulate carriers (e.g. liposomes, red cells, microspherical beads) may be widely used in infectious and neoplastic diseases. Similarly, the conjugation of drugs with antibodies may be useful in the treatment of malignant disease. The more extensive use of prodrugs may also lead to greater target specificity.

Drug distribution

After administration and absorption, drugs are initially present in plasma and may be partly bound to plasma proteins. They subsequently gain access to other tissues and organs, and when distribution is complete their concentration in plasma water and extracellular fluid is equal.

The distribution of drugs in the body is extremely variable; it may be assessed by distribution studies in animals, or by pharmacokinetic methods in humans (i.e. measurement of the total apparent volume of distribution). Some drugs (e.g. warfarin, tolbutamide) are extensively bound to plasma proteins and are predominantly distributed in blood. Similarly, ionized compounds (e.g. lithium, most quaternary amines) cannot readily penetrate most cell membranes, and are largely confined to extracellular fluid. Since these drugs are poorly distributed in tissues, they characteristically have a low apparent volume of distribution (usually 9–20 l in adults). By contrast, lipid-soluble drugs with a relatively low molecular weight are widely distributed in tissues. For instance, ethyl alcohol, urea and some sulphonamides are evenly distributed throughout body water. These drugs usually have a volume of distribution similar to total body water (30–45 l in adults). Other drugs penetrate cells and are extensively bound to tissue proteins, or are sequestered in fat (e.g. morphine, thiopentone, digoxin). In these conditions, the volume of distribution is characteristically greater than total body water (i.e. more than 30–45 l).

Blood–brain barrier

Other drugs are widely distributed in most tissues, but do not readily enter the central nervous system (CNS). In cerebral capillaries, endothelial cells have overlapping tight junctions which restrict passive diffusion, and pinocytotic vesicles are usually absent. The surrounding capillary basement membrane is closely applied to the peripheral processes of astrocytes (neuroglial cells that play an important part in neuronal nutrition). In order to pass from capillary blood to the brain, most drugs have to cross the endothelium, the basement membrane and the peripheral processes of astrocytes by simple diffusion or filtration. Some drugs cannot readily cross these structures, which are collectively referred to as the blood–brain barrier.

In addition to this structural barrier, there is also a metabolic or enzymatic blood–brain barrier, which is mainly associated with the peripheral processes of astrocytes. Many potentially neurotoxic agents (e.g. free fatty acids and ammonia) can readily cross the capillary endothelium, but are metabolized before they reach the CNS. Monoamine oxidase and cholinesterases are also present in capillary endothelium, and some drugs (e.g. noradrenaline, dopamine, local anaesthetic esters, 5-hydroxytryptamine) may be metabolized as they cross the blood–brain barrier.

Consequently, the blood–brain barrier is not simply a passive and immutable structural barrier, but a dynamic membrane interface between the blood and the brain. Both its structure and function are dependent on trophic factors secreted by astrocytes. It develops during the first trimester of fetal life, but is immature at birth and may be less restrictive to poorly lipid-soluble drugs and endogenous substances.

Certain metabolic substrates and hormones (e.g. glucose, insulin, L-amino acids, L-thyroxine, transferrin) cross the blood–brain barrier by endocytosis or carrier transport. In addition, low molecular weight lipid-soluble drugs (e.g. general anaesthetics, local anaesthetics, opioid analgesics) easily cross the barrier and enter the CNS. In contrast, when drugs are highly protein-bound (e.g. tolbutamide, warfarin), only the unbound fraction can readily diffuse from blood to the CNS, so that the concentration of these drugs in the brain may be 1–2% of the total plasma level. Drugs that are highly ionized (e.g. quaternary amines) cannot cross the blood–brain barrier; consequently, muscle relaxants do not enter or affect the brain. Similarly, dyes that are protein-bound (e.g. trypan blue and Evans blue) and drugs with a large molecular weight (e.g. cyclosporin) do not readily cross the blood–brain barrier. Some drugs (e.g. benzylpenicillin) cannot penetrate the barrier or enter the brain unless its permeability is increased by inflammation (e.g. in bacterial meningitis). The normal impermeability of the blood–brain barrier can be modified by pathological changes (e.g. inflammation, oedema and acute and chronic hypertension).

In some parts of the brain (i.e. the area postrema, the median eminence, the pineal gland and the choroid plexus) the blood–brain barrier is deficient or absent. The diffusion of drugs and the exchange of endogenous substrates is not restricted at these sites. For example, in the choroid plexus drugs may freely diffuse from capillary blood to CSF across the relatively permeable choroidal epithelium. Similarly, the ependyma lining the cerebral ventricles does not appear to restrict the diffusion of most drugs. Neuropeptides and certain ionized compounds (e.g. benzylpenicillin, probenecid) may be actively secreted in the opposite direction, i.e. from the cerebral ventricles into capillary blood.

Placental transfer

During late pregnancy, structural changes occur in the placenta, involving the gradual disappearance of the cytotrophoblast and the loss of chorionic connective tissue from placental villi. At term, maternal and fetal blood are separated by a single layer of chorion (the syncytiotrophoblast) in continuous contact with the endothelial cells of fetal capillaries. Consequently, the placental barrier consists of a vasculosyncytial membrane, and from a functional point of view behaves like a typical lipid membrane. Most low molecular weight lipid-soluble drugs are readily transferred across the placenta: their rate of removal from maternal blood is dependent on placental blood flow, the area available for diffusion and the magnitude of the effective diffusion gradient. In contrast, large molecular weight or polar molecules cannot readily cross the vasculosyncytial membrane. Almost all drugs that cross the blood–brain barrier and affect the CNS can also cross the placenta, and their elimination by fetal tissues may be difficult and prolonged.

Some drugs that readily cross the placenta are known to produce fetal abnormalities if taken in pregnancy (e.g. cytotoxic agents, folate antagonists, phenytoin, oestrogens, progestogens, aminoglycoside antibiotics, tetracyclines, antithyroid drugs). Inhalational anaesthetics, intravenous barbiturates, local anaesthetics and many analgesics (including morphine and pethidine) may diffuse from maternal plasma to the fetus, and when used in labour can cause complications. Similarly, some β-adrenoceptor antagonists (e.g. propranolol) can cross the placenta and may cause fetal bradycardia and hypoglycaemia. When diazepam is used in late pregnancy (e.g. in the treatment of pre-eclampsia and eclampsia), it readily crosses the placenta, but is not effectively metabolized by the fetus. Several of its active metabolites (including both desmethyldiazepam and oxazepam) accumulate in fetal tissues, and can cause neonatal hypotonia and hypothermia. By contrast, ionized compounds (e.g. muscle relaxants) cannot readily cross the placenta, and their use during late pregnancy or lactation only rarely produces complications.

Local concentration

Some drugs tend to be localized in certain tissues or organs; for example, bromosulphonphthalein is concentrated in the liver, guanethidine by postganglionic sympathetic nerve endings, iodine in the thyroid gland and tetracyclines in developing teeth and bone. The concentration of drugs in these tissues may be much greater than in plasma. Drugs that are widely distributed in tissues and concentrated in cells have an extremely large volume of distribution, which is usually greater than total body water (e.g. phenothiazines, tricyclic antidepressants).

After intravenous administration, some drugs are initially sequestered by well-perfused tissues, but are subsequently redistributed to other organs as the plasma concentration declines. Approximately 25% of intravenous thiopentone and methohexitone is initially taken up by the brain, due to its extensive blood supply and the high lipid solubility of the barbiturates. As the plasma concentration falls, the drugs are progressively taken up by less well-perfused tissues with a higher affinity for these compounds (e.g. muscle and adipose tissue). In consequence, intravenous barbiturates are rapidly redistributed from brain to muscle, and finally to subcutaneous fat. Redistribution is mainly responsible for the short duration of action of these drugs; their final elimination from the body may be delayed for 24 h.

Protein binding

Drug distribution may be affected by reversible binding to plasma proteins. When drugs are partially bound by albumin or globulins, only the unbound fraction is immediately available for diffusion into tissues. The concentration of drugs in salivary secretions and CSF may reflect the level of the free or unbound drug in plasma. Alternatively, this may be determined by *in vitro* techniques (e.g. equilibrium dialysis, ultracentrifugation or ultrafiltration).

Many drugs are partially bound to albumin or globulins (or sometimes to both proteins). Albumin usually plays the most important role in the binding of drugs. It has a number of distinct binding sites with a variable affinity for drugs, and mainly binds neutral or acidic compounds (e.g. salicylates, phenylbutazone, indomethacin, tolbutamide, carbenoxolone, oral anticoagulants). Some basic drugs and physiological substrates (bilirubin, fatty acids, tryptophan) are also bound by albumin. Globulins bind many basic drugs (e.g. chlorpromazine, bupivacaine, opioid analgesics). These drugs are mainly bound by α_1-acid glycoprotein (one of the plasma globulins that plays an important part in binding many basic compounds). The plasma concentration of α_1-acid glycoprotein is increased by surgery and by certain pathological conditions (e.g. myocardial infarction, malignant disease, ulcerative colitis). Plasma globulins also play an important part in the binding of minerals, vitamins and hormones. Hydrocortisone (cortisol) is mainly transported in plasma by a specific globulin (transcortin) which has a high affinity for the steroid hormone. Thyroxine, oestrogens and hydroxocobalamin are also bound to globulins. Some drugs (e.g. tubocurarine, pancuronium) are bound to both albumin and an immunoglobulin (IgG). Indeed, the resistance to muscle relaxants that is sometimes seen in patients with liver disease is usually attributed to the increased binding of these drugs by plasma globulins.

There is considerable variation in the degree of protein binding, even among closely related drugs. Thus, the binding of the semisynthetic penicillins to plasma albumin at therapeutic concentrations varies from 25% (ampicillin) to 90% (cloxacillin). Protein binding is primarily a method for the rapid distribution of drugs from their site of absorption to their site of action. The binding of extremely lipid-soluble compounds may be essential for their transport in plasma, due to their low inherent solubility in plasma water. During tissue perfusion, the concentration of the unbound drug in plasma falls, and the protein-bound drug dissociates. A continual concentration gradient is therefore provided for the diffusion of drugs from plasma to tissues.

Most of the available evidence suggests that plasma protein binding is only of practical importance when drugs are extensively (i.e. more than 80%) bound at therapeutic plasma concentrations. Drugs that are highly bound to plasma proteins may interact with each other, since they may compete for and be displaced from related sites on plasma albumin (Chapter 5).

Some protein-bound drugs have a long duration of action, and are only slowly eliminated from the body. Nevertheless, their prolonged action may not be related to their binding to plasma proteins. The hepatic clearance of many drugs is limited by liver blood flow, and is not restricted by plasma protein binding (which is a rapidly reversible process). Drug dissociation from binding to plasma proteins probably occurs within microseconds or milliseconds; by contrast, the hepatic perfusion time may be several seconds or more. Thus, binding to plasma proteins is not usually the limiting factor governing the uptake of drugs by the liver. Nevertheless, the elimination of extensively bound drugs with a low hepatic extraction ratio may be sensitive to changes in plasma protein binding, which can increase the amount of drug available for clearance by the liver. Similar principles can be applied to the elimination of drugs by the kidney. Protein binding is unlikely to restrict the renal elimination of drugs, either by the glomerulus or the renal tubule. Although only the unbound drug is secreted by the proximal tubule, the resultant decrease in its plasma concentration leads to the immediate dissociation of protein-bound drug in order to maintain equilibrium. Indeed, a number of protein-bound drugs are completely cleared in a single passage through the kidney (e.g. benzylpenicillin).

Binding to plasma proteins is modified in pathological conditions associated with hypoalbuminaemia (e.g. hepatic cirrhosis, nephrosis, trauma or burns). In these conditions, the concentration of the unbound drug tends to increase, and may result in toxic effects (e.g. with phenytoin and prednisolone). Significant changes are particularly likely when high doses of drugs are used, or when drugs are given intravenously. In these conditions, binding to albumin and other plasma proteins may be saturated, causing a disproportionate increase in the concentration of the unbound drug. Tissues and organs that are well-perfused (e.g. brain, heart and abdominal viscera) may receive a higher proportion of the dose, predisposing them to potential toxic effects. Similar effects may occur in elderly patients and in subjects with renal impairment or uraemia, possibly due to alterations in the affinity of drugs for albumin. In contrast, many basic drugs are bound by the plasma globulin α_1-acid glycoprotein. The plasma concentration of α_1-acid glycoprotein can be modified by a number of pathological conditions (e.g. myocardial infarction, rheumatoid arthritis, Crohn's disease, renal failure and malignant disease), as well as operative surgery. In these conditions, the binding of basic drugs (e.g. propranolol, chlorpromazine) is increased, and the concentration of the free unbound drug is reduced.

Drug metabolism

Hepatic metabolism is usually responsible for the termination of drug action. It decreases the concentration of active drugs in plasma, and thus encourages their diffusion from other tissues and from their site of action. The main purpose of drug metabolism is the conversion of lipid-soluble drugs into water-soluble (polar) compounds, which can be readily filtered by the renal glomerulus or secreted into urine or bile.

Although most agents are primarily metabolized by the liver, a number of drugs used in anaesthesia (e.g. suxamethonium, mivacurium, esmolol) are hydrolysed in plasma by cholinesterase. Alternatively, drugs may be partly or completely metabolized by other tissues, e.g. the gut (chlorpromazine, isoprenaline), the kidney (midazolam, dopamine), or the lung (angiotensin I, prilocaine). Nevertheless, the liver plays the major role in drug metabolism.

After oral administration, drugs are absorbed into portal venous blood and may be extensively removed from hepatic sinusoids and metabolized by the liver before they reach the systemic circulation. As mentioned previously, this phenomenon (the first-pass effect) is an important cause of the failure of some patients to respond to drugs after their oral administration. When lignocaine, propranolol and most opioid analgesics are taken orally, significant amounts are extracted from portal blood by the hepatic sinusoids; all of these drugs have a marked first-pass effect, and their clearance is predominantly dependent on liver blood flow. By contrast, the elimination of other drugs (e.g. warfarin, tolbutamide) is not determined by hepatic blood flow, but is governed by the intrinsic drug-metabolizing capacity of the liver.

Drug metabolism usually reduces biological activity. Most metabolites have less inherent activity than their parent compounds; in addition, their ability to penetrate to receptor sites is limited, due to their enhanced polarity and poor lipid solubility. Nevertheless, some drugs are relatively inactive in the form in which they are administered, and require metabolism to produce or enhance their pharmacological effects (Table 1.3). Other drugs are metabolized to compounds with a different spectrum of pharmacological activity (e.g. pethidine, atracurium). Certain antibiotics (e.g. ampicillin, chloramphenicol) may be administered orally as esters; in this form, they are better absorbed than the parent drugs, and are subsequently hydrolysed to active derivatives. Occasionally, drug metabolism results in the formation of compounds with toxic effects. Paracetamol, for example, is partially converted to a highly reactive electrophilic metabolite (*N*-acetyl-*p*-benzoquinoneimine). Unless this metabolite is rapidly conjugated, it alkylates

Table 1.3 Drugs that require metabolism to produce their pharmacological effects.

Drug	Active metabolite
Prontosil red	Sulphanilamide
Chloral hydrate	Trichlorethanol
Cyclophosphamide	Phosphoramide mustard
Cortisone	Hydrocortisone
Prednisone	Prednisolone
Methyldopa	Methylnoradrenaline
Proguanil	Cycloguanil

macromolecules in the hepatocyte, causing cell necrosis. Similarly, metabolites of halothane are bound covalently by tissue macromolecules, resulting in hepatocellular damage. There is considerable evidence that the breakdown of halothane to reactive intermediate metabolites plays an important role in the phenomenon of 'halothane hepatitis'.

The changes carried out by liver cells during the metabolism of drugs are usually divided into two types. Phase 1 reactions (also known as non-synthetic or functionalization reactions) usually result in drug oxidation, reduction or hydrolysis (Table 1.4). Phase 2 reactions (synthetic or conjugation reactions) subsequently occur, involving the combination of unchanged drugs or the products of phase 1 reactions with other chemical groups (e.g. glucuronide, sulphate, acetate or glycine radicals). Phase 2 reactions enhance the water solubility of drugs or drug metabolites, and thus promote their elimination from the body. Some drugs (e.g. sodium salicylate) are almost entirely metabolized by phase 2 reactions.

Table 1.4 Typical phase 1 reactions resulting in drug oxidation, reduction and hydrolysis.

Reaction	Site	Enzyme	Example
Oxidation	Hepatic endoplasmic reticulum	Cytochrome P-450	Halothane → trifluoracetic acid Thiopentone → pentobarbitone
	Mitochondria	Monoamine oxidase	Dopamine → dihydroxyphenyl-acetaldehyde
	Hepatic cell cytoplasm	Alcohol dehydrogenase	Alcohol → acetaldehyde
Reduction	Hepatic endoplasmic reticulum	Cytochrome P-450	Prontosil → sulphanilamide
	Hepatic cell cytoplasm	Alcohol dehydrogenase	Chloral hydrate → trichlorethanol
Hydrolysis	Hepatic endoplasmic reticulum	Esterase	Pethidine → pethidinic acid
	Plasma	Cholinesterase	Suxamethonium → succinate + choline
	Neuromuscular junction	Acetylcholinesterase	Acetylcholine → acetate + choline
	Hepatic cell cytoplasm	Amidase	Lignocaine → 2,6-xylidine + diethylglycine

Phase 1 reactions

Most phase 1 reactions and glucuronide conjugation are carried out by specific subcellular particles in the liver cell (the smooth endoplasmic reticulum or the microsomes; Fig. 1.5). These can be separated from other subcellular particles in the liver cell by ultracentrifugation. A non-specific enzyme system in the endoplasmic reticulum (cytochrome P-450 or the mixed-function oxidase system) is responsible for most drug oxidations and reductions, and for some hydrolytic reactions. Cytochrome P-450 consists of many different forms of a superfamily of genetically related haemoproteins, which are the terminal oxidases of the mixed-function oxidase system. In the reduced state, cytochrome P-450 enzymes combine with carbon monoxide, forming a complex which maximally absorbs light at a wavelength of 450 nm. During drug oxidation, the oxidized form of the cytochrome combines with the substrate or drug; the complex is subsequently reduced, combines with oxygen, and accepts an electron to form an active oxygen complex. The active

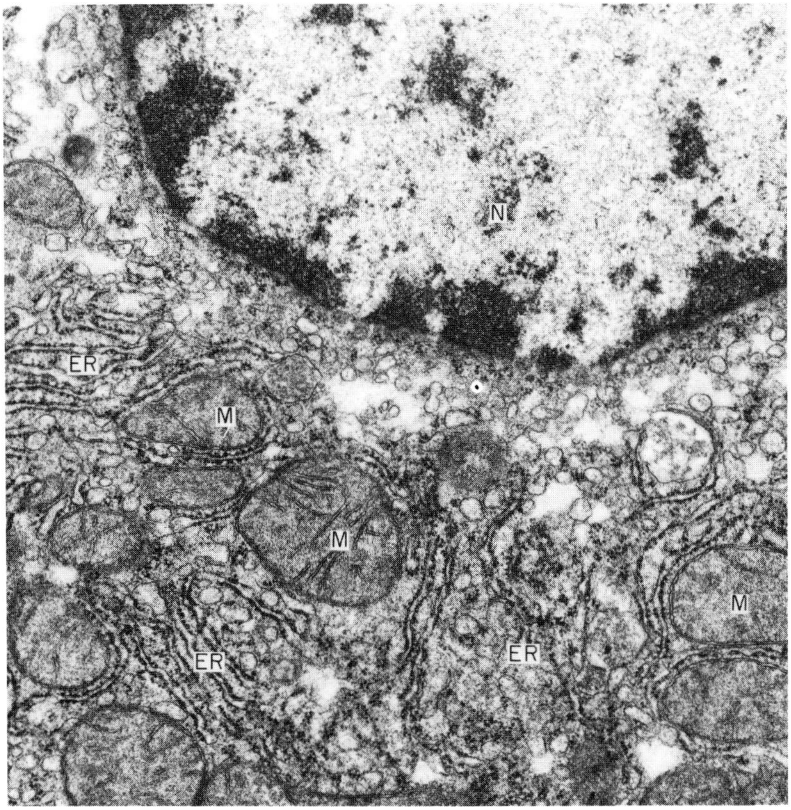

Fig. 1.5 Electron micrograph of part of a mouse liver cell, showing mitochondria (M), endoplasmic reticulum (ER), and the nuclear membrane enclosing the nucleus (N); (× 30 000).

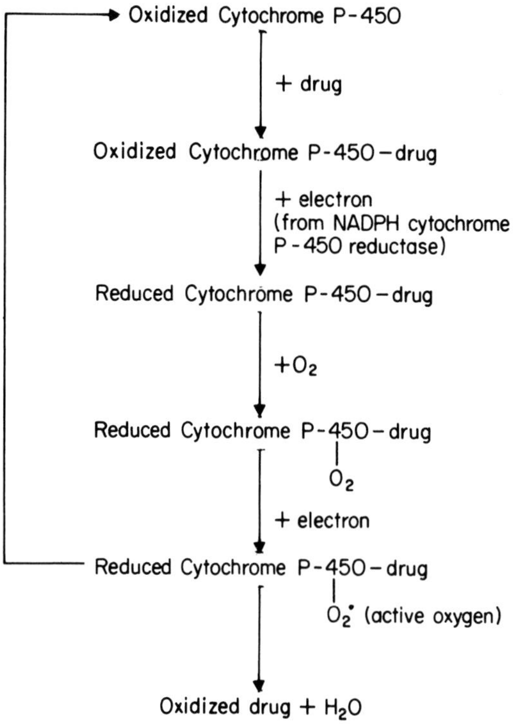

Fig. 1.6 The mixed-function oxidase system (cytochrome P-450).

oxygen then combines with and oxidizes the drug, regenerating cytochrome P-450 in the oxidized form (Fig. 1.6). Cytochrome P-450 enzymes may also mediate the reduction of certain drugs (e.g. the reductive metabolism of halothane, prontosil and chloramphenicol; Table 1.4). The reduction of drugs by cytochrome P-450 enzymes is dependent on their ability directly to accept electrons from the reduced cytochrome P-450–drug complex (Fig. 1.6), and is enhanced by hypoxia.

Many different forms of cytochrome P-450 have been identified in humans; these are usually classified by the similarity in their amino-acid sequences into gene families and gene subfamilies (Table 1.5). The members of each gene family (CYP 1, CYP 2, etc.) have a common amino acid sequence of 40% or more; members of each subfamily (CYP 1A, CYP 1B, etc.) have a sequence similarity of more than 55%. There are 10 different mammalian gene families; six of these families (CYP 7, CYP 11, CYP 17, CYP 19, CYP 21 and CYP 27) are solely concerned with the synthesis of steroids, bile acids and cholesterol, and play no part in drug metabolism. The remaining four gene families (CYP 1, CYP 2, CYP 3 and CYP 4) contain 79 different forms of cytochrome P-450; 14 of these isoforms are responsible for most phase 1 reactions in humans (Table 1.5). The individual isoforms have different but overlapping substrate specificities, and metabolize drugs at different rates; they also differ in their susceptibility to enzyme induction and inhibition. In addition, some of them (e.g. CYP 2C18 and CYP 2D6) are subject to genetic polymorphism, and their expression in different organs is variable.

The P-450 isoform 2E1 is specifically responsible for the defluorination and degradation of many common fluorinated inhalational agents. The rate of anaesthetic defluorination, as assessed by fluoride production, occurs in the order methoxyflurane > sevoflurane > enflurane > isoflurane > desflurane. Other enzyme isoforms (e.g. 1A2, 2C9/10 and 2D6) may also play a part in the metabolism of methoxyflurane. Enzyme induction with ethanol or phenobarbitone increases the rate of defluorination; P-450 2E1 may also be induced by fasting, obesity, diabetes, isoniazid, ketones and isopropyl alcohol. In some cases, it may produce activation of some carcinogens (Table 1.5).

Although most oxidations and reductions are dependent on the isoforms of cytochrome P-450, some drugs (e.g. dopamine, tyramine) are oxidized by monoamine oxidase, which is a mitochondrial enzyme. Ethyl alcohol is oxidized and chloral hydrate is reduced by alcohol dehydrogenase, which is present in the cytoplasm of liver cells (Table 1.4).

The hydrolysis of drugs is a phase 1 reaction that is responsible for the metabolism of esters and amides. Drug hydrolysis may occur in the endoplasmic reticulum and be dependent on microsomal enzyme systems (e.g. the hydrolysis of pethidine to pethidinic acid). Alternatively, it may occur in plasma (e.g. the hydrolysis of suxamethonium and procaine by cholinesterase), at the neuromuscular junction (e.g. the hydrolysis of acetylcholine by acetylcholinesterase), or in the cytoplasm of liver cells (e.g. the hydrolysis of lignocaine and prilocaine by amidases).

Phase 2 reactions

Phase 2 reactions (synthetic reactions) involve the conjugation of other chemical groups with the oxidized, reduced or hydrolysed products of phase 1 reactions. Some relatively polar drugs may only be metabolized by phase 2 reactions. Nevertheless, the metabolic changes that occur during phase 2 reactions usually involve the addition of glucuronide, sulphate, acetate, glycine or methyl groups to the products of phase 1 reactions. The most important of these reactions is glucuronide conjugation.

The conjugation of drugs to glucuronides is mainly dependent on enzyme systems in the hepatic endoplasmic reticulum. The microsomal enzyme glucuronyl transferase catalyses the transference of glucuronide residues from uridine diphosphate (UDP)-glucuronide to unconjugated compounds. This process is responsible for the conjugation of endogenous compounds (e.g. bilirubin, thyroxine) as well as many drugs (e.g. chloramphenicol, morphine, salicylic acid, steroid hormones, sulphonamides, trichlorethanol). Glucuronide conjugation usually results in the formation of acidic drug metabolites with a low pK_a (i.e. relatively strong acids) and consequently increases their water solubility.

Table 1.5 The main forms of cytochrome P-450 that are involved in drug metabolism in humans.

Gene family	Gene subfamily	Enzyme isoform	Substrates	Inhibitors	Biological properties
CYP 1	CYP 1A	CYP 1A1	Benzopyrene (O) 7-Ethoxyresorufin		Widely distributed in extrahepatic tissues Induced by aromatic hydrocarbons Interindividual variation in inducible expression
		CYP 1A2	Phenacetin (D) Caffeine (D) Theophylline (D) Oestrogens (O)	Furafylline α-naphthoflavone	Present in liver but not extrahepatic tissues Induced by cigarette smoking and exercise Marked variability ? due to genetic polymorphism
CYP 2	CYP 2A	CYP 2A6	Coumarin (O) ? Ethoxycoumarin (D) Diethylnitrosamine		Variable concentrations in human liver ? Inactive variant may be present Inducible by pyrazole and other hydrocarbons
	CYP 2B	CYP 2B6	Cyclophosphamide		Major form of cytochrome P-450 induced by barbiturates Marked interindividual variability ? Due to induction or structural mutation
	CYP 2C	CYP 2C8	Retinol; retinoic acid Tolbutamide Benzphetamine		
		CYP 2C9 CYP 2C10	Tolbutamide (O) Hexobarbitone (O) R-mephenytoin (O) Phenytoin (O) S-warfarin (O)	Sulphaphenazole Sulphinpyrazone	Individual variation in expression in human liver Not affected by enzyme-inducing agents Alkylated by tienilic acid metabolites → hepatitis

		CYP 2C18	s-mephenytoin (O) Hexobarbitone (O) Propranolol (O) Diazepam (D)		? Genetic polymorphism (autosomal recessive)
	CYP 2D	CYP 2D6	Debrisoquine (and many other drugs)*	Quinidine	Present in human liver, intestine and kidney Genetic polymorphism (autosomal recessive; C 22) Defective metabolism associated with one of four genetic variants (2D6A, 2D6B, 2D6C and 2D6D)
	CYP 2E	CYP 2E1	*para*-nitrophenol (O) Chlorzoxazone (O) Paracetamol (O) Ethanol (O) Fluorinated anaesthetics	Disulphiram Methoxypsoralen Diethyl-dithiocarbamate	Present in human liver, intestine and leukocytes Induced by fasting, obesity, diabetes and many compounds (pyrazole, isoniazid, ethanol, acetone, ketones, isopropanol) Metabolizes procarcinogens to active compounds
CYP 3	CYP 3A	CYP 3A3 CYP 3A4	Nifedipine (O) Midazolam (O) Lignocaine (D) Cyclosporin	Triacetyl-oleandomycin Gestodene Tacrolimus	Almost identical forms of cytochrome P-450 in liver Induced by glucocorticoids, macrolides, phenobarbitone Metabolize many exogenous and endogenous compounds
		CYP 3A5	Testosterone (O) Midazolam (O)		Present in fetal and adolescent liver, but only 25% of adult livers; expressed in placenta and kidney
CYP 4	CYP 4B	CYP 4B1			Expressed in lung and other non-hepatic epithelial tissues; ? mediates (ω)-oxidation of drugs

* Many other drugs are metabolized by CYP 2D6 in humans, including codeine, dextromethorphan, encainide, flecainide, sparteine, mexiletine, timolol, metoprolol, propranolol, bufuralol, indoramin, guanoxan, perphenazine, trifluoperidol, fluphenazine, thioridazine, clozapine, nortriptyline, amitriptyline, clomipramine, desipramine and imipramine. Metabolism of all these drugs shows genetic polymorphism.

(O), Oxidation or hydroxylation; (D), dealkylation (e.g. demethylation or de-ethylation).

Sulphate conjugation may occur in the gut wall or in the cytoplasm of the liver cell. The enzymes involved are normally concerned with the synthesis of sulphated polysaccharides (e.g. heparin). Sulphate conjugation may be the final step in the metabolism of chloramphenicol, isoprenaline, noradrenaline, paracetamol and certain steroids.

Drug acetylation may take place in several tissues (e.g. spleen, lung and liver). In the liver, Kupffer cells rather than hepatocytes may be responsible for conjugation, which involves the transfer of acetyl groups from coenzyme A to the unconjugated drug. The rate and extent of acetylation in humans are under genetic control. Isoniazid, many sulphonamides, hydralazine and phenelzine are partly metabolized by acetylation.

Conjugation with glycine may occur in the cytoplasm of the liver cell; bromosulphonphthalein is one of several drugs that are partly eliminated in bile as glycine conjugates.

Enzymes that mediate methylation are present in the cytoplasm of many tissues. Methylation plays an important part in the metabolism of catecholamines (e.g. adrenaline and noradrenaline) by the enzyme catechol *O*-methyltransferase.

Enzyme induction

The activity of microsomal enzymes may be enhanced by certain drugs, both *in vivo* and *in vitro*. In these conditions, the rate and extent of drug metabolism is increased. These compounds are known as enzyme-inducing agents (Table 1.6); many of them cause an increase in liver weight, microsomal protein content

Table 1.6 Drugs that induce hepatic microsomal enzymes in humans. Enzyme-inducing agents may have selective effects on one or more isoforms of cytochrome P-450.

Analgesic and anti-inflammatory drugs
Amidopyrine, phenazone, phenylbutazone
Anticonvulsants
Carbamazepine, phenytoin, primidone
Antibacterial and antifungal agents
Rifampicin and griseofulvin
Barbiturates
Amylobarbitone, barbitone, cyclobarbitone, phenobarbitone
Inhalational anaesthetics
Enflurane, halothane, methoxyflurane
Insecticides
Aldrin, chlordane, dicophane
Steroid hormones
Glucocorticoids, androgens
Alcohol
Chronic consumption
Tobacco
Cigarette smoking

and the rate of biliary secretion. Characteristically, enzyme induction increases the activity of oxidative enzymes in the endoplasmic reticulum and enhances glucuronide conjugation by glucuronyl transferase. The activity of other enzymes (e.g. reduced nicotinamide adenine dinucleotide phosphate (NADPH) cytochrome P-450 reductase; Fig. 1.6) may also be increased, although some hepatic enzymes concerned with drug metabolism are unaffected. Enzyme induction usually takes place over several days; the rate of metabolism of the inducing agent and of other drugs may be increased, possibly resulting in drug interactions. Barbiturates have a notorious reputation as enzyme-inducing agents. Nevertheless, there is little or no evidence that the routine use of thiopentone or methohexitone results in enzyme induction, or causes drug interactions in humans.

Many inhalational anaesthetics produce complex effects on microsomal enzymes and the mixed-function oxidase system; most fluorinated agents appear to be metabolized by the isoform cytochrome P-450 2E1 (Table 1.5). The enzyme may be variably affected by inhalational anaesthetics; induction, inhibition or a biphasic response may occur. In addition, the metabolic response to surgery may affect hepatic enzyme systems.

Enzyme inhibition

Conversely, some drugs may inhibit microsomal enzymes, and may prevent or retard the metabolism of other drugs. Isoforms of cytochrome P-450 and other hepatic enzymes concerned with drug metabolism may be inhibited in a competitive or a non-competitive manner by many drugs (Table 1.7). Some of these drugs are imidazoles or substituted imidazoles (e.g. etomidate, metronidazole, cimetidine, omeprazole); the imidazole ring may act as a ligand for the haem in the haemoprotein cytochrome P-450, causing inhibition of oxygenation reactions. Etomidate may

Table 1.7 Drugs that inhibit hepatic microsomal enzymes in humans. Enzyme-inhibiting agents may have selective effects on the activity of one or more isoforms of cytochrome P-450.

Analgesic and anti-inflammatory drugs
Phenylbutazone, oxyphenbutazone
Antibacterial drugs
Chloramphenicol, isoniazid, metronidazole
Cytotoxic drugs
Cyclophosphamide
Monoamine oxidase inhibitors
Phenelzine, tranylcypromine
Other enzyme inhibitors
Allopurinol, disulfiram, metyrapone
Alcohol
Acute intoxication
Other drugs
Etomidate, amiodarone, cimetidine

also suppress steroid synthesis by the adrenal cortex, which is dependent on an isoform of cytochrome P-450 not expressed by the liver (Chapter 7).

Individual differences in drug metabolism

When some drugs are administered in the same dose to different patients, plasma concentrations may vary over a 10-fold range. The phenomenon is partly due to interindividual differences in drug metabolism, which are an important cause of the variability in response to drugs (Chapter 6). Most of the available evidence suggests that the rate and the pattern of drug metabolism are mainly controlled by genetic factors. Some metabolic pathways are subject to polymorphism (e.g. drug acetylation, ester hydrolysis and some hydroxylation and dealkylation reactions). Environmental factors (including diet, cigarette smoking, alcohol consumption, exposure to insecticides and the effects of other inducers and inhibitors on drug metabolism) appear to be of lesser importance.

Drug metabolism may be related to age. Thus, at the extremes of life, the hepatic metabolism of many drugs is modified. Newborn children have impaired drug-metabolizing systems (in particular, some isoforms of cytochrome P-450 and glucuronyl transferase may be relatively immature). In the elderly, drug metabolism is also modified; altered environmental influences may be of more importance.

Pathological changes may affect the metabolism and clearance of drugs in an unpredictable manner. In severe hepatic disease (e.g. cirrhosis or hepatitis), the elimination of drugs that are primarily metabolized may be impaired. The reduction in their clearance may result in drug cumulation, and the urinary elimination of their metabolites may be decreased. Liver disease may also enhance and prolong the effects of drugs that are metabolized by plasma cholinesterase. Any decrease in cardiac output (e.g. due to heart block, myocardial infarction or hypertension) may reduce the elimination of drugs whose clearance is dependent on hepatic blood flow. Renal disease usually has little or no effect on drug metabolism, although polar metabolites may accumulate in plasma and produce toxic effects. Thus, norpethidine (a demethylated metabolite of pethidine) is normally rapidly eliminated in urine; in renal failure, its excretion is impaired, sometimes causing cerebral excitation and convulsions.

Hepatic, renal and cardiac disease are important factors affecting the variable response to drugs (Chapter 6).

Drug excretion

Almost all drugs and their metabolites (with the notable exception of the inhalational anaesthetics) are eventually eliminated from the body in urine or in bile. Small amounts of some drugs are excreted in saliva and in milk.

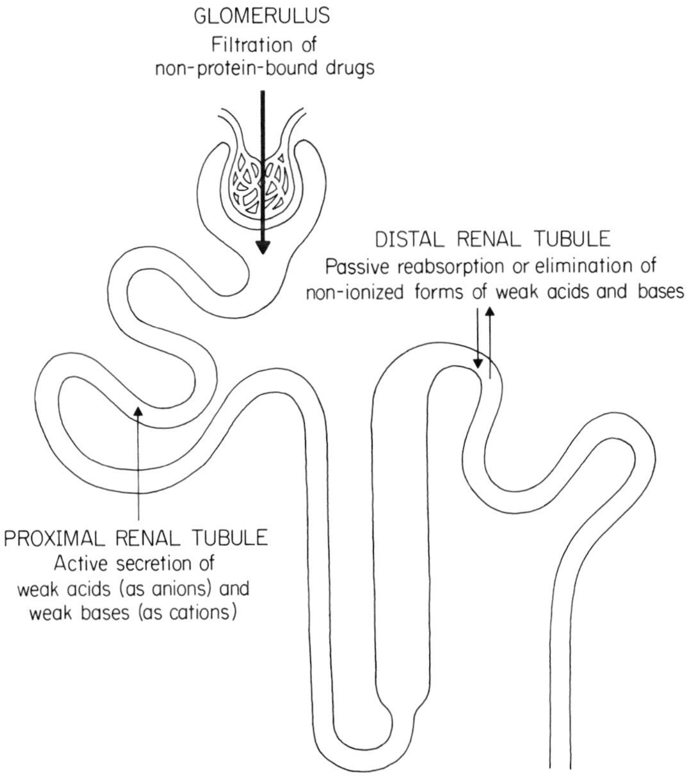

Fig. 1.7 Processes concerned with the renal elimination of drugs by glomerular filtration, proximal tubular secretion and distal tubular reabsorption or excretion. In the distal renal tubule, weak acids and weak bases may be reabsorbed or excreted into urine, depending on their pK_a values and the pH gradient between plasma and urine.

The molecular weight of drugs and their metabolites plays an important part in determining their route of elimination (i.e. in urine or in bile). Most low molecular weight compounds and their metabolites are excreted in urine. By contrast, drugs with a higher molecular weight (above approximately 400–500 in humans) are preferentially eliminated in bile. Thus biliary secretion plays an important part in the elimination of some muscle relaxants, many steroid conjugates and certain antibacterial drugs (Table 1.2).

The renal elimination of drugs is dependent on three separate processes that take place at different sites in the nephron (Fig. 1.7). These are:

1 Glomerular filtration.

2 Proximal tubular secretion.

3 Distal tubular diffusion.

Glomerular filtration

Glomerular filtration is partly responsible for the elimination of poorly lipid-soluble drugs and drug metabolites in urine. Only the free or unbound fraction in plasma water is available for filtration by the renal glomerulus. Nevertheless, since glomerular perfusion time is probably much longer than the dissociation time from the rapidly reversible binding to plasma proteins, significant amounts of protein-bound drugs may be filtered by the glomerulus.

Proximal tubular secretion

The active secretion of drugs by the proximal renal tubule may lead to their rapid elimination from the body. Proximal tubular secretion is an example of carrier transport, requires the expenditure of cellular energy, and may take place against a considerable concentration gradient. A wide number of drugs and drug metabolites are known to be partly eliminated by this process (Table 1.1). Acidic drugs and basic drugs are secreted by two separate and distinct transport systems. These are located in related sites in renal tubule cells, and both have a requirement for cellular energy. Acidic drugs may compete with each other for tubular secretion; conversely, basic drugs may interfere with the elimination of other bases or cations. Acids do not usually compete with or affect the secretion of bases. Occasionally, the competitive inhibition of the tubular transport of acids or bases is of practical significance (e.g. the inhibition of penicillin secretion by probenecid, or the reduction of urate transport by thiazide diuretics).

During tubular secretion, only the unbound drug is transferred from plasma to tubular cells. Nevertheless, protein or red-cell binding does not apparently restrict tubular secretion, and some drugs that are significantly bound to plasma proteins (e.g. phenol red and some penicillins) are completely cleared by the kidney in a single circulation. As discussed above, this probably reflects the rapid dissociation from plasma protein in relation to the time required for renal tubular perfusion.

Distal tubular diffusion

In the distal renal tubule, non-ionic diffusion is partly responsible for the reabsorption and elimination of acids and bases. In this region of the nephron, there is a considerable hydrogen ion gradient between plasma and the normally acid urine. Most acidic drugs are preferentially excreted in alkaline urine, where they are present as non-diffusible anions; in acid urine, they are usually present as non-ionized molecules that can readily back-diffuse into plasma. In these conditions, they are slowly eliminated from the body, and their half-lives may be prolonged. For instance, the weak acid probenecid is actively secreted in the proximal renal tubule as an anion, i.e. $R \cdot COO^-$; in acidic conditions (e.g. in the distal renal tubule) it is partially present in the non-ionized form $R \cdot COOH$, and is extensively reabsorbed. In consequence, its elimination from the body is relatively slow, and its half-life is approximately 6–12 h.

By contrast, basic drugs (e.g. secondary and tertiary amines) are preferentially excreted in acid urine (Fig. 1.3); in these conditions they can readily diffuse from plasma to urine where they are trapped as cations. This provides a gradient for the diffusion of the non-ionized drug from plasma to urine. Many basic drugs are highly lipid-soluble and extensively bound to plasma proteins and may not be significantly eliminated by glomerular filtration or by tubular secretion. Diffusion of the non-ionized fraction from the relatively alkaline plasma to acid urine (Fig. 1.3) may be the only method responsible for the elimination of these drugs.

The effects of changes in urine pH on the elimination of weak acids and weak bases is sometimes used to increase their elimination from the body after drug overdosage.

Biliary excretion

The biliary excretion of drugs and drug metabolites is usually less important than their renal elimination. Nevertheless, almost all drugs or their metabolites can be identified in bile after oral or parenteral administration (although only trace amounts of many compounds may be detected). Biliary excretion is usually the major route of elimination of compounds with a molecular weight of more than 400–500.

Ionized or partly ionized drugs (and drug metabolites) are usually eliminated from liver cells by active transport. High molecular weight anions (including glucuronide and sulphate conjugates) and cations (including quaternary amines) are actively transferred from hepatocytes to the biliary canaliculus by separate transport systems, which are dependent on Na^+/K^+ ATPase. Biliary secretion is relatively non-specific, saturable and can be competitively or non-competitively inhibited by other drugs; thus, anions compete with each other for canalicular transport, while basic drugs interfere with the elimination of other bases or cations. In many respects, the biliary secretion of anions and cations is similar to their active transport in the proximal renal tubule, and accounts for the high concentrations of certain drugs in bile (in some instances, more than 100 times their plasma level).

The phenomenon is sometimes of practical significance. The visualization of contrast media during radiological examination of the biliary tract is dependent on their active secretion and concentration in bile. Similarly, the high concentrations of ampicillin and similar antibacterial drugs that are eliminated in bile may account for their effectiveness in the treatment of carriers of enteric fever. Many muscle relaxants are partly eliminated by biliary secretion, and are present in high concentrations in bile. In general, monoquaternary compounds (e.g. vecuronium, tubocurarine) are more extensively eliminated than their bisquaternary analogues (e.g. pancuronium, dimethyl-tubocurarine), and this may partly account for the differences in their duration of action.

Many compounds that are eliminated in bile as glucuronide conjugates are hydrolysed in the small intestine by bacterial flora which secrete the enzyme

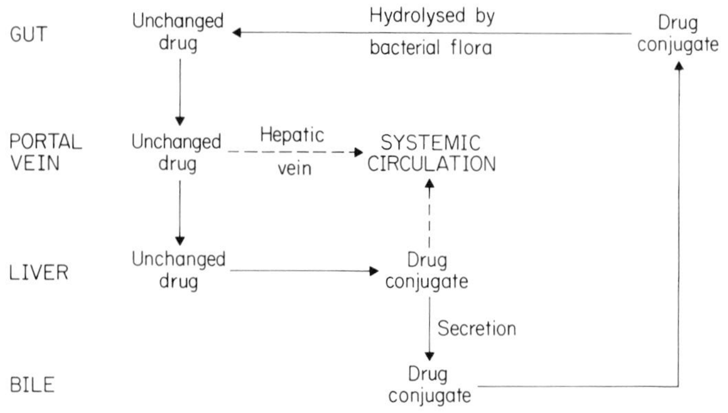

Fig. 1.8 The enterohepatic circulation of drugs. Only small amounts of the absorbed drug and its metabolites (represented by broken arrows) escape recirculation and enter the systemic circulation.

glucuronidase. After hydrolysis, the unchanged drug is reabsorbed, metabolized by the liver, and excreted again as a glucuronide conjugate (Fig. 1.8). This enterohepatic circulation of drugs may occur many times before compounds are finally eliminated from the body, and is often associated with a substantial first-pass effect and a prolonged plasma half-life. Many steroid drugs (e.g. oral contraceptives, oestrogens) have an extensive enterohepatic circulation. During broad-spectrum antibiotic therapy, bacterial flora are inhibited or destroyed, and glucuronide conjugates are no longer extensively hydrolysed in the small intestine; in these circumstances, drug elimination may be enhanced. It has been suggested that this phenomenon is occasionally responsible for the failure of oral contraception in patients taking broad-spectrum antibacterial agents.

The trace amounts of many drugs that are eliminated unchanged in bile are probably directly transferred from hepatic arterial blood to intrahepatic bile ducts via the peribiliary plexus. The transference of drugs may be modified by the hormone secretin, which also increases bile flow by its action at this site.

Excretion in saliva and milk

Small amounts of most drugs are excreted unchanged in saliva and in milk. The elimination of drugs by these routes is usually dependent on simple physical principles. Non-protein-bound, lipid-soluble, small molecular weight drugs can readily diffuse into saliva and milk, where their levels may be similar to the plasma concentration. Since the pH of saliva and milk is slightly acid compared with plasma, the concentration of weak acids will be reduced (although weak bases may be slightly concentrated). Some ions (e.g. chloride, iodide) may be actively secreted into saliva and milk. Nevertheless, drug excretion by these routes is usually of little quantitative significance. Occasionally the elimination of trace amounts of certain drugs in milk (e.g. many opioid analgesics and most hypnotic and tranquillizing drugs) may make breast-feeding inadvisable in patients who are on continual therapy. Muscle relaxants and their antagonists are not significantly eliminated in saliva or in milk.

Further reading

Asling J, Way EL. Placental transfer of drugs. In: La Du BN, Mandel HG, Way EL (eds) *Fundamentals of Drug Metabolism and Drug Disposition*. Baltimore: Williams and Wilkins, 1971; 88–105.

Axelrod J. The metabolism of catecholamines *in vivo* and *in vitro*. *Pharmacological Reviews* 1959; **11**: 402–408.

Bates IP. Permeability of the blood–brain barrier. *Trends in Pharmacological Sciences* 1985; **6**: 447–450.

Berliner RW. Outline of renal physiology. In: Strauss MB, Welt LG (eds) *Diseases of the Kidney*. London: Churchill, 1963; 30–79.

Birkett DJ, Mackenzie PI, Veronese ME, Miners JO. *In vitro* approaches can predict human drug metabolism. *Trends in Pharmacological Sciences* 1993; **14**: 292–294.

Blaschke TF. Protein binding and kinetics of drugs in liver diseases. *Clinical Pharmacokinetics* 1977; **2**: 32–44.

Borzelleca JF, Cherrick HM. The excretion of drugs in saliva; antibiotics. *Journal of Oral Therapeutics and Pharmacology* 1965; **2**: 180–187.

Boyd MR. Evidence for the Clara cell as a site of cytochrome P-450 dependent mixed function oxidase activity in the lung. *Nature* 1977; **269**: 713–715.

Brodie BB, Gillette JR, La Du BN. Enzymatic metabolism of drugs and other foreign compounds. *Annual Review of Biochemistry* 1958; **27**: 427–454.

Calvey TN, Milne LA, Williams NE, Chan K, Murray GR. Effect of antacids on the plasma concentration of phenoperidine. *British Journal of Anaesthesia* 1983; **55**: 535–539.

Cholerton S, Daly AK, Idle JR. The role of individual human cytochromes P450 in drug metabolism and clinical response. *Trends in Pharmacological Sciences* 1992; **13**: 434–439.

Clark AG, Fischer LJ, Millburn P, Smith RL, Williams RT. The role of gut flora in the enterohepatic circulation of stilboestrol in the rat. *Biochemical Journal* 1969; **112**: 17P.

Conney AH. Pharmacological implications of microsomal enzyme induction. *Pharmacological Reviews* 1967; **19**: 317–366.

Csáky TZ. Transport through biological membranes. *Annual Review of Physiology* 1965; **27**: 415–450.

Danielli JF, Davson H. A contribution to the theory of permeability of thin films. *Journal of Cellular and Comparative Physiology* 1935; **5**: 495–508.

Davson H, Danielli JF. *The Permeability of Natural Membranes*, 2nd edn. London: Cambridge University Press, 1952.

Dundee JW, Gray TC. Resistance to *d*-tubocurarine chloride in the presence of liver damage. *Lancet* 1953; **ii**: 16–17.

Dutton GJ. Glucuronic acid, free and combined. In: Dutton GJ (ed.) *Glucuronic Acid: Chemistry, Biochemistry, Pharmacology and Medicine*. New York: Academic Press, 1966.

Eichelbaum M. Defective oxidation of drugs: pharmacokinetic and therapeutic implications. *Clinical Pharmacokinetics* 1982; **7**: 1–22.

Fehrenbach A. Drugs in breast milk. *British Journal of Pharmaceutical Practice* 1987; **9**: 288–290.

Friedman PJ, Cooper JR. The role of alcohol dehydrogenase in the metabolism of chloral hydrate. *Journal of Pharmacology and Experimental Therapeutics* 1960; **129**: 373–376.

George CF. Drug metabolism by the gastro-intestinal mucosa. *Clinical Pharmacokinetics* 1981; **6**: 259–274.

George CF, Shand DG. *Presystemic Drug Elimination*. London: Butterworths, 1982.

Gibaldi M, McNamara PJ. Apparent volumes of distribution and drug binding to plasma proteins. *European Journal of Clinical Pharmacology* 1978; **13**: 373–378.

Gillette JR, Davis DC, Sasame HA. Cytochrome P-450 and its role in drug metabolism. *Annual Review of Pharmacology* 1972; **12**: 57–84.

Goldstein A. The interactions of drugs and plasma proteins. *Pharmacological Reviews* 1949; **1**: 102–165.

Gonzalez FJ. Human cytochromes P450: problems and prospects. *Trends in Pharmacological Sciences* 1992; **13**: 346–352.

Govier WC. Reticuloendothelial cells as the site of sulfanilamide acetylation in the rabbit. *Journal of Pharmacology and Experimental Therapeutics* 1965; **150**: 305–308.

Guengerich FP. Characterization of human microsomal cytochrome P-450 enzymes. *Annual Review of Pharmacology and Toxicology* 1989; **29**: 241–264.

Hasselbalch KA. Die Berechnung der Wasserstoffzahl des Blutes aus der freien und gebundenen Kohlensäure desselben, und die Sauerstoffbindung des Blutes als Funktion der Wasserstoffzahl. *Biochemische Zeitschrift* 1916; **78**: 112–144.

Hawkins RA. Transport of essential nutrients across the blood–brain barrier of individual structures. *Federation Proceedings* 1986; **45**: 2055–2059.

Henderson LJ. Das Gleichgewicht zwischen Basen und Säuren im tierischen Organismus. *Ergebnisse der Physiologie* 1909; **8**: 254–325.

Henry JA. Specific problems of drug intoxication. *British Journal of Anaesthesia* 1986; **58**: 223–233.

Hogben CAM, Tocco DJ, Brodie BB, Schanker LS. On the mechanism of intestinal absorption of drugs. *Journal of Pharmacology and Experimental Therapeutics* 1959; **125**: 275–282.

Inturissi CE, Umans JG. Pethidine and its active metabolite, norpethidine. *Clinics in Anaesthesiology* 1983; **1**: 123–138.

Isherwood CN, Calvey TN, Williams NE, Chan K, Murray GR. Elimination of phenoperidine in liver disease. *British Journal of Anaesthesia* 1984; **56**: 843–847.

Kanto J, Erkkola R, Sellman R. Perinatal metabolism of diazepam. *British Medical Journal* 1974; **1**: 641–642.

Kharasch ED, Thummel KE. Identification of cytochrome P450 2E1 as the predominant enzyme catalysing human liver microsomal defluorination of sevoflurane, isoflurane and methoxyflurane. *Anesthesiology* 1993; **79**: 795–807.

Krakoff IH. Clinical pharmacology of drugs which influence uric acid production and excretion. *Clinical Pharmacology and Therapeutics* 1967; **8**: 124–138.

Lindemann B, Solomon AK. Permeability of luminal surface of intestinal mucosal cells. *Journal of General Physiology* 1962; **45**: 801–810.

McQuay HJ, Moore RA, Paterson GMC, Adams AP. Plasma fentanyl concentrations and clinical observations during and after operation. *British Journal of Anaesthesia* 1979; **51**: 543–550.

Milne MD, Scribner BH, Crawford MA. Non-ionic diffusion and the excretion of weak acids and bases. *American Journal of Medicine* 1958; **24**: 709–729.

Nelson DR, Kamataki T, Waxman DJ et al. The P450 superfamily; update on new sequences, gene mapping, accession numbers, early trivial names of enzymes, and nomenclature. *DNA Cell Biology* 1993; **12**: 1–51.

Nimmo J, Heading RC, Tothill P, Prescott LF. Pharmacological modification of gastric emptying: effects of propantheline and metoclopramide on paracetamol absorption. *British Medical Journal* 1973; **1**: 587–589.

Okey AB. Enzyme induction in the cytochrome P-450 system. *Pharmacology and Therapeutics* 1990; **45**: 241–298.

Omura T, Sato R. The carbon monoxide binding pigment of liver microsomes: I. Evidence for its hemoprotein nature. *Journal of Biological Chemistry* 1964; **239**: 2370–2378.

Orloff J, Berliner RW. Renal pharmacology. *Annual Review of Pharmacology* 1961; **1**: 287–314.

Pappenheimer JR. Passage of molecules through capillary walls. *Physiological Reviews* 1953; **33**: 387–423.

Pardridge WM. Recent advances in blood–brain barrier transport. *Annual Review of Pharmacology and Toxicology* 1988; **28**: 25–39.

Park BK, Breckenridge AM. Clinical implications of enzyme induction and inhibition. *Clinical Pharmacokinetics* 1981; **6**: 1–24.

Park GR, Manara AR, Dawling S. Extra-hepatic metabolism of midazolam. *British Journal of Clinical Pharmacology* 1989; **27**: 634–637.

Peters L. Renal tubular excretion of organic bases. *Pharmacological Reviews* 1960; **12**: 1–35.

Piafsky KM. Disease-induced changes in the plasma binding of basic drugs. *Clinical Pharmacokinetics* 1980; **5**: 246–262.

Prescott LF. Drug conjugation in clinical toxicology. *Biochemical Society Transactions* 1984; **12**: 96–99.

Prescott LF, Nimmo W. *Rate Control in Drug Therapy*. Edinburgh: Churchill Livingstone, 1965.

Rasmussen F. *Studies on the Mammary Excretion and Absorption of Drugs*. Copenhagen: Carl F. Mortensen, 1966.

Renkin EM, Pappenheimer JR. Wasserdurchlässigkeit und Permeabilität der Kapillarwände. *Ergebnisse der Physiologie* 1957; **49**: 59–126.

Reynolds F. Drug transfer across the placenta. In: Chamberlain G, Wilkinson A (eds) *Placenta Transfer*. Tunbridge Wells: Pitman Medical, 1979; 166–181.

Routledge PA. The plasma protein binding of basic drugs. *British Journal of Clinical Pharmacology* 1986; **22**: 499–506.

Runciman WB, Mather LE. Effects of anaesthesia on drug disposition. In: Feldman SA, Scurr CF, Paton WM (eds) *Drugs in Anaesthesia: Mechanisms of Action*. London: Edward Arnold, 1987; 87–122.

Schanker LS. Mechanisms of drug absorption and distribution. *Annual Review of Pharmacology* 1961; **1**: 29–44.

Schanker LS. Passage of drugs across body membranes. *Pharmacological Reviews* 1962; **14**: 501–530.

Scheline RR. Drug metabolism by intestinal micro-organisms. *Journal of Pharmaceutical Sciences* 1968; **57**: 2021–2037.

Siggaard-Andersen O. The first dissociation exponent of carbonic acid as a function of pH. *Scandinavian Journal of Clinical and Laboratory Investigation* 1962; **14**: 587–597.

Singer SJ, Nicolson GL. The fluid mosaic model of the structure of cell membranes. *Science* 1972; **175**: 720–731.

Sjöqvist F, Von Bahr C. Interindividual differences in drug oxidation: clinical importance. *Drug Metabolism and Disposition* 1973; **1**: 469–474.

Smith RL. The biliary excretion and enterohepatic circulation of drugs and other organic compounds. *Progress in Drug Research* 1966; **9**: 299–360.

Somogyi A. New insights into the renal secretion of drugs. *Trends in Pharmacological Sciences* 1987; **8**: 354–357.

Sperber I. Secretion of organic anions in the formation of urine and bile. *Pharmacological Reviews* 1959; **11**: 109–134.

Stoeckel M, Hengstmann JH, Schüttler J. Pharmacokinetics of fentanyl as a possible explanation for recurrence of respiratory depression. *British Journal of Anaesthesia* 1979; **51**: 741–745.

Stoughton RB. Percutaneous absorption of drugs. *Annual Review of Pharmacology and Toxicology* 1989; **29**: 55–69.

Tillement JP, Lhoste F, Giudicelli JF. Diseases and drug protein binding. *Clinical Pharmacokinetics* 1978; **3**: 144–154.

Tomson G, Lunell N-O, Sundwall A, Rané A. Placental passage of oxazepam and its metabolism in mother and newborn. *Clinical Pharmacology and Therapeutics* 1979; **25**: 74–81.

Tucker GT. Drug metabolism. *British Journal of Anaesthesia* 1979; **51**: 603–618.

Tucker GT. The rational selection of drug interaction studies: implications of recent advances in drug metabolism. *International Journal of Clinical Pharmacology, Therapy and Toxicology* 1992; **30**: 550–553.

Wandel C, Böcker R, Böhrer H, Browne A, Rügheimer E, Martin E. Midazolam is metabolized by at least three different cytochrome P450 enzymes. *British Journal of Anaesthesia* 1994; **73**: 658–661.

Warburg E. Carbonic acid compounds and hydrogen ion activities in blood and salt solutions. A contribution to the theory of L.J. Henderson and K.A. Hasselbalch. *Biochemical Journal* 1922; **16**: 153–340.

Weiner IM, Washington JA II, Mudge GH. On the mechanisms of action of probenecid on renal tubular secretion. *Bulletin of Johns Hopkins Hospital* 1960; **106**: 333–346.

Wilkinson GR, Shand DG. A physiological approach to hepatic drug clearance. *Clinical Pharmacology and Therapeutics* 1975; **18**: 377–390.

Williams RL, Mamelok RD. Hepatic disease and drug pharmacokinetics. *Clinical Pharmacokinetics* 1980; **5**: 528–547.

Wrighton SA, Stevens JC. The human hepatic cytochromes P450 involved in drug metabolism. *Critical Reviews in Toxicology* 1992; **22**: 1–21.

Chapter 2
Pharmacokinetics

Pharmacokinetics was originally defined as the quantitative study and mathematical analysis of drug and drug metabolite levels in the body. More recently, the term has been generally applied to the processes of drug absorption, distribution, metabolism and excretion, and to their description in numerical terms; it is sometimes described as 'what the body does to drugs'.

During the past 25 years, a number of extremely sensitive analytical techniques (e.g. gas–liquid chromatography, high performance liquid chromatography, mass spectrometry and radioimmunoassay) have been used to measure the concentration of many drugs and their metabolites in plasma and urine. Changes in drug concentration in relation to time have been measured, and used to derive pharmacokinetic constants that describe the behaviour of drugs in the body. These constants can be used to determine the optimum dosage and frequency of administration (or the loading dose and the rate of infusion) required to maintain steady-state concentrations, and to predict the rate and extent of drug cumulation. They have also been used to provide a rational guide to the modification of drug dosage required in renal and hepatic disease, and to determine the possible effects of other agents and pathological conditions on drug disposition.

The two most important pharmacokinetic constants are the volume of distribution (V) and the clearance (CL). The volume of distribution represents the apparent volume available in the body for the distribution of the drug; the clearance reflects the ability of the body to eliminate the drug. These constants are related to the terminal half-life of the drug ($t_{1/2}$, the time required for the plasma concentration to decrease by 50% during the terminal phase of decline) by the expression:

$$t_{1/2} \propto \frac{V}{\mathrm{CL}}$$

$$= \mathrm{k} \times \frac{V}{\mathrm{CL}}$$

where k is a constant (ln 2; 0.693). Consequently, the terminal half-life is also a constant, which is dependent on the primary pharmacokinetic constants V and CL. A prolonged terminal half-life may reflect an increased volume of distribution, a reduced clearance, or both these changes; similarly, a shorter terminal half-life may represent a decreased volume of distribution, an increased clearance or both phenomena. When the terminal half-lives of drugs are compared, differences between them do not necessarily reflect changes in drug elimination.

Volume of distribution

The volume of distribution represents the relation between the total amount of a drug in the body and its plasma concentration, and thus reflects the process of drug dispersal in the body. It is dependent on the partition coefficient of the drug, regional blood flow to tissues and the degree of plasma protein and tissue binding.

Although the volume of distribution is an apparent volume, and does not correspond to anatomical or physiological tissue compartments, it may be of considerable practical significance. When measured by pharmacokinetic analysis, its value for various drugs in adults may range from 5 to 1000 l. Drugs with a volume of distribution of 5–20 l are predominantly localized in plasma or extracellular fluid (e.g. muscle relaxants and other quaternary amines) or are extensively bound by plasma proteins (e.g. warfarin and phenytoin). Conversely, when the volume of distribution is greater than the presumed values for total body water (i.e. 45 l in adults), there is extensive tissue distribution of drugs (although the specific sites of drug distribution cannot be determined or inferred). In these circumstances, the concentration in tissues is higher than in plasma. The binding of drugs in tissues is common; drugs with high apparent volumes of distribution include digoxin, fentanyl, pethidine, lignocaine, prilocaine, most phenothiazines and most antidepressant drugs. The volume of distribution of drugs may be modified by age and physiological factors, since extracellular fluid volume is greater in infants and during pregnancy than in adults; it may also be affected by disease (e.g. renal and cardiac failure).

An appreciation of the total apparent volume of distribution of potentially toxic drugs may significantly affect the management of drug poisoning. Thus, drugs with a large volume of distribution may take many hours or days to be entirely removed from the body, and cannot be reliably eliminated by forced acid or alkaline diuresis. By contrast, drugs with a relatively small volume of distribution may be eliminated by this method (as long as they are not significantly metabolized or extensively bound by plasma proteins). Theoretical considerations suggest that displacement of drugs from plasma protein binding may produce disproportionate changes in the volume of distribution and the concentration of the unbound drug in tissues (depending on the initial value of the volume of distribution).

Clearance

Clearance represents the volume of blood or plasma from which the drug is completely eliminated in unit time; it is usually measured in ml min^{-1}. It can be considered to represent the sum of the different ways of drug elimination that are carried out by various organs in the body; thus,

$$CL = CL_R + CL_H + CL_X$$

where CL_R is renal clearance, CL_H is hepatic clearance and CL_X is clearance by other routes. Alternatively, clearance can be defined as the rate of drug elimination (in mg min^{-1}) per unit of blood or plasma concentration (in mg ml^{-1}).

In many instances, the renal clearance of drugs can be directly measured by classical methods (or by dividing the total drug eliminated in urine by the area under the plasma concentration–time curve during drug elimination). Consequently, separate estimates may be obtained for renal clearance (CL_R) and extrarenal clearance (CL_{ER}), where $CL_{ER} = CL - CL_R$. These values may be useful in assessing the relative importance of renal and hepatic function in drug elimination. When the total body clearance of drugs is predominantly due to renal excretion (i.e. when $CL_R > 0.7$ CL), drug cumulation may occur in renal failure or during renal transplantation. By contrast, when $CL_R < 0.3$ CL, renal disease has little effect on drug elimination. In these circumstances, drug clearance is predominantly dependent on metabolism or biliary excretion. Although these processes may be affected by liver disease, the effect of hepatic dysfunction on the clearance of drugs is usually less predictable.

Nevertheless, the clearance of most drugs from the body is dependent on the liver (either by hepatic metabolism and/or biliary excretion). In steady-state conditions, the removal of drugs by the liver can be expressed by the extraction ratio (ER). This can be defined as:

$$ER = \frac{C_a - C_v}{C_a} = 1 - \frac{C_v}{C_a}$$

where C_a is the drug concentration in mixed portal venous and hepatic arterial blood, and C_v is the drug concentration in hepatic venous blood. The extraction ratio is an overall measure of the ability of the liver to remove drugs from the hepatic capillaries, and reflects drug metabolism, biliary secretion and similar processes. It is also one of the main factors that governs the hepatic clearance of drugs.

The most generally accepted model of hepatic clearance assumes that the unbound concentration of drugs in hepatic venous blood and in liver cell water is equal. In these conditions, the elimination of drugs by the liver is dependent on: (i) hepatic blood flow; (ii) the proportion of unbound drug in blood; and (iii) the activity of drug-metabolizing enzymes. Hepatic clearance represents the product of hepatic blood flow (Q) and the extraction ratio (ER), i.e.:

$$CL_H = Q \times ER.$$

Hepatic clearance can also be expressed in terms of blood flow and intrinsic clearance ($CL_{intrinsic}$), i.e.

$$CL_H = Q \times \frac{CL_{intrinsic} \times f}{Q + (CL_{intrinsic} \times f)}.$$

$CL_{intrinsic}$ represents the rate at which liver water is cleared of drug (measured in ml min^{-1}) and f is the fraction of the drug unbound in blood. Intrinsic clearance is independent of blood flow, and represents the maximum ability of the liver to irreversibly eliminate drugs by metabolism or biliary excretion. It has a unique value for different drugs, and can be interpreted in terms of enzyme kinetics as the ratio V_{max}/K_m (p. 60).

When intrinsic clearance ($CL_{intrinsic}$) is relatively low compared to blood flow (Q), then

$$Q + (CL_{intrinsic} \times f) \approx Q$$

and

$$CL_H \approx CL_{intrinsic} \times f.$$

In these circumstances, hepatic clearance is only dependent on intrinsic clearance (i.e. enzyme activity) and the fraction of the drug that is unbound in blood. This type of drug elimination (capacity-limited or restrictive elimination) is characteristic of the hepatic elimination of phenytoin, tolbutamide, theophylline, warfarin and most barbiturates and benzodiazepines. These drugs have a limited first-pass effect after oral administration and a low hepatic extraction ratio (i.e. less than 0.3). Their clearance is relatively low and is unaffected by alterations in liver blood flow, but is profoundly influenced by changes in hepatic enzyme activity. These changes may be induced by other drugs or environmental agents, as well as age, malnutrition or disease, which characteristically affect both the total body clearance and the half-life of these compounds. Since $CL_H \approx (CL_{intrinsic} \times f)$, hepatic clearance is also dependent on the fraction of the unbound drug in blood, and may be modified by plasma protein binding. Drugs that are only slightly bound (i.e. 20–30% or less) may be unaffected by changes in protein binding (capacity-limited, binding-insensitive drugs). On the other hand, the clearance and terminal half-life of extensively bound drugs will be modified by changes in protein binding (capacity-limited, binding-sensitive drugs).

When intrinsic clearance ($CL_{intrinsic}$) is relatively large compared to blood flow, then $Q + (CL_{intrinsic} \times f) \approx CL_{intrinsic} \times f$, and the expression

$$CL_H = Q \times \frac{CL_{intrinsic} \times f}{Q + (CL_{intrinsic} \times f)}$$

can be reduced to

$$CL_H \approx Q.$$

In these conditions, hepatic clearance is primarily determined by liver blood flow (flow-limited or non-restrictive elimination). The hepatic clearance of some β-adrenoceptor antagonists, tricyclic antidepressants, opioid analgesics and lignocaine are dependent on this type of elimination. The hepatic extraction ratio is usually high (i.e. 0.7 or more) and there is usually a substantial first-pass effect after oral administration. Characteristically, the clearance of these drugs is relatively high, and is dependent on and determined by liver blood flow (in adults 21 ml kg^{-1} min^{-1}). The half-life may be modified by changes in liver blood flow, but is relatively insensitive to alterations in hepatic enzyme activity or plasma protein binding.

The hepatic elimination of many drugs cannot be readily classified as capacity-limited or flow-limited. Their removal may be partly governed by intrinsic clearance (i.e. enzyme activity and/or biliary secretion) and partly by hepatic blood flow, depending on the conditions in which elimination is assessed. Nevertheless, these concepts provide a physiological approach to the hepatic clearance of drugs, and illustrate the unpredictable relationship between plasma protein binding and drug elimination. When the hepatic clearance of drugs is dependent or partly dependent on intrinsic clearance, significant protein binding may reduce the concentration of the free drug and restrict its elimination. By contrast, when clearance is dependent on hepatic blood flow, protein binding has little or no effect.

Terminal half-life

Although the terminal half-life of a drug is a complex constant (i.e. its value is determined by the primary pharmacokinetic constants *V* and CL), it provides a useful guide to the optimum frequency of drug administration. In general, drugs are usually best given at intervals that are approximately equal to their terminal half-lives. In these conditions, there is often an acceptable compromise between the decline in drug concentrations after successive doses, and the necessity for frequent drug administration in order to maintain an adequate plasma level. The terminal half-lives of drugs that are commonly used in anaesthetic practice are extremely variable (Table 2.1). When drugs are administered at intervals that are equal to their half-lives, they cumulate (i.e. there is a progressive rise in plasma concentration) for 4–5 half-lives until steady-state concentrations are reached (Fig. 2.1). The latent period before the presence of steady-state concentrations can be avoided by the initial administration of a loading dose equal to twice the normal dose. Similarly, when drugs are given by continuous intravenous infusion, steady-state concentrations are reached (to within 5%) after 4–5 terminal half-lives (Fig. 2.2). If the desired plasma concentration (or the level required to produce a given effect) is known, the dose required after oral or intramuscular administration can be calculated from the clearance, using the expression:

$$\text{required dose (mg)} = \frac{C_p \times I \times \text{CL}}{f}$$

where C_p is the desired plasma concentration (mg ml^{-1}), I is the dosage interval (min), CL is the clearance (ml min^{-1}), and f is the fraction of the dose that enters the

Table 2.1 Plasma half-lives (elimination half-lives) of drugs commonly used in anaesthetic practice. Values were obtained in patients with normal renal and hepatic function.

Drug	Plasma half-life (min)
Analgesics	
Alfentanil	73–110
Fentanyl	87–346
Morphine	120–180
Pethidine	160–300
Phenoperidine	15–30
Intravenous anaesthetics	
Etomidate	186–282
Methohexitone	60–134
Propofol	184–382
Thiopentone	360–440
Local anaesthetics	
Bupivacaine	160–240
Lignocaine	100–120
Prilocaine	80–120
Procaine	10–20
Ropivacaine	100–140
Muscle relaxants and their antagonists	
Alcuronium	180–220
Atracurium	18–22
Gallamine	80–220
Mivacurium	2–8
Pancuronium	110–150
Rocuronium	70–140
Suxamethonium	3–5
Tubocurarine	150–230
Vecuronium	36–72
Atropine	90–200
Neostigmine	15–90
Pyridostigmine	15–130
Other drugs	
Adrenaline	5–10
Diazepam	1200–5400
Dobutamine	5–10
Hydrocortisone	90–120
Midazolam	120–250
Nitrazepam	1100–1800
Prednisolone	200–300
Sodium nitroprusside	5–10

systemic circulation (i.e. the proportion that is absorbed and is not subject to first-pass effects).

Unfortunately, after oral or intramuscular administration of many drugs, precise values for f are not available, and calculation of the required dose may be relatively inaccurate. By contrast, when drugs are given intravenously, the loading dose (mg)

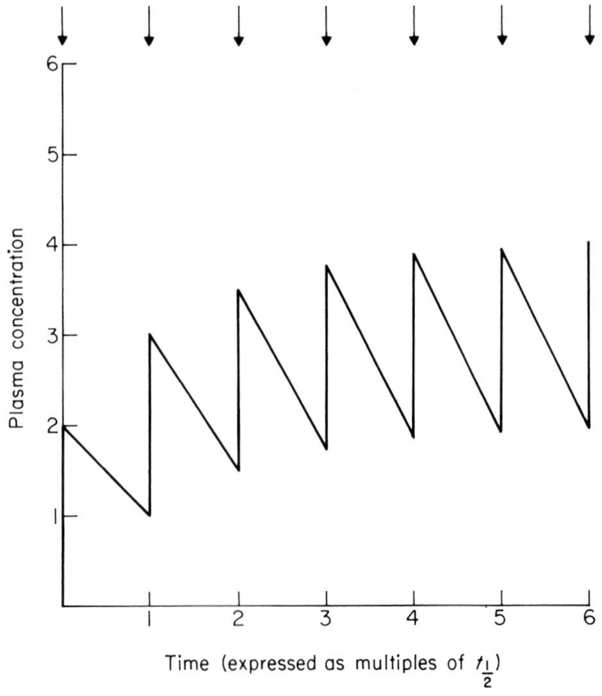

Fig. 2.1 The cumulation of drugs when they are administered (arrows) at intervals that are equal to their half-lives.

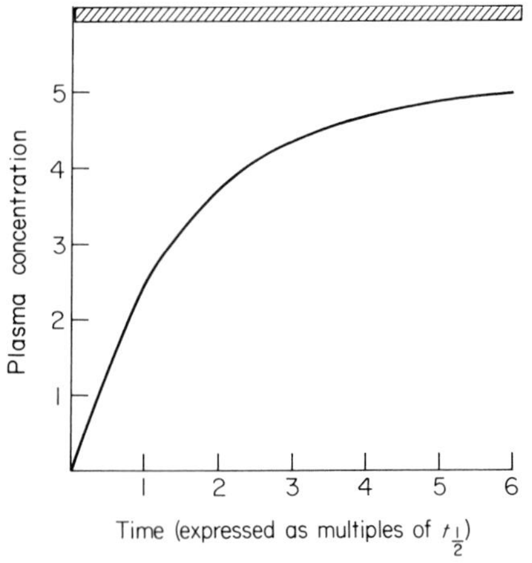

Fig. 2.2 Drug cumulation during continuous intravenous infusion (shaded box).

is given by $C_p \times V$, and the rate of infusion (mg min^{-1}) by $C_p \times$ CL, where C_p is the desired steady-state plasma concentration (mg ml^{-1}), V is the volume of distribution at steady-state (ml), and CL is the clearance (ml min^{-1}). When drugs are given intravenously over prolonged periods (e.g. opioid analgesics, non-depolarizing muscle relaxants, antibiotics), this method can be used to produce accurate, constant

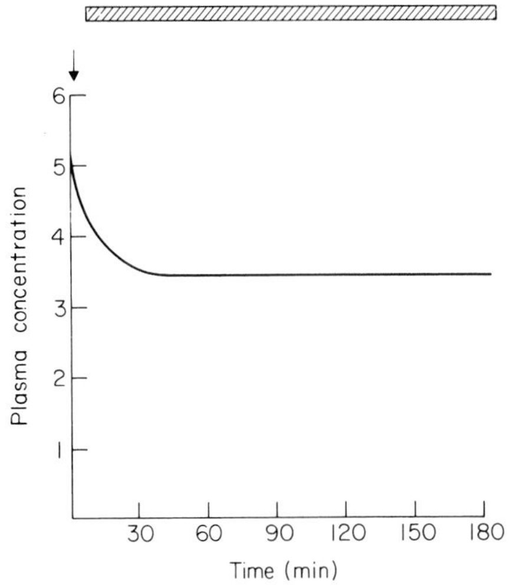

Fig. 2.3 Maintenance of a constant plasma concentration C_p based on the equations: loading dose (arrow) = volume of distribution × C_p and infusion rate (shaded box) = clearance × C_p.

plasma concentrations (Fig. 2.3). Unfortunately, it depends on the determination of the volume of distribution and the clearance, which may be subject to considerable interindividual variability. In addition, the loading dose may result in transiently high plasma concentrations above the acceptable range, and may therefore require modification (e.g. by the use of an initial rapid rate of infusion).

Pharmacokinetic constants can also be used to predict the effects of altered hepatic and renal function on the plasma concentration of drugs. Chronic renal disease causes a reduction in creatinine clearance and the renal elimination of many drugs. In particular, the clearance of drugs that are almost entirely eliminated unchanged by the kidney (e.g. aminoglycoside antibiotics, chlorpropamide and digoxin) is reduced. In these conditions, the dosage required to produce a given plasma level in patients with reduced renal clearance can be calculated from the equation:

$$\text{required dose} = \frac{C_p \times I \times \text{CL}}{f} \quad \text{(see p. 40).}$$

Chronic renal failure reduces the clearance and increases the half-life of most non-depolarizing muscle relaxants (Table 2.2). Although the modification in drug dosage required to produce the plasma concentration associated with neuromuscular blockade can be calculated, in practice this is rarely carried out. Most of the clinical evidence suggests that the action of large single doses or multiple doses of alcuronium, gallamine, pancuronium and tubocurarine is prolonged in renal failure, since the plasma concentration of the drug mainly determines the extent and the duration of neuromuscular blockade. In contrast, the effects of atracurium,

Table 2.2 Terminal half-lives and total body clearance of non-depolarizing muscle relaxants in patients with normal and impaired renal function.

	$t_{1/2}$ (min)		Clearance (ml min^{-1})	
Muscle relaxant	Normal patients	Renal failure	Normal patients	Renal failure
Atracurium	18–22	18–22	300–400	340–470
Gallamine	80–220	400–1300	50–100	5–25
Mivacurium*	2–8	2–8	2100–8400	2100–8400
Pancuronium	110–150	280–490	75–125	20–50
Rocuronium	70–140	70–180	170–420	100–320
Tubocurarine	150–230	250–330	80–120	50–70
Vecuronium	36–72	42–94	150–350	130–500

* Values for the two most active isomers (*cis–trans* mivacurium and *trans–trans* mivacurium).

mivacurium and vecuronium are not prolonged, and these drugs do not cumulate in patients with renal failure.

When drugs act in a reversible manner, their activity and duration of action are usually related to the decline in their plasma concentration, which is in turn dependent on their terminal half-lives. Consequently, the duration of action of some drugs (e.g. local anaesthetics and muscle relaxants) are related to their terminal half-lives. In contrast, when drugs act irreversibly (e.g. many cholinesterase inhibitors, monoamine oxidase inhibitors, some cytotoxic drugs and phenoxybenzamine) they may act for days or even weeks, and their duration of action is unrelated to their plasma concentration or their terminal half-lives. Similarly, when the effects of drugs are terminated by redistribution (e.g. intravenous barbiturates, benzodiazepines, and some opioids) their duration of action is not predictably related to their terminal half-lives.

Exponential changes

Changes in the plasma concentration of drugs in relation to time can usually be expressed as mathematical equations containing one or more exponential terms. In the mathematical expression

$$10^3 = 1000,$$

10^3 is an exponential term; the number 10 must be raised to the power or exponent of 3 in order to equal 1000. Equations of this type can be conveniently considered in terms of the common logarithms of numbers, which are defined as the power or exponent to which the base must be raised in order to give the number. Consequently, the logarithm of 1000 to base 10 is 3. Since

$$10^a \times 10^b = 10^{a+b}$$

and

$10^a \div 10^b = 10^{a-b}$,

the multiplication of numbers can be carried out by summating their logarithms, and the division of numbers by subtracting their logarithms, followed by an antilogarithmic transformation. Logarithms to base 10 ($\log_{10}$) are commonly used for this purpose.

Natural or Napierian* logarithms ($\log_e$ or ln) are similar to common logarithms, but use the mathematical constant e (2.718) as their base. In numerical terms, e can be expressed as the limiting sum of an infinitely convergent series:

$$e = 1 + 1 + \frac{1}{2 \cdot 1} + \frac{1}{3 \cdot 2 \cdot 1} + \frac{1}{4 \cdot 3 \cdot 2 \cdot 1} \text{ etc.}$$

and

$$e^x = 1 + x + \frac{x^2}{2 \cdot 1} + \frac{x^3}{3 \cdot 2 \cdot 1} + \frac{x^4}{4 \cdot 3 \cdot 2 \cdot 1} \text{ etc.}$$

convergent for all finite values of x.

Alternatively e can be considered as an irrational number which can be expressed as the sum of a series:

$$e = \left(1 + \frac{1}{n}\right)^n \qquad (n \to \infty).$$

The importance of the constant e is related to the mathematical interpretation of exponential changes, in which the rate of change in a variable is proportional to its magnitude. Many processes concerned with the absorption, distribution and elimination of drugs result in exponential changes in drug concentration in relation to time. In these exponential changes, the increase or decrease in the concentration of a drug is directly proportional to its magnitude; in mathematical terms,

$$\pm \frac{dX}{dt} \propto X$$

$$\pm \frac{dX}{dt} = kX$$

where dX/dt is the rate of increase or decrease of the variable X during an infinitesimal moment of time t, k is a constant and X is the value of the variable at time t.

On integration of this expression between $t = 0$ and $t = \infty$:

$$X = X_0 \cdot e^{kt} \qquad \text{(for exponential growth)}$$

* John Napier of Merchiston, Edinburgh (1550–1617); Napier's original base depended on e^{-1} (0.36788) rather than e.

$X = X_0 \cdot e^{-kt}$ (for exponential disappearance)

where X is the value of X at any time t; X_0 is the initial value of X at zero time; e is the base of natural logarithms (2.718), and k is a constant.

In these conditions, X can be described as an exponential function of time.

Consider the equation for exponential disappearance:

$$X = X_0 \cdot e^{-kt}.$$

On taking natural logarithms:

$$\ln X = \ln X_0 - kt$$

and

$$\ln\left(\frac{X}{X_0}\right) = -\,kt.$$

Consequently $k = -\ln(X/X_0)/t$; in this equation k can be considered as a rate constant, and represents the proportional change in X in unit time. Alternatively, the rate of exponential change can be represented as the half-time (half-life) or as a time constant.

Since

$$k = \frac{-\ln\left(\dfrac{X}{X_0}\right)}{t}$$

$$t = \frac{\ln\left(\dfrac{X}{X_0}\right)}{-k}.$$

If $(X/X_0) = 1/2$, t represents the time for X to decline to half its original value; consequently:

$$t = \frac{\ln\left(\dfrac{1}{2}\right)}{-k}$$

$$= \frac{\ln 2}{k}$$

$$= \frac{0.693}{k}.$$

In these conditions, t represents the half-time (half-life) of the exponential change.

Alternatively, if

$$\frac{X}{X_0} = \frac{1}{2.718} = \frac{1}{e},$$

t represents the time required for *X* to decline to 1/e (37%) of its original value; thus:

$$t = \frac{\ln\left(\frac{1}{e}\right)}{-k}$$

$$= \frac{\ln\left(e^{-1}\right)}{-k}$$

$$= \frac{-\ln e}{-k}$$

$$= \frac{1}{k}.$$

In these conditions *t* represents the time constant of the exponential change; it is the reciprocal of the rate constant k.

Determination of volume of distribution and clearance

Compartmental models have been widely used to determine the volume of distribution and the clearance of drugs. Nevertheless, the choice of a suitable pharmacokinetic model may be difficult, and can depend on technical, analytical and sampling factors. The behaviour of some drugs (e.g. tubocurarine) has been described by different pharmacokinetic models, and in these conditions the interpretation of the results may be complex. The calculation of the volume of distribution and the clearance is critically dependent on the choice of model (and on the accuracy with which plasma concentration–time data can be represented by it).

Consequently, in recent years non-compartmental methods have been widely used to determine the volume of distribution and the clearance of drugs. Nevertheless, the distribution and elimination of many drugs in the body can be adequately characterized by simple pharmacokinetic models.

One-compartment model

The decline in the plasma concentration of many drugs after intramuscular administration is consistent with a simple one-compartment pharmacokinetic model. For example, in one study neostigmine (2 mg) was given by intramuscular injection to five patients with myasthenia gravis, and blood samples were removed at 30, 60, 90, 120, 150 and 180 min. The concentration of neostigmine in plasma was then measured. Table 2.3 shows the results obtained in one patient.

When the logarithm or the natural logarithm ($\log_e$ or ln) of the plasma concentration of neostigmine is plotted against time (Fig. 2.4), a straight line is

Table 2.3 Concentration of neostigmine in plasma after intramuscular injection in a patient with myasthenia gravis.

Time after intramuscular injection (min)	Concentration of neostigmine (ng ml^{-1})
30	19
60	14
90	11
120	9
150	7
180	6

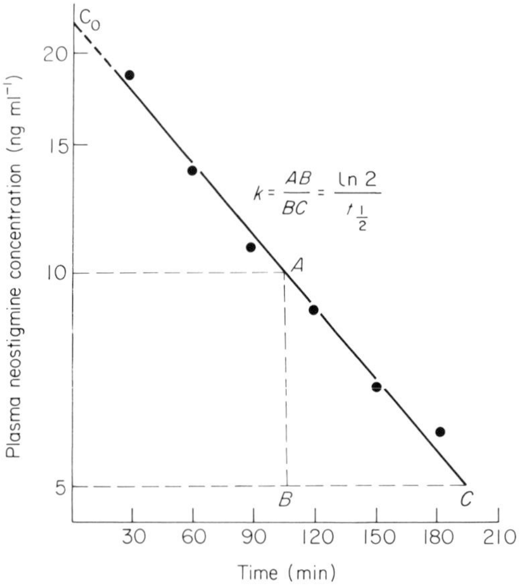

Fig. 2.4 Monoexponential decline in the plasma concentration on neostigmine after intramuscular injection. Data points (black circles) correspond to the concentration of neostigmine at different times after administration, expressed on a logarithmic (ln) scale. *BC* corresponds to the half-life of neostigmine; the slope of the regression line relating the data points = k = *AB*/*BC* = ln 2/ $t_{1/2}$ C_0 is the extrapolated concentration of neostigmine at time $t = 0$.

obtained, indicating that the decline in the plasma concentration of the drug is an exponential function of time (p. 46). The decrease in the plasma concentration of neostigmine is greatest initially (i.e. between 30 and 60 min), and then gradually declines, although a constant proportion of the drug is removed during each time interval.

The slope of the monoexponential decline in the plasma concentration of neostigmine reflects the half-life of the drug. The plasma half-life is defined as the time required for the concentration of a drug in plasma to decline by 50% (i.e. to one-half of its initial value). Since there is a linear relationship between the logarithm of plasma concentration and time (Fig. 2.4), the plasma half-life can be measured from any point on the line. In Fig. 2.4, the plasma half-life is given by:

$$t_{1/2} = BC = 93 \text{ min}$$

as measured by graphical estimation. This corresponds to the time required for the plasma concentration to fall from 10 to 5 ng ml^{-1}. Since the natural logarithm of the plasma concentration of neostigmine was plotted against time, the slope of the monoexponential decline in plasma concentration is equal to:

$$\frac{AB}{BC} = \frac{\ln 10 - \ln 5}{t_{1/2}} = \frac{\ln 2}{t_{1/2}} = \frac{0.693}{t_{1/2}}.$$

The gradient of the line can be used to predict or determine the plasma concentration of neostigmine (C_p) at any time (t) after administration of the drug. It can be shown that the equation relating the decline in plasma concentration to time is

$$C_p = C_0 \cdot e^{-kt}$$

where C_p is the plasma concentration at time t; C_0 is the extrapolated concentration of the drug at $t = 0$; e = 2.718 (the base of natural logarithms); and k is the gradient of the decline in plasma concentration:

$$k = \frac{\ln 2}{t_{1/2}}$$

In this instance, the decline in the plasma concentration of neostigmine after intramuscular injection is consistent with a one-compartment, pharmacokinetic model. According to this model, the body is considered in a highly simplified manner as a single homogeneous entity or compartment (Fig. 2.5). Drugs are administered into, and eliminated from, this compartment (either by metabolism or renal and biliary excretion). The rate of drug elimination is assumed to be proportional to the amount of drug in the body (X) at any time (t), i.e. it decreases exponentially with time and is consistent with first-order kinetics. When expressed as a differential equation:

$$\frac{dX}{dt} \propto X$$

and:

$$\frac{dX}{dt} = -kX$$

where X is the amount of drug in the body at time t; and k is the elimination rate

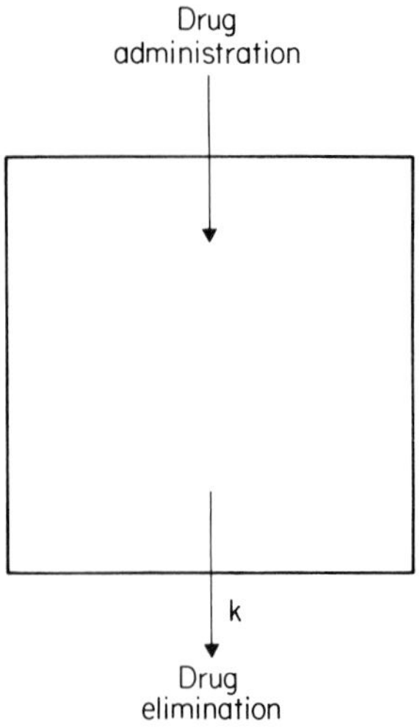

Fig. 2.5 A one-compartment, open pharmacokinetic model. The constant k corresponds to the elimination rate constant, and is measured in units of reciprocal time (e.g. min^{-1}).

constant measured in units of reciprocal time (i.e. per min or min^{-1}). The negative sign reflects the removal of the drug from the body. Integration of this expression with respect to time gives the expression:

$$X = X_0 \cdot e^{-kt}$$

where X_0 is the amount of drug initially present in the body (i.e. the intravenous dose or the fraction of the dose that is absorbed) and e = 2.718.

The division of this equation by the volume of the compartment (the volume of distribution or *V*) gives the expression

$$C = C_0 \cdot e^{-kt}$$

which is identical to the equation that describes the plasma concentration of the drug at different times after its administration. The constant k defines the slope of the drug concentration–time relationship obtained from plasma levels (Fig. 2.4); it also represents the elimination rate constant when the data are interpreted by a one-compartment open model. The elimination rate constant k is estimated from the equation:

$$k = \frac{\ln 2}{t_{1/2}} = \frac{0.693}{t_{1/2}}.$$

The volume of distribution can be calculated from the expression:

$$V = \frac{X_0}{C_0}.$$

It corresponds to the volume of the compartment, and represents the relationship between the total amount of drug in the body and the plasma concentration.

The clearance of the drug is given by:

$$CL = V \cdot k.$$

Thus, clearance corresponds to the volume of the compartment multiplied by the rate of drug elimination (i.e. the volume that is cleared of the drug in unit time). It represents the sum of all the processes of drug clearance that occur in different organs of the body (p. 37). The estimation of renal clearance is simplified by the measurement or calculation of the total area subtended by the plasma concentration–time curve between $t = 0$ and $t = \infty$ (infinity). The area under the curve (AUC) is given by:

$$AUC = \frac{C_0}{k}$$

and the renal clearance (CL_R) by the expression:

$$CL_R = \frac{\text{total drug eliminated in urine}}{AUC}.$$

When the pharmacokinetics of intramuscular neostigmine was studied, the plasma concentration data did not exactly correspond to a monoexponential decline (Fig. 2.4). Differences between the data points and the plasma concentration–time regression line were probably due to unavoidable analytical and sampling errors. Although estimates of some pharmacokinetic values (e.g. $t_{1/2}$, k, and C_0) can be made by graphical methods, and other parameters (e.g. V, CL and AUC) derived from them, this method is time-consuming and relatively inaccurate.

More commonly, plasma concentrations are converted to logarithms, and the linear relation between these values and time (see Fig. 2.4) is derived by least-squares regression analysis. The other constants are usually generated by computer programs. In the example given, when the decline in the plasma concentration of neostigmine after intramuscular injection was interpreted in terms of a one-compartment open model, the following results were obtained, using a computer program:

$$t_{1/2} = 91 \text{ min}$$
$$k = 0.0077 \text{ min}^{-1}$$
$$C_0 = 23 \text{ ng ml}^{-1}$$
$$V = 58\,700 \text{ ml}$$
$$CL = 450 \text{ ml min}^{-1}$$
$$AUC = 2967 \text{ ng ml}^{-1} \cdot \text{min}.$$

After oral or intramuscular administration, drugs are usually absorbed by first-order processes, and their absorption can be defined and expressed as an absorption rate constant. In the postabsorptive phase, the decline in their plasma concentration can usually be interpreted by a one-compartment open model (as in the example of intramuscular neostigmine). The behaviour of a minority of drugs after intravenous administration (e.g. bromosulphonphthalein, suxamethonium and possibly inulin) can also be described by this simple model, since their plasma concentration usually declines in a monoexponential manner.

It should be emphasized that compartments in kinetic models do not necessarily have any physiological meaning. A one-compartment model is primarily defined by the behaviour of the drug in the body, and not by anatomical or physiological considerations; the model merely implies that the drug does not pass from one part of the body to another at a measurable rate. Although drug concentrations in plasma are probably different from levels in other tissues, a one-compartment model implies that differences in concentration within the body bear a constant relationship to each other. By contrast, the behaviour of many other drugs after intravenous injection cannot be realistically interpreted in terms of a one-compartment open model. In these conditions, paradigms of greater complexity provide a more accurate description of the decline in plasma concentration. In particular, the two-compartment open model has been widely used to account for the behaviour of many drugs that are used in anaesthetic practice and administered by intravenous injection.

Two-compartment model

After intravenous injection, most drugs are initially present in a restricted volume, and are then rapidly distributed throughout the body. During the phase of distribution, there is a rapid decline in plasma concentration; its rate and extent are primarily dependent on the physicochemical characteristics of the drug (e.g. molecular weight and lipid solubility). When distribution is complete and a state of equilibrium has been established, the subsequent decline in plasma concentration reflects the elimination of the drug.

The decrease in the plasma concentration of many drugs after intravenous injection is consistent with this concept. Thus, after the intravenous injection of phenoperidine, there is a biexponential decline in the plasma level of the drug (Fig. 2.6). An initial rapid fall in concentration (due to drug distribution) is followed by a slower phase of exponential decline (due to drug elimination). The decrease in the plasma concentration of phenoperidine can be resolved into two exponential components by extrapolation. The terminal phase of the decline in plasma concentration (β, slow disposition, or elimination phase) is extended to the ordinate (y axis), which it intersects at point B. Subtraction of the extrapolated values from the initial data points gives a series of residual values, which represent the initial phase of exponential decline. This initial phase (α, rapid disposition or distribution phase) is defined by a regression line that intercepts the ordinate at A. Both the α

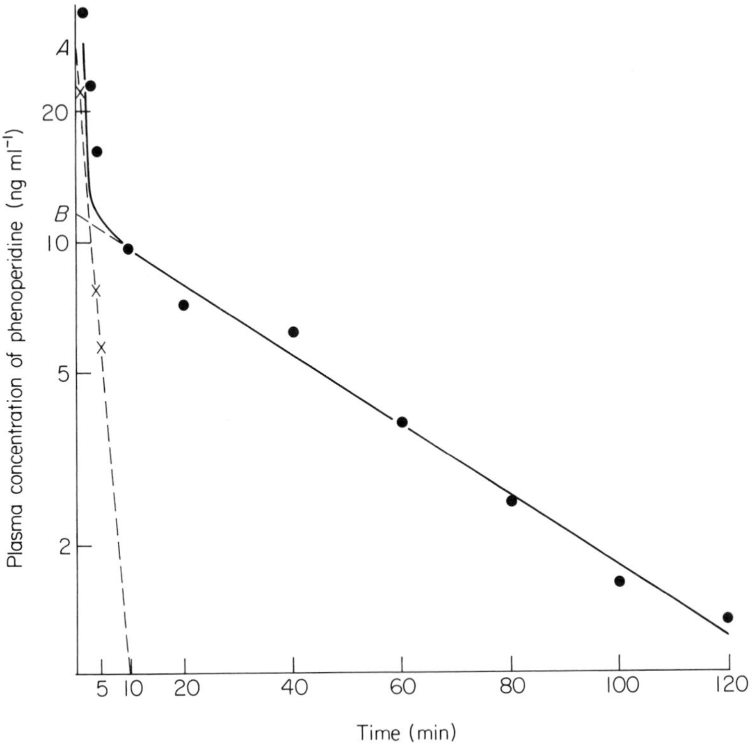

Fig. 2.6 Biexponential decline in the plasma concentration of phenoperidine after intravenous injection. The abscissa (*x* axis) shows the time in minutes; the ordinate (*y* axis) represents the logarithm of the plasma concentration of phenoperidine; data points (black circles) correspond to the plasma concentration of the drug at different times. *B* represents the initial concentration of the slower phase of exponential decline, extrapolated to zero time. Extrapolated values on this line were subtracted from the data points to give a series of residual values (*x*); the least-squares regression line through these points corresponds to the rapid disposition phase.

and the β phases have characteristic slopes (α and β) and half-lives ($t_{1/2\alpha}$ and $t_{1/2\beta}$). Numerical values for the slopes α and β can be estimated from the equations:

$$\alpha = \frac{\ln 2}{t_{1/2\alpha}}$$

$$\beta = \frac{\ln 2}{t_{1/2\beta}}$$

and the concentration C_p at time *t* is given by the expression

$$C_p = A \cdot e^{-\alpha t} + B \cdot e^{-\beta t}$$

where *A* and *B* are intercepts on the ordinate (Fig. 2.6) and e = 2.718. The constants α and β are hybrid constants, since they are determined by, and are dependent on, other constants. Values for *A*, *B*, α and β can be derived by graphical methods, or more accurately determined by digital computer programs. Analysis of the decline in the plasma concentration of phenoperidine (Fig. 2.6) gave the following expression:

$$C_p = 30e^{-0.276t} + 12e^{-0.019t}$$

where C_p is measured in ng ml^{-1} and t in min.

The biexponential decline in the plasma concentration of phenoperidine was interpreted in terms of a two-compartment open pharmacokinetic model (Fig. 2.7). This model consists of a relatively small central compartment, into which the drug is administered and from which it is eliminated, and a peripheral compartment. The rate of drug elimination is governed by the rate constant k_{10}. The peripheral compartment usually has a larger apparent volume than the central compartment; bidirectional (reversible) drug transfer between the two compartments is governed by the rate constants k_{12} and k_{21} (Fig. 2.7). As in the one-compartment model (p. 47), the central and the peripheral compartment have no direct physiological meaning, and their parameters and constants are solely determined by the behaviour of the drug in the body.

The two-compartment model is essentially a theoretical concept which accounts for the observed biexponential decline in plasma concentration (Fig. 2.6). In the case of phenoperidine (and many other drugs), the central compartment probably consists of the blood, interstitial fluid and some of the intracellular water of highly perfused organs (e.g. the heart, lungs, liver, kidneys). The peripheral compartment consists of the brain and less well-perfused tissues (e.g. most skeletal muscle, fat, skin, connective tissue). During the distribution phase, the plasma concentration of phenoperidine falls rapidly as the drug is distributed from the central compartment

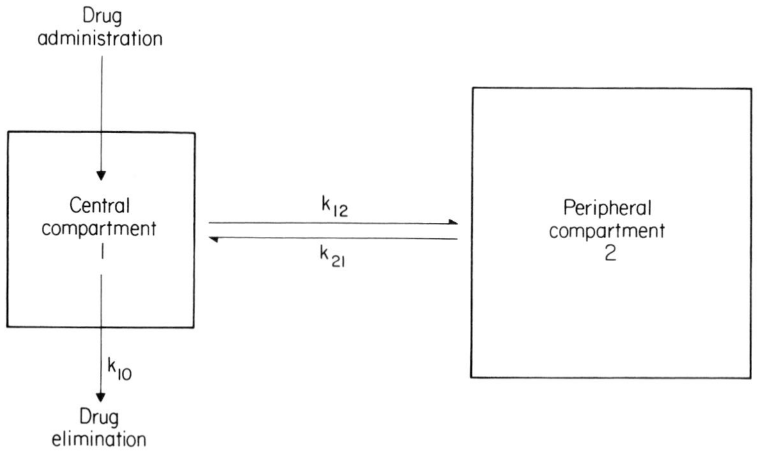

Fig. 2.7 A two-compartment, open model, consisting of a central compartment 1 and a peripheral compartment 2. The constants k_{12} and k_{21} govern drug transfer between the central and peripheral compartments; k_{10} is the elimination rate constant.

to the peripheral compartment (Fig. 2.7). After the occurrence of distribution equilibrium between the two compartments, removal of the drug is solely dependent on elimination, which is governed by the rate constant k_{10}.

As in the one-compartment model, resolution is dependent on the assumption that both distribution and elimination are exponential first-order processes (i.e. that the rate at which they occur is proportional to the amount of drug in each compartment). Differential equations can then be derived that express the rate of change of drug in each compartment (i.e. dX_1/dt and dX_2/dt, where X_1 and X_2 are the amounts of drug in each compartment at time t). The solution of these first-order differential equations for dX_1/dt and dX_2/dt, and the conversion of X_1 and X_2 to concentrations, gives expressions that relate the concentration of the drug in the central compartment (C_1) and the peripheral compartment (C_2) to time.

In the case of the central compartment:

$$C_1 = A \cdot e^{-\alpha t} + B \cdot e^{-\beta t}$$

where A, α, B, β are constants, and e = 2.718. This is identical to the equation that describes the biexponential decline in the plasma concentration of drugs after their intravenous injection. Consequently, values for A, α, B, β can be derived from the measured plasma concentrations. These constants can then be used to derive other parameters of the two-compartment open model (e.g. the area under the plasma concentration–time curve (AUC), the clearance (CL), the volume of distribution (V), as well as the rate constants k_{21}, k_{10} and k_{12}), using the following formulae:

$$\mathrm{AUC} = \frac{A}{\alpha} + \frac{B}{\beta}$$

$$\mathrm{CL} = \frac{\mathrm{dose}}{\mathrm{AUC}} = \frac{\mathrm{dose}}{\frac{A}{\alpha} + \frac{B}{\beta}}$$

$$k_{21} = \frac{A\beta + B\alpha}{A + B}$$

$$k_{10} = \frac{\alpha\beta}{k_{21}}$$

$$k_{12} = \alpha + \beta - (k_{21} + k_{10})$$

$$V_{\mathrm{area}} = \frac{\mathrm{dose}}{\beta(\mathrm{AUC})} = \frac{\mathrm{dose}}{\beta\left(\frac{A}{\alpha} + \frac{B}{\beta}\right)}$$

$$V_{\mathrm{ss}} = \frac{\mathrm{dose}}{A + B} \times \frac{k_{12} + k_{21}}{k_{21}}.$$

Analysis of the plasma concentration of phenoperidine after intravenous injection gave the following values, using a digital computer program:

$A = 30$ ng ml^{-1}
$\alpha = 0.276$ min^{-1}
$t_{\frac{1}{2}\alpha} = 2.5$ min
$B = 12$ ng ml^{-1}
$\beta = 0.019$ min^{-1}
$t_{\frac{1}{2}\beta} = 37.0$ min
AUC = 725 ng ml^{-1} · min
CL = 2511 ml min^{-1}
$k_{21} = 0.090$ min^{-1}
$k_{10} = 0.057$ min^{-1}
$k_{12} = 0.147$ min^{-1}
$V_{area} = 134$ l
$V_{ss} = 117$ l.

As shown above, two expressions for the volume of distribution can be derived — V_{area} and V_{ss}. V_{area} expresses the relation between the total amount of phenoperidine in the body and its concentration in the central compartment during the terminal or slow disposition phase (i.e. when distribution equilibrium has been established). V_{area} may overestimate the true volume of distribution when rapid drug elimination occurs and clearance is high. V_{ss} is not dependent on the rate of drug elimination, and therefore provides a more objective and accurate estimate of the volume of distribution.

The pharmacokinetics of drugs whose distribution and elimination are consistent with a two-compartment open model are often determined after rapid intravenous injection, using a bolus dose. In these conditions, the accurate measurement of some kinetic parameters may be relatively difficult. For instance, the estimation of both the clearance (CL) and the volume of distribution (V) are critically dependent on the area under the plasma concentration–time curve between $t = 0$ and $t = \infty$ (AUC). The AUC is determined from the relationship $A/\alpha + B/\beta$; since A is usually large and α is relatively small, any errors or inaccuracy in the determination of these constants may significantly affect the estimation of the AUC. Unfortunately, after the bolus injection of drugs, measurement of A and α may be extremely inaccurate since: (i) they are dependent on derived rather than measured concentration; (ii) they are usually determined from a relatively small number of points; and (iii) the plasma concentration of drugs is rapidly decreasing during the distribution phase, so that minor difficulties in the timing or removal of blood samples may lead to considerable errors.

In consequence, pharmacokinetic parameters that are based on measurements of plasma concentrations after the bolus injection of drugs should be interpreted with circumspection. These values can usually be measured more accurately when drugs are administered by intravenous infusion. In these conditions, pharmacokinetic parameters are best assessed after the administration of drugs for several half-lives.

Unfortunately, this is rarely possible, and shorter periods of infusion are usually employed. Pharmacokinetic constants applicable to a two-compartment open model can be derived from the postinfusion plasma concentration data by appropriate mathematical techniques. It should be recognized that when drugs are given by continuous intravenous infusion, the subsequent decline in their plasma concentration (and the α or fast disposition phase) is attenuated, since rapid distribution or redistribution no longer occurs. The slower decline in the plasma concentration after intravenous infusion may be clinically significant, and can prolong the effects of short-acting drugs (particularly when their effects are usually terminated by distribution).

Three-compartment models

The kinetics of most drugs after intravenous injection are consistent with a two-compartment open model. Nevertheless, in some circumstances models of greater complexity provide a better interpretation of the results. Thus, the decline in the plasma concentration of drugs after intravenous injection can sometimes be resolved into three exponential components, and the plasma concentration C_p after time t is defined by the expression:

$$C_p = Pe^{-\pi t} + Ae^{-\alpha t} + Be^{-\beta t}.$$

Values for the intercepts (P, A and B) and the slopes (π, α and β) of the three components can then be obtained either graphically or by the use of a digital computer program.

The decline in the plasma concentration of the drug can be interpreted in terms of a three-compartment open model, with drug administration into and elimination from the central compartment (Fig. 2.8). Alternatively, the decrease in plasma concentration can be interpreted by a three-compartment model in which elimination occurs from one of the peripheral compartments (Fig. 2.9). The parameters of these models (i.e. clearance, volume of distribution, individual compartmental volumes and the rate constants governing transfer between compartments) can then be determined.

In some instances, the decline in the plasma concentration of drugs is apparently consistent with both a two-compartment and a three-compartment model. The most appropriate pharmacokinetic model can be selected in the following manner. A semilogarithmic curve relating plasma concentration to time is resolved into both two and three exponential components, using a digital computer program. In each case, the residual variation between the experimental points and the computer-derived curves is calculated. If there is no significant reduction in variation when the results are analysed as a triexponential equation, then the biexponential solution (consistent with a two-compartment open model) is assumed to be correct. Although this does not prove that the two-compartment model is authentic, it does suggest

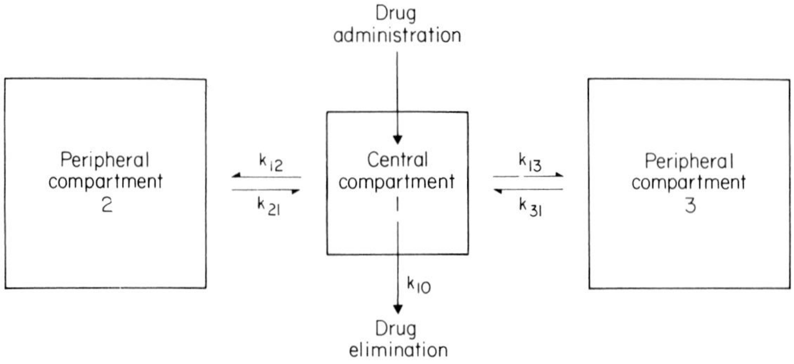

Fig. 2.8 A three-compartment, open model, consisting of a central compartment 1 and two peripheral compartments, 2 and 3. Drug administration occurs into, and elimination occurs from, the central compartment. The constants k_{12}, k_{21}, k_{13} and k_{31} govern drug transfer between the central and peripheral compartments; k_{10} is the elimination rate constant.

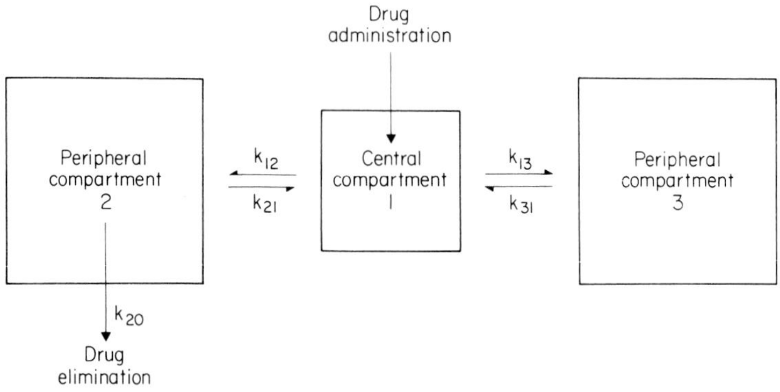

Fig. 2.9 A three-compartment, open model, consisting of a central compartment 1 and two peripheral compartments, 2 and 3. Drug administration occurs into the central compartment; drug elimination occurs from peripheral compartment 2. The constants k_{12}, k_{21}, k_{13} and k_{31} govern drug transfer between the central and the peripheral compartments; k_{20} is the elimination rate constant.

that the model provides a better interpretation of the results. In practice, the distinction between two-compartment and three-compartment models is small and of little importance. The difference between the experimental points and the computer-derived values may well be less than the accuracy of the analytical method used to measure drug concentrations. Similarly, the timing of the removal of blood samples may influence the choice of a pharmacokinetic model; inappropriate sampling times may fail to identify the initial phase or the terminal phase of exponential decline. In consequence, technical, analytical and sampling factors may play a disproportionate role in determining the type of pharmacokinetic model that is chosen. For instance, the decline in the plasma concentration of most non-depolarizing relaxants has been analysed by different authors using both two- and three-compartment models; these differences probably reflect the variability in the analytical measurement of plasma concentrations, different sampling times and possibly other technical factors.

Non-compartmental methods of pharmacokinetic analysis

The various problems associated with the resolution of plasma concentration data into specific compartmental models have led to the use of non-compartmental methods of pharmacokinetic analysis. These methods do not depend on the assumption of a specific pharmacokinetic model, although they can be used to estimate drug clearance (CL) and the volume of distribution at steady state (V_{ss}). The terminal half-life can also be derived by non-linear least-squares regression analysis, using a digital computer program; if necessary, the data can be weighted (usually by the reciprocal of the squares of the individual plasma concentrations).

Clearance can be derived from the relationship:

$$CL = \frac{\text{dose}}{\text{AUC}}$$

where AUC is the area under the plasma concentration–time curve between $t = 0$ and $t = \infty$. The AUC can be estimated by the trapezoidal rule, which depends on the measurement and summation of the area of each trapezoid between successive sampling times and the corresponding plasma concentrations. The area between the plasma concentration and time of the final sample and $t = \infty$ is estimated from the expression: final plasma concentration × terminal half-life ÷ 0.693.

Volume of distribution at steady state is given by the equation:

$$V_{ss} = \text{dose} \times \frac{\text{AUMC}}{(\text{AUC})^2}$$

where AUMC is the total area under the first moment of the plasma concentration–time curve (i.e. the area under the plasma concentration × time versus time curve, extrapolated to infinity).

Non-linear pharmacokinetics

When drug behaviour is analysed by pharmacokinetic models, it is usually assumed that distribution and elimination are first-order processes. In these conditions, the rate of drug transfer from compartment to compartment is always proportional to drug concentration. This presumption is not necessarily correct. Many physiological processes concerned with drug distribution and elimination are dependent on carrier transport, and are potentially saturable (i.e. they have a maximum finite transport capacity). Similarly, many reactions concerned with drug metabolism are saturable, and proceed at a maximal rate in the presence of high substrate concentrations. In these circumstances, drug transport and metabolism occur at a high but constant rate that is not dependent on drug concentration; in mathematical terms, $dX/dt = -k$, where X is the amount of drug in the body or compartment at time t, and k is a constant. This type of kinetics is called non-linear or saturation kinetics, and occurs with the capacity-limited elimination of drugs. Metabolic reactions that are subject to saturation kinetics are consistent with Michaelis–Menten kinetics; when saturation occurs, metabolism changes from a first-order process ($dX/dt = -kX^1 = -kX$) to a zero-order process ($dX/dt = -kX^0 = -k$), and is constant and independent of drug concentration.

These relationships can be derived from the Michaelis–Menten equation for enzyme kinetics as expressed in the form:

$$v = \frac{V_{max} \cdot C_p}{K_m + C_p}$$

where v is the rate of drug elimination; V_{max} is the maximum rate of drug elimination; K_m is an affinity constant (the Michaelis constant) and C_p is the plasma concentration. When the plasma concentration C_p is much less than K_m, then $v \approx (V_{max}/K_m) \times C_p$; since V_{max} and K_m are both constants, $v \propto C_p$, so that the rate of drug elimination is consistent with first-order kinetics. On the other hand, at higher plasma concentrations C_p may be greater than K_m, so that $v \approx (V_{max} \times C_p)/C_p$ and $v \approx V_{max}$. Thus the rate of drug elimination becomes constant at high concentrations, and is consistent with zero-order kinetics. The affinity constant K_m represents the affinity of the drug for the enzyme, carrier or transport system; it corresponds to the plasma concentration at which drug elimination is half its maximal rate (i.e. $v/V_{max} = 0.5$).

In practice, the phenomenon of non-linear or saturation kinetics is relatively uncommon, since the capacity of carrier transport systems and metabolic reactions is normally much greater than effective drug concentrations. Nevertheless, in some instances (particularly with drugs that are primarily or predominantly eliminated by hepatic metabolism), non-linear or zero-order kinetics occurs *in vivo*. In these conditions, increases in drug dosage and plasma concentration may cause prolongation in the half-life of drugs, and the area under the plasma concentration–time curve is disproportionately raised. (By contrast, when drugs are distributed and eliminated by first-order processes, all kinetic parameters are by definition independent of the dose.) Non-linear pharmacokinetics may occur during the metabolism of ethanol, salicylates and phenytoin, due to saturation of hepatic metabolic pathways. In the case of phenytoin, saturation may occur at subtherapeutic or therapeutic concentrations (40–80 μmol l^{-1}), so that subsequent increments in dosage cause a disproportionate increase in plasma concentration. Saturation kinetics may also occur during the elimination of large or repeated doses of thiopentone; in these circumstances, the terminal half-life of the drug is increased and its pharmacological effects are prolonged, possibly due to zero-order hepatic metabolism.

Non-linear pharmacokinetics also occurs in many patients during drug overdosage. It is uncertain whether this reflects saturation of hepatic metabolism, the toxic effects of drugs, or both phenomena. When drugs are eliminated by saturable processes (e.g. after the administration of phenytoin or during drug overdosage), the subsequent decrease in plasma concentration is associated with reversion from zero-order to first-order kinetics. Consequently, the plasma half-life becomes progressively shorter during drug elimination, and the logarithm of the plasma concentration versus time curve is bell-shaped, rather than monoexponential or biexponential.

Compartmental analysis and pharmacological effects

When drugs produce reversible effects at their site of action, there is usually a close correlation between their concentration and their pharmacological effects. When the site of action is in the central compartment, there may be a close correlation between the amount of drug in the compartment and the intensity or magnitude of its effects. Thus, in some studies the serum concentration of tubocurarine (and the amount of the drug in the central compartment) was closely correlated with its effects on neuromuscular transmission, suggesting that the action of the drug is in this compartment. More recent evidence suggests that a better interpretation of the pharmacokinetics and pharmacodynamics of muscle relaxants may be obtained when a separate effect compartment is added to a pharmacokinetic model. Thus, when non-depolarizing muscle relaxants are infused intravenously, there is a short latent period between the rise in their plasma concentration and the onset of neuromuscular blockade; when the infusion ceases, the fall in plasma concentration occurs slightly earlier than the recovery in neuromuscular transmission. This phenomenon of hysteresis or temporal disequilibrium can be rationalized by the addition of a separate effect compartment (with distinct rate constants) to the central compartment of a pharmacokinetic model.

Hysteresis or temporal disequilibrium occurs with other drugs, and can be interpreted and analysed by statistical techniques. When plasma concentration (abscissa) is plotted against pharmacological effect (ordinate), a hysteresis loop is obtained by sequentially joining the points relating concentration to effect at different times (Fig. 2.10). When changes in plasma concentration have a close temporal correlation with pharmacological effects, the area enclosed by the hysteresis loop is relatively small, suggesting that the drug may act in the same compartment as plasma. In other circumstances, there may be a considerable latent period between the rise in plasma concentration and the onset of a pharmacological response, or drug action may persist for some time after the decline in plasma concentration. In these conditions, the area enclosed by the hysteresis loop relating concentration to effect is significantly greater than zero (Fig. 2.10). This may suggest that the drug is acting in a compartment that is different from plasma, or that its effects on drug receptors are not readily reversible.

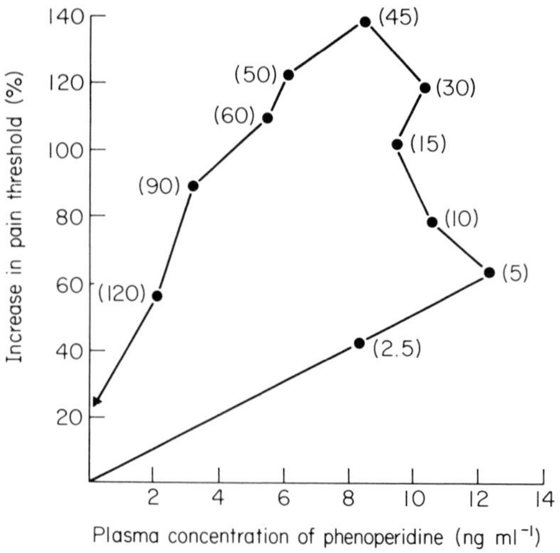

Fig. 2.10 Relation between the plasma concentration of phenoperidine and its analgesic effects. Values in parentheses represent the time (min) after intravenous injection of phenoperidine.

The value and limitations of pharmacokinetic analysis

The clinical use of anaesthetic agents is primarily based on their fundamental biological properties and pharmacodynamic effects, i.e. by their intrinsic ability to affect and modify cellular and subcellular processes. In comparison, pharmacokinetics is a subject of lesser importance and little practical significance. Nevertheless, pharmacokinetic models can be used to design acceptable dosage regimes for the intravenous administration of anaesthetic agents; in some instances, automatic control systems based on pharmacokinetic models have been designed to produce predetermined plasma concentrations of drugs. More recently, feedback devices that monitor drug responses have been used to produce closed-loop control of infusion systems. Unfortunately, there are several difficulties involved in the consistent application of these pharmacokinetic regimes in humans.

In the first place, the pharmacokinetic models used may not accurately predict or reflect *in vivo* conditions in anaesthetized patients. The choice of an appropriate pharmacokinetic model may be influenced by sampling times, or reflect technical, analytical or procedural factors. Although the distinction between two- and three-compartment models is often based on relatively small differences in plasma concentrations, it may result in large differences in derived kinetic values. In addition, determination of the parameters of the rapid disposition phase after the bolus administration of drugs is extremely difficult, and may lead to considerable inaccuracies in the determination of model parameters. In many instances, pharmacokinetic parameters are based on sampling for less than the ideal period of 6–10 half-lives; in other cases, accepted values for the terminal half-life have to be modified as the sensitivity of analytical methods increases. In addition, the use of a mean or average pharmacokinetic model may not reflect the physiological or ethnic variability between patients, or the changes induced by pathological conditions. In these circumstances, the determination of pharmacokinetic parameters with an accuracy of several places of decimals is entirely unjustified.

Second, the value of pharmacokinetic methods in clinical anaesthesia depends on the presence of a definite and measurable relationship between the plasma concentration of drugs and their pharmacological effects in humans. Pharmacokinetic analysis is of little practical use unless drug activity is a predictable function of plasma concentration. Unfortunately, in many instances the relationship between plasma concentration and biological effects is uncertain or unpredictable; indeed, in some circumstances, there are theoretical or a priori reasons for supposing that the relationship between these variables is complex or unquantifiable. Thus, anaesthetic agents may not act in a reversible manner (e.g. neostigmine, pyridostigmine); others have active metabolites with similar effects (e.g. diacetylmorphine, morphine, diazepam, thiopentone); while some have an onset and duration of action independent of their pharmacokinetics (e.g. some opioids and local anaesthetics). In all of these instances, pharmacokinetic methods will be of little use in the accurate prediction of drug activity.

Finally, approximately 60% of anaesthetic drugs are administered as chiral agents, which are usually given as racemic mixtures of two stereoisomers (Chapter 4). These drugs include many inhalational anesthetics, intravenous anaesthetics and local anaesthetics, as well as some muscle relaxants and agents that act on the cardiovascular system. In most instances, their plasma concentrations have been determined by non-stereoselective methods after administration of the racemic drug. In these conditions, the proportion of stereoisomers in the racemic mixture (originally 50% : 50%) may rapidly change to an unknown ratio in the body, and the pharmacokinetic interpretation of the derived kinetic constants may be extremely inaccurate and misleading. In addition, the plasma concentrations of both enantiomers may be declining in a monoexponential manner characterized by different rate constants, resulting in an apparent but erroneous biexponential decline in plasma concentration. It is also extremely unlikely that the unresolved plasma concentrations of the chiral mixture will reflect the pharmacodynamic effects of the more active isomer. In these circumstances, pharmacokinetic interpretation of the decline in plasma concentration may lead to incorrect conclusions. Indeed, the generation of pharmacokinetic data on racemates by methods that do not distinguish between the enantiomers has been described as a waste of money on unscientific, sophisticated nonsense.

Bioavailability

When drugs are administered orally, the concept of bioavailability is frequently used to indicate the proportion of the dose that is present in the systemic circulation.

Bioavailability (or biological availability) has been defined as the rate and extent to which a drug is absorbed and becomes available at its site of action. Nevertheless, the total amount of drug that is present in the systemic circulation is usually more important than its rate of absorption, and bioavailability is usually defined by reference to the area under the plasma concentration–time curve (AUC). After intravenous administration, drugs can be presumed to have a bioavailability of 100%; consequently, the absolute bioavailability (%) of drugs can be defined as:

$$\frac{(\mathrm{AUC}_{0-\infty}\text{ after oral administration})}{(\mathrm{AUC}_{0-\infty}\text{ after intravenous administration})}\times 100.$$

Alternatively, the absolute bioavailability of drugs can be measured from the total excretion of unchanged drug in urine after oral and intravenous administration. Occasionally, absolute bioavailability can be determined without intravenous administration, for example, with drugs that show pH-dependent renal clearance. When intravenous administration is not possible, the relative bioavailability can be measured by reference to a different standard (e.g. an alternative dosage form). Sometimes relative bioavailability is defined by reference to a different route of administration (e.g. subcutaneous or intramuscular injection); in these conditions, it may not be identical with the absolute bioavailability.

Some drugs have a high oral bioavailability (e.g. diazepam, digoxin, phenytoin, warfarin). These compounds are stable in gastrointestinal secretions, are well-absorbed from the small intestine, and are not significantly metabolized by the gut wall or the liver before they gain access to the systemic circulation. In contrast, other drugs have a low oral bioavailability, which may be due to several factors. In the first place, some drugs are unstable or are broken down in the gastrointestinal tract (e.g. benzylpenicillin, heparin, many polypeptide hormones). Second, drugs may be absorbed to a limited extent, due to physicochemical factors (e.g. relatively poor lipid solubility and a high molecular weight). Drugs that are poorly absorbed from the small intestine include neostigmine, glycopyrrolate and aminoglycoside antibiotics. Finally, drugs with a high first-pass effect have a low systemic bioavailability, due to their extensive metabolism by the gut and the liver (e.g. morphine, propranolol, lignocaine). This reduces the amount of unchanged drug which gains access to the systemic circulation.

The cause of the reduced oral bioavailability of drugs can often be determined by the isolation and identification of drug metabolites in plasma or urine. When high concentrations of drug metabolites are present, poor systemic bioavailability is usually due to an extensive first-pass effect and flow-limited hepatic clearance. On the other hand, if significant amounts of drug metabolites are not identified in plasma or urine, poor absorption (or gastrointestinal breakdown) is probably responsible.

Differences in the oral bioavailability of drugs may be due to several causes. Numerous pharmaceutical factors can influence the dissolution of tablets and capsules. In these conditions, proprietary or generic preparations of the same drug may have different dissolution characteristics and thus produce a range of plasma concentrations after oral administration. These variations in drug dissolution mainly occur with relatively insoluble drugs that are administered orally, and the subsequent differences in bioavailability may be clinically significant (p. 9). Interindividual differences in hepatic blood flow and first-pass metabolism can also lead to variations in bioavailability. With flow-limited hepatic clearance, any reduction in hepatic blood flow may lead to an increase in bioavailability. Drugs that induce or inhibit hepatic microsomal enzymes may also affect systemic bioavailability; for instance, cimetidine can increase the bioavailability of propranolol. Similarly, physiological changes (old age) and pathological factors (hepatic cirrhosis) can impair drug metabolism and increase bioavailability.

Physiological perfusion models

Although the systemic pharmacokinetics of many drugs have been investigated, the precise interpretation of many of these studies may be difficult or obscure. Consequently, the distribution and elimination of a small number of drugs (e.g. thiopentone, digoxin, lignocaine, methotrexate, inhalational anaesthetics) have been described in terms of physiological perfusion models. These depend on the interpretation of drug distribution in terms of anatomical or physiological spaces, which have defined volumes, perfusion characteristics and partition coefficients that are specific for each drug. Models, or individual compartments, may have either flow-limited or membrane-limited characteristics (depending on whether blood flow or transmembrane transport is the limiting factor governing drug uptake).

One of the best-known examples of a physiological perfusion model is concerned with the distribution and disposition of thiopentone. The concentration of the drug in blood, skeletal muscle and subcutaneous fat at various times after its administration was shown to be consistent with a relatively simple model (consisting of a central blood pool and six tissue compartments). This suggested that thiopentone was primarily removed from the brain by lean body tissues (e.g. muscle) and that subcutaneous fat only played a subsidiary role. The model was subsequently refined by the inclusion of compartments representing drug metabolism, plasma protein binding and tissue binding.

Physiological perfusion models have a number of distinct advantages. They can be used to predict drug concentrations at the site of action in tissues. Distribution and elimination can be precisely described, and they can also take account of local or general physiological changes during anaesthesia (e.g. alterations in cardiac output, regional blood flow and renal function). In some instances, they recognize intrasubject variability in drug disposition. Unfortunately, a number of problems may be associated with their use. They depend on the detailed measurement and analysis of a large number of physiological and pharmacological data, and the collection of appropriate tissue samples from anaesthetized patients may be difficult or impossible. In addition, the models may be described by complex differential equations, and their solution may require access to a digital computer.

Further reading

Allott PR, Steward A, Mapleson WW. Pharmacokinetics of halothane in the dog. *British Journal of Anaesthesia* 1976; **48**: 279–295.

Ariens EJ. Stereochemistry, a basis for sophisticated nonsense in pharmacokinetics and clinical pharmacology. *European Journal of Clinical Pharmacology* 1984; **26**: 663–668.

Ariens EJ. Chirality in bioactive agents and its pitfalls. *Trends in Pharmacological Sciences* 1986; **7**: 200–205.

Aziz NS, Gambertoglia JG, Lin ET, Grausz H, Benet LZ. Pharmacokinetics of cephamandole using a HPLC assay. *Journal of Pharmacokinetics and Biopharmaceutics* 1978; **6**: 153–164.

Benet LZ, Galeazzi RL. Noncompartmental determination of the steady-state volume of distribution. *Journal of Pharmaceutical Sciences* 1979; **68**: 1071–1074.

Benet LZ, Massoud N, Gambertoglio JG. *Pharmacokinetic Basis for Drug Treatment*. New York: Raven Press, 1984.

Benet LZ, Ronfeld RA. Volume terms in pharmacokinetics. *Journal of Pharmaceutical Sciences* 1969; **58**: 639–641.

Bennett WM, Porter GA, Bagby SP, McDonald WJ. *Drugs and Renal Disease*. New York: Churchill Livingstone, 1978.

Bevan DR, Bevan JC, Donati F. Pharmacokinetic Principles. In: Bevan DR, Donati F (eds) *Muscle Relaxants in Clinical Anesthesia*. Chicago: Year Book Medical Publishers, 1988; 100–132.

Bischoff KB, Dedrick RL. Thiopental pharmacokinetics. *Journal of Pharmaceutical Sciences* 1968; **57**: 1346–1351.

Blaschke TF. Protein binding and kinetics of drugs in liver diseases. *Clinical Pharmacokinetics* 1977; **2**: 32–44.

Boobis AR, Davies DS. Pharmacokinetics. *Hospital Update* 1981; **7**: 453–460.

Calvey TN, Williams NE, Muir K, Barber HE. Plasma concentration of edrophonium in man. *Clinical Pharmacology and Therapeutics* 1976; **19**: 813–820.

Dost FH. *Der Blutspiegel: Kinetic der Konzentrations-Ablaufe in der Kreisaufflussigkeit*. Leipzig: Thieme, 1953.

Evans AM, Nation RL, Sansom LN, Bochner F, Somogyi AA. Stereoselective drug disposition: potential for misinterpretation of drug disposition data. *British Journal of Clinical Pharmacology* 1988; **26**: 771–780.

Galeazzi RL, Benet LZ, Sheiner LB. Relationship between the pharmacokinetics and pharmacodynamics of procainamide. *Clinical Pharmacology and Therapeutics* 1979; **20**: 278–289.

Gibaldi M. *Biopharmaceutics and Clinical Pharmacokinetics*, 3rd edn. Philadelphia: Lea & Febiger, 1984.

Gibaldi M, Levy G, Hayton W. Kinetics of the elimination and neuromuscular blocking effect of *d*-tubocurarine in man. *Anesthesiology* 1972; **36**: 213–218.

Gibaldi M, McNamara PJ. Tissue binding of drugs. *Journal of Pharmaceutical Sciences* 1977; **66**: 1211–1212.

Gibaldi M, McNamara PJ. Apparent volumes of distribution and drug binding to plasma proteins and tissues. *European Journal of Clinical Pharmacology* 1978; **13**: 373–378.

Gibaldi M, Perrier D. *Pharmacokinetics*, 2nd edn. New York: Marcel Dekker, 1982.

Gillis PP, De Angelis RJ, Wynn RL. Nonlinear pharmacokinetic model of intravenous anesthesia. *Journal of Pharmaceutical Sciences* 1976; **65**: 1001–1006.

Greenblatt DJ, Koch-Weser J. Clinical pharmacokinetics. *New England Journal of Medicine* 1975; **293**: 702–705, 964–970.

Greenblatt DJ, Smith TW, Koch-Weser J. Bioavailability of drugs: the digoxin dilemma. *Clinical Pharmacokinetics* 1976; **1**: 36–51.

Himmelstein KJ, Lutz RJ. A review of the applications of physiologically based pharmacokinetic modeling. *Journal of Pharmacokinetics and Biopharmaceutics* 1979; **7**: 127–145.

Hunter JM, Jones RS, Utting JE. Use of atracurium in patients with no renal function. *British Journal of Anaesthesia* 1982; **54**: 1251–1258.

Hunter JM, Jones RS, Utting JE. Comparison of vecuronium, atracurium, and tubocurarine in normal patients and in patients with no renal function. *British Journal of Anaesthesia* 1984; **56**: 941–951.

Jusko WJ, Gibaldi M. Effects of change in elimination on various parameters of the two-compartment open model. *Journal of Pharmaceutical Sciences* 1972; **61**: 1270–1273.

Kaplan SA, Jack ML, Alexander K, Weinfeld RE. Pharmacokinetic profile of diazepam in man following single intravenous and oral and chronic oral administrations. *Journal of Pharmaceutical Sciences* 1973; **62**: 1789–1796.

Klotz U. Pathophysiological and disease-induced changes in drug distribution volume; pharmacokinetic implications. *Clinical Pharmacokinetics* 1976; **1**: 204–218.

Koch-Weser J. Serum drug concentrations as therapeutic guides. *New England Journal of Medicine* 1972; **287**: 227–231.

Labaune J-P. *Textbook of Pharmacokinetics*. Chichester: Ellis Horwood, 1989.

Lalka D, Feldman H. Absolute drug bioavailability. Approximation without comparison to parenteral dose for compounds exhibiting perturbable renal clearance. *Journal of Pharmaceutical Sciences* 1974; **63**: 1812.

Levy G. Pharmacokinetics of salicylate elimination in man. *Journal of Pharmaceutical Sciences* 1965; **54**: 959–967.

Levy G. Kinetics of pharmacological activity of succinylcholine in man. *Journal of Pharmaceutical Sciences* 1967; **56**: 1687–1688.

Levy G. Pharmacokinetics of succinylcholine in newborns. *Anesthesiology* 1970; **32**: 551–552.

Levy G, Tsuchiya T, Amsel LP. Limited capacity for salicyl phenolic glucuronide formation and its effects on the kinetics of salicylate elimination in man. *Clinical Pharmacology and Therapeutics* 1970; **13**: 258–268.

Loo JCK, Riegelman S. Assessment of pharmacokinetic constants from post-infusion blood curves obtained after IV infusion. *Journal of Pharmaceutical Sciences* 1970; **59**: 53–55.

Lundquist F, Wolthers H. The kinetics of alcohol elimination in man. *Acta Pharmacologica et Toxicologica* 1958; **14**: 265–289.

Michaelis M, Menten ML. Die Kinetic der Invertinwirkung. *Biochemische Zeitschrift* 1913; **49**: 333–369.

Milne L, Williams NE, Calvey TN, Murray GR, Chan K. Plasma concentration and metabolism of phenoperidine in man. *British Journal of Anaesthesia* 1980; **52**: 537–540.

Nagashima R, Levy G, O'Reilly RA. Comparative pharmacokinetics of coumarin anticoagulants. IV. Application of a three compartment model to the analysis of the dose-dependent kinetics of bishydroxycoumarin elimination. *Journal of Pharmaceutical Sciences* 1968; **57**: 1888–1895.

Notari E. *Biopharmaceutics and Clinical Pharmacokinetics: An Introduction*, 3rd edn. New York: Marcel Dekker, 1980.

Paxton JW. Elementary pharmacokinetics in clinical practice: 3. Practical pharmacokinetic applications. *New Zealand Medical Journal* 1981; **94**: 381–384.

Peck CC, Barrett BB. Nonlinear least squares regression programs for microcomputers. *Journal of Pharmacokinetics and Biopharmaceutics* 1979; **5**: 537–541.

Price HL, Kovnat PJ, Safer JN, Conner EH, Price ML. The uptake of thiopental by body tissues and its relation to the duration of narcosis. *Clinical Pharmacology and Therapeutics* 1960; **1**: 16–22.

Prys-Roberts C, Hug CC. (eds) *Pharmacokinetics of Anaesthesia*. Oxford: Blackwell Scientific Publications, 1984.

Riegelman S, Loo JCK, Rowland M. Shortcomings in pharmacokinetic analysis by conceiving the body to exhibit properties of a single compartment. *Journal of Pharmaceutical Sciences* 1968; **57**: 117–123.

Riegelman S, Loo J, Rowland M. Concept of a volume of distribution and possible errors in evaluation of this parameter. *Journal of Pharmaceutical Sciences* 1968; **57**: 128–133.

Riggs DS. *The Mathematical Approach to Physiological Problems*. Baltimore: Williams and Wilkins, 1963.

Rowland M, Benet LZ, Graham GG. Clearance concepts in pharmacokinetics. *Journal of Pharmacokinetics and Biopharmaceutics* 1973; **1**: 123–136.

Rowland M, Tozer TN. *Clinical Pharmacokinetics: Concepts and Applications*. Philadelphia: Lea & Febiger, 1980.

Saidman LJ, Eger EI II. The effect of thiopental metabolism on duration of anesthesia. *Anesthesiology* 1966; **27**: 118–126.

Shaw TRD, Howard MR, Hamer J. Variation in the biological availability of digoxin. *Lancet* 1972; **ii**: 303–307.

Sheiner LB, Stanski DR, Vozeh S, Miller RD, Ham J. Simultaneous modeling of pharmacokinetics and pharmacodynamics: application to *d*-tubocurarine. *Clinical Pharmacology and Therapeutics* 1979; **215**: 358–371.

Somani SM, Chan K, Dehghan A, Calvey TN. Kinetics and metabolism of intramuscular neostigmine in myasthenia gravis. *Clinical Pharmacology and Therapeutics* 1980; **28**: 64–68.

Stanski DR, Mihm FG, Rosenthal MH, Kalman SM. Pharmacokinetics of high-dose thiopental used in cerebral resuscitation. *Anesthesiology* 1980; **53**: 169–171.

Stanski DR, Watkins WD. *Drug Disposition in Anesthesia*. New York: Grune & Stratton, 1982.

Teorell T, Dedrick RL, Condliffe PG. (eds) *Pharmacology and Pharmacokinetics*. New York: Plenum Press, 1974.

Tozer TN. Concepts basic to pharmacokinetics. *Pharmacology and Therapeutics* 1981; **12**: 109–131.

Tyrer JH, Eadie MJ, Sutherland JM, Hooper WD. Outbreak of anticonvulsant intoxication in an Australian city. *British Medical Journal* 1970; **4**: 271–273.

Walle T, Walle UK. Pharmacokinetic parameters obtained in racemates. *Trends in Pharmacological Sciences* 1986; **7**: 112–116.

Ward S, Boheimer N, Weatherley BC, Simmonds RJ, Dopson TA. Pharmacokinetics of atracurium and its metabolites in patients with normal renal function and in patients in renal failure. *British Journal of Anaesthesia* 1987; **59**: 697–706.

Waud BE, Waud DR. Dose–response curves and pharmacokinetics. *Anesthesiology* 1986; **65**: 355–358.

Westlake WJ. Problems associated with the analysis of pharmacokinetic models. *Journal of Pharmaceutical Sciences* 1971; **60**: 882–885.

Wilkinson GR. Clearance approaches in pharmacology. *Pharmacological Reviews* 1987; **39**: 1–47.

Wilkinson GR, Shand DG. A physiologic approach to hepatic drug clearance. *Clinical Pharmacology and Therapeutics* 1975; **18**: 377–390.

Wood AJJ. Drug disposition and pharmacokinetics. In: Wood M, Wood AJJ (eds) *Drugs and Anesthesia: Pharmacology for Anesthesiologists*. Baltimore: Williams and Wilkins, 1982.

Chapter 3
Drug Action

Drugs produce a wide range of responses in humans. These usually depend on the modification of cellular or subcellular function by agents with a relatively simple chemical structure. In some instances (e.g. with inhalational anaesthetics, local anaesthetics and non-depolarizing muscle relaxants) there is a reasonably close relationship between chemical structure or physicochemical properties and the effects of drugs. By contrast, compounds that are closely related chemically (e.g. promazine and promethazine) may produce quite different pharmacological effects (Chapter 4). The relation between chemical structure and biological activity was a central theme of experimental research for many years; indeed, this relationship played an important part in the development of the concept of drug receptors by John Newport Langley and Paul Ehrlich.

Relation between drug dosage and response

Pharmacological effects or responses are usually related to drug dosage or concentration by means of dose–response curves. In intact animals and in humans, the concentration of drugs at their site of action is dependent on the processes of absorption, distribution, metabolism and excretion, and it may be difficult to determine the precise relationship between the concentration of drugs in tissues and the pharmacological response. In experimental animals, the observation and analysis of the effects of drugs can be simplified by the use of isolated preparations (for instance, the frog rectus abdominis muscle, the rat phrenic nerve-diaphragm preparation, and the guinea-pig ileum). In these isolated tissue preparations, a defined concentration of the drug can be added to a tissue bath, and the response obtained can be directly measured by appropriate techniques. In some conditions, cumulative responses to drugs are studied (i.e. the tissue is not washed between successive doses of the drug). Many of the effects of drugs that produce observable and measurable responses (agonists) were originally assessed in these experimental conditions. Isolated human tissues removed during surgical operations are sometimes used to obtain dose–response curves in humans.

In these *in vitro* preparations, the relationship between drug dosage and the biological response obtained is usually shown by a dose–response curve. In most experimental situations, this curve has a hyperbolic shape. When the dose–response curve is converted to or expressed as a log dose–response relationship, the hyperbolic

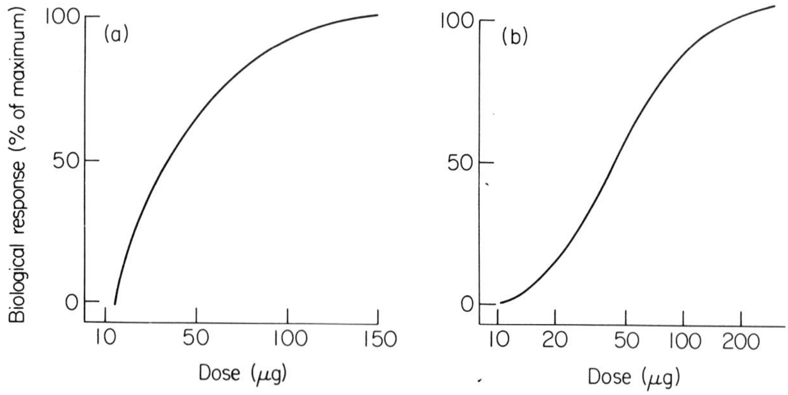

Fig. 3.1 The relation between drug dosage and response. In (a) the dose is plotted on a linear scale, giving a hyperbolic curve. In (b) the dose is plotted on a logarithmic scale, giving a sigmoid curve that is linear for most of its length.

dose–response curve usually becomes sigmoid or S-shaped (Fig. 3.1). The use of a sigmoid log dose–response curve (rather than the hyperbolic dose–response relationship) has a number of advantages; in particular, it is linear for most of its course (i.e. between 20% and 80% of the maximum response), and it permits the simultaneous comparison and assessment of drugs with large differences in potency. As shown in Fig. 3.1, incremental dosage progressively increases the responses obtained; as the dose is further increased, the proportional response diminishes, and eventually a maximum effect is obtained which cannot be exceeded irrespective of the dose. Highly potent agents (i.e. drugs that produce a given biological response at a relatively low dose level) have a log dose–response curve which is displaced to the left (i.e. towards the ordinate or *y* axis). By contrast, drugs of lower potency have a log dose–response curve that is displaced to the right.

The relationship between drug concentration and response can also be represented by the Hill plot. This method was first used by A.V. Hill at the turn of the century, during his studies on the relation between the partial pressure of oxygen and the percentage saturation of haemoglobin. In the Hill plot, the logarithm of drug dosage or concentration (*x* axis) is related to the value:

$$\log \frac{E}{E_{max} - E}$$

(*y* axis), where E_{max} is the maximum effect observed and E is the response obtained at different dose levels or concentrations (Fig. 3.2). If the relation between drug concentration and response is represented by a hyperbolic curve (Fig. 3.1), the Hill plot is usually linear and has a slope of approximately +1 (the Hill coefficient). The linear relationship between the variables in the Hill plot considerably simplifies the statistical analysis of the results.

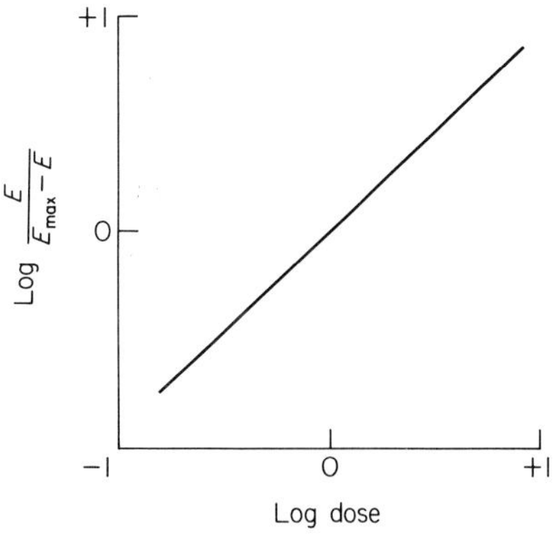

Fig. 3.2 A Hill plot relating the logarithm of drug dosage to the logarithm of $E \div (E_{max} - E)$, where E_{max} is the maximum effect and E is the observed effect at different dose levels. The Hill coefficient in the example shown is +1.0.

Many dose–response relationships are hyperbolic, and give rise to sigmoid log-dose–response curves, and Hill plots with a coefficient of +1. Nevertheless, other types of concentration–effect relationship are sometimes observed. Thus, dose–response curves for agonists at nicotinic, glutamate and γ-aminobutyric acid receptors are frequently sigmoidal rather than hyperbolic. In some experimental situations, log dose–response curves are biphasic (e.g. the effects of noradrenaline and adrenaline on the rabbit heart) or even bell-shaped (e.g. the effects of histamine on vascular smooth muscle in the guinea-pig pulmonary artery; Fig. 3.3). In these conditions, Hill plots can produce non-linear curves, or Hill coefficients that are significantly greater than 1.

In intact animals or in humans, the relation between drug dosage and response is more complex, and may be modified by homeostatic reflexes and pharmacokinetic

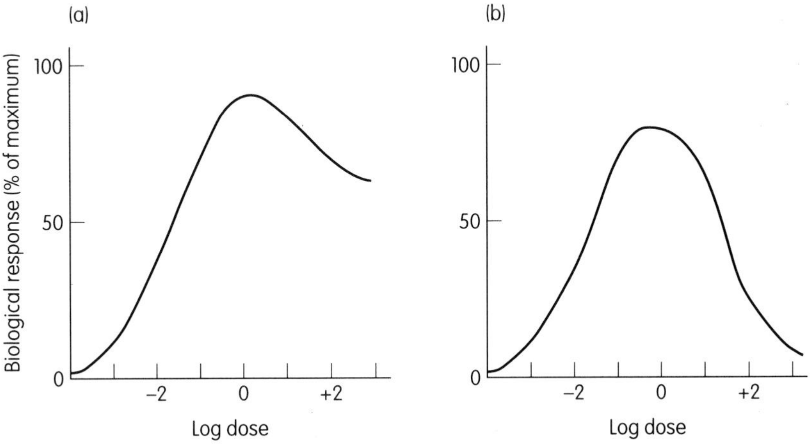

Fig. 3.3 Examples of atypical log dose–response relationships. (a) Biphasic log dose–response curve; (b) bell-shaped log dose–reponse curve.

processes (e.g. plasma protein binding and the presence of active metabolites). Consequently, the plasma concentrations of drugs (rather than their dosage) is usually related to their pharmacological effects. In these conditions, the slope of the plasma concentration–response curve may indicate the potential safety margin of a drug. When a relatively steep plasma level response relationship is present, toxic effects may be produced after small increments in dosage. By contrast, if drugs have more gradual plasma concentration–response relationships, incremental increases in dosage are usually less hazardous.

This type of dose–response relationship measures the response to incremental doses of the drug in isolated tissue preparations, rather than an all-or-none (quantal) response. At one time, quantal responses were widely used in experimental pharmacology, in order to estimate the median effective dose (ED_{50}) and the median lethal dose (LD_{50}) of drugs and the relation between their effectiveness and toxicity. In recent years their use has greatly declined.

The basis of drug action

In general, drugs produce their pharmacological effects in three ways. In the first place, the effects of drugs may be related to their physicochemical properties, or to their chemical combination with other agents or trace elements. Secondly, they may act by inhibiting enzymes concerned with normal metabolic processes. Finally, drugs may act on receptor sites in cells or subcellular structures. In recent years, studies of many drug–receptor reactions suggest that a relatively small number of cellular and molecular mechanisms may mediate a wide range of different responses to drugs, hormones and other endogenous compounds.

Actions dependent on chemical or physicochemical properties

The effects of some drugs may be directly dependent on their chemical properties. Antacids, for example, act primarily by neutralizing gastric acid, and may produce minor changes in systemic pH and acid–base status. Alterations in systemic or urinary pH are commonly produced by many acids and bases, due to the addition or removal of hydrogen ions from body fluids. The effects of chelating agents are also due to their chemical properties. These drugs combine with certain metallic ions (e.g. arsenic, lead, copper, zinc, mercury, silver, gold), and are sometimes used to remove these elements from the body. Chelating agents that are used in medicine include penicillamine, sodium calcium edetate, dicobalt edetate, desferrioxamine and the tetracyclines.

Penicillamine (dimethylcysteine) increases the elimination of lead, copper and mercury by combining with these elements and enhancing their urinary excretion. Consequently, the drug is used in the management of heavy-metal poisoning, and in the treatment of Wilson's disease (in which copper deposition occurs in the liver, the basal ganglia and the cornea). Although it has other therapeutic applications (e.g. in rheumatoid arthritis and cystinuria), its effectiveness in these conditions is not dependent on chelation. Penicillamine is a normal breakdown product of penicillin.

Sodium calcium edetate chelates lead (and certain other heavy metals), and is used in the treatment of lead poisoning and encephalopathy. It is usually administered by slow intravenous infusion; the use of the calcium salt prevents the development of hypocalcaemia. A related drug (calcium trisodium pentetate) has a greater affinity for heavy metals, and is sometimes used in lead or iron poisoning. Sodium edetate preferentially removes calcium ions from extracellular fluid; when injected or infused intravenously it may cause significant hypocalcaemia, but is commonly used *in vitro* as an anticoagulant (sequestrene). Sodium hydrogen citrate (acid citrate) also chelates calcium ions (forming a calcio-citrate), and is used to prevent coagulation in stored blood. When large amounts of blood are given (or the rate of infusion is rapid) hypocalcaemia may occur; this complication can be prevented by calcium gluconate (1 g intravenously).

Dicobalt edetate chelates cyanide ions, and is used in the treatment of cyanide poisoning. It has also been used to remove cyanide ions after the infusion of large doses of sodium nitroprusside. Dicobalt edetate is a relatively toxic drug, and may cause bradycardia and cardiac arrhythmias.

Desferrioxamine is a specific binding agent for iron, and is used in the treatment of iron poisoning and in the management of haemochromatosis. This drug has a high affinity for the iron in ferritin and haemosiderin; it has little effect on iron that is bound to transferrin or contained in myoglobin, haemoglobin or the cytochrome enzymes.

The tetracyclines are potent chelating agents, and readily combine with iron, calcium, magnesium and aluminium ions; when given orally with compounds containing these elements (e.g. iron salts and antacids), the absorption of tetracyclines may be impaired. The ability of tetracyclines to chelate calcium and magnesium ions may be partly responsible for their bacteriostatic effects.

The action of other drugs may be dependent on their physicochemical properties. Both local anaesthetics and inhalational anaesthetics may act by producing non-specific changes in the lipid or protein components, which affect the diameter of ion channels in the neuronal membrane. Nevertheless, recent evidence suggests that local and inhalational anaesthetics may affect the nervous system in a more specific manner. Local anaesthetics may combine with receptors at the internal aspect of sodium channels, causing a decrease in their diameter. In these conditions, sodium conductance is reduced below the threshold required for depolarization. Inhalational anaesthetics have been generally considered to interact with non-polar sites associated with membrane proteins or phospholipids; nevertheless, current views suggest that they affect neuronal proteins in the brain in a relatively selective manner (Chapter 8).

Actions dependent on enzyme inhibition

The action of many drugs is dependent on the inhibition of enzymes concerned with normal metabolic processes (Table 3.1). Drugs that act by enzyme inhibition are often chemically related to natural substrates that are normally metabolized by the enzyme. For example, allopurinol (a xanthine oxidase inhibitor) is a chemical analogue of the naturally occurring purine bases xanthine and hypoxanthine, which are normally converted by xanthine oxidase to uric acid.* Similarly, many sulphonamides are closely related to *para*-aminobenzoic acid, and prevent its conversion to folic acid by the bacterial enzyme folate synthetase.

Drugs may inhibit enzymes in a reversible or an irreversible manner. Reversible enzyme inhibitors (e.g. edrophonium, allopurinol and the sulphonamides) generally compete with natural substrates for enzymes, and their effects do not depend on the formation of stable chemical bonds.

Table 3.1 Commonly used drugs whose effects are partly or totally due to enzyme inhibition.

Drug	Enzyme inhibited
Allopurinol	Xanthine oxidase
Aminophylline Enoximone Milrinone	Phosphodiesterases
Acetylsalicylic acid (and other NSAIDs)	Prostaglandin synthetase (cyclo-oxygenase)
Captopril Enalapril Lisinopril	Angiotensin-converting enzyme
Benserazide	Dopa decarboxylase
Chlorophenylalanine	Tryptophan hydroxylase
Disulfiram	Aldehyde dehydrogenase
Methotrexate Trimethoprim Pyrimethamine	Dihydrofolate reductase
Methyldopa	Amino acid decarboxylase
Edrophonium Neostigmine Pyridostigmine Organophosphates	Acetylcholinesterase Plasma cholinesterase
Benzylpenicillin	Bacterial wall transpeptidase
Moclobemide Phenelzine Tranylcypromine	Monoamine oxidase
Sulphonamides	Folate synthetase

In some instances, enzyme inhibition is dependent on the formation of drug metabolites.
NSAIDs, Non-steroidal anti-inflammatory drugs.

* A related drug, the antimetabolite mercaptopurine, is also metabolized to thio-uric acid by the enzyme.

The reaction can be expressed as:

inhibitor + enzyme $\rightleftharpoons$ enzyme–inhibitor complex.

The plasma or tissue concentration of reversible inhibitors may be related to the degree of enzyme inhibition. As reversible enzyme inhibitors are eliminated from the body, their plasma concentration falls and inhibition decreases. Since their action is not dependent on the formation of stable chemical bonds, their effects are usually brief and evanescent, and probably reflect the presence of drugs or their active metabolites in the immediate environment of the enzyme. Neostigmine, pyridostigmine and physostigmine are also usually classified as reversible enzyme inhibitors; nevertheless, this is only partially correct. Although they initially combine in a reversible manner with plasma cholinesterase and acetylcholinesterase, their action is dependent on the formation of a covalent chemical bond resulting in carbamylation of the enzyme. This covalent bond is slowly hydrolysed in the body, and the enzyme is gradually regenerated (Chapter 10).

Irreversible enzyme inhibition usually depends on the formation of a stable chemical complex between the inhibitor and the enzyme. In these conditions, regeneration of the inhibited enzyme is often impossible and a latent period is required for resynthesis of the enzyme before its function is restored. Drugs that act by irreversible enzyme inhibition include organophosphorus compounds, methotrexate and most potent monoamine oxidase inhibitors. These drugs have an extremely long duration of action, and they may produce effects for days or weeks after they are eliminated from the body.

In some instances, inhibitors that are closely related to natural substrates are metabolized by enzyme systems to compounds that interfere with or prevent normal cellular function. For instance, the cytotoxic drug fluorouracil competes with uracil for enzymes that normally synthesize ribonucleic acid (RNA); metabolites of fluorouracil are formed and incorporated into RNA, preventing protein synthesis. Similarly, methyldopa is converted to methyldopamine and methylnoradrenaline by both central and peripheral sympathetic neurones. These drug metabolites replace the physiological neurotransmitter (noradrenaline) in sympathetic nerve endings.

Actions dependent on combination with receptors

Many drugs produce their effects by combining with macromolecular sites in cells known as drug receptors. These receptor sites are closely related to the tissue cells that mediate the effects of drugs (effector cells). The concept of receptors was originally introduced by J.N. Langley, in order to account for the remarkable specificity and antagonism of certain drugs on physiological systems (e.g. the effects of pilocarpine and atropine on salivary secretion, and the action of nicotine and curare on neuromuscular transmission). The German physician Paul Ehrlich also played an important part in the development and acceptance of the concept of chemoreceptors associated with cells. Ehrlich was clearly influenced by the work of Langley, and by his own studies concerned with the development of cross-resistance to antitrypanosomal drugs with a similar chemical structure. The mathematical and quantitative aspects of drug–receptor reactions and drug responses were developed later by A.J. Clark and J.H. Gaddum.

In subsequent work between 1930 and 1960, the nature and properties of drug receptors were mainly inferred from the investigation of structure–activity relationships. In these studies, the response of isolated tissues to a series of drugs with related chemical structures was analysed (e.g. the response of smooth-muscle preparations to a series of choline esters). Although this work was of considerable value, it represented a relatively indirect approach to the structure and properties of receptors.

Since 1965, it has been possible to isolate receptors from tissues, or to study their properties in cell membrane preparations *in vitro*. More recently, the structure, function and organization of many receptors have been determined by molecular biological techniques. Intact receptors have been solubilized from cellular membranes, and subsequently purified by affinity chromatography or related techniques; the amino acid sequences of the purified receptors have then been established, using recombinant DNA technology. In some studies, messenger RNA (mRNA) has been generated by transcription of complementary DNA (cDNA), and injected into cultured cells *in vitro* (e.g. *Xenopus* oocytes or neuroblastoma–glioma hybrid cells), and the properties of the expressed receptors have been studied. In some instances, receptors expressed in stable cultured cells have been reconstituted with their transcription systems, and the molecular mechanisms underlying their physiological and biochemical effects have been studied. Similarly, many receptor variants and subtypes have been cloned from cDNA libraries and expressed in cultured cells; some of these receptor subtypes have no known physiological function and are not present in humans.

The distribution and heterogeneity of receptors in mammalian and human tissues have also been extensively studied, using radiolabelled compounds (radioligands) with a high affinity for specific receptors. For instance, the neurotoxins α-bungarotoxin (a polypeptide present in sea-snake venom) and cobra toxin are selectively bound by nicotinic receptors at the motor endplate. These radiolabelled neurotoxins have been widely used to isolate acetylcholine receptors from the synaptic junctions of many different species. Muscarinic receptors in the heart, the small intestine, sympathetic ganglia and the brain have also been identified by radiolabelled irreversible antagonists (e.g. ^{3}H-quinnuclidinyl benzilate). Similarly, dopamine receptors have been identified and isolated from a number of sites in the central nervous system (CNS) (e.g. the substantia nigra, the corpus striatum, the limbic system, the chemoreceptor trigger zone and the pituitary gland), using radiolabelled dopamine antagonists (e.g. ^{3}H-haloperidol, ^{3}H-spiperone, ^{3}H-flupenthixol). Dopamine receptors can also be identified in vascular smooth muscle (e.g. in the renal and the mesenteric circulation), and in sympathetic ganglia.

Similarly, both α- and β-adrenoceptors can be specifically labelled and identified by different radioligands, which may be agonists (e.g. ^{3}H-hydroxybenzylisoprenaline) or antagonists (e.g. ^{3}H-prazosin or ^{3}H-dihydroalprenolol). The binding of radioligands to adrenergic receptors has been extensively studied *in vitro*; in these conditions, radiolabelled drugs have a high receptor affinity and their binding to receptors is saturable, specific and competitive (i.e. they can be readily displaced by other agonists or antagonists). Adrenergic receptors are widely distributed in the body; in some instances (e.g. α_2-receptors in platelets, or β_2-receptors in vascular smooth muscle) their presence is not associated with a nerve supply. Adrenergic receptor density is modified in various pathological conditions (e.g. bronchial asthma, congestive cardiac failure, thyrotoxicosis). In general, high catecholamine concentrations reduce the number and density of adrenergic receptors (down-regulation). This phenomenon is partly due to the sequestration (internalization) of receptors within cells, although receptor affinity may also be modified. By contrast, any fall in circulating adrenaline and noradrenaline, either produced by drugs or by sympathetic denervation, increases the number of receptors (up-regulation). Similar changes in receptor density are probably produced by most neurotransmitters that act at synapses and neuroeffector junctions.

In some situations, an increase in the number of receptors may be partly responsible for the phenomenon of denervation supersensitivity. After peripheral denervation or damage to skeletal muscle, the response to acetylcholine and other depolarizing agents is increased, due to up-regulation. Extrajunctional receptors develop on the surface of the muscle fibre outside the motor endplate; the total number of nicotinic acetylcholine receptors may increase 100 times. In these conditions, the ionic changes associated with depolarization and repolarization may produce significant hyperkalaemia (e.g. when suxamethonium is given to patients with burns or some neurological conditions). Sympathetic denervation by surgical or pharmacological methods also increases peripheral responses to noradrenaline (and, to a lesser extent, to adrenaline). In these circumstances, the increased response is mainly related to impairment of the neuronal uptake of the sympathetic neurotransmitter. Any increase in the number of adrenergic receptors due to up-regulation probably plays a less important part.

The identification of macromolecular sites in cells as drug receptors depends on their association with a pharmacological effect or response. In addition, many receptor systems demonstrate the properties of sensitivity, specificity and saturability. Most receptors are extremely sensitive to naturally occurring agonists, and only small concentrations are required to produce a significant response. Consequently, considerable amplification or enhancement of the initial stimulus by intracellular mechanisms may be required to generate pharmacological effects. In addition, many receptor systems show considerable selectivity; they characteristically respond to a limited range of chemical agents with a defined structure, which are often closely related to naturally occurring neurotransmitters or hormones. Finally, drug receptors usually have a finite binding capacity. The number of receptors associated with cells is usually constant (although it can be modified by physiological or pharmacological factors). In consequence, the binding of many radiolabelled ligands and drugs by authentic receptors is a competitive and saturable process. Drug receptors characteristically show a high affinity and a low capacity for specific agonists and antagonists; by contrast, non-specific binding is a low-affinity, high-capacity phenomenon.

Most receptors that have been studied and isolated are present on the external surface of cells. An important exception are receptors for steroid hormones, which are present in the cytoplasm or nuclear membrane of certain cells (target cells). Steroid hormones are bound by specific receptor proteins; receptor activation modifies mRNA, and indirectly affects ribosomal protein synthesis.

The reversible combination of an agonist with the receptor (i.e. receptor occupancy) is the primary event that initiates a sequence of biophysical and biochemical reactions (e.g. ion transport, enzyme activation and protein synthesis) which results in the response. These reactions may be expressed in the following manner:

Drug + receptor
⇅
Drug–receptor complex
↓
Drug–activated receptor complex → drug + receptor
↓
Biophysical or biochemical change
↓
Drug response.

In general, there are three main types of biophysical or biochemical changes produced by receptor activation:

1. Direct changes in ionic permeability.
2. Accumulation of intermediate messengers.
3. Modification of nucleic acid synthesis.

Direct changes in ionic permeability

In some instances, receptor activation directly affects ion channels in synaptic membranes, resulting in a selective or non-selective increase in ionic permeability. In these conditions, receptors and ion channels usually form part of the same macromolecular complex (i.e. the receptor and the ion channel are identical). The increase in ionic permeability produced by receptor activation is usually rapid and evanescent; a maximal response may occur within microseconds, and only last for several milliseconds. Some neurotransmitters (e.g. acetylcholine, γ-aminobutyric acid, glutamate and glycine) act in this manner, and directly increase the ionic permeability of the postsynaptic membrane.

Neuromuscular transmission is a well-known example of a direct response to receptor activation. Acetylcholine is released from the motor nerve terminal and combines with receptors associated with non-selective ion channels. The nicotinic receptor at the neuromuscular junction is an integral membrane protein with a molecular weight or approximately 250 kDa; it consists of five subunits (α_1, α_2, β, γ and δ) which traverse the postsynaptic membrane and surround the ion channel or ionophore. Two of these subunits (the α units) have a molecular weight of approximately 40 kDa and contain acetylcholine binding sites (at Cys 192–Cys 193). Combination of the neurotransmitter with these binding sites results in conformational changes that open the ion channel; the probability of this occurring is considerably increased when both sites are occupied by acetylcholine. Ion channel opening is an extremely rapid all-or-none phenomenon which lasts for 1–3 ms, and causes a non-specific increase in permeability to small ions (mainly sodium, potassium and calcium ions). In experimental conditions, it has been estimated that acetylcholine causes the transfer of 10 000 ions per ionophore during each millisecond that the channel is open. These changes result in a localized endplate potential; if this reaches a threshold amplitude, an action potential is conducted along the muscle fibre (Chapter 10).

Other neurotransmitters also activate receptors that are directly linked to ion channels. Gamma-aminobutyric acid (GABA) is the main inhibitory neurotransmitter in the CNS, and mediates presynaptic (axoaxonal) and postsynaptic (axodendritic or axosomatic) inhibition at approximately 40% of all synapses. Many responses that are mediated by GABA depend on a directly induced, selective increase in permeability to chloride ions (rather than the non-selective response that occurs at the motor endplate). Receptor activation allows ions to diffuse from the external environment into the neurone, resulting in hyperpolarization and decreased neuronal excitability.

Accumulation of intermediate messengers

In many cells, receptor activation does not directly produce changes in ionic permeability or other drug responses. Many drugs are extremely potent substances, and amplification of the initial stimulus is essential in order to produce a biological response. In these conditions, receptor activation increases or decreases the activity of specific enzymes, resulting in the accumulation of intracellular metabolites that act as intermediate messengers. (They are more commonly known as second messengers; nevertheless, intermediate messengers is a better term, since more than one agent may be involved in drug responses.)

The most important intermediate messengers are: (i) cyclic adenosine monophosphate (cAMP); (ii) cyclic guanosine monophosphate (cGMP); (iii) nitric oxide; (iv) phosphoinositides and calcium ions.

Cyclic adenosine monophosphate

cAMP is synthesized from adenosine triphosphate (ATP) by the enzyme adenylyl cyclase (Fig. 3.4). Many drugs and hormones combine with receptors on the external aspect of cells, affect the activity of adenylyl cyclase, and thus modify the synthesis of cAMP. Receptor systems are coupled to adenylyl cyclase by regulatory G proteins (guanosine triphosphate (GTP)-binding proteins), which can stimulate (G_s) or inhibit

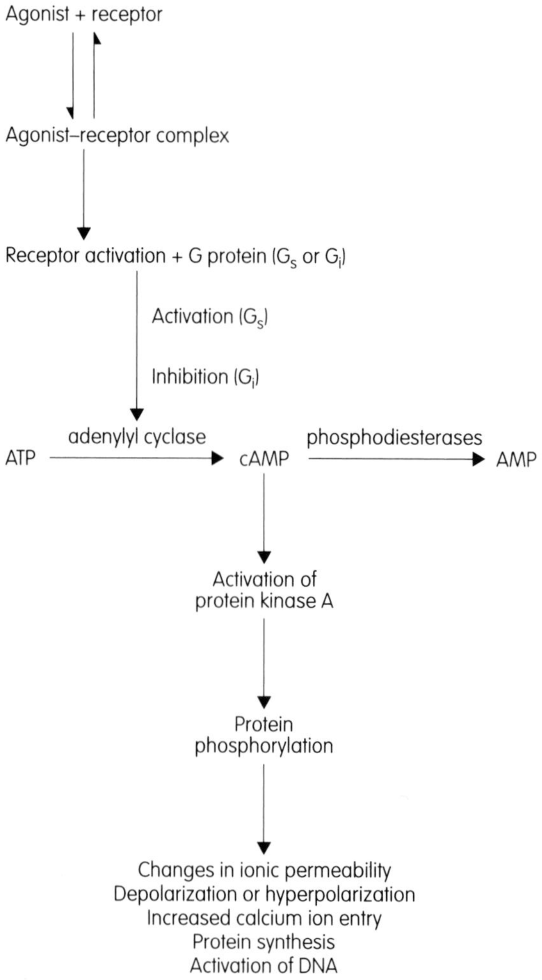

Fig. 3.4 The synthesis of cyclic adenosine monophosphate (cAMP) by adenylyl cyclase.

(G_i) the activity of the enzyme. When the regulatory protein is G_s, receptor agonists activate adenylyl cyclase and increase the synthesis of cAMP; if the regulatory protein is G_i, receptor agonists inhibit adenylyl cyclase and decrease the synthesis of cAMP. Regulatory G proteins have a heterotrimeric structure (i.e. they consist of three different subunits, α, β and γ). Receptor activation results in the binding of GTP by the α subunits of the regulatory protein, which is then transferred from the receptor to adenylyl cyclase (Fig. 3.5). G proteins play an important role in many other cellular systems; for example, the regulatory protein G_q controls the receptor-mediated activation of phospholipase C and the breakdown of phosphoinositides (p. 89). They are also involved in the phenomenon of desensitization, may control the gating of ion channels, and are closely related to *ras* proteins that are concerned with cell division. Regulatory G proteins are affected by some bacterial exotoxins;

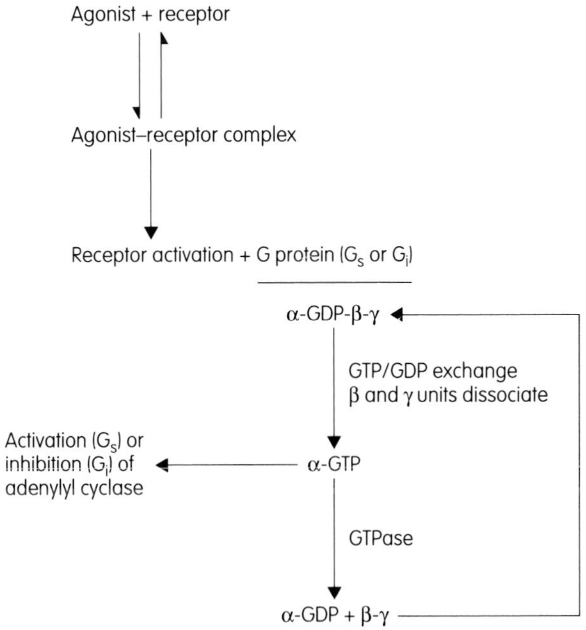

Fig. 3.5 The role of regulatory proteins (G proteins) in the activation (by G_s) or inhibition (by G_i) of adenylyl cyclase. The regulatory proteins G_s and G_i consist of three subunits, α, β and γ: in the inactive state, the α subunit is bound to guanosine diphosphate (GDP). Receptor activation results in the binding of G_s or G_i by the receptor, followed by guanosine triphosphate (GTP)/GDP exchange (i.e. GDP dissociates from the α subunits, and is replaced by GTP); the β and γ subunits of the G protein also dissociate. The α subunit–GTP complex then combines with adenylyl cyclase, producing activation (G_s) of inhibition (G_i) of the enzyme. The α subunit–GTP complex is subsequently broken down by its inherent GTPase activity to an α subunit–GDP complex, which recombines with the β and γ subunits to reform the inactive G protein. The activation of different receptor sites by agonists may result in competition for G_s and G_i, which will be reflected by the activity of adenylyl cyclase and the subsequent production of cyclic adenosine monophosphate (cAMP).

for example, cholera toxin activates G_s (by adenosine diphosphate (ADP)-ribosylation of its α subunit), while pertussis toxin blocks the receptor-mediated activation of G_i in a similar manner.

The effects of many drugs and endogenous compounds are mediated by receptors coupled to the regulatory protein G_s and adenylyl cyclase; consequently, receptor activation results in increased enzyme activity and enhanced synthesis of cAMP. All the β-adrenergic effects of catecholamines are mediated by an increase in cAMP; indeed, its significance was first recognized by Sutherland and Rall during their studies of the effects of adrenaline on glycogenolysis in isolated liver cells. More recently, it has been recognized that increases in intracellular cAMP mediate effects at many other receptor sites, including adenosine A_2-receptors, histamine H_2-receptors, and some dopamine, 5-hydroxytryptamine, vasopressin and prostanoid receptors (Table 3.2).

In addition, it has been suggested that adenylyl cyclase may play a crucial role in neuromuscular transmission. Increased synthesis of cAMP in the neuronal membrane may activate protein kinases that are coupled to a calcium ionophore. The subsequent entry of calcium ions into the nerve terminal results in the release of acetylcholine from synaptic vesicles (Chapter 10).

In contrast, the effects of other drugs and hormones are dependent on the activation of receptors coupled to the regulatory protein G_i and adenylyl cyclase, resulting in enzyme inhibition and decreased synthesis of cAMP. The effects of noradrenaline on α_2-receptors (e.g. in postganglionic sympathetic nerve terminals and platelets), the degranulation of mast cells induced by type I hypersensitivity and the effects of acetylcholine on some muscarinic receptors (M_2 and M_4 receptors) are dependent on this mechanism. In addition, some of the effects of adenosine, dopamine, glutamate, opioids and somatostatin are mediated by the attenuation of adenylyl cyclase activity (Table 3.2).

In some instances, opposing or complementary physiological responses may be dependent on the activation and inhibition of adenylyl cyclase (e.g. the effects of sympathetic and vagal tone on heart rate and cardiac contractility). An increase in cardiac sympathetic tone causes β_1-receptor activation, resulting in enhanced synthesis of cAMP; in contrast, increased vagal tone activates myocardial muscarinic M_2 receptors, reducing cAMP.

Intracellular cAMP is rapidly bound by the regulatory units (R units) of protein kinase A; the free catalytic C units of the enzyme are then activated, resulting in the phosphorylation of membrane proteins (Fig. 3.4). These changes lead to other biophysical or biochemical effects (e.g. the phosphorylation of ion channels; alterations in ionic permeability resulting in the depolarization or hyperpolarization of effector cells; increased diffusion of calcium ions from extracellular fluid; protein synthesis; or activation of DNA). During these changes, there is considerable amplification of the biological stimulus due to receptor occupation, and many drugs whose action is mediated by cAMP are extremely potent substances.

Table 3.2 Primary receptor sites where effector pathways are dependent on modification of the synthesis of intermediate messengers.

Receptor type	Main effector pathway
ACTH receptors	G_s, A : AC, ↑ cAMP
Adenosine receptors	
A_1, A_3	G_i, I : AC, ↓ cAMP
A_2	G_s, A : AC, ↑ cAMP
Adrenergic receptors	
α_1	G_q, A : PLC, ↑ IP_3
α_2	G_i, I : AC, ↓ cAMP
β_1, β_2, β_3	G_s, A : AC, ↑ cAMP
Angiotensin receptors	
AT_1	G_q, A : PLC, ↑ IP_3
AT_2	G_i, I : GC, ↓ cGMP
ANP receptors	
ANP_A, ANP_B	G_s, A : GC, ↑ cGMP
Dopamine receptors	
D_1, D_5	G_s, A : AC, ↑ cAMP
D_2, D_4	G_i, I : AC, ↓ cAMP
Endothelin receptors	
ET_A, ET_B	G_q, A : PLC, ↑ IP_3
Glucagon receptors	G_s, A : AC, ↑ cAMP
Glutamate receptors	
$mGlu_1$, $mGLu_5$	G_q, A : PLC, ↑ IP_3
$mGlu_{2-4}$, $mGlu_6$, $mGlu_7$	G_i, I : AC, ↓ cAMP
$GABA_B$ receptors	G_i, I : AC, ↓ cAMP
Histamine receptors	
H_1	G_q, A : PLC, ↑ IP_3
H_2	G_s, A : AC, ↑ cAMP
Hydroxytryptamine (5-HT) receptors	
$5\text{-}HT_1$	G_i, I : AC, ↓ cAMP
$5\text{-}HT_2$	G_q, A : PLC, ↑ IP_3
$5\text{-}HT_4$, $5\text{-}HT_6$, $5\text{-}HT_7$	G_s, A : AC, ↑ cAMP
Muscarinic receptors	
M_1, M_3, M_5	G_q, A : PLC, ↑ IP_3
M_2, M_4	G_i, I : AC, ↓ cAMP
Opioid receptors	
μ, κ, δ	G_i, I : AC, ↓ cAMP
Vasopressin receptors	
V_1	G_q, A : PLC, ↑ IP_3
V_2	G_s, A : AC, ↑ cAMP

ACTH, Adrenocorticotrophic hormone; GABA, γ-aminobutyric acid; G_s, G_i, G_q, G proteins; A, activation; I, inhibition; AC, adenylyl cyclase; ANP, atrial natriuretic peptide; GC, guanylyl cyclase; PLC, phospholipase C; cAMP, cyclic adenosine monophosphate; cGMP, cyclic guanosine monophosphate; IP_3, inositol (1,4,5)-trisphosphate.

After the activation of adenylate cyclase by G_s, increased intracellular concentrations of cAMP rapidly return to their basal levels, due to its metabolism by phosphodiesterase enzymes; in this process, cAMP is converted to AMP (Fig. 3.4). At least five different families of phosphodiesterase isoenzymes are present in mammalian cells, with different specificities, tissue distributions and sensitivity to enzyme inhibition by drugs (Table 3.3). In these conditions, phosphodiesterase III (and to a lesser extent, phosphodiesterase IV) play an important part in the hydrolysis of cAMP.

When phosphodiesterase enzyme systems are inhibited, the effects of cAMP may be prolonged, producing similar effects to the activation of receptors linked to G_s (i.e. an increase in intracellular cAMP). Several drugs primarily act by the reversible inhibition of one or more forms of the enzyme. For example, many methylxanthines (e.g. aminophylline, caffeine) non-selectively inhibit phosphodiesterase isoenzymes in most tissues, producing widespread effects on the heart, blood vessels, bronchial smooth muscle and the central nervous system; other non-selective phosphodiesterase inhibitors include pentoxifylline and papaverine. In contrast, other drugs with a structural relationship to the natural substrate cAMP (e.g. enoximone, peroximone, milrinone) selectively inhibit phosphodiesterase III, which is mainly localized in the heart and vascular smooth muscle (Table 3.3). Consequently,

Table 3.3 The classification of phosphodiesterase isoenzymes.

Isoenzyme family	Affinity cAMP	: cGMP	Tissue distribution	Selective inhibitors
I Ca^{2+}-calmodulin -dependent	*	High	Brain Heart Liver Kidney	Phenothiazines Vinpocetine
II cGMP-stimulated	Low	Low	Heart Adrenal cortex	
III cGMP-inhibited	High	High	Heart Blood vessels Airways Platelets	Pimobendan Milrinone Enoximone Peroximone
IV cAMP-specific	High	Low	Brain Heart Kidney Inflammatory cells	Rolipram Denbufylline
V cGMP-specific	*	*	Retina Platelets	Dipyridamole Zaprinast Sildenafil

* Different isoforms may have high or low affinities for the substrate.
cAMP, Cyclic adenosine monophosphate; cGMP, cyclic guanosine monophosphate.

their effects are mainly restricted to the cardiovascular system, and these agents are principally used for their positive inotropic effects. Similarly, selective inhibitors of phosphodiesterase IV (e.g. rolipram) have anti-inflammatory and bronchodilator effects, while inhibitors of phosphodiesterase V (e.g. zaprinast and dipyridamole) are potent inhibitors of platelet aggregation (Table 3.3).

Cyclic guanosine monophosphate (cGMP)

In some conditions, the cyclic nucleotide cGMP has a restricted role as an intermediate messenger, and changes in its intracellular concentration may mediate the effects of some hormones and neurotransmitters. In many ways, the synthesis and degradation of cGMP and cAMP are similar (Figs 3.4 and 3.6). Thus, cGMP is

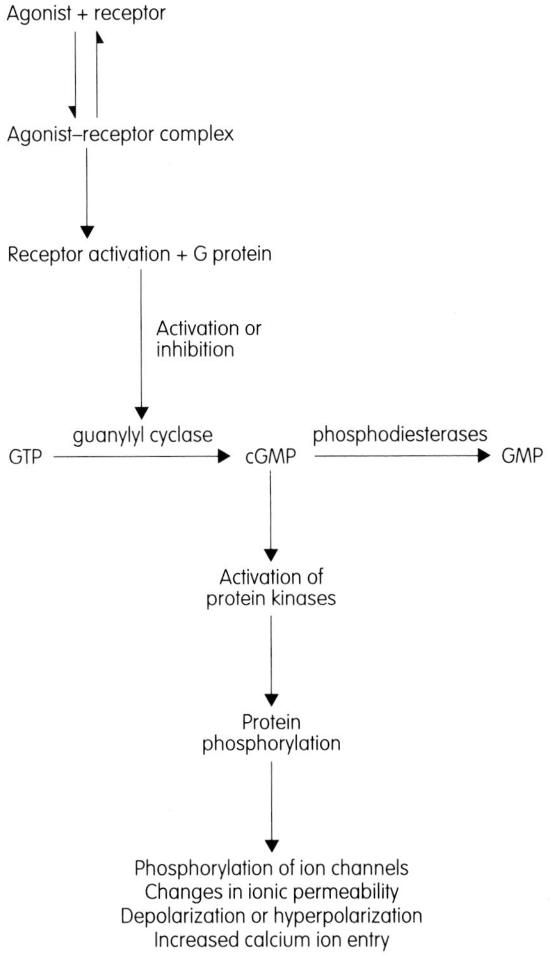

Fig. 3.6 The synthesis of cyclic guanosine monophosphate (cGMP) by guanylyl cyclase.

synthesized from GTP by the enzyme guanylyl cyclase, which is present in most cellular membranes. The synthesis of cGMP (like cAMP) is dependent on receptor activation and is mediated by regulatory, heterotrimeric G proteins whose α units can stimulate (G_s) or inhibit (G_i) guanylyl cyclase (Fig. 3.6). The cyclic nucleotide cGMP is rapidly metabolized by one or more of the phosphodiesterase family of isoenzymes; some forms of the enzyme (e.g. phosphodiesterase I and phosphodiesterase V) have a high affinity for cGMP and play an important part in its hydrolysis (Table 3.3). The synthesis of cGMP causes activation of specific protein kinases, resulting in changes in cellular function (e.g. the phosphorylation of ion channels or alterations in ionic permeability).

The response to some hormones and neurotransmitters is mediated by changes in cGMP; for instance, the effects of atrial natriuretic peptide and related agonists are produced by an increase in intracellular cGMP. Conversely, the action of angiotensin II and angiotensin III at AT_2 receptors is associated with a reduction in cGMP (Table 3.2). Similarly, reduced concentrations of cGMP mediate the effects of light on the visual pigment rhodopsin. In other systems, the role of the cyclic nucleotide in signal transduction is less clear.

Nitric oxide

Nitric oxide (previously known as endothelium-derived relaxing factor) and drugs that are metabolized or converted to nitric oxide by blood vessels (e.g. glyceryl trinitrate and sodium nitroprusside) cause vasodilatation by the activation of soluble (cytoplasmic) guanylyl cyclase in vascular smooth muscle cells, thus increasing the synthesis of cGMP (Fig. 3.7).

In endothelial cells, the amino acid L-arginine is metabolized to nitric oxide and L-citrulline by a constitutive calcium-dependent enzyme, nitric oxide synthase. Nitric oxide subsequently diffuses from the endothelium to vascular smooth muscle, where it combines with iron in the haem moiety of soluble (cytoplasmic) guanylyl cyclase; the enzyme is activated and cGMP synthesis is increased. Subsequently, cGMP-dependent protein kinases are activated, causing phosphorylation of membrane proteins, decreased Ca^{2+} entry, and relaxation of vascular smooth muscle (Fig. 3.7). Nitric oxide also reacts with intracellular sulphydryl groups in cysteine, albumin and tissue-type plasminogen activator; the *S*-nitrosothiol compounds formed are potent vasodilators. Both acetylcholine and bradykinin, and the shear stress of blood flow, increase the synthesis of nitric oxide by endothelial cells and cause cGMP-dependent relaxation of vascular smooth muscle. In addition, nitric oxide may act in conjunction with prostacyclin as an inhibitor of platelet aggregation and adhesion, and has negative inotropic effects; its continuous synthesis and release by endothelial cells play an important functional role in the control of peripheral resistance and vascular smooth-muscle tone. In physiological conditions, vasodilatation may be dependent on the continual synthesis of nitric oxide, and deficiencies in its production may play an important part in the genesis of essential hypertension.

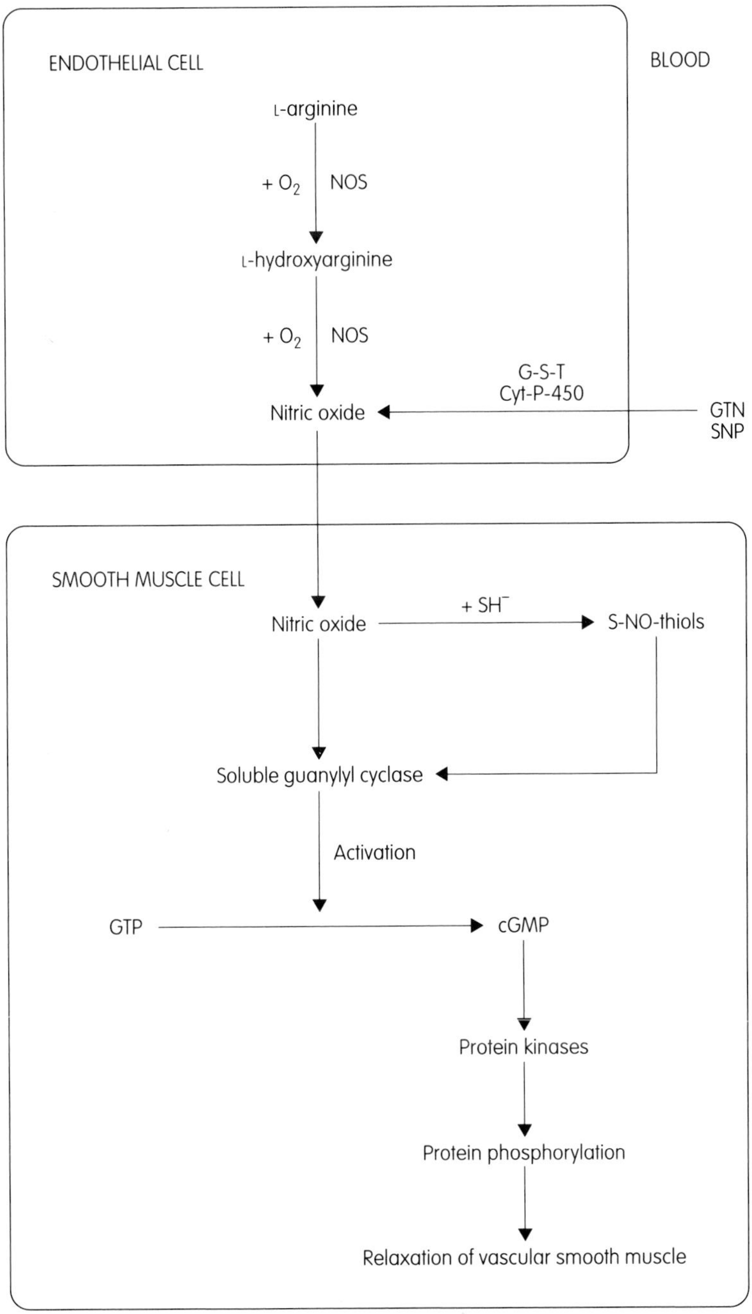

Fig. 3.7 The synthesis, release and actions of nitric oxide in vascular smooth muscle. NOS = Nitric oxide synthase; GTN = glyceryl trinitrate; SNP = sodium nitroprusside; G-S-T = glutathione *S*-transferase; Cyt-P-450 = cytochrome-P-450; SH = sulphydryl groups; S-NO-thiols = *S*-nitrosothiols.

Nitric oxide is also involved in the regulation of the pulmonary circulation. Low concentrations of inhaled nitric oxide (50–80 p.p.m.) have been used in the management of acute and chronic pulmonary hypertension, with encouraging results.

It may also inhibit the release of a vasoconstrictor polypeptide (endothelin) which is synthesized by vascular smooth muscle. Nitric oxide is rapidly degraded by blood vessels, and has a circulatory half-life of approximately 5–7 s.

Nitric oxide is also a neurotransmitter, and is synthesized and released by many peripheral and central neurones. In the peripheral nervous system, it is formed by non-adrenergic, non-cholinergic (NANC) nerves in the adventitial wall of blood vessels, and regulates the neuronal control of smooth-muscle function in many organs and tissues (e.g. the stomach, the small intestine and the uterus). In the penis, the release of nitric oxide from NANC nerves causes relaxation of the corpus cavernosum and erection. In the CNS, activation of *N*-methyl-D-aspartate (NMDA)-type glutamate receptors in granular cells increases intracellular calcium (and the binding of Ca^{2+} by calmodulin); in these conditions, Ca^{2+}-dependent nitric oxide synthase is stimulated, increasing the formation of nitric oxide and cGMP. The transmitter subsequently diffuses into Purkinje cells (which contain high concentrations of guanylate cyclase). Nitric oxide may also mediate retrograde neurotransmission and regulate synaptic plasticity.

In some pathological conditions (e.g. bacterial sepsis, endotoxaemia and ulcerative colitis) nitric oxide synthesis is greatly increased, due to the induction of a non-constitutive, calcium-independent isoform of nitric oxide synthase by immune and inflammatory cells. In these and other cells (e.g. endothelial cells and microglia), enzyme synthesis is induced by bacterial endotoxins, tumour necrosis factor α, interleukin-1β and other cytokines. During pyrexia, nitrate excretion is frequently increased due to the induction of nitric oxide synthase. Similar changes occur in bacterial sepsis and endotoxaemia, and nitric oxide is a major cause of delayed hypotension in shocked patients. Similarly, in ulcerative colitis, synthesis by macrophages and neutrophil leukocytes is increased; nitric oxide is an important effector of the cytotoxicity induced by activated macrophages. Cell toxicity may be due to the generation of superoxides, the formation of peroxynitrites and other breakdown products, the nitrosylation of nucleic acids, or other changes.

Induction of the Ca^{2+}-independent enzyme is inhibited by anti-inflammatory glucocorticoids; some of the anti-inflammatory and antiallergic effects of these drugs may be due to the inhibition of nitric oxide synthase.

Drugs that are metabolized to nitric oxide produce relaxation of vascular smooth muscle in a related manner (Fig. 3.7). Glyceryl trinitrate and sodium nitroprusside are highly lipid-soluble drugs, which readily diffuse from blood vessels into vascular smooth muscle. They are metabolized or converted intracellularly to nitric oxide and nitroso-thiols by glutathione-*S*-transferases and cytochrome P-450 enzyme systems, resulting in the activation of soluble guanylyl cyclase and increased synthesis of cGMP. In some conditions, sulphydryl-containing compounds (e.g. cysteine) are required for the metabolism of nitrates to nitric oxide.

Tolerance to the vascular effects of nitrates is associated with an attenuation of the increase in guanylyl cyclase activity and the rise in cGMP. Nitrate tolerance is sometimes delayed or prevented by the infusion of drugs containing sulphydryl groups (e.g. acetylcysteine).

Phosphoinositides and calcium ions

The phosphoinositides are a group of relatively minor membrane phospholipids containing inositol (a structural isomer of glucose). In many cells, receptor activation and the hydrolysis of membrane phosphoinositides result in the mobilization of calcium ions from intracellular and extracellular stores.

Receptor occupation by agonists activates the enzyme phospholipase C (phosphoinositidase C; Fig. 3.8). As in the case of adenylyl cyclase and guanylyl cyclase, the activation of phospholipase C is dependent on a regulatory protein that can bind guanine nucleotides (G_p, G_q or G_x). Phospholipase C hydrolyses a membrane

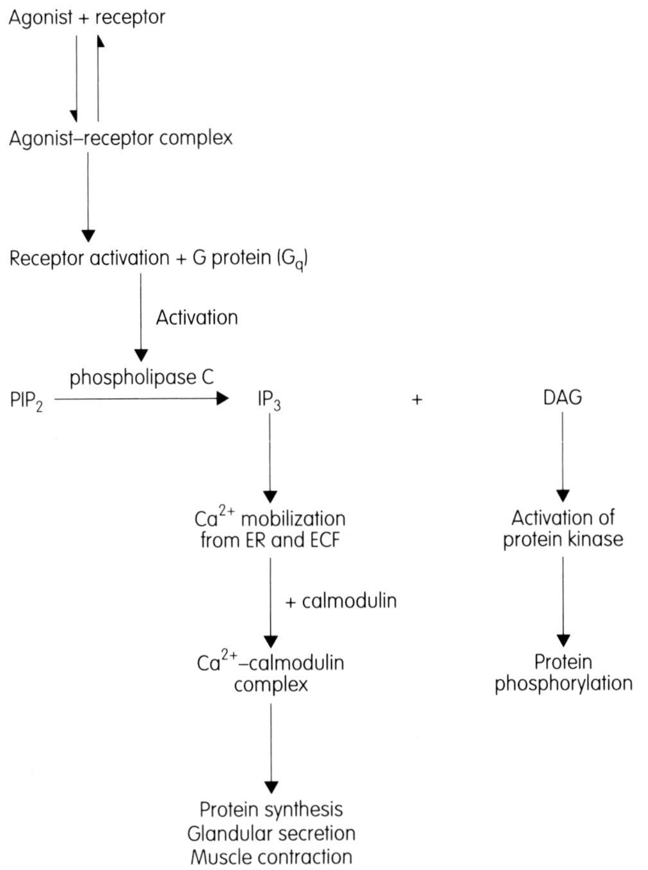

Fig. 3.8 The phosphatidylinositol pathway. PIP_2 = Phosphatidylinositol 4,5-bisphosphate; IP_3 = inositol 1,4,5-trisphosphate; DAG = diacylglycerol; ER = endoplasmic reticulum; ECF = extracellular fluid. In skeletal and cardiac muscle, released Ca^{2+} ions are bound by troponin C.

phospholipid (phosphatidylinositol 4,5-bisphosphate; PIP_2), to diacylglycerol (DAG) and inositol 1,4,5-trisphosphate (IP_3). Both of the products of this reaction act as intermediate messengers. DAG (in the presence of Ca^{2+} and phosphatidylserine) activates a protein kinase (protein kinase C) resulting in the phosphorylation of intracellular proteins. On the other hand, IP_3 combines with receptors in the endoplasmic reticulum, causing the opening of calcium channels, intracellular release of Ca^{2+} and increased Ca^{2+} influx from extracellular fluid (Fig. 3.8). Both DAG and IP_3 are rapidly metabolized; IP_3 is broken down to phosphatidylinositol and inositol, which are used to resynthesize PIP_2. Lithium salts may interfere with this process by inhibiting the metabolism and degradation of the phosphatidylinositols, and thus prevent the recycling and recirculation of inositol in the brain.

The action of many drugs and neurotransmitters depends on receptor mechanisms that are mediated by the activation of phospholipase C, the hydrolysis of PIP_2 to IP_3 and DAG, and the release of Ca^{2+} ions from the endoplasmic reticulum (Table 3.2). Other phosphoinositides may also be involved in the release of Ca^{2+} from intracellular stores (e.g. 1,3,4,5-IP_4 and 1,3,4-IP_3). In addition, activation of ryanodine receptors in the endoplasmic reticulum of many cells can open calcium channels and increase intracellular Ca^{2+}. Ryanodine receptors may be activated by Ca^{2+}-induced Ca^{2+} release mechanisms, by caffeine or by cyclic ADP-ribose (a possible physiological intermediate messenger).

Nevertheless, the intermediate messenger IP_3 normally plays a crucial role in the control of cellular Ca^{2+}. Intracellular Ca^{2+} concentrations are normally extremely low (approximately 100 nmol l^{-1}); any increase in internal Ca^{2+} causes profound changes in cellular activity. IP_3 (and other mediators) cause the release of Ca^{2+} from the endoplasmic reticulum, which then combines with specific intracellular calcium-binding proteins (which can be considered as internal receptors for Ca^{2+}). Calmodulin is the main calcium-binding protein in smooth muscle and all non-muscular tissue; the related protein troponin C plays a comparable role in cardiac and skeletal muscle. The combination of calcium ions with calmodulin causes conformational changes in the protein, and can modify the activity of many enzymes (e.g. Ca^{2+}/calmodulin-dependent kinase, Ca^{2+} ATPase, phosphorylase kinase, adenylyl cyclase and the phosphodiesterase isoenzymes). Consequently, the Ca^{2+}–calmodulin complex can produce a wide range of pharmacological responses (e.g. protein synthesis, and changes in ionic permeability, glandular secretion and muscle contraction; Fig. 3.8).

In skeletal and cardiac muscle, the sequestration of released Ca^{2+} by troponin C plays a crucial role in excitation and contraction. Electromechanical coupling between dihydropyridine receptors in the T-tubular membrane and ryanodine receptors in the sarcoplasmic reticulum membrane results in receptor activation, Ca^{2+} channel opening and Ca^{2+}-induced Ca^{2+} release. Subsequently, released Ca^{2+} is bound by the troponin–tropomyosin complex, myosin ATPase is activated and ATP is hydrolysed. Cross-bridges form between the myosin and actin filaments in the myofibril, resulting in muscle contraction. IP_3 may be involved in the release of calcium from the sarcoplasmic reticulum in skeletal muscle; in addition, the intermediate mediator may regulate calcium entry into cells.

Although cAMP, cGMP, IP_3, DAG and calcium ions are commonly considered as independent intermediate messengers, there is considerable evidence that many of their effects are interrelated. For example, activation of a single receptor or receptor subtype can be mediated by multiple G proteins (or different subunits of a single G protein) that are concerned with several intermediate messengers. In addition, both cAMP and cGMP increase intracellular Ca^{2+}, and modify responses to calcium ions; thus, phosphorylation of many enzymes and proteins by cAMP or cGMP often results in a significant increase in their Ca^{2+} sensitivity. Indeed, Ca^{2+} is generally considered to be the universal messenger in mediating the response of cells to receptor activation, and is responsible for the regulation of all forms of cellular activity.

Modification of nucleic acid synthesis

Steroid hormones and their synthetic analogues produce their effects by combining with intracellular receptors and indirectly affecting protein synthesis. Consequently, their onset of action is usually relatively slow. Steroid receptors are discrete cytoplasmic proteins that are expressed in most cells, although their density is extremely variable; they are bound in a large molecular weight complex with other proteins (e.g. the heat shock protein, Hsp 90), which prevents their translocation to the nucleus. Lipid-soluble steroids (e.g. oestrogens, progestogens, androgens and glucocorticoids) readily diffuse across cellular membranes and are bound by unoccupied steroid receptors in the cytoplasm, forming activated steroid–receptor complexes. The activated complexes then dissociate from other proteins, translocate to the nucleus and are bound by specific high-affinity binding sites on DNA (steroid regulatory/response elements). The transcription of 10–100 target genes in the immediate vicinity of the steroid-regulatory elements is modified, resulting in changes in mRNA and ribosomal protein synthesis.

The diverse and widespread effects of many steroids are dependent on the modification of protein synthesis in target cells. Thus, the anti-inflammatory effects of glucocorticoids are mainly due to their combination with intracellular steroid receptors. The activation of steroid receptors by glucocorticoids modifies DNA and RNA synthesis, and indirectly increases the formation of an intracellular glycoprotein (lipocortin-1). This protein inhibits the enzyme phospholipase A_2, which normally mediates the conversion of membrane phospholipids to arachidonic acid (Fig. 3.9). In addition, the transcription of phospholipase A_2 may be inhibited; consequently, the formation of lipid mediators (e.g. prostaglandins, leukotrienes and platelet-activating factor) by inflammatory cells is reduced. Glucocorticoids also inhibit the transcription and modify the synthesis of many other proteins,

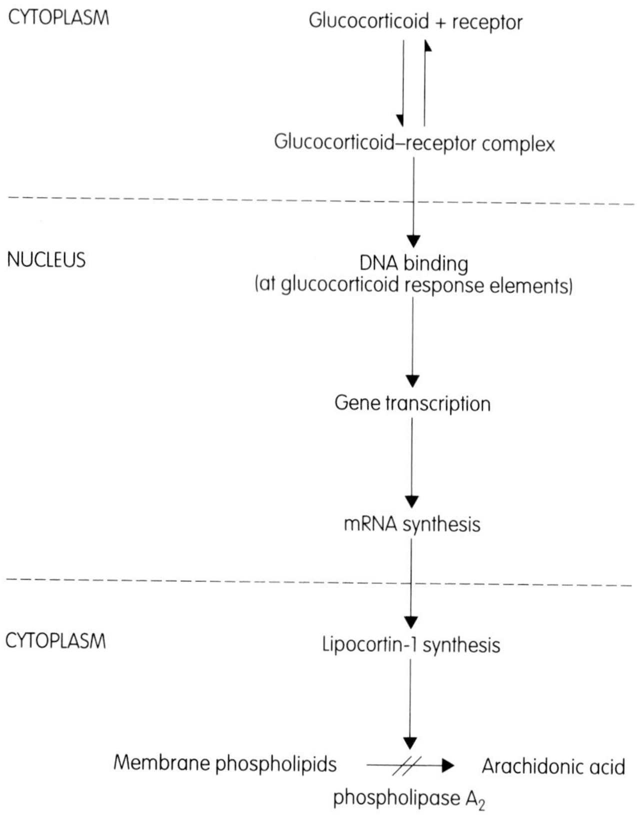

Fig. 3.9 The effect of glucocorticoids on the formation of lipocortin-1 and the synthesis of arachidonic acid by phospholipase A_2. −//→ represents enzyme inhibition.

including many cytokines, cyclooxygenase 2, inducible nitric oxide synthase and vasocortin.

Kinetics of drug–receptor reactions

The classical analysis of drug responses in terms of the combination of agonists with receptors (occupation theory) was introduced by A.J. Clark in the 1930s. It depends on the assumption that each drug molecule combines with a receptor in a reversible manner, forming a drug–receptor complex, i.e.:

$$D + R \underset{k_2}{\overset{k_1}{\rightleftharpoons}} DR$$

where D is the number of free (unbound) drug molecules, R is the number of free receptors, DR is the number of occupied receptor sites, k_1 the association rate constant and k_2 the dissociation rate constant. At equilibrium, the rates of association and dissociation are equal; if D, R and DR are expressed as molar concentrations (i.e. $[D]$, $[R]$ and $[DR]$), then:

$$k_1[D]\,[R] = k_2[DR]$$

and

$$\frac{k_2}{k_1} = \frac{[D][R]}{[DR]} = K_d$$

where K_d is the dissociation constant at equilibrium, and reflects the affinity with which drugs bind to receptors. When K_d is high, there is a low affinity for drug receptors; when K_d is low, there is high receptor affinity. In numerical terms, K_d represents the concentration of the drug required to occupy half the receptor sites at equilibrium.

If R_t is the total number of receptors:

$$[R_t] = [R] + [DR]$$

and

$$[R] = [R_t] - [DR]$$

thus

$$K_d = \frac{[D][R]}{[DR]} = \frac{[D]\left([R_t]-[DR]\right)}{[DR]}$$

and

$$[D]\,([R_t] - [DR]) = K_d\,[DR]$$

thus

$$[D]\,[R_t] - [D]\,[DR] = K_d\,[DR]$$

and

$$\begin{aligned}[D]\,[R_t] &= K_d\,[DR] + [D]\,[DR]\\ &= [DR]\,(K_d + [D])\end{aligned}$$

consequently

$$\frac{[DR]}{[R_t]} = \frac{[D]}{K_d+[D]}$$

and

$$f = \frac{[D]}{K_d+[D]}$$

since the fraction of receptors occupied (f) is given by:

$$f = \frac{[DR]}{[R_t]}.$$

This equation (the Langmuir equation, or the Langmuir absorption isotherm) was originally derived by A.V. Hill in 1909; a similar relationship was used by Langmuir to characterize the absorption of gases to metal surfaces.

If the total number of receptors remains constant, the Langmuir equation corresponds to a rectangular hyperbola; as the concentration of the drug is increased, the fraction of receptors that are occupied will rise progressively and approach the asymptote $f = 1$ at high drug concentrations (Fig. 3.10). If it is assumed that the pharmacological response is proportional to the fraction of receptors occupied, there will also be a hyperbolic relationship between drug dosage and response. As previously mentioned (p. 70), this type of relationship may be observed (Fig. 3.1), and in these circumstances the Hill plot (Fig. 3.2) has a coefficient of +1. If the number of drug-binding sites on each unit of the receptor macromolecule is represented by n, a Hill plot with a coefficient n should be obtained.

Until the 1950s, it was generally considered that the pharmacological responses of tissues to drugs were directly proportional to the number or the fraction of total receptors that were occupied by the agonist. This concept was known as occupation theory, and was based on the work of A.J. Clark. In 1956, Stephenson identified certain apparent anomalies in these concepts, and suggested three important modifications to classical occupation theory.

In the first place, it was proposed that maximal responses could be produced by a small degree of receptor occupation, and that spare receptors (i.e. receptors in excess of the proportion required to generate a maximal response) were present at

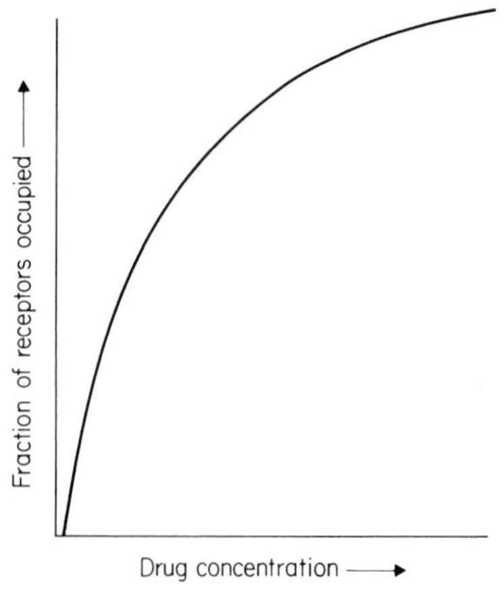

Fig. 3.10 The hyperbolic relationship between drug concentration and the fraction of receptors occupied by the drug. It is assumed that each drug molecule combines with a receptor in a non-cooperative manner.

many sites. Thus, when highly potent drugs produce a maximal response, they may also occupy a relatively small proportion of the total receptor population (e.g. 1% or even less). The presence of spare receptors in excess of the numbers required to produce a maximum response ensures that adequate pharmacological effects can be produced by relatively low concentrations of drugs or transmitters. It is generally considered that spare receptors are present at the neuromuscular junction; only 25% of the receptor population may be required to produce a maximal twitch response to indirect stimulation, and only 50% may be required to produce a sustained tetanic response. Consequently, non-depolarizing blockade may depend on the occupation of significant numbers of receptors before effects on neuromuscular function are observed.

Second, Stephenson suggested that drugs could have quite different properties, distinct from their receptor affinity, that defined their ability to induce a biological response. This property was known as efficacy. Agonists that could only produce a half-maximal response were considered to have an efficacy of unity, while full agonists had an efficacy that was greater than one.

Intrinsic activity is a similar, but slightly different concept. The ability of drugs to combine with receptors (receptor affinity) is determined by simple intermolecular forces. This property is usually considered to be distinct from the capacity to produce receptor activation (intrinsic activity, on a scale from 0 to 1). Agonists combine with receptors and induce a pharmacological response, i.e. they possess both receptor affinity and intrinsic activity.

Finally, it was considered that drug responses were not necessarily proportional to the number or fraction of receptors combined with the agonist, as predicted by occupation theory. Since 1960, it has been widely recognized that classical occupation theory is a simplistic approach to drug action, and that many pharmacological effects are complex and non-linear functions of receptor occupation. Thus, the relation between concentration and response is not always hyperbolic (p. 71); in some instances the relationship is sigmoidal (S-shaped). In these conditions, a Hill plot relating the logarithm of drug concentration to the logarithm [observed effect/(maximum effect – observed effect)] often produces a non-integral coefficient greater than unity.

This phenomenon is characteristically produced by drugs that act at nicotinic, glutamate and γ-aminobutyric acid receptors, and is believed to be due to the presence of multiple agonist binding sites on a single macromolecular complex. The binding of a drug molecule by a single receptor site may produce conformational (allosteric) changes, and alter the affinity of the remaining receptor sites for the drug. In these conditions, the affinity of the remaining receptor sites for agonists may be increased or decreased. This concept (cooperativity) was originally advanced by Monod, Wyman and Changeux in the mid 1960s in order to explain the allosteric properties of enzymes. Certain protein molecules (e.g. haemoglobin) are known to combine with their substrates (oxygen) in this manner. Thus, the combination of haemoglobin with oxygen affects its affinity for additional molecules of oxygen. Other substances (e.g. 2,3-diphosphoglycerate) may also bind to haemoglobin at different sites and significantly decrease its affinity for oxygen.

A comparable phenomenon probably occurs at the neuromuscular junction. When the effects of acetylcholine or other agonists on nicotinic receptors at the neuromuscular junction are studied, the relationship between drug concentration and response is usually sigmoid, and the Hill plot characteristically has a slope (the Hill coefficient) of 1.5 or more. This is consistent with the presence of two agonist binding sites on each receptor macromolecule, which are present on the two α subunits of the nicotinic receptor (Chapter 10). The Hill coefficient may reflect the increased probability of ion channel opening when both these sites are occupied (positive cooperativity).

In other experimental situations, log dose–response curves are biphasic (e.g. the effects of noradrenaline and adrenaline on the rabbit heart) or even bell-shaped (e.g. the effects of histamine on vascular smooth muscle in the guinea-pig pulmonary artery; Fig. 3.3). In these conditions, Hill plots can produce non-linear curves, or Hill coefficients that are significantly different from unity. Both biphasic and bell-shaped log dose–response curves may be due to agonists acting on two opposing receptor populations that mediate different effects (e.g. activation and inhibition of vascular smooth muscle). Alternatively, these atypical dose–response curves may be due to other phenomena (e.g. autoinhibition or desensitization). Complex dose–response curves of this type can usually be unmasked by selective antagonists.

Drug antagonism

Drug antagonists characteristically prevent or decrease pharmacological responses to agonists. Drug antagonism can be classified as:

1 Competitive reversible antagonism.
2 Competitive irreversible antagonism.
3 Non-competitive antagonism.

Competitive antagonism implies that the antagonist competes for and combines with the same binding site as the agonist; it may either be reversible (competitive reversible antagonism) or irreversible (competitive irreversible antagonism). In contrast, non-competitive antagonism does not depend on competition between agonists and antagonists for the same binding sites on receptors.

Competitive reversible antagonism

The ability of drugs to combine with receptors (affinity) is determined by simple intermolecular forces; it is usually considered to be distinct from the capacity to produce receptor activation (intrinsic activity). Since agonists combine with receptors and induce pharmacological responses, they possess both receptor affinity and intrinsic activity.

In contrast, competitive reversible antagonists combine reversibly with the same receptors as agonists but do not induce pharmacological responses, i.e. they possess receptor affinity but no intrinsic activity. Consequently, they do not cause receptor activation and induce the sequence of biochemical and biophysical changes that result in drug responses. Competitive reversible antagonists can be completely displaced from receptors by a sufficiently high concentration of any agonist that acts on the same receptors. They typically displace the log dose–response curve to the right in a parallel manner, although the maximum response obtained is unaffected (Fig. 3.11). This is the essential feature of competitive reversible antagonism.

A number of competitive reversible antagonists are commonly used in anaesthetic practice (Table 3.4). In experimental conditions, they can be characterized by the dose ratio (i.e. the ratio or factor by which the dose of the agonist must be raised to produce an equivalent response in the presence of the antagonist). It can be shown that:

$$\text{Dose ratio} - 1 = \frac{[A]}{K_d}$$

where $[A]$ is the molar concentration of the antagonist and K_d is the dissociation constant of the antagonist–receptor complex at equilibrium. It is comparable with the dissociation constant of the drug–receptor complex (p. 93), and reflects the affinity with which antagonists bind to receptors. Alternatively, this expression can be transformed to:

$$\text{Dose ratio} - 1 = K_a\,[A]$$

where K_a is the affinity constant of the antagonist–receptor complex (since the

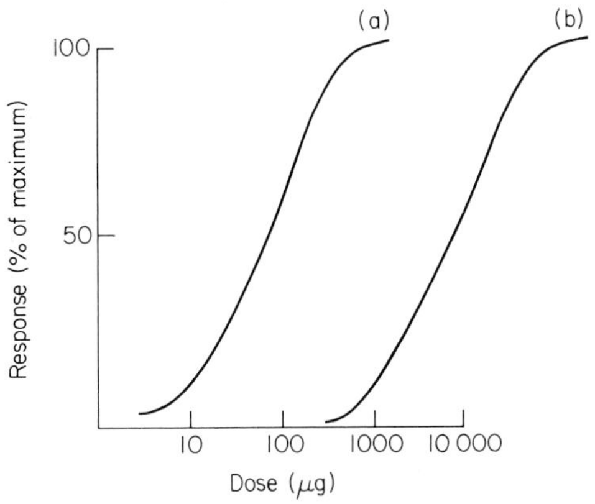

Fig. 3.11 The effect of competitive reversible antagonists on the log dose–response relationship (a) in the absence of an antagonist; (b) in the presence of an antagonist. The log dose–response relationship is displaced to the right in a parallel manner, although the maximum response is unaffected.

Table 3.4 Competitive reversible antagonists used in anaesthetic practice.

Drug	Endogenous compound antagonized
Atropine Glycopyrrolate Hyoscine	Acetylcholine (at muscarinic sites)
Alcuronium Atracurium *cis*-atracurium Gallamine Pancuronium Rocuronium Tubocurarine Vecuronium	Acetylcholine (at the motor endplate)
Trimetaphan Tubocurarine	Acetylcholine (at autonomic ganglia)
Atenolol Esmolol Propranolol	Adrenaline and noradrenaline (β-effects)
Chlorpromazine Domperidone Metoclopramide Perphenazine Prochlorperazine	Dopamine
Chlorpheniramine Promethazine Trimeprazine Cimetidine Ranitidine	Histamine
Granisetron Ondansetron Tropisetron	5-Hydroxytryptamine
Naloxone Naltrexone Nalmefene	Endorphins
Flumazenil	? Endogenous benzodiazepines

affinity constant is the reciprocal of the dissociation constant). This equation is known as the Schild equation; when log [*A*] (abscissa) is plotted against log (dose ratio – 1) (ordinate) a straight-line relationship is usually obtained, from which values for K_d (or K_a) can be easily derived.

The relationship between log [*A*] and log (dose ratio – 1; the Schild plot) can be used to compare the potency of competitive reversible antagonists, using their pA_2 values. The pA_2 value represents the negative logarithm of the molar dose of antagonist required to produce a dose ratio of 2; in these conditions, $K_d = [A]$, and $K_a = 1/K_d = 1/[A]$. The pA_2 values of some anticholinergic (antimuscarinic) drugs,

Table 3.5 The pA_2 values of some drugs with anticholinergic properties (guinea-pig ileum preparation).

Drug	pA_2 value
Hyoscine	9.5
Glycopyrrolate	9.5
Atropine	9.0
Promethazine	7.7
Chlorpromazine	7.5
Amitriptyline	6.7
Pethidine	5.3
Sotalol	5.1
Propranolol	5.0
Imipramine	3.4

obtained from experiments in which acetylcholine was used as an agonist in isolated tissue preparations, are shown in Table 3.5. Determination of the pA_2 value is a convenient way of comparing the potency of a series of competitive reversible antagonists; the most potent compounds have the highest pA_2 values. These values are entirely independent of the characteristics and the relative potency of the agonist, as long as the different antagonists compete with the agonist for the same receptor population.

Competitive irreversible antagonism

Competitive irreversible antagonists compete with agonists for receptors but only slowly dissociate from receptor sites, so that the total number of receptors available for combination with agonists is reduced. This type of antagonism is usually due to the formation of stable chemical bonds between the agonist and the receptor, or to disorientation and distortion of the receptor molecule. Competitive irreversible antagonists characteristically displace the log dose–response curve to the right in a non-parallel manner, and also decrease the maximal response produced by the agonist. They often have a long duration of action, and their effects are usually unrelated to their plasma concentration. Examples of competitive irreversible antagonism include the effects of phenoxybenzamine on α-adrenoceptors, and the action of α-bungarotoxin on acetylcholine receptors at the neuromuscular junction.

In spite of these differences, the precise distinction between reversible and irreversible antagonism is not always clear. As mentioned previously, many tissues contain significant numbers of 'spare receptors' (i.e. a receptor reserve that allows a maximum response to be obtained at a relatively low receptor occupancy). In these conditions, an irreversible decrease in the total number of receptor sites may not initially reduce the maximal response, and may displace the log dose–response curve to the right in a parallel manner. Low concentrations of competitive irreversible antagonists may therefore produce initial effects that are consistent with reversible antagonism. Higher concentrations, and prolonged exposure, may be required to produce the unequivocal features of irreversible antagonism.

In other instances, irreversible antagonism may be preceded by a reversible, competitive phase. When neostigmine or pyridostigmine is exposed to acetylcholinesterase *in vitro*, enzyme inhibition is initially reversible and competitive, and can be entirely reversed by dilution or exposure of the enzyme to acetylcholine. Relatively prolonged exposure is required to produce covalent chemical bonding (dimethylcarbamylation) at the esteratic site, which is only reversed by slow spontaneous hydrolysis (half-time = 36 min).

Non-competitive antagonism

Other types of drug antagonism do not depend on competition between agonists and antagonists for the same receptor binding sites, and are usually described as non-competitive antagonism. Non-competitive antagonism is sometimes mediated by receptor systems or receptor mechanisms; for instance, the effects of gallamine on heart rate are mainly due to the reduction in the affinity of cardiac muscarinic receptors for acetylcholine, resulting in tachycardia.

Alternatively, non-competitive antagonism may be dependent on direct chemical combination between the antagonist and the agonist, so that the effects of the agonist are prevented or diminished. For instance, the effects of some metallic ions (e.g. arsenic, copper, gold, lead, mercury, silver and zinc) can be neutralized by various chelating agents, and this type of chemical antagonism is widely used in the management of heavy-metal poisoning. Similarly, heparin can be neutralized by protamine, resulting in the formation of a stable salt; the large number of acidic sulphate groups in heparin (on which its activity depends) are neutralized by basic arginine residues in the protamine.

Other types of non-competitive antagonism include functional antagonism (physiological antagonism); these terms are sometimes used to describe the effects of drugs on two independent receptor systems that normally mediate opposing responses. Thus, histamine causes contraction of bronchial smooth muscle, while adrenaline causes relaxation; adrenaline can therefore be considered to be a functional antagonist of histamine. In some instances, this type of antagonism occurs in physiological conditions, and is responsible for the opposite effects of sympathetic and parasympathetic tone in effector systems.

Finally, pharmacokinetic interactions may reduce the plasma concentration and activity of other drugs by affecting their absorption, distribution, metabolism or excretion, and can therefore be considered as a form of non-competitive antagonism.

Partial agonists

In 1954, Ariens showed that some drugs (dualists) possessed both agonist and antagonist activity, depending on the experimental conditions that were used. The concept of intrinsic activity was developed to provide an explanation for this phenomenon. Agonists were considered to have two properties or characteristics: first, the capacity to combine with receptors (receptor affinity) and second, the ability, when combined with receptors, to cause receptor activation (intrinsic activity). Competitive reversible antagonists possess a variable receptor affinity, as reflected in their pA_2 values, but little or no intrinsic activity. Partial agonists, or dualists, are also drugs with receptor affinity, and they can therefore compete with both agonists and competitive antagonists; they also have some intrinsic activity, which is rather greater than competitive antagonists (zero), but less than full agonists (unity). In consequence, partial agonists can produce either agonist or antagonist effects, depending on the circumstances in which they are used (Fig. 3.12). In low doses or concentrations, they usually produce agonist effects; in the presence of small concentrations of a full agonist, additive effects are observed. When the response to the full agonist equals the maximum response to the partial agonist, the latter has no apparent action; in the presence of the full agonist, it produces neither

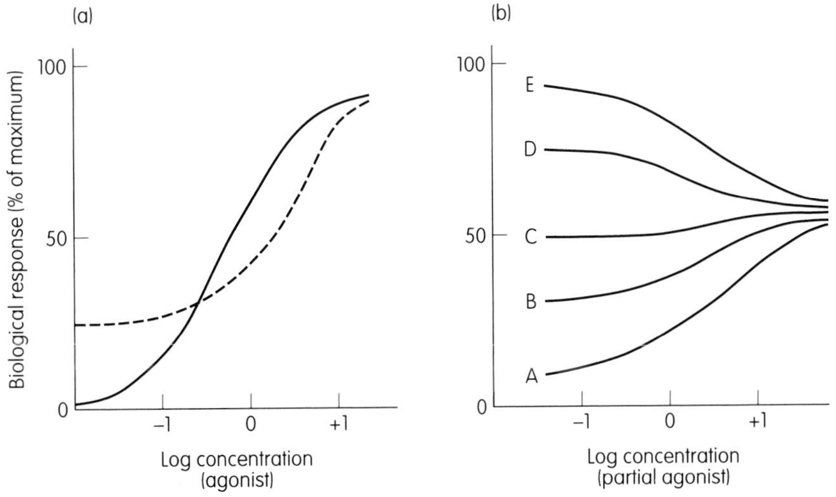

Fig. 3.12 (a) Dose–response relationship for a full agonist in the presence of a constant concentration of a partial agonist. Solid line, response to full agonist alone; broken line, response to full agonist in presence of partial agonist. At low concentrations of the full agonist, the partial agonist increases the response, due to their combined intrinsic activities. At higher concentrations of the full agonist, the response is reduced, since the partial agonist (intrinsic activity < 1) competes with the full agonist (intrinsic activity = 1) for receptor occupancy. At extremely high concentrations, the partial agonist is completely displaced from receptors, so the maximal responses are identical.

(b) Dose–response relationship for a partial agonist in the presence of increasing concentrations of a full agonist (represented by the curves A–E). At lower concentrations of the full agonist (A and B) the partial agonist has additive effects, due to their combined intrinsic activities; at higher concentrations of the full agonist (D and E), the partial agonist has antagonist effects, since it competes with the full agonist for receptor occupancy. When the response to the full agonist equals the maximal response to the partial agonist alone (C), little or no effect is observed.

agonist nor antagonist effects. When high concentrations of the full agonist are present, the partial agonist acts as a competitive reversible antagonist and reduces the response to the agonist (Fig. 3.12).† Partial agonism can be interpreted in terms of the drug–receptor complex (*DR*), and its subsequent conformational change to the activated drug–receptor complex (DR^*). These two forms are in equilibrium, so that all bound receptors are in the inactive form *DR*, or the activated form DR^*, i.e.

$$DR \rightleftharpoons DR^*.$$

In these conditions, the equilibrium constant determines the presence of agonist, partial agonist or antagonist activity. Full agonists have an increased affinity for DR^* and stabilize receptors in this form; competitive antagonists do not preferentially stabilize either form. Partial agonists tend to favour the formation of *DR* rather than DR^* (depending on their intrinsic activity). Consequently, the activity of different partial agonists may be distributed along a spectrum, depending on the value of the equilibrium constant. It can be shown that partial agonist activity is dependent on receptor expression, receptor density and the efficiency of effector mechanisms, which may vary in different tissues. Consequently, drugs that are partial agonists in one tissue or system may be full agonists or antagonists in another.

At least two groups of drugs are known to have some partial agonist activity which may be of clinical significance in humans. These are β-adrenoceptor antagonists and opioid analgesics.

β-Adrenoceptor antagonists possess a variable degree of partial agonist activity (which is often referred to as intrinsic sympathomimetic activity). Propranolol has no partial agonist activity and primarily causes β-adrenoceptor blockade; by contrast, pindolol possesses significant partial agonist activity and may produce sympathomimetic effects (Table 3.6). Other drugs that are partial agonists at β-adrenoceptors (e.g. xamoterol) have been used as positive inotropic agents in patients with cardiac failure, and in intensive care. Unfortunately, in patients with high sympathetic tone and enhanced noradrenaline release, xamoterol may act as a β-adrenoceptor antagonist; in these conditions, cardiac output is reduced and clinical deterioration may occur. The partial agonist activity of other β-adrenoceptor antagonists may be important when these drugs are used in the management of patients with borderline congestive cardiac failure.

Some synthetic opioid analgesics are partial agonists at opioid receptors (Table 3.7). In consequence, they may show either agonist or antagonist activity, depending on the circumstances in which they are used. They are sometimes referred to as

† Although these relationships are produced by partial agonists, they do not uniquely define partial agonist activity. For example, they may be produced by drugs acting on receptors that mediate opposing effects, mixtures of enantiomers with different pharmacodynamic activities, or by desensitization.

Table 3.6 The partial agonist activity (intrinsic sympathomimetic activity) of some β-adrenoceptor antagonists.

Drug	Partial agonist activity
Acebutolol	+
Alprenolol	++
Atenolol	–
Esmolol	–
Metoprolol	–
Oxprenolol	++
Pindolol	+++
Propranolol	–
Sotalol	–
Timolol	+

–, Absent or minimal; +, slight; ++, moderate; +++, marked.

Table 3.7 Opioid analgesics with partial agonist activity at μ or κ receptors.

	Partial agonist activity at opioid receptors	
Drug	μ receptors	κ receptors
Nalorphine		+
Levallorphan		+
Pentazocine		++
Cyclazocine		++
Butorphanol		+++
Nalbuphine		++
Buprenorphine	++	

agonist/antagonists (although this term is also applied to drugs with agonist and antagonist effects at different types of opioid receptor). The partial agonist effects of drugs at opioid receptors may have clinical implications. Thus, the analgesic effects of full agonists (e.g. morphine, pethidine, fentanyl) may not be enhanced by partial agonists; indeed, their effects may be antagonized.

Inverse agonists

Inverse agonists can be considered as drugs with receptor affinity but negative intrinsic activity (as compared with competitive antagonists, which have affinity but little or no intrinsic activity). Inverse agonists can be shown to compete with full agonists, partial agonists and competitive antagonists for receptors; their displacement and binding depend on their relative affinity. Inverse agonists also produce pharmacological effects that are opposite to those of the full agonist. Thus, simple esters of β-carboline-3-carboxylate (β-CCM, β-CCE and β-CCP) are competitive antagonists of benzodiazepines, and can be shown to antagonize the anticonvulsant, anxiolytic, sedative and muscle relaxant effects of these drugs. Nevertheless, when given alone, β-CCM and β-CCE have excitatory, proconvulsant or overtly convulsant effects. Similarly, the competitive antagonist flumazenil occasionally causes anxiety, or precipitates convulsions in susceptible patients (Chapter 13), possibly due to its inverse agonist activity. In some experimental systems (particularly in cultured cells with variable degrees of receptor expression), many drugs appear to possess inverse agonist activity.

Desensitization

Desensitization can be defined as a decrease in cellular sensitivity or responsiveness due to continuous or repeated exposure to agonists. It is usually observed in *in vitro* conditions (e.g. in isolated tissues or cultured cells).

Acute desensitization usually occurs rapidly, and is readily reversible. It was first described in 1957 by Katz and Thesleff, in relation to the effects of agonists on the motor endplate and skeletal muscle. In humans, it is sometimes produced by large or repeated doses of suxamethonium (a phenomenon more commonly referred to as tachyphylaxis or rapid tolerance; Chapter 6). This type of acute desensitization can be explained by the conversion of the activated drug–receptor complex (DR^*) to an inactivated and desensitized form (DR^-); only the activated complex can increase ionic permeability and cause depolarization at the motor endplate. Many agonists, and some antagonists, may have a preferential affinity for the desensitized receptor (metaphilic antagonists). Acute desensitization may also occur with receptors that are linked to GTP-binding proteins and adenylyl cyclase.

Chronic desensitization usually develops more slowly and is less readily reversible. It is often associated with the loss or sequestration of receptors from effector cells by endocytosis (internalization), irreversible conformational changes or receptor degradation. Chronic increases in hormonal or transmitter release may cause receptor down-regulation or loss; this can occur at both cholinergic and adrenergic synapses. Thus, receptor loss occurs when effector cells are exposed to excess concentrations of agonists (e.g. when bronchial smooth-muscle cells are exposed to sympathomimetic amines with β_2-adrenergic effects). Chronic desensitization due to receptor loss may also occur in pathological conditions associated with autoimmune processes (e.g. myasthenia gravis).

Further reading

Ariens EJ. Affinity and intrinsic activity in the theory of competitive inhibition. Part I. Problems and theory. *Archives Internationales de Pharmacodynamie et de Therapie* 1954; **99**: 32–49.

Ariens EJ. Receptors: from fiction to fact. *Trends in Pharmacological Sciences* 1979; **1**: 11–15.

Ariens EJ, van Rossum JM, Simonis AM. A theoretical basis of receptor pharmacology. Part II. Interactions of one or two compounds with two interdependent receptor systems. *Arzneimittel Forschungen* 1956; **6**: 611–621.

Axelrod J, Gordon E, Hertting G, Kopin IJ, Potter LT. On the mechanism of tachyphylaxis to tyramine in the isolated rat heart. *British Journal of Pharmacology* 1962; **19**: 56–63.

Barnes PJ. Radioligand binding studies of adrenergic receptors and their clinical relevance. *British Medical Journal* 1981; **282**: 1207–1210.

Barnes PJ, Adcock I. Anti-inflammatory actions of steroids: molecular mechanisms. *Trends in Pharmacological Sciences* 1993; **14**: 436–441.

Beavo JA, Reifsnyder DH. Primary sequence of cyclic nucleotide phosphodiesterase isozymes and the design of selective inhibitors. *Trends in Pharmacological Sciences* 1990; **11**: 150–155.

Bennett BM, McDonald BJ, Nigam R, Simon WC. Biotransformation of organic nitrates and vascular smooth muscle function. *Trends in Pharmacological Sciences* 1994; **15**: 245–249.

Berridge MJ. Inositol trisphosphate and diacylglycerol as second messengers. *Biochemical Journal* 1984; **220**: 345–360.

Berridge MJ. Inositol trisphosphate and diacylglycerol: two interacting second messengers. *Annual Review of Biochemistry* 1987; **56**: 159–193.

Boughton-Smith NK. Pathological and therapeutic implications for nitric oxide in inflammatory bowel disease. *Journal of the Royal Society of Medicine* 1994; **87**: 312–314.

Budd K. Clinical use of opioid antagonists. *Clinics in Anaesthesiology* 1987; **1**: 993–1011.

Butler AR, Flitney FW, Williams DLH. NO, nitrosonium ions, nitroxide ions, nitrosothiols and iron-nitrosyls in biology: a chemist's perspective. *Trends in Pharmacological Sciences* 1995; **16**: 18–22.

Calvey TN. Side-effect problems of μ and κ agonists in clinical use. *Clinics in Anaesthesiology* 1987; **1**: 803–827.

Calvey TN, Williams NE, Muir KT, Barber HE. Plasma concentration of edrophonium in man. *Clinical Pharmacology and Therapeutics* 1976; **19**: 813–820.

Changeux J-P, Giraudat J, Dennis M. The nicotinic acetylcholine receptor; molecular architecture of a ligand-regulated ion channel. *Trends in Pharmacological Sciences* 1987; **8**: 459–465.

Changeux J-P, Thiery J, Tung Y, Kittel C. On the cooperativity of biological membranes. *Proceedings of the National Academy of Sciences* 1967; **57**: 335–341.

Chenoweth MB. Clinical uses of metal-binding drugs. *Clinical Pharmacology and Therapeutics* 1968; **9**: 365–387.

Chuang DM, Costa E. Evidence for internalization of the recognition site of β-adrenergic receptors during receptor subsensitivity induced by (–) isoproterenol. *Proceedings of the National Academy of Sciences of the USA* 1979; **76**: 3024–3028.

Clark AJ. *Mode of Action of Drugs on Cells.* London: Edward Arnold, 1933.

Clark AJ. General pharmacology. In: *Heffter's Handbuch der Experimentellen Pharmakologie, Ergänzuungswerk*, vol. 4. Berlin: Springer-Verlag, 1937: 1–223.

Clark BJ, Menninger K, Bertholet A. Pindolol — the pharmacology of a partial agonist. *British Journal of Clinical Pharmacology* 1982; **13**: 149–158S.

Cooper JR, Bloom FE, Roth RH. *The Biochemical Basis of Neuropharmacology*, 3rd edn. New York: Oxford University Press, 1978.

Dretchen KL, Standaert FG, Skirboll LR, Morgenroth VH III. Evidence for a prejunctional role of cyclic nucleotides in neuromuscular transmission. *Nature* 1976; **264**: 79–91.

Erhlich BE, Kaftan E, Bezprozvannaya S, Bezprozvanny I. The pharmacology of intracellular Ca^{2+}-release channels. *Trends in Pharmacological Sciences* 1994; **15**: 145–149.

Ehrlich P. Chemotherapeutics: scientific principles, methods and results. *Lancet* 1913; **ii**: 445–451.

Endo M. Calcium release from the sarcoplasmic reticulum. *Physiological Reviews* 1977; **57**: 71–108.

Fambrough DM. Control of acetylcholine receptors in skeletal muscle. *Physiological Reviews* 1979; **59**: 165–216.

Flower RJ. Lipocortin and the mechanism of action of the glucocorticoids. *British Journal of Pharmacology* 1988; **94**: 987–1015.

Gaddum JH. Theories of drug antagonism. *Pharmacological Reviews* 1957; **9**: 211–218.

Galant SP, Duriseti L, Underwood S, Insel PA. Decreased β-adrenergic receptors on polymorphonuclear leukocytes after adrenergic therapy. *New England Journal of Medicine* 1978; **299**: 933–936.

Galione A. Ca^{2+}-induced Ca^{2+} release and its modulation by cyclic ADP-ribose. *Trends in Pharmacological Sciences* 1992; **13**: 304–306.

Garland CJ, Plane F, Kemp BK, Cocks TM. Endothelium-dependent hyperpolarisation: a role in the control of vascular tone. *Trends in Pharmacological Sciences* 1995; **16**: 23–30.

Gilman AG. G proteins: transducers of receptor-generated signals. *Annual Review of Biochemistry* 1987; **56**: 615–649.

Goldberg LI. Monoamine oxidase inhibitors. Adverse reactions and possible mechanisms. *Journal of the American Medical Association* 1964; **190**: 456–462.

Graziano MP, Gilman AG. Guanine nucleotide-binding regulatory proteins: mediators of transmembrane signaling. *Trends in Pharmacological Sciences* 1987; **8**: 478–481.

Griffiths TM, Edwards DH, Lewis MJ, Henderson AH. Evidence that cyclic guanosine monophosphate (cGMP) mediates endothelium-dependent relaxation. *European Journal of Pharmacology* 1985; **112**: 195–202.

Helmreich EJM, Pfeuffer T. Regulation of signal transduction by β-adrenergic hormone receptors. *Trends in Pharmacological Sciences* 1985; **6**: 438–442.

Hill AV. The possible effect of the aggregation of the molecules of haemoglobin on its dissociation curves. *Journal of Physiology* 1910; **40**: iv–vii.

Holmstedt B. Pharmacology of organophosphorus cholinesterase inhibitors. *Pharmacological Reviews* 1959; **11**: 567–688.

Huganir RL, Greengard P. Regulation of receptor function by protein phosphorylation. *Trends in Pharmacological Sciences* 1987; **8**: 472–477.

Karlin A, Kao PN, DiPaola M. Molecular pharmacology of the nicotinic acetylcholine receptor. *Trends in Pharmacological Sciences* 1986; **7**: 304–308.

Katz B, Thesleff S. A study of the 'desensitization' produced by acetylcholine at the motor endplate. *Journal of Physiology* 1957; **138**: 63–80.

Langley JN. On the physiology of the salivary secretion. Part II. On the mutual antagonism of atropin and pilocarpin, having especial reference to their relations in the sub-maxillary gland of the cat. *Journal of Physiology* 1878; **1**: 339–369.

Langley JN. On the reaction of cells and of nerve-endings to certain poisons, chiefly as regards the reaction of striated muscle to nicotine and to curari. *Journal of Physiology* 1905; **33**: 374–413.

Michell RH. Inositol phospholipids and cell surface receptor function. *Biochemica et Biophysica Acta* 1975; **415**: 81–147.

Miller KW. The nature of the site of general anesthesia. *International Review of Neurobiology* 1985; **27**: 1–60.

Milligan G. Mechanisms of multifunctional signalling by G-protein-linked receptors. *Trends in Pharmacological Sciences* 1993; **14**: 239–244.

Milligan G, Bond RA, Lee M. Inverse agonism: pharmacological curiosity or potential therapeutic strategy? *Trends in Pharmacological Sciences* 1995; **16**: 10–13.

Moncada S, Palmer RMJ. Inhibition of the induction of nitric acid synthase by glucocorticoids: yet another explanation for their anti-inflammatory effects? *Trends in Pharmacological Sciences* 1991; **12**: 130–131.

Monod J, Wyman J, Changeux J-P. On the nature of allosteric transitions: a plausible model. *Journal of Molecular Biology* 1965; **12**: 88–118.

Mukherjee C, Caron MG, Lefkowitz RJ. Regulation of β-adrenergic receptors by β-adrenergic agonists *in vivo*. *Endocrinology* 1976; **99**: 343–353.

Nahorski SR, Ragan CI, Challiss RAJ. Lithium and the phosphoinositide cycle: an example of uncompetitive inhibition and its pharmacological consequences. *Trends in Pharmacological Sciences* 1991; **12**: 297–303.

Nicholson CD, Challiss RAJ, Shahid M. Differential modulation of tissue function and therapeutic potential of selective inhibitors of cyclic nucleotide phosphodiesterase isoenzymes. *Trends in Pharmacological Sciences* 1991; **12**: 19–27.

Oleson J, Thomsen LL, Iversen H. Nitric oxide is a key molecule in migraine and other vascular headaches. *Trends in Pharmacological Sciences* 1994; **15**: 149–153.

Olsen RW. Drug interactions at the GABA receptor–ionophore complex. *Annual Review of Pharmacology* 1982; **22**: 245–277.

Palmer RMJ, Ferrige AG, Moncada S. Nitric oxide accounts for the biological activity of endothelium-derived relaxing factor. *Nature* 1987; **327**: 524–526.

Parascandola J. Origins of the receptor theory. In: Lamble JW (ed) *Towards Understanding Receptors*. Amsterdam: Elsevier/North-Holland Biomedical Press, 1981; 1–7.

Paton WDM, Waud DR. The margin of safety of neuromuscular transmission. *Journal of Physiology* 1967; **191**: 59–90.

Putney JW. Calcium-mobilizing receptors. *Trends in Pharmacological Sciences* 1987; **8**: 481–486.

Rance MJ. Multiple opiate receptors — their occurrence and significance. *Clinics in Anaesthesiology* 1983; **1**: 183–200.

Rees DD, Palmer RMJ, Hodson HF, Moncada S. A specific inhibitor of nitric oxide formation from L-arginine attenuates endothelium-dependent relaxation. *British Journal of Pharmacology* 1989; **96**: 418–424.

Ringold GM. Steroid hormone regulation of gene expression. *Annual Review of Pharmacology and Toxicology* 1985; **25**: 529–566.

Rovati GE, Nicosia S. Lower efficacy: interaction with an inhibitory receptor or partial agonism? *Trends in Pharmacological Sciences* 1994; **15**: 140–144.

Schild HO. pA, a new scale for measurement of drug antagonism. *British Journal of Pharmacology* 1947; **2**: 189–206.

Schleimer RP. The mechanisms of anti-inflammatory steroid action in allergic diseases. *Annual Review of Pharmacology and Toxicology* 1985; **25**: 381–412.

Schulz R, Triggle CR. Role of NO in vascular smooth muscle and cardiac muscle function. *Trends in Pharmacological Sciences* 1994; **15**: 255–259.

Snyder SM, Bredt DS. Nitric oxide as a neuronal messenger. *Trends in Pharmacological Sciences* 1991; **12**: 125–128.

Sorrentino V, Volpe P. Ryanodine receptors: how many, where and why? *Trends in Pharmacological Sciences* 1993; **14**: 98–103.

Stephenson RP. A modification of receptor theory. *British Journal of Pharmacology* 1956; **11**: 379–393.

Study RE, Barker JL. Cellular mechanisms of benzodiazepine action. *Journal of the American Medical Association* 1982; **247**: 2147–2151.

Sutherland EW, Rall TW. The relation of adenosine-3′,5′-phosphate and phosphorylase to the actions of catecholamines and other hormones. *Pharmacological Reviews* 1960; **12**: 265–299.

Szabadi E. A model of two functionally antagonistic receptor populations activated by the same agonist. *Journal of Theoretical Biology* 1977; **69**: 101–112.

Vane JR, Gryglewski RJ, Botting RM. The endothelial cell as a metabolic and endocrine organ. *Trends in Pharmacological Sciences* 1987; **8**: 491–496.

Whittaker VP. The storage and release of acetylcholine. *Trends in Pharmacological Sciences* 1986; **7**: 312–315.

Wildsmith JAW. Peripheral nerve and local anaesthetic drugs. *British Journal of Anaesthesia* 1986; **58**: 692–700.

Wilson IB, Hatch MA, Ginsburg S. Carbamylation of acetylcholinesterase. *Journal of Biological Chemistry* 1960; **235**: 2312–2315.

Chapter 4
Isomerism and Anaesthetic Drugs

Isomers are different compounds with an identical atomic content. Consequently, they have the same molecular formula,* the same molecular weight and the same elementary chemical composition. They are difficult to define in terms of their physical, chemical or biological properties, since these may be almost identical or quite different (depending on the type of isomerism that is involved).

In general, there are two main types of isomerism — structural isomerism and stereoisomerism.

Structural isomerism

Structural isomers have the same molecular formula but different chemical structures, because their atoms are not arranged in the same manner. The inhalation agents isoflurane and enflurane are the best-known example of structural isomerism in anaesthetic drugs (Fig. 4.1). Both drugs have the same molecular formula ($C_3H_2ClF_5O$), and contain five fluorine atoms; however, these are not arranged in the same manner in relation to the common carbon atom structure of the two agents. There are many other examples of structural isomerism involving drugs that have been used in anaesthetic practice (Table 4.1).

In some instances, isomerism involves a relatively small change in chemical structure which profoundly affects the pharmacological activity of the individual isomers. For instance, promethazine and promazine are both phenothiazine derivatives and structural isomers, and have a similar chemical structure (Fig. 4.2). Nevertheless, promethazine is primarily a competitive antagonist at H_1 histamine receptors, and is used clinically in motion sickness and allergic disorders. A minor alteration in its phenothiazine side-chain (i.e. the simple translocation of a methyl group) produces the compound promazine, with a much greater spectrum of pharmacological activity. Promazine is a major tranquillizer and a competitive antagonist of many endogenous neurotransmitters (e.g. histamine, 5-hydroxytryptamine, acetylcholine, adrenaline and dopamine); in some countries, it has been used in the treatment of schizophrenia.

* The molecular formula simply shows the numbers of different kinds of atom in a molecule; for example, the molecular formula of ethyl alcohol (ethanol) is C_2H_6O.

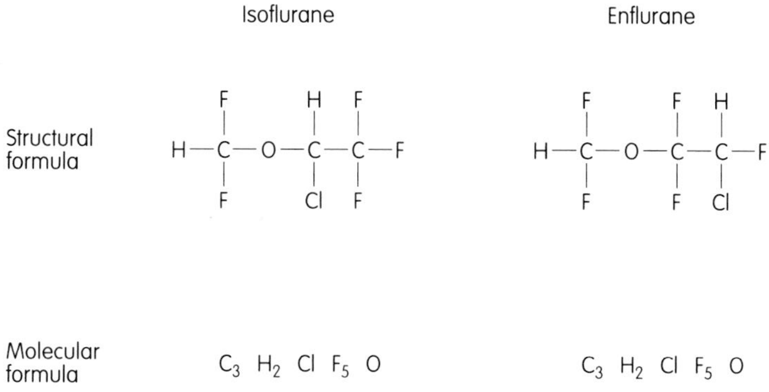

Fig. 4.1 The structural and molecular formulae of isoflurane and enflurane.

Table 4.1 Structural isomers of drugs that have been used in anaesthetic practice.

Molecular formula	Structural isomers
$C_3H_2ClF_5O$	Isoflurane; enflurane
$C_7H_8N_4O_2$	Theophylline; theobromine
$C_8H_{11}NO$	Tyramine; phenylethanolamine
$C_8H_{11}NO_2$	Dopamine; octopamine
$C_{10}H_{16}ClNO$	Edrophonium chloride; ephedrine hydrochloride
$C_{11}H_{17}NO_3$	Isoprenaline; orciprenaline; methoxamine
$C_{11}H_{18}N_2O_3$	Amylobarbitone; pentobarbitone
$C_{12}H_{16}N_2O_3$	Cyclobarbitone; hexobarbitone
$C_{13}H_{20}N_2O_2$	Procaine; monocaine
$C_{14}H_{20}N_2O_2$	Pindolol; piridocaine
$C_{14}H_{21}ClNO_2$	Amylocaine; meprylocaine
$C_{14}H_{22}N_2O_3$	Atenolol; practolol
$C_{15}H_{23}NO_3$	Oxprenolol; parethoxycaine
$C_{15}H_{25}NO_3$	Metoprolol; butoxamine
$C_{16}H_{13}ClN_2O$	Diazepam; mazindol
$C_{17}H_{19}NO_3$	Morphine; hydromorphine; norcodeine
$C_{17}H_{20}N_2S$	Promethazine; promazine
$C_{17}H_{21}NO$	Diphenhydramine; tofenacin
$C_{17}H_{21}NO_4$	Scopolamine (hyoscine); cocaine; fenoterol
$C_{18}H_{22}N_2$	Cyclizine; desipramine
$C_{18}H_{22}N_2S$	Trimeprazine; diethazine
$C_{18}H_{23}NO_3$	Dihydrocodeine; dobutamine; isoxsuprine
$C_{18}H_{25}NO$	Cyclazocine; dextromethorphan
$C_{21}H_{28}O_5$	Cortisone; prednisolone; aldosterone

Structural isomerism played an important part in the development of β-adrenoceptor antagonists (β-blockers). Approximately 25 years ago, practolol was widely use as a cardioselective β_1-adrenoreceptor antagonist. Unfortunately, its prolonged use resulted in a number of adverse effects (notably, systemic lupus erythematosus, fibrosing peritonitis and various cutaneous, ocular and aural reactions). In some patients, antinuclear antibodies and impaired lymphocyte

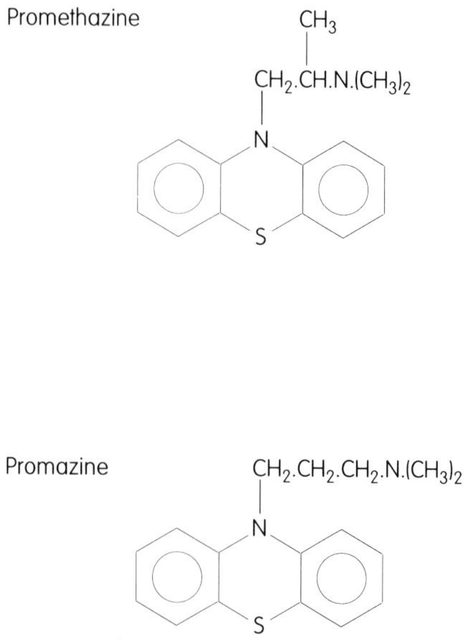

Fig. 4.2 The chemical formulae of promethazine and promazine. Both drugs are phenothiazine derivatives and structural isomers.

migration were observed; these changes were generally considered to be due to an abnormal immunological response to the drug in susceptible patients. The hypersensitivity response to practolol appeared to be induced by a secondary amine group (CH_3—CO—NH—) in the terminal side-chain of the drug (Fig. 4.3), which could combine with amide (—CO—NH—) groups in proteins. The replacement of this substituent by an isomeric primary amine group (NH_2—CO—CH_2—) produced a structural isomer of practolol (atenolol), which does not induce these complications. Atenolol is now widely used as a β_1-adrenoceptor antagonist in the treatment of hypertension, angina and cardiac arrhythmias.

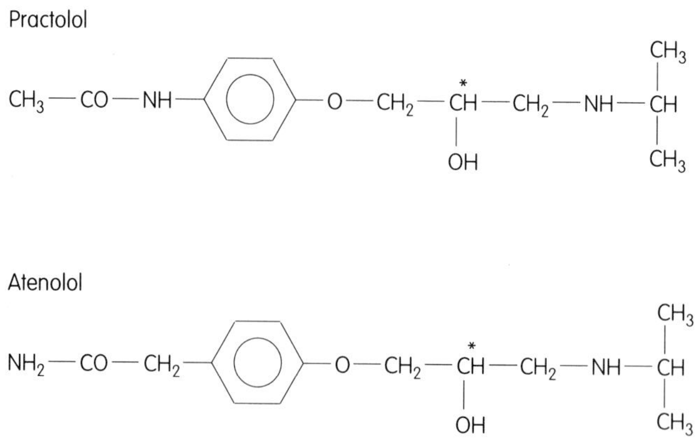

Fig. 4.3 The chemical formulae of practolol and atenolol. Both drugs are β-adrenoceptor antagonists and structural isomers. The asterisks denote the presence of a chiral centre in the structure of both drugs.

The pharmacological properties of structural isomers may be relatively similar (e.g. isoflurane and enflurane, or practolol and atenolol); alternatively, their actions and uses may be quite different (e.g. edrophonium chloride and ephedrine hydrochloride). Structural isomers do not usually present problems of identity or identification, since they are easily recognized as entirely different drugs, with distinctive names. Consequently, isomerism of this type is not of great interest or importance.

Nevertheless, other types of structural isomerism may be of considerable significance in anaesthetic practice. In tautomerism or dynamic isomerism, two unstable structural isomers are present in equilibrium; one isomer can be reversibly and rapidly converted to the other by physical changes (notably, by alterations in pH). Tautomerism occurs with a number of anaesthetic agents, including thiopentone, methohexitone and other barbiturates.

In alkaline solution (pH 10.5), sodium thiopentone is ionized and water-soluble, due to the presence of an ionized sulphide group; on injection into plasma (pH 7.4), the sulphide anion attracts hydrogen ions and the drug becomes non-ionized. This structure rapidly undergoes tautomerism, due to the transfer of a hydrogen atom from the undissociated acid to the barbiturate ring (Fig. 4.4). Tautomerism alters the physical properties of thiopentone, and considerably increases its lipid solubility. Thus, although thiopentone is injected intravenously as an ionized, water-soluble agent, its subsequent tautomerism in plasma converts the compound to a highly lipid-soluble drug that rapidly crosses the blood–brain barrier.

Tautomerism also occurs with many other barbiturates, including methohexitone, and increases their lipid solubility after intravenous administration. In alkaline solution (pH 11), methohexitone is ionized and water-soluble; on injection into plasma (pH 7.4) it attracts hydrogen ions and becomes non-ionized. In the subsequent tautomeric change, hydrogen atoms are transferred from the side-chain to the barbiturate ring (Fig. 4.5), greatly increasing its lipid solubility. This is an example of keto-enol isomerism (more correctly, lactam-lactim isomerism), which occurs with many chemical compounds.

In a similar manner, the structure of midazolam is reversibly modified (and its lipid solubility significantly increased) by the change in pH produced by intravenous administration. At pH 4, midazolam is almost completely ionized and highly water-soluble, since the drug contains a primary amine group ($—CH_2—NH_2$) that exists in an ionized form ($—CH_2—NH_3^+$) in acid conditions (Fig. 4.6). After injection into plasma (pH 7.4), the primary amine group is incorporated in a non-ionized benzodiazepine nucleus (ring closure). This change significantly increases the lipid solubility of midazolam; consequently, at pH 7.4 the drug readily crosses the blood–brain barrier.†

† Purists may consider that this is not a true example of tautomerism, since a molecule of water (H_2O) is eliminated when midazolam is converted from an ionized form (pH 4) to a non-ionized form (pH 7.4). Nevertheless, in the authors' view its inclusion is justified, since: (i) it is reversible; (ii) it is induced by changes in pH; and (iii) it markedly increases the lipid solubility of midazolam.

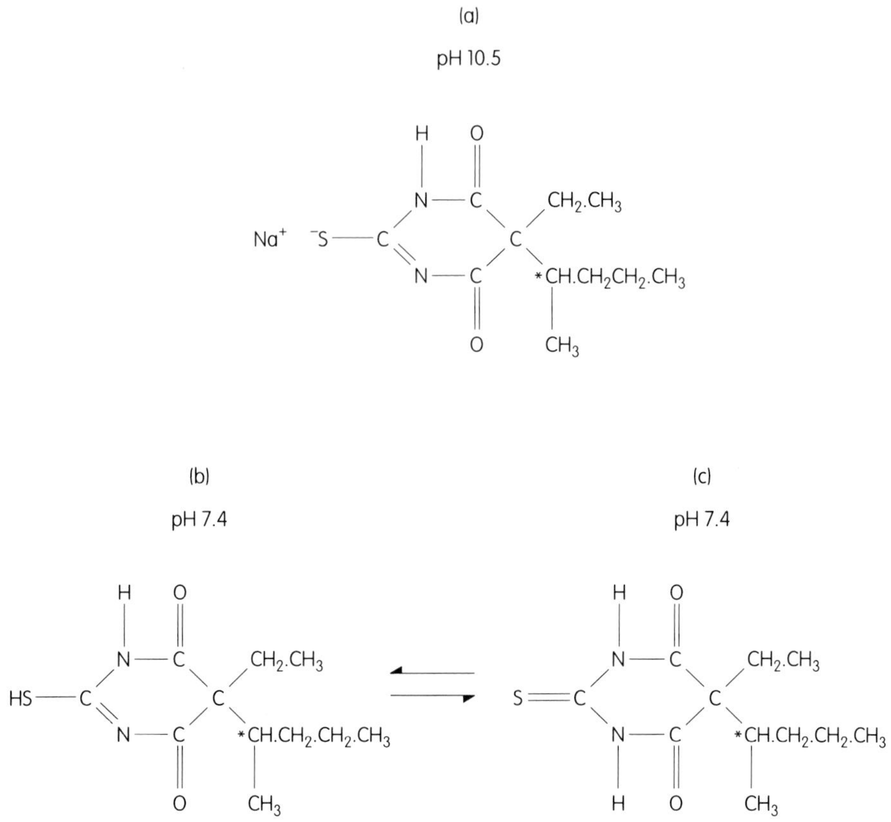

Fig. 4.4 The tautomerism (dynamic isomerism) of sodium thiopentone. (a) In alkaline solution (pH 10.5), sodium thiopentone is highly water-soluble, due to the ionization of its S–Na group. (b) In plasma (pH 7.4), thiopentone anions attract hydrogen ions and are present in a transient, undissociated, non-ionized form. (c) The undissociated thiopentone acid rapidly isomerizes to its tautomer, a highly lipid-soluble compound which readily crosses the blood–brain barrier. An asterisk represents the presence of a chiral centre (an asymmetric carbon atom).

Stereoisomerism

Stereoisomers are two or more different substances with the same molecular formula and chemical structure as each other, but a different configuration (i.e. their atoms or chemical groups occupy different positions in space, and thus differ in their spatial arrangements). Stereoisomerism has a remarkable and fascinating history; its existence was first recognized during studies of optical isomerism in the early 19th century (Appendix I). Stereoisomers can be classified into two main groups — enantiomers and diastereomers.

Enantiomers

Enantiomers (literally, substances of opposite shape) are pairs of stereoisomers

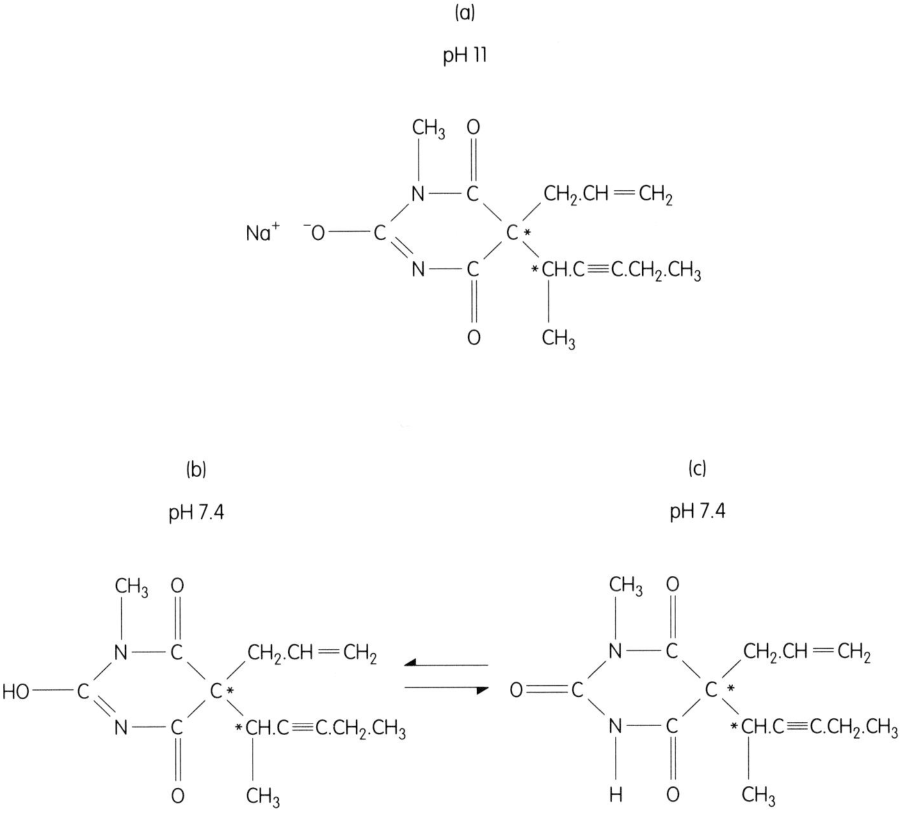

Fig. 4.5 The tautomerism (dynamic isomerism) of sodium methohexitone. (a) In alkaline solution (pH 11), sodium methohexitone is water-soluble, due to the ionization of its O–Na group. (b) In plasma (pH 7.4), methohexitone anions attract hydrogen ions, and are converted to a transient, undissociated, non-ionized form. (c) Undissociated methohexitone acid rapidly isomerizes to its tautomer; hydrogen atoms are transferred from the hydroxyl group to the oxybarbiturate ring, producing a highly lipid-soluble compound which readily crosses the blood–brain barrier. This type of isomerism is an example of keto-enol (or lactam-lactim) tautomerism. An asterisk represents the presence of a chiral centre (an asymmetric carbon atom).

that are non-superimposable mirror images of each other. This type of stereo-isomerism is dependent on chirality, i.e. the presence of an asymmetric, chiral centre in the molecular structure of certain drugs.

Chirality literally means 'having handedness'. Our right and left hands are mirror images of each other, but cannot be superimposed when the palms are facing the same direction. Similarly, many chemical structures and drugs can exist in right-handed and left-handed forms, which have almost identical physical and chemical properties. These two forms are non-superimposable mirror images of each other, and are usually known as R and S enantiomers (from the Latin words *rectus* and *sinister*). The R and S enantiomers can be defined by their absolute configurations, i.e. by the position that is occupied by their groups in space.‡ Both the R and S

‡ The distinction between R- and S- isomers is based on the priority (according to atomic number) of their substituent groups.

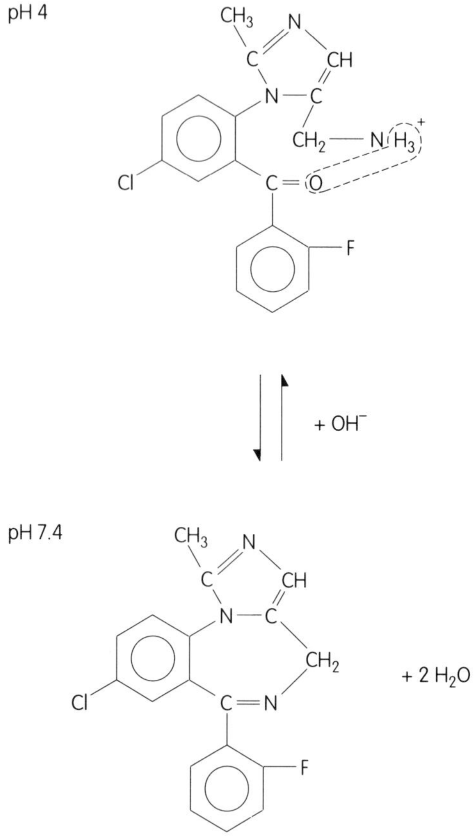

Fig. 4.6 The structure of midazolam at pH 4 and pH 7.4.

enantiomers are also optically active, i.e. they can rotate the plane of polarized light; consequently, this type of isomerism is also known as optical isomerism. One of the enantiomers (which may be either the R or the S isomer) rotates polarized light to the right; this form is known as the (+), (*d*), or (dextro) form. The other enantiomer (similarly, either the R or the S isomer) rotates polarized light to the left; this form is the (–), (*l*), or (levo) form. Equal mixtures of the two forms (racemic mixtures), with the prefixes (±) or (*dl*), have no optical activity. Consequently, enantiomers can be defined by their absolute configuration (R or S) or by their optical rotation [(+) (*d*) (dextro) or (–) (*l*) (levo)]; however, there is no relationship or correlation between the two classifications.

Chirality is due to the presence of a centre of molecular asymmetry (a chiral centre) in the chemical structure of drugs. This centre is usually a single carbon atom with four different substituent atoms or groups (Fig. 4.7); it is often incorrectly referred to as an asymmetric carbon atom. Drugs with this type of structure (chiral drugs) have a mirror image that cannot be superimposed on their original

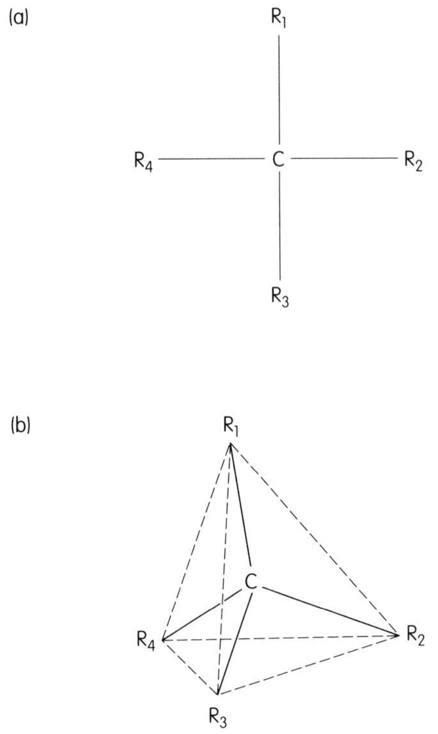

Fig. 4.7 General structure of a chiral centre (a centre of molecular asymmetry),. R_1–R_4 represent four different chemical groups attached to a single carbon atom. (a) Two-dimensional representation of an asymmetric carbon atom. (b) Three-dimensional (steric) representation of an asymmetric carbon atom, situated at the centre of a regular tetrahedron, with its valencies directed towards the four vertices.

configuration, and they therefore exist as R and S isomers that are optically active. Other agents that do not possess a chiral centre are known as achiral drugs.

The presence of chirality and the existence of drug enantiomers can be demonstrated in many anaesthetic agents with chiral centres, e.g. halothane (2-bromo-2-chloro-1,1,1-trifluoroethane). Halothane clearly has an asymmetric, chiral centre in its structure, since its CF_3, Br, Cl and H groups are attached to the four valencies of a single carbon atom (Fig. 4.8). A molecular model of R-halothane is present in the left foreground, with atoms of carbon, fluorine, chlorine, bromine and hydrogen. A mirror in the background shows the reflected image of the molecular structure; in the right foreground is an exact model of the mirror image. Clearly, halothane and its mirror image are not superimposable, since two of its atoms (chlorine and hydrogen) do not occupy the same position in space (i.e. their configuration is different; Fig. 4.8). The molecule of halothane can be rotated internally about its carbon–carbon bond, or the molecule as a whole can be turned; nevertheless, the model of the mirror image does not have the same configuration as the original structure, since two of its groups always occupy different positions in space (Fig. 4.8). Consequently, halothane exists as two enantiomers (R-halothane

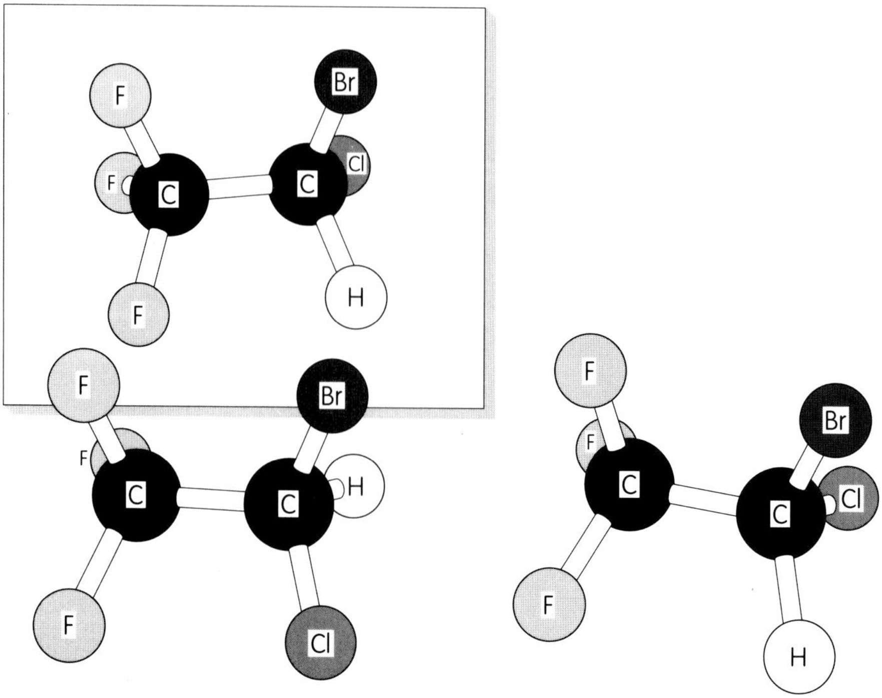

Fig. 4.8 The presence of chirality in the structure of halothane. A molecular model of R-halothane (2-bromo-2-chloro-1,1,1-trifluoroethane) is shown in the left foreground, with atoms of carbon, fluorine, chlorine, bromine and hydrogen. The mirror in the background shows the mirror image of the drug; in the right foreground is an exact model of the mirror image (S-halothane). Clearly, R-halothane and its mirror image (S-halothane) are not superimposable, since the atoms of chlorine and hydrogen occupy different positions in space. No matter how the model of the mirror image is rotated, two of its groups always occupy different positions in space. (Differences in bond lengths and bond angles have been ignored.)

and S-halothane); these are the only two possible configurations that are consistent with the structure of the drug.

Diastereomers

Diastereomers are pairs of stereoisomers that are not enantiomers (i.e. not mirror images). Diastereomers characteristically have different physical and chemical properties; for example, they do not have the same melting point or solubility, and they do not take part in chemical reactions in the same manner.

In general, diastereomerism in drugs arises in two main circumstances: (i) when drugs have more than one chiral centre; and (ii) when drugs show geometric isomerism.

Drugs with more than one chiral centre

When drugs have more than one chiral centre, individual stereoisomers may not be non-superimposable mirror images. Methohexitone, for example, has two chiral centres; one of these centers (C5) is in position 5 in the barbiturate ring, while the other (C1) is the initial carbon atom in the 1-methyl-2-pentynyl side-chain (Fig. 4.5). Each of these centers can exist in a right-handed form (R) or a left-handed form (S); consequently, the structure of methohexitone is consistent with two pairs of enantiomers [(1R, 5R)- and (1S, 5S)-methohexitone; and (1R, 5S)- and (1S, 5R)-methohexitone]. However, (1R, 5R)-methohexitone and (1R, 5S)-methohexitone are not mirror images (i.e. they are not enantiomers). Consequently, this pair of stereoisomers are classified as diastereomers.

Similarly, the analgesic tramadol has two chiral centres, in positions 1 and 2 in the cyclohexanol ring (Fig. 4.9). Each of these centres can exist in a right-handed form (R) or a left-handed form (S); consequently, the chemical structure of tramodol is consistent with two pairs of enantiomers [(1R, 2R)- and (1S, 2S)-tramodol; and (1R, 2S)- and (1S, 2R)-tramodol]. However, (1R, 2R)-tramodol and (1R, 2S)-tramodol are not mirror images, and are classified as diastereomers.

When a drug has a number (*n*) of different, non-equivalent chiral centres, the maximal number of possible stereoisomers is usually 2^n. Thus, both methohexitone and tramodol both have two chiral centres and can exist in four different stereoisomeric forms, as described above.§ However, when two chiral centres in a compound are identical (equivalent), the number of possible stereoisomers is reduced.

For example, although tartaric acid has two identical chiral centres (Fig. 4.10), it is internally symmetrical (congruent), and only exists in three different stereoisomeric forms (two of which are optically active). In theory, there are four possible isomers (1R, 2R; 1S, 2S; 1R, 2S; and 1S, 2R). In practice, the (1R, 2S)- and the (1S, 2R)-forms have the same structure and configuration; if the (1R, 2S)-form is inverted (i.e. rotated through 180°), it is identical to the (1S, 2R)-form (Fig. 4.10). Consequently, although tartaric acid has two chiral centres, it can only exist in three different forms [(1R, 2R)-tartaric acid; (1S, 2S)-tartaric acid); and (1R, 2S)-tartaric

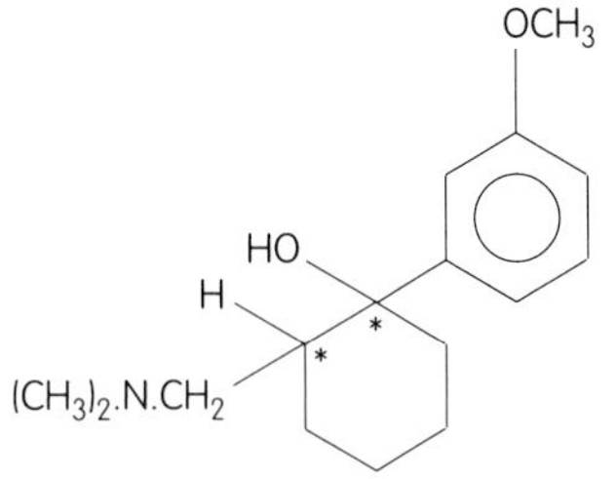

Fig. 4.9 The chemical structure of tramodol. The asterisks represent the presence of chiral centres (asymmetric carbon atoms), in positions 1 and 2 in the cyclohexanol ring.

§ In practice, methohexitone is administered as an equal mixture of the two least excitatory isomers. Similarly, tramodol is administered as a chiral mixture of two enantiomers.

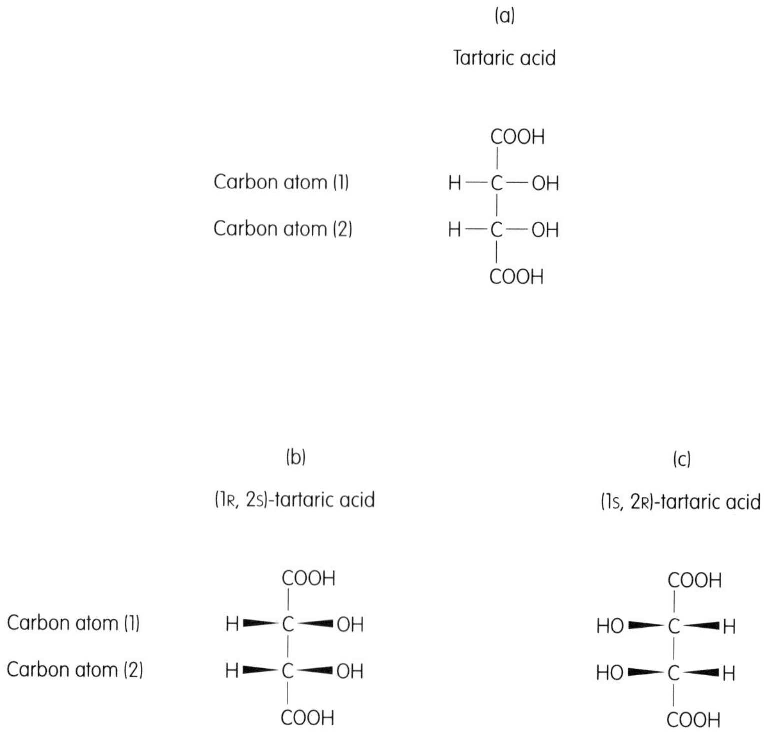

Fig. 4.10 The stereoisomerism of tartaric acid. (a) Chemical structure of tartaric acid. Both carbon atoms (1) and (2) are chiral; but both are equivalent, and have exactly the same constituent groups (–H, –OH, –COOH and –CH(OH)·COOH). In (b) and (c) ► ◄ represent bonds that are projecting from the plane of the paper towards the viewer. (b) The configuration of (1R, 2S)-tartaric acid. (c) The configuration of (1S, 2R)-tartaric acid. When (1R, 2S)-tartaric acid is inverted (rotated through 180°), it has the same configuration as (1S, 2R)-tartaric acid, due to the equivalence of the chiral centres.

acid (meso-tartaric acid)]. Meso-tartaric acid is optically inactive due to internal compensation by the two chiral centres.

Similarly, atracurium has four stereoisomeric centres, at positions 1 (carbon atom) and 2 (nitrogen atom) of the two tetrahydropapaverine units (see Fig. 4.11; Appendix II). The structure of the drug is therefore theoretically consistent with 16 possible stereoisomers. However, the chiral carbons and nitrogen atoms in the two tetrahydropapaverine units are equivalent to each other, and have the same substituent groups. Due to the internal symmetry (congruence) of its molecular structure, the number of possible stereoisomers is reduced to 10 (four pairs of enantiomers and one pair of diastereomers). The stereoisomerism of atracurium and mivacurium is discussed in more detail in Appendix II.

Consequently, the presence of internal molecular symmetry may reduce the number of possible stereoisomers associated with drugs (and other chemical structures). Clearly, the number of stereoisomers that occur with drugs that have more than one chiral centre cannot be predicted unless their chemical structure is considered.

Geometric isomers

Geometric isomerism usually occurs in drugs containing a carbon–carbon double bond (i.e. C═C), or a rigid carbon–carbon single bond (e.g. a C—C bond in a heterocyclic ring). When both carbon atoms have the same dissimilar substituent groups (i.e. compounds of the type *ab*C═C*ba* or *ab*C—C*ba*, where *a* and *b* are dissimilar), geometrical isomerism can occur. In the *cis* isomer, the two identical groups (*a* and *a*, or *b* and *b*) are on the same side of the rigid C═C or C—C plane; in the *trans* isomer, the groups *a* and *b* are on opposite sides of the plane. This type of stereoisomerism occurs in muscle relaxants (e.g. atracurium and mivacurium; Appendix II) as well as other drugs (e.g. the retinoic acids, oestrogens, antihistamines, thioxanthenes).

Geometric isomers are not usually optically active (unless they also have chiral centres); they have different physical and chemical properties, and can be separated from each other by physical techniques (e.g. chromatography). Individual *cis* and *trans* isomers are usually directly superimposable on their mirror images, although they exist as distinct stereoisomers with different configurations. However, *cis* and *trans* stereoisomers are not enantiomers, and geometric isomers are therefore usually classified as diastereomers.

Stereoisomerism and anaesthetic agents

In terms of stereoisomerism, anaesthetic agents can be divided into four main groups (Table 4.2):

1 Achiral drugs.
2 Drugs administered as single stereoisomers.
3 Drugs administered as mixtures of two stereoisomers.
4 Drugs administered as mixtures of more than two stereoisomers.

Achiral drugs

Approximately 40% of common anaesthetic agents are achiral; the remaining 60% are chiral (Table 4.2). Achiral anaesthetic drugs do not have centres of molecular asymmetry (chiral centres); they have directly superimposable mirror images, and are not optically active. Since they can exist only in one possible configuration, they are not present in different stereoisomeric forms. Consequently, all of their molecules interact with receptors, enzymes and other proteins in an identical manner.

Table 4.2 Some achiral and chiral drugs that are currently used in anaesthetic practice. Although some chiral drugs are administered as single isomers or as mixtures of more than two isomers, most of them are used as equal, racemic mixtures of two enantiomers.

	Chiral		
Achiral	One isomer	Two isomers	More than two isomers
Propofol	Etomidate	Methohexitone	Atracurium
Nitrous oxide	Ropivacaine	Thiopentone	Mivacurium
Sevoflurane	Alcuronium	Ketamine	
Amethocaine	Cisatracurium	Desflurane	
Lignocaine	Pancuronium	Enflurane	
Gallamine	Rocuronium	Halothane	
Fentanyl	Tubocurarine	Isoflurane	
Pethidine	Hyoscine	Bupivacaine	
Edrophonium	Morphine	Etidocaine	
Neostigmine		Mepivacaine	
Dopamine		Prilocaine	
		Adrenaline	
		Noradrenaline	
		Dobutamine	
		Atropine	
		Glycopyrrolate	

Drugs administered as single stereoisomers

A minority of chiral anaesthetic agents (e.g. etomidate and ropivacaine) are synthesized and used clinically as single enantiomers, which may either be R or S isomers (Table 4.2). In addition, most anaesthetic drugs that are derived from plants or organisms are synthesized as single stereoisomers, which are usually optically active. Naturally occurring enzymes and proteins are themselves chiral and stereoselective, and can only synthesize drugs in a single, specific configuration. Consequently, many naturally occurring drugs are administered as single stereoisomers (e.g. *l*-morphine, *l*-hyoscine, *d*-tubocurarine). The clinical use of these agents has no stereochemical implications, since all their molecules have the same configuration and will form the same three-dimensional relationships with L-amino acids in receptors, enzymes and other proteins.

In other instances, drugs that are naturally synthesized as single isomers are converted to chiral mixtures during extraction, or undergo spontaneous racemization (e.g. atropine, adrenaline, noradrenaline). Although these drugs are synthesized as single isomers, they may be administered as racemic mixtures of two stereoisomers.

Drugs administered as mixtures of two stereoisomers

Most synthetic chiral drugs used in anaesthetic practice are administered as mixtures of two stereoisomers. They are usually equal, racemic mixtures of R- and S-enantiomers, since most chiral drugs are synthesized in this form from achiral compounds. Approximately 60% of anaesthetic drugs are administered as chiral mixtures, including most inhalational anaesthetics, some intravenous agents and local anaesthetics, and a number of autonomic drugs (Table 4.2). The use of these drugs as mixtures of stereoisomers has important implications, since the pharmacodynamics and pharmacokinetics of the individual enantiomers may be different.

Drugs administered as mixtures of more than two stereoisomers

Some anaesthetic agents are administered as mixtures of more than two stereoisomers (Table 4.2). For example, atracurium is administered as a mixture of 10 different stereoisomers, while mivacurium consists of a mixture of three geometric isomers (Appendix II). Methohexitone was originally synthesized and used as a mixture of four stereoisomers (i.e. two pairs of enantiomers); the drug is now commonly used as a chiral mixture of the two least excitatory isomers. In all of these instances, there are important differences in the properties of the individual stereoisomers.

General differences between stereoisomers

When drugs are administered as mixtures of two or more stereoisomers, there may be differences in the activity and the pharmacokinetics of the individual isomers. These biological differences have been mainly described with drugs that are administered as chiral mixtures of two enantiomers (Table 4.2).

Although the R and S enantiomers have the same structure, they have a different configuration (i.e. their substituent groups occupy different positions in space). Consequently, the two enantiomers may form different three-dimensional relationships in the asymmetric environment of receptors and enzymes, which are almost entirely composed of chiral amino acids (i.e. L-amino acids) with stereoselective properties. In these conditions, there may be significant differences in the biological properties of the enantiomers, since the same complementary relationship may not be present between individual R and S isomers and specific receptor sites or enzymes. These pharmacological differences will also apply to stereoisomers that are present in more complex isomeric mixtures (e.g. atracurium and mivacurium). In many ways, the administration of drugs as mixtures of stereoisomers is comparable with the simultaneous use of two or more agents with different pharmacodynamic and pharmacokinetic properties.

Pharmacodynamic activity

There are quantitative differences in the pharmacodynamic activity of the R and S enantiomers of many chiral drugs, which are usually apparent as differences in potency. For instance, in many experimental preparations and conditions S(+)-isoflurane is approximately 50% more potent than its R(−)-enantiomer. More extreme differences in potency are not uncommon (e.g. S(+)-ketamine and R(−)-ketamine; see Table 4.3). Occasionally, one stereoisomer is almost inactive; thus *d*-atropine, *d*-noradrenaline and *d*-adrenaline are approximately 50–100 times less potent than their *l*-enantiomers. When differences in potency are present, the relation between the activity of the more active isomer (the eutomer) and its less active enantiomer (the distomer) can be expressed by the stereospecific index (the eudismic ratio), which represents the stereoselectivity of the individual isomers. Stereospecific indices of 100 or more are not uncommon (e.g. atropine, noradrenaline) and may be due to differences in either the affinity or intrinsic activity of the individual enantiomers at receptor sites. An inverse relationship may be present between the stereospecific index and the average clinical dose of the racemic compound (on the rationale that high stereospecific indices suggest that one enantiomer has a highly complementary relationship with the receptor site, and is therefore likely to be extremely potent). This generalization (Pfeiffer's rule) has a number of limitations, and takes no account of the molecular flexibility of organic molecules.

Alternatively, there may be important differences in the type of pharmacological activity produced by the enantiomers. For example, one isomer may be an agonist, while its enantiomer is a competitive antagonist. In some experimental conditions, R(−)-isoprenaline is an agonist at α_1-adrenergic receptors, while S(+)-isoprenaline is a competitive antagonist. Similarly, R(+)-picenadol is an agonist at opioid receptors, while its enantiomer is a competitive antagonist. When individual enantiomers have different intrinsic activities at receptor sites (e.g. when one is an agonist and the other is an antagonist), their racemic mixtures may behave as partial agonists (pseudopartial agonists). In other instances, isomers produce opposing pharmacological effects that are unrelated to agonism or antagonism at receptor sites.

Other differences in the pharmacological activity of individual enantiomers are sometimes present. Occasionally, the isomers have distinct effects that can be used for different therapeutic purposes; thus, levorphanol (R(−)-3-hydroxy-*N*-methylmorphinan) is an opioid analgesic while its enantiomer, dextromethorphan (S(+)-3-hydroxy-*N*-methylmorphinan) is a cough suppressant. The individual R and S enantiomers of chiral local anaesthetics (e.g. prilocaine, mepivacaine, bupivacaine) have different effects on the tone of vascular smooth muscle; only enantiomers with the S configuration have significant vasoconstrictor activity. In some conditions, one isomer in a racemic mixture may be predominantly responsible for the undesirable effects of chiral drugs. When ketamine is used clinically, emergence reactions, agitated behaviour, postoperative pain and inadequate intraoperative amnesia are predominantly related to the administration of one enantiomer (see Table 4.3).

Drug disposition

There are differences in the disposition of the enantiomers of many chiral drugs which may affect their absorption, distribution, metabolism or excretion.

Absorption

The absorption of most drugs from the upper small intestine is dependent on passive transport. In these circumstances, differences between the absorption of drug enantiomers are unlikely to be present. Nevertheless, the absorption of some chiral drugs is dependent on active transport (e.g. L-dopa and S-cephalexin). In these conditions, differences between the absorption of individual enantiomers may occur. In addition, the S-isomers of chiral local anaesthetics all tend to produce vasoconstriction; this reduces the absorption of both enantiomers, and prolongs the duration of local anaesthesia.

Plasma protein binding

Most drugs are bound to plasma proteins, particularly albumin or α_1-acid glycoprotein. In many instances, the binding of drugs to both these plasma proteins is stereoselective. L-Tryptophan is the endogenous substrate of one of the principal binding sites on serum albumin (the diazepam binding site); its binding affinity at this site is approximately 100 times greater than its enantiomer, D-tryptophan. Nevertheless, differences in the protein-binding of most R and S enantiomers are usually relatively small (usual range = 1.0–1.5); the protein binding of the S enantiomers is generally greater than their antipodes. In some cases (e.g. (R, S)-propranolol) the S enantiomer is more highly bound to α_1-acid glycoprotein, but less bound than its enantiomer to albumin. Differential binding of R and S enantiomers to tissue proteins may also occur. In some instances, stereoisomers that are selectively bound to proteins have been used to induce specific chiral antibodies which have been used for the enantiomer-specific assay of racemic drugs by radioimmunoassay techniques.

Drug metabolism

There may be important quantitative differences in the metabolism of drug enantiomers. One isomer may be more rapidly metabolized than its antipode; for example, both R(+)-propranolol and R(–)-prilocaine are more rapidly metabolized than their enantiomers, and have a greater intrinsic hepatic clearance. Consequently, after oral administration of (R, S)-prilocaine, plasma concentrations of S(+)-prilocaine are almost seven times greater than R(–)-prilocaine. These differences are not present after parenteral or perineural administration of racemic prilocaine; in these circumstances, drug clearance is largely dependent on hepatic blood flow (rather than intrinsic hepatic clearance).

The enantiomers of many other drugs are metabolized by hepatic enzyme systems in a stereoselective manner. For example, S(+)-hexobarbitone is more rapidly metabolized than its R(–)-enantiomer; similarly, the demethylation of S(+)-ketamine to norketamine is approximately 20% greater than its antipode. In addition, R(–)-ketamine can inhibit the metabolism of its S(+)-enantiomer, and may account for the more prolonged action of the racemate. Consequently, S(+)-ketamine has a higher plasma clearance and a shorter duration of action than the racemic mixture. Similar metabolic interactions are known to occur with other chiral drugs; for example, the analgesic activity of levomethorphan is significantly enhanced and prolonged by its enantiomer (dextromethorphan), due to metabolic inhibition. In other metabolic reactions, achiral drugs may be converted to chiral metabolites in a stereoselective manner. Thus, para-hydroxylation of a benzene group in the achiral drug phenytoin results in a chiral centre, with preferential formation of the S-enantiomer. Similarly, the reduction or conjugation of chiral drugs may introduce additional asymmetric centres, with the formation of at least two pairs of enantiomers.

Finally, drugs may undergo unidirectional metabolic conversion (inversion) of one enantiomer to another. Thus, the inactive R(–) enantiomers of some non-steroidal anti-inflammatory drugs (NSAIDs), such as ibuprofen and fenoprofen, are metabolically converted to their active S(+) enantiomers in the body; this conversion can occur at various sites, including the intestine, the liver and the kidney. When R(–)-ibuprofen is used in humans, there is a rapid appearance of the S(+) enantiomer in the blood; in contrast, after administration of S(+)-ibuprofen, the R(–) enantiomer is not present. Consequently, in *in vitro* conditions, S(+)-ibuprofen is some 160 times more potent than the R(–) enantiomer in inhibiting prostaglandin synthetase; *in vivo*, their potencies are almost identical, since the inactive R(–)-ibuprofen is almost completely converted to its S(+) enantiomer. Concentrations of the active S(+) isomer must be measured in order to predict the pharmacological response to the racemic compound, which is widely used as an anti-inflammatory drug. In the near future, the active enantiomer S(+)-ibuprofen may be available for clinical use in the UK.

Renal elimination

The renal elimination of drugs depends on glomerular filtration, tubular secretion and passive reabsorption in the distal renal tubule. Differences in the plasma protein binding of drugs may modify glomerular filtration and passive reabsorption; consequently, the plasma protein binding of individual enantiomers may influence their renal excretion. Differences in the intrinsic renal elimination of enantiomers can be demonstrated by measurement of the clearance of unbound drug; in these conditions, there may be slight differences in the renal secretion of the enantiomers of some basic drugs.

Pharmacokinetics

Differences in the disposition of the R and S enantiomers of many chiral drugs have important pharmacokinetic implications. Drug enantiomers may have different pharmacokinetic constants which describe their behaviour in the body (e.g. terminal half-life, clearance and volume of distribution). Unfortunately, in many cases the pharmacokinetic constants of chiral mixtures (Table 4.2) have been determined after the administration of racemic drugs, and their plasma concentrations have been measured by methods that are unable to distinguish between the enantiomers. In these conditions, the proportion of stereoisomers in the racemic mixture (50% : 50%) may rapidly change to an unknown ratio in the body, and the interpretation and meaning of kinetic constants is extremely questionable. In addition, the plasma concentrations of both enantiomers may be declining in a monoexponential manner, characterized by different rate constants; this can result in an apparent biexponential decline in the concentration of the unresolved, racemic drug. Pharmacokinetic interpretation of the decline in plasma concentration by compartmental methods may clearly lead to incorrect conclusions. Indeed, the generation of pharmacokinetic data on racemates by methods that do not distinguish between the enantiomers has been described as a waste of money on unscientific, sophisticated nonsense.

Differences between the stereoisomers of anaesthetic agents

There are important differences in the pharmacodynamic properties and pharmacokinetic behaviour of the enantiomers of many anaesthetic agents. Many of these drugs are normally administered as racemic mixtures (Table 4.2). In some instances, the relative activity of individual stereoisomers provides an important insight into the mechanism of action of the chiral mixtures. In particular, there may be differences between the activity and properties of the enantiomers of intravenous anaesthetics, inhalational anaesthetics, local anaesthetics, muscle relaxants, analgesics and drugs that act on the adrenergic nervous system.

Intravenous anaesthetics

Pharmacodynamic and pharmacokinetic differences are present between the enantiomers of all chiral intravenous anaesthetics (i.e. thiopentone, methohexitone, etomidate and ketamine). Most oral and intravenous barbiturates are administered as chiral mixtures, and there are important differences between the individual enantiomers. In general, the S(–) isomers are some two to three times more potent than their R(+) enantiomers; they also have shorter terminal half-lives, due to their rapid metabolism and clearance. Thiopentone is administered as a racemic mixture; the S(–) isomer is more potent, but has a shorter half-life than its enantiomer, due to its more rapid metabolism and clearance. These differences are also present with the stereoisomers of its metabolite pentobarbitone, which is at least partly responsible for the prolonged after-effects of thiopentone anaesthesia.

Methohexitone possesses two non-equivalent chiral centres, and can therefore exist as four stereoisomers (i.e. two pairs of enantiomers). In experimental studies, one of these isomers was up to five times more potent than the others. Originally, methohexitone was used clinically as a mixture of all four stereoisomers, but was found to produce unacceptable excitatory effects. For the past 30 years, the drug has been generally used as a racemic mixture of the two least excitatory stereoisomers.

Etomidate is administered as a single stereoisomer (R(+)-etomidate); the S(–) enantiomer has only slight sedative and hypnotic activity.

Ketamine is commonly used clinically as a racemic mixture ((R, S)-ketamine). Nevertheless, there are important clinical and pharmacological differences between the enantiomers of ketamine (Table 4.3), which were first identified in experimental animals, and subsequently studied in unpremedicated outpatients undergoing elective surgical procedures. It was shown that S(+)-ketamine was approximately three times as potent as R(–)-ketamine, and produced adequate anaesthesia in a higher proportion of patients. In addition, the S(+) enantiomer caused significantly less psychotic emergence reaction, agitated behaviour and postoperative pain, and better intraoperative amnesia. It is now generally accepted that ketamine would be a more useful and a more commonly used drug if it were available as the S(+) isomer, rather than as a racemic mixture.

Studies of this type provide an important insight into the nature of intravenous anaesthesia. Most intravenous anaesthetic agents are administered as racemic mixtures; the activity of the more active eutomers is approximately three to five times greater than their less active distomers. The stereoselectivity of the enantiomers of most intravenous agents strongly suggests that anaesthesia is due to an action on chiral receptors or enzymes in the central nervous system (CNS), rather than to physicochemical effects, non-specific actions or effects on cellular lipids (which are mainly achiral in nature). Differences between the pharmacodynamic activity of the stereoisomers of intravenous anaesthetics are quite consistent with their probable effects on γ-aminobutyric $acid_A$ ($GABA_A$) or *N*-methyl-D-aspartate (NMDA) receptor complexes in the CNS (Chapter 7).

Inhalational anaesthetics

Most fluorinated inhalational anaesthetics in current clinical use are chiral drugs, and are administered as equal, racemic mixtures of two enantiomers. Halothane,

Table 4.3 Clinical and pharmacological differences between S(+)-ketamine and R(−)-ketamine.

	S(+)-ketamine		R(−)-ketamine
Clinical differences			
Relative potency	3–4		1
Adequate anaesthesia (%)	95		68
Emergence reactions (%)	5		37
Agitated behaviour (%)	0		26
Postoperative pain (%)	0		16
Operative amnesia (%)*	24		5
Recovery of vigilance*	Faster		Slower
Pharmacological differences			
Analgesia (ischaemic pain)	S(+)	>	R(−)
Impaired psychomotor function	R(−)	>	S(+)
EEG slowing	S(+)	>	R(−)
Non-competitive antagonism of NMDA receptors	S(+)	>	R(−)
Blockade of NMDA receptor current	S(+)	>	R(−)
Affinity for PCP-binding sites†	S(+)	>	R(−)
Affinity for σ-binding sites‡	R(−)	>	S(+)
Dissociation from binding sites	R(−)	>	S(+)
Inhibition of neuronal catecholamine uptake ($Uptake_1$)	S(+)	>	R(−)
Inhibition of extraneuronal catecholamine uptake ($Uptake_2$)§	S(+)	>>>	R(−)
Inhibition of neuronal 5-hydroxytryptamine transport	R(−)	>	S(+)
Acetylcholinesterase inhibition**	R(−)	>	S(+)
Rapid disposition half-life	S(+)	>	R(−)
Clearance	S(+)	>	R(−)
Volume of distribution	S(+)	>	R(−)
Hepatic *N*-demethylation††	S(+)	>	R(−)
Hepatic norketamine hydroxylation	S(+)	>	R(−)

* Assessed in unpremedicated subjects.
† Defined by displacement of specific binding of radiolabelled thienylphencyclidine.
‡ Defined by displacement of specific binding of radiolabelled *N*-allylnormetazocine (SKF 10047).
§ R(−)-ketamine does not inhibit extraneuronal uptake.
** Ketamine has approximately 1/1000 of the potency of neostigmine. There are also stereoselective differences in the prophylaxis of organophosphorus inhibition, effects on oxime reactivation and the prophylaxis of enzyme 'ageing' by dealkylation.
†† In the racemic mixture, R(−)-ketamine inhibits the demethylation of its enantiomer.
EEG, Electroencephalogram; NMDA, *N*-methyl-D-aspartate; PCP, phencyclidine.

enflurane, isoflurane and desflurane all contain a centre of molecular asymmetry, and can exist in two enantiomeric forms. Initial studies with R- and S-halothane suggested that the enantiomers had similar physical properties (e.g. in relation to optical rotatory dispersion and electron spin resonance in lipid environments). Nevertheless, until recently, little was known of the differential effects of the individual enantiomers of inhalational anaesthetics.

Recent work has shown that the enantiomers of isoflurane have stereoselective effects on neuronal ion channels in the great pond snail (*Lymnaea stagnalis*). An identified neurone in the right parietal ganglion was extremely sensitive to volatile anaesthetics, due to the presence of a reversible, anaesthetic-activated potassium current ($I_{K(An)}$); exposure of the neurone to anaesthetic agents resulted in potassium efflux, hyperpolarization and neuronal inexcitability. The two enantiomers of isoflurane activated $I_{K(An)}$ in a stereoselective manner; S(+)-isoflurane was approximately twice as effective as R(−)-isoflurane.

Acetylcholine-induced (nicotinic) chloride currents in the pond snail were also inhibited in a stereoselective manner; similarly, S(+)-isoflurane was approximately twice as potent as its R(−) enantiomer. Inhibition of the acetylcholine-induced chloride current by both enantiomers was consistent with the predictions of a simple model, in which two molecules of isoflurane are independently bound to the receptor/chloride channel (although only one molecule is required for inhibition). The binding affinity of each molecule of S(+)-isoflurane was approximately 50% greater than each molecule of the R(−) enantiomer.

In experimental animals, *in vivo* studies with the enantiomers of isoflurane have confirmed that anaesthesia is stereoselective; S(+)-isoflurane was approximately 50–60% more potent than its antipode. As anticipated, the anaesthetic potency of the racemic (R, S) mixture was less than S(+)-isoflurane, but greater than R(−)-isoflurane. Both enantiomers produced a dose-dependent increase in anaesthetic sleep time, associated with the absence of a righting reflex and the inability to respond to painful stimuli; the potency of S(+)-isoflurane, as measured by anaesthetic sleep times, was significantly greater than its R(−) enantiomer.

The effects of the enantiomers of isoflurane on $GABA_A$-receptor-mediated responses has also been studied. In cultured hippocampal neurones, both enantiomers of isoflurane stereoselectively increase the duration of inhibitory postsynaptic currents; similarly, the enantiomers also modulate the binding of radiolabelled benzodiazepines, muscimol and GABA to $GABA_A$ receptors in a stereoselective manner. In both instances, the effects of S(+)-isoflurane are greater than its antipode (although the concentrations of isoflurane are higher than those that are present during inhalational anaesthesia).

At some receptor sites and ion channels, the effects and protein binding of the enantiomers of isoflurane may not be stereoselective or stereospecific. For instance, S(+)- and R(−)-isoflurane appear to be equally bound by slow L-type calcium channels in the CNS and the myocardium. Indeed, it has been suggested that S(+)-isoflurane may have significant therapeutic advantages when compared with the racemic agent, since its enhanced potency may not be associated with any increase in cardiovascular depression.

The effects of isoflurane on the CNS appear to be mainly mediated by its actions on chiral receptor channel proteins, rather than by physicochemical effects on the surrounding, relatively achiral lipids. Although the enantiomers of isoflurane have identical effects on pure lipid bilayers, they stereoselectively inhibit many biological processes that are dependent on protein function, and have different anaesthetic potencies in mammals. Consequently, integral proteins rather than membrane phospholipids appear to be the primary site of action of inhalational anaesthetics (Chapter 8).

Local anaesthetics

Some local anaesthetics (i.e. mepivacaine, prilocaine and bupivacaine) are chiral, and are used clinically as racemic mixtures of two enantiomers. In most instances, their R and S isomers appear to have approximately equal local anaesthetic activity. The absence of significant stereoselectivity suggests that these drugs may act in a non-specific manner (e.g. by Na^+ channel blockade, or by producing physicochemical changes in the lipid environment of the channel). Other evidence supports this interpretation; thus, many tertiary amines with pK_a values of approximately 8.0 possess local anaesthetic properties (Chapter 9). In contrast, some recent studies suggest that R(+)-bupivacaine may be approximately two to three times more potent than its S(–) enantiomer. Differences in potency may reflect the action of local anaesthetics on specific receptor sites within the Na^+ channel; in these conditions, some degree of stereoselectivity would be anticipated.

Any differences in the intrinsic activity or potency of local anaesthetic enantiomers may be modified by their stereoselective effects on vascular tone. Local anaesthetics with the S configuration produce enhanced and prolonged vasoconstriction, when compared with their R enantiomers. Thus, S(+)-prilocaine, S(+)-mepivacaine, and S(–)-bupivacaine have a longer duration of action after subcutaneous administration than their antipodes, due to enhanced vasoconstriction and the subsequent reduction in their systemic absorption.

In addition, R(–)-prilocaine is more rapidly metabolized than its S(+) enantiomer; in experimental conditions, plasma concentrations of both *o*-toluidine and methaemoglobin are increased. After oral administration of (R, S)-prilocaine, plasma concentrations of S(+)-prilocaine are almost seven times greater than R(–)-prilocaine, reflecting differences in presystemic metabolism and greater intrinsic clearance of the R(–) enantiomer. These differences are not present after parenteral or perineural administration of (R, S)-prilocaine; in these circumstances, drug clearance is largely dependent on hepatic blood flow (rather than intrinsic hepatic clearance).

There are also differences in toxicity between the R and S isomers of local anaesthetics. In particular, there are clear differences in cardiotoxicity between the two enantiomers of bupivacaine. After intravenous or subcutaneous injection, the toxicity of R(+)-bupivacaine is approximately 30–40% greater than its S(–) enantiomer; in addition, R(+)-bupivacaine produces more pronounced frequency-dependent blockade in isolated guinea-pig papillary muscle. It has been suggested that the increased toxicity of R(+)-bupivacaine may be due to its enhanced affinity for calcium and/or potassium channels in cardiac muscle. Studies in humans with racemic bupivacaine, its s(–) enantiomer, and the s(–) enantiomer of related local anaesthetics suggest that both s(–) enantiomers may have a reduced potential for cardiotoxicity, when compared with the racemic drug.

Clearly, local anaesthetic enantiomers with the s configuration may have considerable advantages. At the present time, at least two single isomer preparations of local anaesthetics are under clinical development. One of these compounds (ropivacaine) is the s(–) enantiomer of the propyl analogue of mepivacaine and bupivacaine; ropivacaine appears to have considerable clinical advantages when compared to racemic bupivacaine. Although its local anaesthetic activity is similar to racemic bupivacaine, it has a longer duration of action (due to enhanced vasoconstriction) and a reduced risk of cardiotoxicity. It may also decrease the incidence of motor paralysis at a comparable level of sensory blockade. In addition, the s(–) enantiomer of bupivacaine has been recently studied; it appears to have similar advantages to ropivacaine, although its duration of action may be longer. Both of these single isomer preparations may be available for clinical use in the near future.

Muscle relaxants

Some muscle relaxants (e.g. gallamine) are achiral; some (e.g. tubocurarine, alcuronium, pancuronium and vecuronium) are used as single stereoisomers; while others (e.g. atracurium and mivacurium) have more than one chiral centre, and are administered as complex mixtures of more than two stereoisomers (Table 4.2).

Both tubocurarine and alcuronium [(*N*, *N′*)-diallyl-nortoxiferine] contain several asymmetric centres in their molecular structure, and are obtained (or derived semisynthetically) from natural sources. Consequently, they are synthesized in a stereoselective manner by naturally occurring chiral enzymes and proteins, which can only synthesize compounds in a single, specific configuration (p. 120). Both tubocurarine and alcuronium are therefore synthesized and administered as single stereoisomers.

In contrast, pancuronium and vecuronium are synthetic aminosteroid derivatives; in common with some other steroids, both drugs contain as many as 10 asymmetric centres. Consequently, their molecular structure is consistent with more than 100 possible stereoisomers. Nevertheless, both drugs are synthesized with a unique, predetermined configuration at each of their asymmetric centres, and both pancuronium and vecuronium can be considered as single isomer preparations with definitive spatial relationships.

Atracurium and mivacurium are both complex examples of stereoisomerism. Both drugs contain four isomeric centres, at positions 1 (carbon atom) and 2 (nitrogen atom) of the two tetrahydropapaverine units. Consequently, the structure of both atracurium and mivacurium is theoretically consistent with 16 possible stereoisomers (Appendix II). Atracurium is synthesized in a non-selective manner; however, the number of possible isomers is reduced by the internal symmetry (congruence) of the drug. Mivacurium is synthesized with a defined (R) configuration at the two isomeric carbon atoms; consequently, the drug consists of a mixture of three geometrical stereoisomers (Appendix II).

Atracurium consists of a mixture of 10 stereoisomers, which have different activities and pharmacokinetics. Each stereoisomer can be classified by its configuration at the two carbon atoms (R or S), and by its relative configuration at the two carbon–nitrogen bonds (as *cis* or *trans*). The isomers can be divided (and separated by chromatography) into three groups of geometrical isomers: (i) *cis–cis* isomers (58%); (ii) *cis–trans* isomers (36%); and (iii) *trans–trans* isomers (6%; Appendix II). There are considerable differences in their breakdown (*in vitro*) and in their pharmacokinetics (*in vivo*). The *cis–cis* isomers have a half-life of 20–25 min, and a clearance of 5–6 ml min^{-1} kg^{-1}; the half-life of the *cis–trans* isomers is slightly less and their clearance is rather greater (9 ml min^{-1} kg^{-1}). The *cis–trans* group contains isomers with different rates of degradation, while the *trans–trans* isomers are eliminated extremely rapidly. There are also differences in the phamacodynamic activity of the stereoisomers of atracurium. The R-*cis*, R-*cis* isomer (cisatracurium) is the most active and potent isomer, and is some 3.3 times as potent as the parent isomeric mixture. Although neuromuscular blockade is qualitatively similar to atracurium, cisatracurium has only slight autonomic effects; it produces little or no histamine release, and significantly lower laudanosine levels than atracurium. Consequently, cisatracurium has considerable advantages when compared with atracurium, and has been recently introduced into clinical practice.

Mivacurium consists of three geometrical isomers: *cis–cis* (6%), *cis–trans* (36%) and *trans–trans* (58%). The predominant (94%) *cis–trans* and *trans–trans* isomers are equipotent and have similar pharmacokinetic characteristics (terminal half-life = 1–3 min; clearance = 70–100 ml min^{-1} kg^{-1}; volume of distribution = 200–220 ml kg^{-1}). In contrast, the *cis–cis* isomer has a prolonged terminal half-life (50–60 min) and a low clearance (5–6 ml min^{-1} kg^{-1}), but has only 5–10% of the potency of the *cis–trans* or *trans–trans* isomers. Consequently, almost all the neuromuscular blockade induced by mivacurium is due to the *cis–trans* and *trans–trans* isomers.

The least potent isomer of mivacurium is synthesized as an R-*cis*, R-*cis* stereoisomer (Appendix II). Consequently, the most active isomer of atracurium and the least active isomer of mivacurium both have the same R-*cis*, R-*cis* configuration (in spite of the chemical similarity between the two quaternary amine groups in the two drugs).

Simple analgesics

Some simple analgesics and NSAIDs are achiral compounds (e.g. acetylsalicylic acid, paracetamol and diclofenac). In contrast, many other NSAIDs are chiral compounds; although some (e.g. S(+)-naproxen) are administered as single stereoisomers, most are used as racemic mixtures of two enantiomers. In many instances, the R(−) enantiomers are inactive or almost inactive *in vitro* (e.g. R(−)-ibuprofen, R(−)-fenoprofen, R(−)-flurbiprofen). However, many R(−) enantiomers are partly or completely converted to their active S(+) enantiomers *in vivo*; this metabolic conversion occurs at many sites in the body (e.g. the intestine, the liver and the kidney). Thus, when R(−)-ibuprofen is used in humans, its S(+) enantiomer is rapidly detected in plasma; in contrast, after administration of S(+)-ibuprofen, metabolic inversion does not occur. In *in vitro* conditions, S(+)-ibuprofen is some 160 times more potent than the inactive R(−) enantiomer; *in vivo* their potencies are almost identical (since the inactive R(−)-ibuprofen is almost completely converted to its active S(+) enantiomer). In the UK, racemic (R, S)-ibuprofen is widely used as an anti-inflammatory drug; its replacement by the single enantiomer S(+)-ibuprofen may have significant advantages.

Opioid analgesics

Some synthetic opioids that are used in anaesthetic practice (e.g. pethidine and fentanyl) are achiral drugs. In contrast, morphine and many of its synthetic analogues and semisynthetic derivatives (e.g. buprenorphine, codeine, phenoperidine, propoxyphene) are chiral drugs. Almost all of these drugs are used as single stereoisomers.

The naturally occurring analgesic (*l*)-morphine has five asymmetric centres, and its structure is consistent with as many as 32 possible stereoisomers; like most other naturally occurring drugs, (*l*)-morphine is synthesized in a stereoselective manner, and has a unique and defined configuration that is essential for analgesic activity. Opioid receptors have highly specific stereochemical requirements; thus, the enantiomer of (*l*)-morphine has no opioid or analgesic effects.

Similarly, the activity of other agonists or antagonists at opioid receptors often depends on their specific stereochemical configuration. Thus, the enantiomers of many potent analgesics have little or no affinity or activity at opioid receptors (i.e. the drugs have a high stereospecific index). The opioid antagonist activity of (*l*)-naloxone is approximately 10 000 greater than (*d*)-naloxone and, although methadone is usually given as a chiral mixture, its analgesic effects are mainly due to its R(−) enantiomer. In some instances, opioid enantiomers have qualitatively different effects on opioid receptors, due to differences in their intrinsic activities; thus, R(+)-picenadol is an agonist at opioid receptors, while its S(−) enantiomer is a competitive antagonist. In these conditions, the racemic mixture may behave as a partial agonist (pseudopartial agonism). In other circumstances, the enantiomers have distinct effects that can be used for different therapeutic purposes; thus, levorphanol (R(−)-3-hydroxy-*N*-methylmorphinan) and levomethorphan (R(−)-3-methoxy-*N*-methylmorphinan) are potent analgesics, while their enantiomers dextrorphan (S(+)-3-hydroxy-*N*-methylmorphinan) and dextromethorphan (S(+)-

3-methoxy-*N*-methylmorphinan) have antitussive activity and are used as cough suppressants. Similarly, the active α-stereoisomers of propoxyphene are used for different purposes; dextropropoxyphene (S(+)-α-propoxyphene) is an analgesic, while levopropoxyphene (R(–)-α-propoxyphene) is an antitussive.

The opioid analogue tramadol has two asymmetric centres (Fig. 4.9), and its structure is therefore consistent with the presence of two pairs of enantiomers ((1R, 2R)- and (1S, 2S)-tramadol; and (1R, 2S)- and (1S, 2R)-tramadol). The drug used clinically is a chiral mixture of the first pair of enantiomers (i.e. (1R, 2R) (+)-tramadol and (1S, 2S) (–)-tramadol), which have different pharmacological effects. (1R, 2R) (+)-Tramadol has a greater affinity for μ- and δ-receptors, and is a more potent inhibitor of 5-hydroxytryptamine uptake, as well as an enhancer of its release; in contrast (1S, 2S) (–)-tramadol has a lower affinity for μ- and δ-receptors, but is a more potent inhibitor of noradrenaline uptake and a differential enhancer of its stimulus-evoked release. Both enantiomers produce centrally mediated antinociception, and may have supra-additive effects. The isomers of tramadol also have active and stereoselective metabolites; thus, (1R, 2R) (+)-desmethyl-tramadol activates μ-receptors, while (1S, 2S) (–)-desmethyl-tramadol acts at α_2-receptors. Consequently, both the (1R, 2R) and the (1S, 2S) enantiomers and their metabolites appear to be make independent and complementary contributions to the effects of the chiral mixture.

Drugs that act on the adrenergic nervous system

In the UK and the USA, both adrenaline and noradrenaline are commonly administered as the naturally occurring R(–) stereoisomers (i.e. as (*l*)-adrenaline and (*l*)-noradrenaline). Although both (*d*)-adrenaline and (*d*)-noradrenaline have sympathomimetic effects, their potency is some 50–500 times less than their enantiomers (depending on the experimental preparation on which they are assessed). Consequently, racemic (*dl*)-adrenaline and (*dl*)-noradrenaline have approximately 50% of the activity of the (*l*) enantiomers; the naturally occurring and more potent isomers [(*l*)-adrenaline and (*l*)-noradrenaline] are therefore generally used. Nevertheless, (*dl*)-adrenaline may have certain advantages, particularly when used in the management of croup and upper respiratory obstruction in children. When (*dl*)-adrenaline is administered into the respiratory tract as a nebulized solution, it appears to have a longer duration of action than (*l*)-adrenaline; while the (*l*) enantiomer acts for only 1–2 h, the racemic mixture may act for up to 6 h. It is possible that (*d*)-adrenaline in the racemic mixture may compete for and saturate uptake mechanisms or enzyme systems in submucosal sympathetic nerve endings, and thus prolong the action of the (*l*) enantiomer in racemic preparations.

Some inotropic agents, e.g. dopamine, are achiral compounds. In contrast, its chemical analogue dobutamine is a chiral drug, and is usually administered as a racemic mixture of R(+)-dobutamine and S(–)-dobutamine; the enantiomers have complementary effects, and both play an essential part in the pharmacological activity of the drug. R(+)-dobutamine acts on β_1- and β_2-receptors, increasing heart rate, stroke volume, cardiac output and myocardial contractility, as well as causing peripheral vasodilatation. In contrast, S(–)-dobutamine is a potent agonist at postsynaptic myocardial α_1-adrenoceptors, increasing myocardial contractility with little or no change in heart rate. Consequently, the relatively selective inotropic effects of dobutamine are mainly due to the action of the S(–) enantiomer on α_1-receptors in the myocardium; the inotropic selectivity is attenuated or abolished by α_1-adrenoceptor blockade (e.g. with prazosin). Both R(+)- and S(–)-dobutamine increase cardiac contractility, and the complementary effects of the combination of both enantiomers is essential for the clinical effectiveness of the drug.

Many other drugs that affect adrenergic receptors (either directly or indirectly) are chiral, and show a high degree of stereoselectivity. Thus, the α_2-agonist medetomidine has a high stereoselectivity index, and almost all its activity is due to its (+) enantiomer (dexmedetomidine). In general, R(–) enantiomers are more active at sympathetic receptors than their S(+) antipodes, and drugs that act on β-adrenergic receptors show greater stereoselectivity than those that affect α-adrenergic receptors. Consequently, many drugs that affect the heart and the circulation (e.g. β-adrenoceptor antagonists, calcium antagonists, sympathomimetic agents and antiarrhythmic drugs) are also chiral. In many instances (e.g. β-adrenergic antagonists) the drugs are administered as racemic mixtures, although only one enantiomer is active.

Chirality and the development of new drugs

In some instances (e.g. with tramadol and dobutamine) the enantiomers of chiral drugs have different but complementary actions, and both stereoisomers make an important contribution to the overall pharmacological profile of the drug. In these conditions, the use of drugs as chiral mixtures is clearly essential.

In other cases, the use of chiral drugs in stereoisomeric mixtures has been widely accepted, although their use appears to have few practical advantages. Until recently, it was not generally appreciated that drug enantiomers could have different biological effects, or that one of the stereoisomers could be mainly responsible for their undesirable actions. In addition, the chemical technology for the separation of individual isomers from chiral mixtures on an industrial scale was not generally available (or was extremely expensive).

During the past decade, there has been a significant change in this position. Progress in chemical technology has greatly simplified the separation and preparation of individual stereoisomers (e.g. by asymmetric chemical syntheses, or by the chiral inversion of one enantiomer). In addition, the disadvantages inherent in the use of drugs as isomeric mixtures has been more widely appreciated (particularly in instances where one enantiomer is much more active than its antipode, or is responsible for adverse effects). In these conditions, the distomer (i.e. the less active isomer) has been regarded by some as an impurity, or 'therapeutic ballast'; it does not contribute to the required pharmacological actions, but is an additional and unnecessary metabolic imposition on the body. In addition, drug regulatory authorities in many countries have encouraged the introduction of new drugs as single stereoisomers. According to one authority, 'the pharmaceutical industry is facing ever-increasing demands made by regulatory agencies concerning the optical purity of drugs; and the time is near when regulatory agencies will not permit the development or marketing of drugs that are not optically pure unless there is a valid pharmacological and/or medical reason to have mixtures of isomers present in the preparation'. Consequently, since 1990 many new drugs have been introduced as single enantiomers, and in some instances previously available chiral mixtures have been reintroduced as single stereoisomers.

These considerations suggest that most chiral anaesthetic drugs should be prepared and administered as the most active and safest enantiomer, rather than as isomeric mixtures. In most instances, methods can be developed for their chemical synthesis as single, pure and specific stereoisomers. In practice, the position is more complex. Some anaesthetic drugs that are currently used as chiral mixtures have been used in this form for many years (e.g. intravenous barbiturates and most fluorinated anaesthetics); it is doubtful whether much would be gained by the development of single enantiomers of these drugs. In other instances (notably ketamine, bupivacaine and some muscle relaxants), the development and introduction of single isomer preparations would have considerable practical clinical advantages; indeed, it seems likely that single enantiomer preparations of these drugs will be introduced before the new millennium.

Further reading

Aberg G. Toxicological and local anaesthetic effects of optically active isomers of two local anaesthetic compounds. *Acta Pharmacologica et Toxicologica* 1972; **31**: 273–286.

Akerman B. Uptake and retention of the enantiomers of a local anaesthetic in isolated nerve in relation to different degrees of blocking of nervous conduction. *Acta Pharmacologica et Toxicologica* 1973; **32**: 225–236.

Akerman B, Persson H, Tegner C. Local anaesthetic properties of the optically active isomers of prilocaine (Citanest). *Acta Pharmacologica et Toxicologica* 1967; **25**: 233–241.

Akerman B, Ross S. Stereospecificity of the enzymatic biotransformation of the enantiomers of prilocaine Citanest). *Acta Pharmacologica et Toxicologica* 1970; **28**: 445–453.

Andrews PR, Mark LC. Structural specificity of barbiturates and related drugs. *Anesthesiology* 1982; **57**: 314–320.

Aps C, Reynolds F. An intradermal study of the local anaesthetic and vascular effects of the isomers of bupivacaine. *British Journal of Clinical Pharmacology* 1978; **6**: 63–68.

Ariens EJ. Stereochemistry, a basis for sophisticated nonsense in pharmacokinetics and clinical pharmacology. *European Journal of Clinical Pharmacology* 1984; **26**: 663–668.

Ariens EJ. Chirality in bioactive agents and its pitfalls. *Trends in Pharmacological Sciences* 1986; **7**: 200–205.

Ariens EJ, Wuis EW, Veringa EJ. Stereoselectivity of bioactive xenobiotics. *Biochemical Pharmacology* 1988; **37**: 9–18.

Birkett DJ. Racemates or enantiomers: regulatory approaches. *Clinical and Experimental Pharmacology and Physiology* 1989; **16**: 479–483.

Brockway M, Bannister J, McKeown D, Wildsmith JAW. Double-blind comparison of extradural bupivacaine and ropivacaine. *British Journal of Anaesthesia* 1990; **64**: 388.

Calvey TN. Chirality in anaesthesia. *Anaesthesia* 1992; **47**: 93–94.

Calvey TN. Isomerism and anaesthetic drugs. *Acta Anaesthesiological Scandinavica* 1995; **39** (suppl. 106): 83–90.

Christensen HD, Lee IS. Anesthetic potency and acute toxicity of optically active disubstituted barbituric acids. *Toxicology and Applied Pharmacology* 1973; **26**: 495–503.

Cooper MJ, Anders MW. Metabolic and pharmacodynamic interactions of enantiomers of propoxyphene and methorphan. *Life Sciences* 1974; **15**: 1665–1672.

Degkwitz E, Ullrich V, Staudinger H, Rummel W. Metabolism and cytochrome-P450 binding spectra of (+) and (–)-hexobarbital in rat liver microsomes. *Hoppe-Seyler's Zeitschrift fur Physiologische Chemie* 1969; **350**: 547–553.

Doenicke A, Kugler J, Mayer M, Angster R, Hoffman P. Ketamin-Razemat oder S-(+)-Ketamin und Midazolam. *Anaesthetist* 1992; **41**: 610–618.

Drayer DE. Pharmacodynamic and pharmacokinetic differences between drug enantiomers in humans: an overview. *Clinical Pharmacology and Therapeutics* 1986; **40**: 125–133.

Dundee JW, Wyant GM. *Intravenous Anaesthesia*. Edinburgh: Churchill Livingstone, 1988.

Eggers KA, Power I. Tramodol. *British Journal of Anaesthesia* 1995; **74**: 247–249.

Evans AM, Nation RL, Sansom LN, Bochner F, Somogyi AA. Stereoselective drug disposition: potential for misinterpretation of drug disposition data. *British Journal of Clinical Pharmacology* 1988; **26**: 771–780.

Fairley JW, Reynolds F. An intradermal study of the local anaesthetic and vascular effects of the isomers of mepivacaine. *British Journal of Anaesthesia* 1981; **53**: 1211–1216.

Fessenden RJ, Fessenden JS. *Organic Chemistry*, 4th edn. Pacific Grove, California: Brooks/Cole, 1990.

Finar IL. *Organic Chemistry*, 6th edn. Harlow, Essex: Longman, 1973.

Finucane BT. Ropivacaine — a worthy replacement for bupivacaine? *Canadian Journal of Anaesthesia* 1990; **37**: 722–725.

Franks NP, Lieb WR. Stereospecific effects of inhalational general anesthetic optical isomers on nerve ion channels. *Science* 1991; **254**: 427–430.

Franks NP, Lieb WR. Selective actions of volatine general anaesthetics at molecular and cellular levels. *British Journal of Anaesthesia* 1993; **71**: 65–76.

Furner RW, McCarthy JS, Stitzel RE, Anders MW. Stereoselective metabolism of the enantiomers of hexobarbital. *Journal of Pharmacology and Experimental Therapeutics* 1969; **169**: 153–158.

Gibson WR, Doran WJ, Wood WC, Swanson EE. Pharmacology of stereoisomers of 1-methyl-5-(1-methyl-2-pentynyl)-5-allyl-barbituric acid. *Journal of Pharmacology and Experimental Therapeutics* 1959; **125**: 23–27.

Gristwood R, Bardsley H, Baker H, Dickens J. Reduced cardiotoxicity of levobupivacaine compared with racemic bupivacaine (Marcaine): new clinical evidence. *Experimental Opinions and Investigations of Drugs* 1994; **3**: 1209–1212.

Haley TJ, Gidley JT. Pharmacological comparison of R(+), S(–) and racemic thiopentone in mice. *European Journal of Pharmacology* 1976; **36**: 211–214.

Harris B, Moody E, Skolnick P. Isoflurane anesthesia is stereoselective. *European Journal of Pharmacology* 1992; **217**: 215–216.

Hutt AJ, Caldwell J. The metabolic chiral inversion of 2-arylpropionic acids — a novel route with pharmacological consequences. *Journal of Pharmacy and Pharmacology* 1983; **35**: 693–704.

Jones RM. Volatile anaesthetic agents. In: Nimmo WS, Rowbotham DJ, Smith G, (eds). Anaesthesia, 2nd edn. Oxford: Blackwell Scientific Publications, 1994; 43–74.

Kharasch ED, Labroo R. Metabolism of ketamine stereoisomers by human liver microsomes. *Anesthesiology* 1992; **77**: 1201–1207.

Klepstad P, Maurset A, Moberg ER, Øye I. Evidence of a role for NMDA receptors in pain perception. *European Journal of Pharmacology* 1990; **187**: 513–518.

Lee-Son S, Wang GK, Concus A, Crill E, Strichartz G. Stereoselective inhibition of neuronal sodium channels by local anesthetics. Evidence for two sites of action. *Anesthesiology* 1992; **77**: 324–335.

Luduena FP. Duration of local anaesthesia. *Annual Review of Pharmacology* 1969; **9**: 503–520.

Lundy PM, Lockwood PA, Thompson G, Frew R. Differential effects of ketamine isomers on neuronal and extraneuronal catecholamine uptake mechanisms. *Anesthesiology* 1986; **64**: 359–363.

Mason S. *Molecular Optical Activity and the Chiral Discriminations*. Cambridge: Cambridge University Press, 1982.

Mason S. The origin of chirality in nature. *Trends in Pharmacological Sciences* 1986; **7**: 20–23.

Mather LE. Disposition of mepivacaine and bupivacaine enantiomers in sheep. *British Journal of Anaesthesia* 1991; **67**: 239–246.

Mather LE, Rutten AJ. Stereochemistry and its relevance in anesthesiology. *Current Opinion in Anaesthesiology* 1991; **4**: 473–479.

Meretoja OA, Taivainen T, Wirtavuori K. Pharmacodynamic effects of 51W89, an isomer of atracurium, in children during halothane anaesthesia. *British Journal of Anaesthesia* 1995; **74**: 6–11.

Miller RD. Is 51W89 an improvement compared with atracurium? *British Journal of Anaesthesia* 1995; **74**: 1–2.

Mirakhur RK. Anticholinergic drugs. *British Journal of Anaesthesia* 1979; **51**: 671–679.

Moody EJ, Harris BD, Skolnick P. The potential for safer anaesthesia using stereoselective anaesthetics. *Trends in Pharmacological Sciences* **15**: 387–391.

Pasteur L. In: Richardson GM (ed) *Memoirs by Pasteur, van't Hoff, Le Bel and Wislicenus*. New York: American Book Company, 1901.

Pfeiffer CC. Optical isomerism and pharmacological action, a generalisation. *Science*1956; **124**: 29–30.

Portoghese PS. Relationships between stereostructure and pharmacological activities. *Annual Review of Pharmacology* 1970; **10**: 51–76.

Puu G, Koch M, Artursson E. Ketamine enantiomers and acetylcholinesterase. *Biochemical Pharmacology* 1991; **41**: 2043–2045.

Raffa RB, Friderichs E, Reimann W et al. Complementary and synergistic antinociceptive interaction between the enantiomers of tramadol. *Journal of Pharmacology and Experimental Therapeutics* 1993; **267**: 331–340.

Reynolds F. Ropivacaine. *British Journal of Anaesthesia* 1991; **46**: 339–340.

Ruffolo RR. Review: The pharmacology of dobutamine. *American Journal of the Medical Sciences* 1987; **294**: 244–248.

Ruffolo RR. Signs of support. *Trends in Pharmacological Sciences* 1990; **11**: 61.

Ruffolo RR, Messick K. Inotropic selectivity of dobutamine enantiomers in the pithed rat. *Journal of Pharmacology and Experimental Therapeutics* 1985; **235**: 344–348.

Sallustio BC, Purdie YJ, Whitehead AG, Ahern MJ, Meffin PJ. The disposition of ketoprofen enantiomers in man. *British Journal of Clinical Pharmacology* 1988; **26**: 765–770.

Schüttler J. *S*-(+)-Ketamin. Beginn einer neuen Ketamin-Aera? *Anaesthetist* 1992; **41**: 585–587.

Simonyi M. On chiral drug action. *Medicinal Research Reviews* 1984; **4**: 359–413.

Simonyi M, Fitos I, Visy J. Chirality of bioactive agents in protein binding storage and transport processes. *Trends in Pharmacological Sciences* 1986; **7**: 112–116.

Smith DJ, Azzaro AJ, Zaldivar SB, Palmer S, Lee HS. Properties of the optical isomers and metabolites of ketamine on the high affinity transport and catabolism of monoamines. *Neuropharmacology* 1981; **20**: 391–396.

Stenlake JB, Waigh RD, Dewar GH et al. Biodegradable neuromuscular blocking agents. Part 6. Stereochemical studies on atracurium and related polyalkylene di-esters. *European Journal of Medicinal Chemistry* 1984; **19**: 441–450.

Testa B. Chiral aspects of drug metabolism. *Trends in Pharmacological Sciences* 1986; **7**: 60–64.

Thiel A, Adams HA, Fengler G, Hempelmann G. Untersuchungen mit *S*-(+)-Ketamin an Probanden. *Anaesthetist* 1992; **41**: 604–609.

Tsui D, Graham GG, Torda TA. The pharmacokinetics of atracurium isomers *in vitro* and in humans. *Anaesthesiology* 1987; **67**: 722–728.

Tucker GT. Chirality and drug development — a clinical pharmacologist's perspective. *Biochemical Society Transactions* 1991; **19**: 460–462.

Tucker GT, Lennard MS. Enantiomer specific pharmacokinetics. *Pharmacology and Therapeutics* 1990; **45**: 309–329.

Tucker GT, Mather LE, Lennard MS, Gregory A. Plasma concentrations of the stereoisomers of prilocaine after administration of the racemate: implications for toxicity. *British Journal of Anaesthesia* 1990; **65**: 333–336.

Vanhoutte F, Vereecke J, Verbeke N, Carmeliet E. Stereoselective effects of the enantiomers of bupivacaine on the electrophysiological properties of the guinea-pig papillary muscle. *British Journal of Pharmacology* 1991; **103**: 1275–1281.

Walle T, Walle UK. Pharmacokinetic parameters obtained in racemates. *Trends in Pharmacological Sciences* 1986; **7**: 155–158.

Weissinger J. Considerations in the development of stereoisomeric drugs: FDA viewpoint. *Drug Information Journal* 1989; **23**: 663–667.

White PF, Ham J, Way WL, Trevor AJ. Pharmacology of ketamine isomers in surgical patients. *Anesthesiology* 1980; **52**: 231–239.

White PF, Schuttler J, Shafer A, Stanski DR, Horai Y, Trevor AJ. Comparative pharmacology of the ketamine isomers. *British Journal of Anaesthesia* 1985; **57**: 197–203.

White PF, Way WL, Trevor AJ. Ketamine — its pharmacology and therapeutic uses. *Anesthesiology* 1982; **56**: 119–136.

Zeilhofer HU, Swandulla D, Geisslinger G, Brune K. Differential effects of ketamine enantiomers on NMDA currents in cultured neurones. *European Journal of Pharmacology* 1992; **213**: 155–158.

Appendix I: The history and nomenclature of stereoisomerism

Stereoisomerism has a remarkable and fascinating history, which profoundly affected the development of current concepts of chemical structure. The recognition of the phenomenon of stereoisomerism gradually developed from studies of optical isomers during the early 19th century. In the 1820s, it was shown that quartz crystals occurred naturally in two different forms, which could be distinguished from each other by their hemihedral facets (minor faces in the crystal structure). These two forms of quartz were mirror images, and had equal but opposite optical activity; thus, one of the crystal forms rotated plane-polarized light to the left, while the other rotated plane-polarized light to the right. The optical activity of quartz was clearly due to its crystal structure, since it was lost if the crystals were fused or dissolved.

Within several years, solutions of some naturally occurring compounds were also shown to rotate plane-polarized light, including one of the tartaric acids (organic acids isolated from the tartars deposited by maturing wine). The main tartaric acid in wine was shown to rotate polarized light to the right [(*d*)- or (+)-tartaric acid]; in contrast, a minor component (racemic acid) had no optical activity. Subsequently Louis Pasteur, while still a student in Paris (1843–1848), showed that racemic acid (*para*-tartaric acid) was an equal mixture of two different optically active compounds. Recrystallization of sodium ammonium racemate resulted in two different mirror-image forms (which he separated by hand, using a microscope and a pair of tweezers). Solutions of these forms were shown to rotate polarized light to the same extent, but in opposite directions; one form rotated light to the right, the other to the left (i.e. the forms were optical isomers). Pasteur concluded that the individual molecules and their crystals were non-superimposable mirror-image forms of the same chemical substance; consequently, the optically inactive racemic acid was an equal 'racemic' mixture of two optical isomers.

Although Louis Pasteur clearly recognized that optical isomers were different forms of a single chemical compound, he was unable to explain their occurrence in terms of the contemporary chemistry of the 1850s. At that time, organic molecules were generally considered to be flat, planar structures; consequently, their two-dimensional formulae could not account for the existence of different forms of a single chemical compound. The precise explanation of optical isomerism was obscure until 1874, when Le Bel and van't Hoff independently advanced similar theories of molecular structure. They proposed that the tetravalent carbon atom was situated at the centre of a regular tetrahedron, with its valencies directed towards the four vertices (Fig. 4.7). In these conditions, molecules containing a single carbon atom with four different substituent groups are asymmetric, and can exist in two different forms, one of which is the non-superimposable mirror image of the other.

After 1874, it became generally accepted that molecular asymmetry was the cause of optical isomerism, and resulted in two enantiomers (substances of opposite shape) that were not directly superimposable on their mirror images. Pasteur originally referred to this phenomenon as dissymmetry (*la dissymétrie*); in 1884, Kelvin introduced the term chirality ('having handedness'), from the analogy between the right and left hands, which are non-superimposable mirror images of each other. Consequently, centres of molecular asymmetry or optical activity were described as chiral or handed centres. In subsequent years, the number of stereoisomers associated with more than one chiral centre was shown to be generally consistent with these concepts. Other types of stereoisomerism, e.g. geometric (*cis–trans*) isomerism, were also described in optically inactive compounds containing double bonds.

During the late 19th century, the stereochemical configuration of simple sugars presented a particularly difficult problem. Simple monosaccharides with the molecular formula $C_6H_{12}O_6$ (e.g. glucose) have four inequivalent chiral centres, and therefore give rise to 16 different stereoisomers (including glucose, galactose and mannose), as well as a number of structural isomers (e.g. fructose). It was shown that the terminal chiral centre in all the naturally occurring sugars had the same configuration as (+)-glyceraldehyde; these sugars were therefore defined as (D)-isomers (since they had the same configuration as dextrorotatory glyceraldehyde). Similarly, the configuration of all the naturally occurring chiral amino acids was related to levorotatory (–)-glyceraldehyde, resulting in their classification as (L)-amino acids. The German chemist Emil Fischer established the stereochemical configuration of glucose in 1891, and subsequently showed that its methylated isomers were stereoselectively hydrolysed by specific enzymes. Consequently, Fischer concluded that the reactions of chiral compounds with endogenous proteins were governed by the 'key-and-lock' principle (i.e. that an exact and precise stereochemical relationship was an essential requirement for many biological processes).

Nevertheless, until 1950 it was impossible to determine the absolute configuration of stereoisomers; their classification in terms of the (presumed) configuration of glyceraldehyde was completely arbitrary. The (D) and (L) classification was therefore invariably widely used to define the relative configuration of many chemical compounds, including naturally occurring substances and drugs. Unfortunately, it has several limitations, and it can only be reliably used with drugs that have structural similarities to glyceraldehyde. In 1951, the absolute configuration of (+)-tartaric acid was established by J.M. Bijvoet in Utrecht, using X-ray diffraction techniques, and (+)-tartaric acid was therefore used as an independent standard. These developments led to the introduction of a new system of stereochemical nomenclature, based on the priority of the chemical groups attached to the chiral carbon atom. The (R) and (S) system (the Cahn, Ingold, Prelog or CIP system) allows the absolute configuration of groups around a chiral carbon atom to be independently defined, and is now invariably used to specify the stereochemistry of chemical compounds. It is also widely used to define and identify the stereoisomers of many drugs, although its use for this purpose is not universally accepted.

Stereochemical nomenclature

A complex and confusing nomenclature is used to identify the enantiomers of chiral drugs and natural products, reflecting the long history of stereoisomerism. At least three systems of classification are in current use, and the individual enantiomers of drugs can be identified by:

1 Their direction or sign of optical rotation.
2 Their relative stereochemical configuration.
3 Their absolute stereochemical configuration.

These three systems are entirely distinct and bear no relationship to each other, and there is no simple or predictable connection between the relative or absolute configuration of drugs and their optical rotation. In recent years, it has also been suggested that the stereochemical status of drugs can be represented by one of seven prefixes to their generic names. It is unclear whether this system of classification (SIGNS) will be widely adopted.

All these systems of nomenclature are commonly used in different circumstances; consequently, the classification of individual stereoisomers can result in problems in the identity and identification of the individual enantiomers.

Optical rotation

Enantiomers are specified as (+) and (–), (*d*) and (*l*), or (dextro) and (levo), depending on the direction of rotation of polarized light by their solutions. This may be to the right (denoted by (+), (*d*), or (dextro)), or to the left (denoted by (–), (*l*), or (levo).

This nomenclature dates from the time of Pasteur, but has many disadvantages:

1 The direction of optical rotation bears no relationship to stereochemical configuration; for example, the configuration of glyceraldehyde is not affected by the oxidation of (+)-glyceraldehyde to (–)-glyceric acid.

2 The optical activity of some compounds slowly alters in the course of time; the activity of many simple sugars in solution slowly changes to a constant value, due to their isomerism (mutarotation).

3 The optical rotation of some drugs (e.g. chloramphenicol) depends on the solvent used for its measurement. Solutions of chloramphenicol in ethyl alcohol rotate polarized light to the right; in contrast, solutions of the drug in ethyl acetate rotate light to the left.

4 The direction of optical rotation of many drugs is reversed when acid salts are converted to their bases (e.g. when drugs administered as hydrochloride or sulphate salts are injected or neutralized); consequently, enantiomeric drug salts and their neutralized, biologically active bases may rotate polarized light in opposite directions.

For these reasons, the use of optical rotation as a basis for the classification of stereoisomers is completely unacceptable to most organic chemists. Nevertheless, in the biological sciences and in medicine, stereoisomers are commonly classified by their optical rotation. Indeed, the commonly used names of some monosaccharides (e.g. dextrose and laevulose) as well as many drugs (e.g. levodopa, dilevalol, levallorphan, levorphanol, levophed, dexamphetamine and dextropropoxyphene) are based on their optical rotation.

Relative configuration

Simple sugars and amino acids are commonly classified as D or L isomers (e.g. D-glucose; L-alanine), depending on the relationship of their configuration to D(+)-glyceraldehyde. All naturally occurring sugars are D isomers, while most physiological amino acids are L isomers. Although this system of nomenclature is widely used for simple sugars, aminoacids and their derivatives, its application to drugs can result in a number of difficulties.

In the first place, D and L are often confused with (*d*) and (*l*), which usually refer to optical rotation and therefore have an entirely different meaning. Consequently, problems may occur with the identity and identification of many drugs, including naturally occurring catecholamines and their derivatives. For example, (*l*)-adrenaline and L-adrenaline are not the same isomer; they are enantiomers, and only (*l*)-adrenaline (i.e. the D-configuration) has any biological activity. Similarly, (*l*)-noradrenaline and L-noradrenaline are not the same enantiomer, and only (*l*)-noradrenaline (D-noradrenaline) is biologically active.

Second, it can only be reliably used to identify the stereoisomers of drugs that are structurally related to glyceraldehyde. It is therefore difficult or impossible to define the enantiomers of most drugs as D or L isomers, since they have little or no structural relationship to glyceraldehyde.

Finally, it is difficult to classify some compounds as D or L isomers; for example, naturally occurring (+)-tartaric acid can be classified as a D or an L stereoisomer (depending on whether its synthesis or degradation is considered).

At the present time, only sugars and amino acids are commonly classified as D and L isomers; when applied to these compounds, the nomenclature is universally accepted and causes little or no ambiguity.

Absolute configuration

Since 1950, it has been possible to determine and define the absolute configuration of chemical compounds and drugs as right-handed (R) or left-handed (S), using the CIP sequence rules. This nomenclature does not depend on spatial relationships with other compounds, and can only be applied to drugs whose absolute stereochemistry has been determined. During the past 20 years, it has been widely used to specify the configuration of chiral drugs.

The nomenclature of other types of stereoisomerism

When stereoisomers contain more than one chiral centre, the isomers can be defined by their configuration at each of the asymmetric atoms. Thus, the analgesic tramadol is a chiral mixture of (1R, 2R)-tramadol and (1S, 2S)-tramodol (where 1 and 2 refer to the position of the asymmetric carbon atoms in the cyclohexanol ring; Fig. 4.9).

In geometric isomerism, an entirely different type of nomenclature is used. Geometric isomerism usually occurs when two different groups are attached to adjacent atoms linked by a rigid chemical bond (e.g. a double bond or a single bond in a heterocyclic ring). Thus, geometric isomerism can occur between the carbon atom (C1) and the nitrogen atom (N2) in the tetrahydropapaverine rings in atracurium and mivacurium (Fig. 4.11). When two identical groups are on the same side of the bond, the stereoisomer is defined as *cis*; when they are on opposite sides of the bond, the isomer is called *trans*. Occasionally, the letters *Z*- (for zusammen, together) or *E*- (for entgegen, across) are used instead of *cis* and *trans*; however, *Z*- and *E*- usually have a more general applicability.

Appendix II: Stereoisomerism of atracurium and mivacurium

The muscle relaxants atracurium and mivacurium are complex examples of stereoisomerism. The structure of both drugs contains four isomeric centres, in positions 1 (carbon atom) and 2 (nitrogen atom) of the two tetrahydropapaverine units (Fig.

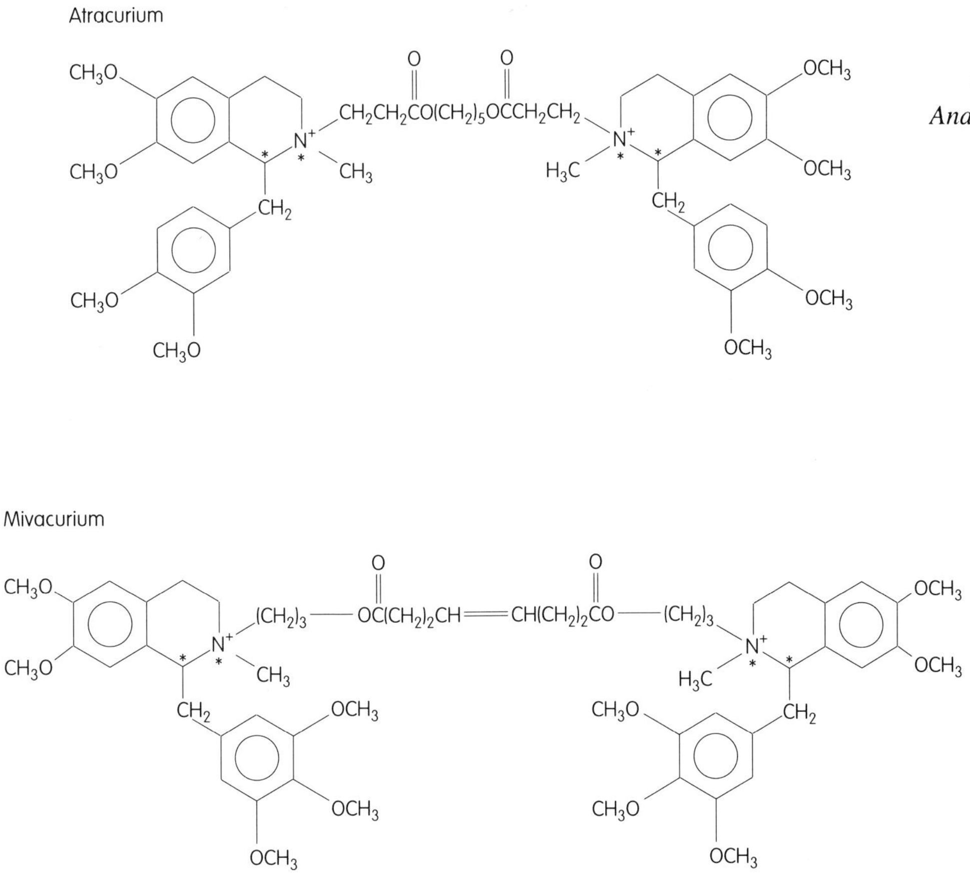

Fig. 4.11 The chemical structure of atracurium and mivacurium. The asterisks denote the presence of four centres of stereoisomerism in each molecule.

4.11). Consequently, the structure of both atracurium and mivacurium is theoretically consistent with a maximum of 16 (2^4) possible stereoisomers. Each isomer can be classified by its configuration at the two carbon atoms (as R or S), and by its relative configuration at the two carbon–nitrogen bonds (as *cis* or *trans*). When the two large substituent groups are on the same side of the C—N bond, the isomer is arbitrarily defined as *cis*; when they are on opposite sides of the C—N bond, the isomer is defined as *trans*. Consequently, the configuration of the 16 possible stereoisomers in both chemical structures (from left to right of the molecule) are:

(1) R-*cis*, R-*cis*
(2) R-*cis*, R-*trans*
(3) R-*cis*, S-*cis*
(4) R-*cis*, S-*trans*
(5) R-*trans*, R-*cis*

(6) R-*trans*, R-*trans*
(7) R-*trans*, S-*cis*
(8) R-*trans*, S-*trans*
(9) S-*cis*, R-*cis*
(10) S-*cis*, R-*trans*
(11) S-*cis*, S-*cis*
(12) S-*cis*, S-*trans*
(13) S-*trans*, R-*cis*
(14) S-*trans*, R-*trans*
(15) S-*trans*, S-*cis*
(16) S-*trans*, S-*trans*.

In practice, the number of possible stereoisomers is reduced from 16 to 10, due to the internal symmetry of the molecule (congruence). The structure of both atracurium and mivacurium is internally symmetrical (i.e. the left and right halves of the molecule are identical). Consequently, both molecules can be rotated by 180° (i.e. turned back-to-front, so that the right and left halves of the molecule are reversed) without altering the structure or configuration of the stereoisomers). In these conditions, configuration (2) (R-*cis*, R-*trans*) and configuration (5) (R-*trans*, R-*cis*) are identical (i.e. they have equivalent isomeric centres). Similarly, configurations (3) and (9), (4) and (13), (7) and (10), (8) and (14), and (12) and (15) are equivalent, and the unique 10 configurations are:

(1) R-*cis*, R-*cis*
(2) R-*cis*, R-*trans*
(3) R-*cis*, S-*cis*
(4) R-*cis*, S-*trans*
(6) R-*trans*, R-*trans*
(7) R-*trans*, S-*cis*
(8) R-*trans*, S-*trans*
(11) S-*cis*, S-*cis*
(12) S-*cis*, S-*trans*
(16) S-*trans*, S-*trans*.

Atracurium is synthesized in a non-selective manner; consequently the drug used clinically consists of a mixture of these 10 stereoisomers. They can be divided (and separated by chromatographic techniques) into three groups of geometrical isomers: *cis–cis* isomers (58%; (1), (3) and (11)); *cis–trans* isomers (36%; (2), (4), (7) and (12)); and *trans–trans* isomers (6%; (6), (8) and (16)). The stereoisomers consist of four enantiomeric pairs ((1) and (11); (2) and (12); (6) and (16); and (4) and (7)) and two diastereomers ((3) and (8)).

In contrast, mivacurium is synthesized with both chiral carbon atoms in the two tetrahydropapaverine units in the R configuration; in these conditions, there are four possible stereoisomeric configurations:

(1) R-*cis*, R-*cis*

(2) R-*cis*, R-*trans*

(3) R-*trans*, R-*cis*

(4) R-*trans*, R-*trans*.

Due to the internal symmetry of the molecular structure of mivacurium, configurations (2) and (3) are equivalent; consequently mivacurium consists of a mixture of the three geometrical isomers, R-*cis*, R-*cis* (6%), R-*cis*, R-*trans* (36%), and R-*trans*, R-*trans* (58%).

Chapter 5
Drug Interaction

Drug interaction is the modification of the effects of one drug by another. Many of these reactions are clinically unimportant or harmless, while others form an integral part of medical or anaesthetic practice. A familiar example is the use of neostigmine to antagonize the effects of non-depolarizing neuromuscular blocking agents at the motor endplate and the concomitant use of atropine to prevent muscarinic activity due to the anticholinesterase. However, a small minority of interactions are hazardous or potentially fatal, and it is therefore important for the anaesthetist to be aware of their possible occurrence. Interactions may occur between drugs which are administered concurrently during anaesthesia; alternatively, reactions may occur with prescribed drugs or self-medication. It is thus essential for a full drug history to be available prior to the administration of anaesthesia.

Nevertheless, the assessment of drug interactions in humans must be undertaken with a sense of balance. Reports of adverse effects based on single case histories or circumstantial and anecdotal evidence are of little value, particularly when the mechanisms involved are obscure or poorly understood.

It would appear that the incidence of adverse drug reactions and presumably interactions increases with the number of drugs a patient receives. One hospital study showed that the rate was 7% in those taking 6–10 drugs and 40% in those taking 16–20 drugs. Comparable figures for anaesthetic practice, where the patient may receive as many as 9–10 drugs as part of the anaesthetic regimen, are not available. However, most of the interactions that may occur in anaesthesia are well-known and are usually predictable from an appreciation of the pharmacology of the drugs concerned.

In this chapter, a general account is given of the pharmacological mechanisms that are usually responsible for drug interactions in humans. Reactions with specific groups of drugs that are commonly used in anaesthetic practice are then considered in detail.

Mechanisms of drug interactions may be described in three groups.

1 Pharmaceutical interactions which can occur *in vitro*.

2 Pharmacokinetic interactions which are due to the alteration of the disposition of one drug by another.

3 Pharmacodynamic interactions which are due to interference with the effects of drugs at tissue sites.

Nomenclature

Some confusion exists in the literature regarding the precise meanings of the terms used to describe drug interactions, namely, summation (or additive effects), antagonism, potentiation and synergism.

Summation

Summation (or an additive effect) is not a true drug interaction and merely reflects the combination of two drugs producing the same effects as if each drug were given separately (e.g. nitrous oxide and halothane).

Antagonism

Antagonism can occur with pharmacokinetic interference (e.g. reduced drug absorption or enzyme induction), chemical antagonism (e.g. heparin and protamine; heavy metals and chelating agents) or interactions at receptor sites. Receptor antagonism is usually competitive and reversible (e.g. opioid analgesics and naloxone; propranolol and β-adrenoceptor agonists) but may be potentially irreversible (e.g. phenoxybenzamine and noradrenaline) due to the slow dissociation of the antagonist from the receptor site.

Potentiation

Potentiation may be best defined as the enhancement of the effects of one drug by another drug, usually by mechanisms either involving pharmacokinetic parameters or changes in acid–base and electrolyte balance. In general, the potentiating drug has no similar pharmacological activity (e.g. penicillin and probenecid; digoxin and certain diuretics).

Synergism

Synergism (alternatively described as supra-additive effects) refers to the administration of two drugs with similar pharmacological properties and closely related sites of action which produce an effect in combination which is greater than would have been expected from summation of the contributions of each component. This can be exemplified by observations of the hypnotic effects of benzodiazepines and concomitantly administered intravenous induction agents. Synergism between vecuronium and atracurium has also been described and attributed to differing affinities of drugs with diverse molecular structure on the two α subunits of the receptor. The results of these studies are often interpreted using isoboles, which are graphs showing equieffective combinations of drugs. They were first used approximately 120 years ago to illustrate the antagonism between physostigmine and atropine. Each axis on the graph corresponds to the dosage of a drug, whose individual values for a given effect (e.g. hypnosis) have previously been determined by probit analysis of the dose–response relationship. The median effective dose (ED_{50}) of each agent is plotted on the coordinates of the graph, which are then joined by a straight line between the axes. When equieffective combinations of two drugs approximate to this line, the effects of the drugs are merely additive. This is demonstrated by an isobole showing the interaction between nitrous oxide and halothane (Fig. 5.1). However, when equieffective combinations lie below this line, the interaction is considered to be synergic. In contrast, when the reference point to the combination of two drugs lies above this line an antagonist effect is assumed (Fig. 5.2).

The analysis of interactions between drugs by the use of isoboles has been viewed with considerable circumspection. The method has been regarded as rather empirical and intuitive and appears to take little account of any differences in the dose–response relationships of the two drugs. Nevertheless, current evidence suggests that isoboles can be used to distinguish between additive and synergic effects when the drugs concerned are mutually exclusive, i.e. when they act at (or are bound by) the same receptor or enzyme site. However, combinations of drugs that act at different sites (mutually non-exclusive) cannot be analysed by isoboles, since agents with purely additive effects may give rise to isoboles that are incorrectly

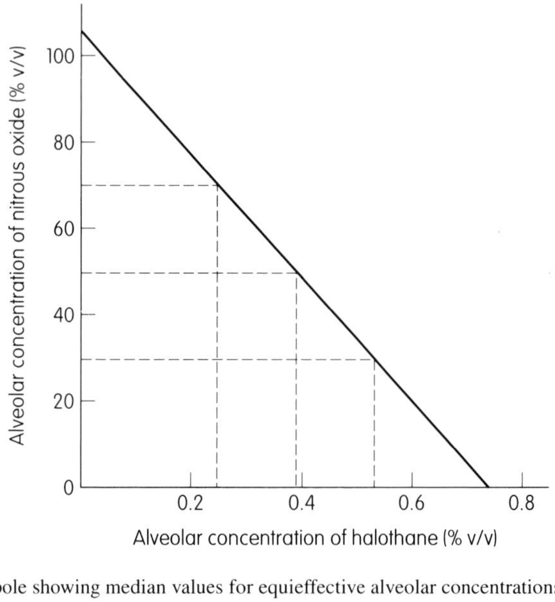

Fig. 5.1 An isobole showing median values for equieffective alveolar concentrations of halothane and nitrous oxide. The effect of the inhalation agents in combination is additive; any point on the additive line subtends approximately equipotent combinations of the two agents. When expressed in a common form (i.e. as minimum alveolar concentration (MAC) values) the potency of individual inhalation agents is additive.

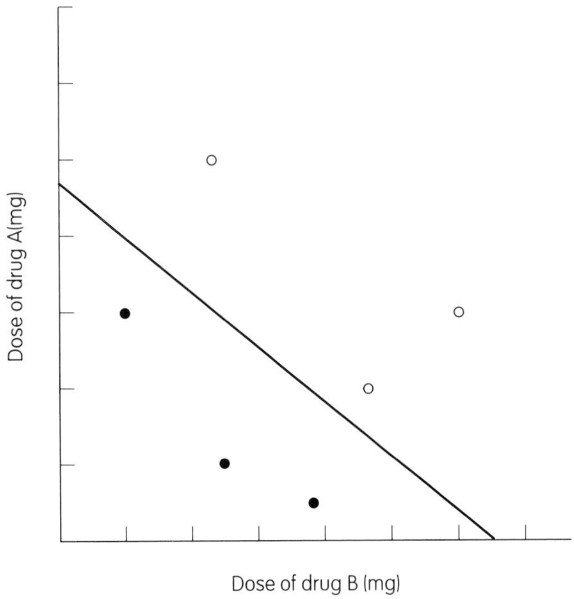

Fig. 5.2 Diagrammatic illustration of an isobole. The two axes show the required median effective dose (ED_{50}) values for each individual drug required to produce a specific pharmacological effect (e.g. loss of response to command, onset of neuromuscular blockade). Points falling below this line (black circles) reflect synergism whilst points above the line (open circles) suggest drug antagonism.

attributed to synergism. Consequently, problems of interpretation may arise when combinations of mutually non-exclusive drugs are analysed by isoboles and they may not be an appropriate way to investigate synergic reactions between anaesthetic drugs with dissimilar mechanisms of action. Nevertheless, they are a convenient method of demonstrating the coexistent effects of two drugs so that the lowest dose combination which is necessary to produce the desired effect can be defined.

Pharmaceutical interactions

Some drug interactions are due to the mixing of drugs or incompatible solutions outside the body. These interactions may be responsible for the loss of activity of drugs, or for their aggregation or precipitation in solution, and this occasionally has serious consequences. Pharmaceutical interactions are divided into two groups — chemical and physical.

Chemical

Most drugs, including anaesthetic agents, inevitably have to be stored before use and in many instances may undergo deterioration during storage. When stored in a powder or solid form, decomposition tends to occur more slowly. The addition of water or a mixing agent may accelerate the rate of decomposition of a drug (e.g. barbiturates for intravenous (i.v.) use), particularly when more concentrated solutions are formed, or when dextrose or saline is used as a solvent. Other drugs (e.g. halothane, catecholamines) are decomposed by light or are sensitive to changes in temperature (e.g. isoflurane, enflurane).

Mixing of solutions with different pH values may result in drug precipitation. Weak acids (e.g. i.v. barbiturates and thiobarbiturates) are usually administered as their sodium salts and are only ionized and water-soluble in alkaline conditions (pH 10–11). Similarly, many other drugs (e.g. local anaesthetics, analgesics, most sympathomimetic amines) are weak bases which can only exist in aqueous solutions as acid salts (e.g. sulphates or hydrochlorides with a pH 4–5). Mixing such dissimilar solutions in the same syringe or in an infusion set usually causes precipitation of free acid and base. The addition of drugs such as suxamethonium to a solution of thiopentone results in rapid alkaline hydrolysis and thus inactivation of the muscle relaxant.

Direct chemical combination may also produce drug interaction *in vitro*. The use of trichlorethylene in anaesthetic circuits incorporating soda lime may lead to the production of the potentially neurotoxic vapour dichloracetylene. There is now considerable evidence that carbon monoxide may be produced in circle systems (resulting in significant levels of carboxyhaemoglobin in anaesthetized patients) when enflurane, isoflurane or desflurane is administered in the presence of warm and dry soda lime. Sevoflurane may also undergo some decomposition when used with warm soda lime (Chapter 8).

The addition of calcium salts to infusion lines containing bicarbonate solutions will result in significant precipitation of the insoluble salt, calcium carbonate. When penicillin derivatives are added to infusion fluids containing amino acids, drug–protein complexes are formed that can induce the formation of cytophilic antibodies (immunoglobulin E; IgE). Alternatively, the individual components of mixtures of drug solutions may be precipitated. Thus, the addition of drugs or electrolytes to fat emulsions (e.g. intralipid) or concentrated solutions (e.g. 20% mannitol) may result in the aggregation or precipitation of the mixture.

Epimerization or racemization of molecules in solutions also occurs. This may involve a change in the steric configuration of the molecule, as in the conversion of adrenaline from an (*l*) to a (*d*) form, which occurs with a pH change in solution. The Maillard reaction involves an interaction between dextrose and amino acid solutions. This results in a colour change and precludes the storage of combined parenteral nutrition mixtures. Although this reaction is minimal at room temperature, it becomes important if the mixture is heat treated.

Physical

A difference in the osmolarity of infusion fluids may lead to interactions which occur during administration. The concurrent infusion of blood with either 5% dextrose or mannitol may result in significant damage to the blood. Solvent system polarity (the solubility of a drug in aqueous solution) may be important when relatively insoluble agents such as diazepam or propofol are presented in organic solvents which are subsequently added to aqueous solutions. The degree of precipitation will depend upon relative volume and concentration of both drug and aqueous solution.

Drugs may also interact with administration sets through which they are given. Sorption is best exemplified by nitroglycerine and refers to the lipophilicity and polarity of the solution which causes the subsequent binding to different types of plastic. Adsorption refers to the tendency of a drug to adhere to the surface of a container, as may occur with insulin in glass or plastic syringes.

Other physical phenomena which may occur include 'salting out', which results when electrolytes are added to supersaturated solutions such as mannitol, and 'emulsion cracking' which can ensue when calcium salts are added to fat emulsions. In the latter instance the surface charge on the fat globules which repels similar particles (the ζ or zeta potential) is reduced in the presence of additional cations and this will allow the globules to coalesce.

Pharmaceutical interactions are often predictable and are not usually an important cause of complications in anaesthetic practice. Their occurrence can be minimized by a number of simple precautions. If possible, only one drug should be added to each unit of a crystalloid solution, except in special circumstances. No additives should be incorporated in infusions of blood, blood products, lipid emulsions, amino acid preparations or hypertonic fluids. The addition of drugs to acid or alkaline solutions should be avoided. Solutions must be thoroughly mixed before administration and this is particularly important when potassium salts are added to intravenous fluids. Solutions containing additives are preferably prepared in the pharmacy and should be clearly labelled. When additives are used in the wards or theatre, the manufacturers' data sheet or a table of drug incompatibilities should be consulted. Cases of doubt can usually be resolved by a pharmacist or drug information centre.

Pharmacokinetic interactions

Pharmacokinetic interactions occur in the body and are due to an alteration in the disposition of one drug by another. In these circumstances, the concentration of a drug at its site of action may be modified. According to the mechanisms involved, these interactions can be classified as those affecting:

1 Dissolution or absorption.
2 Distribution (including protein binding).
3 Metabolism.
4 Elimination.

Dissolution or absorption

These drug interactions usually occur in the stomach or upper intestine, and may concern the anaesthetist when premedicant drugs are given by this route. When drugs are administered by mouth in the form of capsules, they must be present in solution before absorption can occur. Drug dissolution usually takes place in the stomach, and the solubility of some drugs such as the tetracyclines is critically dependent on acid conditions. In these circumstances, drugs which affect gastric pH (e.g. antacids and H_2-receptor antagonists) will influence the degree of absorption. Most drugs, however, are absorbed in the more alkaline medium of the small intestine; thus agents which affect the speed of gastric emptying will alter the rate of delivery of other drugs to the site of absorption and consequently influence uptake. Metoclopramide stimulates gastric emptying and increases the speed of uptake of many drugs administered by mouth, whereas opioid analgesics and anticholinergic agents will exert a converse effect. In most instances involving drugs which affect gastric motility the total amount of an orally administered drug absorbed remains unaltered. However, the bioavailability of digoxin is reduced by metoclopramide and increased by propantheline; conversely, the absorption of levodopa is reduced in the presence of an anticholinergic drug, presumably because of an increased exposure time to metabolism by the intestinal mucosa.

Drug interactions in the small intestine may decrease absorption when chelates or other insoluble complexes are formed. Thus the absorption of tetracyclines is reduced by the simultaneous administration of calcium, magnesium or iron salts, and the resin cholestyramine may decrease the absorption of many other drugs (e.g. warfarin, digoxin, thyroxine).

The absorption of drugs administered by subcutaneous or intramuscular injection is determined by the aqueous solubility of the drug at tissue sites, the extent of biotransformation locally and by the efficiency of peripheral blood flow. Drugs which are prepared in solvents (e.g. diazepam, phenytoin) may precipitate out in tissues, and this may account for the decrease in bioavailability (compared to that attained by oral administration). Various drugs exhibiting autonomic activity (e.g. sympathomimetic amines, α-adrenoceptor antagonists) can significantly modify skin and muscle blood flow. If tissue blood flow is modified by these mechanisms and extensive biotransformation of the parenterally administered drug occurs at tissue sites, bioavailability will be affected.

Distribution

Following administration and absorption, drugs are present in plasma either in simple solution or bound to carrier proteins or erythrocytes, whence they are conveyed to organs and tissues by the vascular system. The uptake and subsequent distribution of inhalational agents are primarily influenced by minute ventilation and cardiac output. The rate of rise of alveolar concentration, which correlates with the induction of anaesthesia, is largely determined by ventilatory activity; thus, respiratory depressants (e.g. opioid analgesics, barbiturates) may slow the rate of onset of anaesthesia. Conversely, drugs which reduce cardiac output (e.g. intravenous induction agents, β-adrenoceptor antagonists) will allow an increased rate of rise of alveolar concentration and by reflex vasoconstrictor effects will lead to enhanced cerebral perfusion; the rate of induction of anaesthesia may thus be increased (Chapter 8).

Protein binding

In many instances, the transport of drugs in the circulation necessitates binding to plasma proteins. Most acidic drugs (e.g. penicillins, salicylates, barbiturates) bind to albumin, whilst in general basic drugs (e.g. opioid analgesics, local anaesthetic agents) bind to other plasma protein constituents such as lipoproteins, α_1-acid glycoprotein and γ-globulin.

Some drugs (e.g. oral anticoagulants) are extensively bound by albumin at therapeutic concentrations, so that only 1–2% of the total in plasma is available for diffusion into tissues. In consequence, drugs that displace oral anticoagulants from plasma proteins (e.g. phenylbutazone, mefenamic acid, some sulphonamides) may significantly increase the unbound fraction of the anticoagulant present in plasma and could enhance its therapeutic and toxic effects. It would appear that problems are only likely to be encountered in relation to acidic drugs with a low volume of distribution which are essentially confined to plasma, and where the ratio between the effective and toxic dose is small (i.e. the drug has a narrow therapeutic index). Basic drugs may have a wider availability of binding sites and plasma levels of α_1-acid glycoprotein may be considerably elevated following surgery and in many disease processes.

However, it is doubtful whether displacement from plasma proteins alone is an important factor in the causation of drug interactions in humans. Enhanced effects are likely to be small and transient, as any increase in the concentration of unbound drug in plasma will usually be counteracted by increased renal and hepatic clearance. A new steady state is thus established (total amount of drug in plasma is reduced, whilst free fraction remains the same) and drug distribution to the site of action is not significantly enhanced. Theoretically, a drug which may be given intravenously and which has a high hepatic extraction ratio (e.g. lignocaine) should be more vulnerable to drug interactions of this nature.

Drugs that lead to clinical interactions with warfarin, such as phenylbutazone, may also affect its metabolism, presumably by competing at enzymatic sites, whose protein configuration may be important.

Certain sulphonamides have been considered to prolong the action of thiopentone by competing for binding on albumin, although it is extremely doubtful whether this interaction is of any clinical significance; it has also been suggested that pretreatment with aspirin or probenecid may reduce the dosage requirements of thiopentone by a similar mechanism.

Some drugs are also extensively bound by proteins in tissues. The antimalarial drugs mepacrine and pamaquin are both bound by hepatic proteins, and may displace each other into extracellular fluid. It is unclear whether this phenomenon is responsible for clinically significant drug interactions in humans. In general, little is known of the possible importance of the binding of drugs to cell and tissue proteins.

Metabolism

Drug interactions affecting metabolism mainly occur in the liver (although drug metabolism may also occur in the intestinal mucosa, plasma and lung parenchyma), and may be due to interference with several different physiological or biochemical processes. Following oral administration, some drugs are highly extracted and extensively metabolized by the liver before they gain access to the systemic circulation. This first-pass effect may be an important cause of the diminished response to certain drugs (e.g. opioid analgesics) when given by the oral route. In the case of drugs which are extensively cleared by the liver (i.e. those with a high extraction ratio), the magnitude of the first-pass effect is dependent on liver blood flow; in consequence, drugs that modify hepatic perfusion may affect the proportion of the oral dose that enters the systemic circulation. Thus, the oral bioavailability of drugs such as lignocaine and some opioid analgesics may be increased by drugs that reduce liver blood flow (e.g. propranolol, volatile anaesthetic agents). Cimetidine, which is a potent inhibitor of liver enzymes, has also been shown to enhance the systemic bioavailability of propranolol by a reduction in hepatic blood flow.

Alternatively, drug interaction in the liver may be due to effects on enzymes that are responsible for drug metabolism. The oxidative metabolism of many drugs and some endogenous hormones is dependent on the activity of microsomal enzyme systems associated with the smooth endoplasmic reticulum of liver cells. Of prime importance is the cytochrome P-450 system, a 'superfamily' of haem-containing mono-oxygenases (Chapter 1). Ten families have been identified in humans, six of which are involved in bile acid and steroid biosynthesis, whilst four (CYP1–CYP4) contain numerous individual enzymes responsible for the metabolism of exogenous substances (e.g. CYP 2D6 produces *O*-demethylation of codeine). The activity of some of the cytochrome P-450 enzymes can be enhanced by many drugs (e.g. barbiturates, some anticonvulsants), insecticides and polycyclic hydrocarbons. In some instances, the activity of other microsomal enzymes (e.g. glucuronyltransferase) is also increased.

The phenomenon of enzyme induction is a common and important cause of drug interaction in humans. Barbiturates, for example, may increase the metabolism of many other drugs (e.g. oral anticoagulants, anticonvulsants, antidepressants, glucocorticoids); enzyme induction reduces the plasma concentration and the pharmacological effects of these drugs. Conversely, withdrawal of the inducing drug will lead to a regression of the enzyme system to its original state. The serum concentration and plasma half-life will thus increase and toxicity will result if appropriate adjustment of dosage is not made. Phenobarbitone may induce enzymes and alter the rate of metabolism of other drugs within 2 days of commencing administration, with further increasing effects over the following weeks. As yet it is not clear whether the repeated use of barbiturates as intravenous anaesthetic agents can lead to significant enzyme induction.

In addition to inducing and enhancing enzyme activity in the liver, some drugs inhibit enzymes that are concerned with drug metabolism. Thus monoamine oxidase inhibitors, *para*-aminosalicylate, isoniazid, verapamil, chloramphenicol and cimetidine may inhibit some enzyme systems and thus increase the activity of other drugs. Some compounds (e.g. suxamethonium, procaine) are not metabolized by hepatic enzymes but are broken down by a cholinesterase (ChE) present in plasma. Drugs that react with this enzyme (e.g. neostigmine, trimetaphan) or inhibit its synthesis (e.g. cyclophosphamide) may prolong the effect of the depolarizing agent or possibly of a local anaesthetic ester.

Elimination

The principal sites at which drugs are eliminated from the body are the liver, kidney, lungs and gastrointestinal tract. Drug interactions are possible when any of these routes are involved.

Compounds that alter the pH of urine may influence the rate and extent of elimination of other drugs. The duration of drug action and the proportion of the dose metabolized by the liver may also be modified. In general, drugs that are weak acids or weak bases may be present in solution in both ionized and non-ionized forms and the relative proportions of the two forms are dependent on pH. In alkaline urine, significant amounts of some weak acids are ionized; in this state, they cannot readily diffuse back into the plasma across the renal tubule, and are therefore eliminated in the urine (Fig. 5.3). By contrast, in neutral or acid urine a higher proportion of the acidic drug is non-ionized; diffusion back into plasma is thus facilitated and excretion accordingly reduced. Conversely, weak bases (e.g. tricyclic antidepressants, opioid analgesics, local anaesthetics) are more highly ionized in acidic urine and their elimination under these circumstances is enhanced, whereas the presence of an alkaline urine will promote reuptake of the basic drug in the renal tubule.

These effects may be of value in the treatment of drug overdosage. Forced alkaline diuresis is useful in the management of salicylate or phenobarbitone poisoning, whilst an acid diuresis is sometimes used in the treatment of amphetamine, quinine, fenfluramine and phencyclidine poisoning. Although modification of the pH of urine may lead to other interactions, these are not usually of clinical significance.

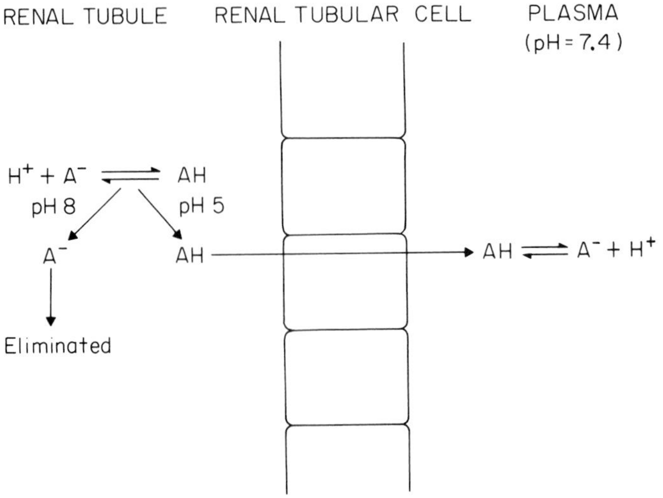

Fig. 5.3 Elimination of weak acids in alkaline and acidic urine. Weak acids are present in plasma and the renal tubule in two forms (A^- and AH); only AH can diffuse across renal tubular cell membranes. At pH 8, most of the drug in the renal tubule is present as A^- and is eliminated in urine. At pH 5, more of the drug is present in a non-ionized form (AH), which can back-diffuse across the renal tubule and is eliminated to a lesser extent. Similar factors apply to the elimination of weak bases.

Alternatively, drug interaction in the kidney may be related to competition for active transport. Both acid and basic drugs and their metabolites are partially eliminated from plasma by secretion in the proximal renal tubule. This process is competitive and may be subject to interference by other drugs. Thus, benzylpenicillin is a weak acid that is actively secreted by the proximal renal tubule; in consequence, it has a relatively short half-life (30–40 min) which can be prolonged by other drugs competing for active transport mechanisms (e.g. probenecid, non-steroidal anti-inflammatory drugs (NSAIDs), most diuretics). The elimination of endogenous substances can similarly be inhibited by drugs. Many thiazide diuretics compete for tubular secretion; in these conditions, the plasma urate concentration may be raised and acute gout can be precipitated.

Similarly, drug interactions in the liver may be due to competition for biliary excretion. Both anions (e.g. ampicillin) and cations (e.g. tubocurarine) are concentrated and excreted in the bile by transport mechanisms which require cellular enzymes; these are saturable systems at which other anions and cations may compete and reduce their transport. This interaction is rarely of practical significance. A number of drugs (e.g. morphine, oestrogens) are excreted in the bile as water-soluble conjugates (glucuronides, sulphates). Some of these compounds are metabolized to the parent compound by the gut flora and subsequently reabsorbed (enterohepatic shunt). If the bacterial flora are inhibited by the presence of an antibiotic this recycling will not occur. This may explain the rare failure of oral contraceptives in association with the use of penicillins or tetracyclines.

Some highly basic and lipid-soluble drugs (e.g. pethidine, fentanyl) may diffuse from plasma into the stomach, and subsequent reabsorption from the small intestine may result in a secondary peak effect. This gastroenteric recirculation process may be modified by drugs which either influence splanchnic blood flow or produce changes in gastric pH.

The rate of removal of inhalational anaesthetic agents is principally determined by minute ventilation and cardiac output; drugs which affect either of these factors (e.g. respiratory depressants, some antiarrhythmic drugs) can reduce the rate of elimination and thus prolong the effects of volatile and gaseous agents.

Pharmacodynamic interactions

Pharmacodynamic interactions are due to interference with the effects of drugs at their sites of action in tissues. Drug interactions of this type may produce additive, synergistic, potentiating or antagonistic effects. Such interactions are frequently beneficial (e.g. the use of protamine to reverse the anticoagulant effects of heparin or the use of anticholinesterase drugs to antagonize the action of muscle relaxants at the neuromuscular junction). Alternatively, adverse interactions can occur; for instance, chlorpromazine and related drugs block α-adrenoceptors, and may therefore enhance the hypotensive effect of other drugs (e.g. tubocurarine, halothane). Some pharmacodynamic interactions are related to the additive effects of drugs on the central nervous system (e.g. barbiturates, benzodiazepines and phenothiazines), the autonomic nervous system (e.g. atropine, tricyclic antidepressants antiparkinsonian drugs) or the cardiovascular system (e.g. β-adrenoceptor antagonists, calcium-channel blockers and other antiarrhythmic agents). A number of important interactions relate to interference with the active transport of drugs to their sites of action (e.g. antagonism of guanethidine and potentiation of noradrenaline by tricyclic antidepressants).

Not all adverse interactions can be attributed to effects on drug absorption, distribution, metabolism and excretion or to reactions at receptor sites. Disturbances of fluid and electrolyte balance may also play a role in some interactions (e.g. digoxin and frusemide; lithium and thiazide diuretics). In some instances, the pharmacological basis of a drug interaction is unknown or obscure. From the anaesthetist's point of view, it is often more important to be aware of the more common established interactions that may be encountered or anticipated in the course of anaesthetic practice.

Drug interactions in anaesthetic practice

Drug interactions in anaesthetic practice may occur between pre-existing drug therapy and general or local anaesthetic agents, muscle relaxants, analgesics and drugs used in premedication. Interactions between anaesthetic agents and their

Table 5.1 Interactions between the main groups of drugs.

General anaesthetics	Local anaesthetics	Muscle relaxants and their antagonists	Analgesics	Hypnotics and tranquillizers
Incompatible drugs in solution	Tricyclic antidepressants	General anaesthetics	Central depressants	Central depressants
Other centrally acting drugs	Muscle relaxants and their antagonists	Local anaesthetics	Monoamine oxidase inhibitors	Enzyme-inducing and inhibiting agents
Cardiovascular drugs	Sulphonamides	Drugs which modify electrolytes	Opioid antagonists	Anticholinergic drugs
Drugs which modify electrolytes		Drugs that modify acid–base balance	Oral anticoagulants	Antiparkinsonian drugs
Muscle relaxants		Cholinesterase inhibitors	Hypoglycaemic agents	
Enzyme-inducing effects		Antibiotics	Uricosuric agents	
Nephrotoxic agents		Calcium-channel blockers	Antihypertensive drugs Diuretics	

adjuvants may also occur and are similarly discussed. The principal interactions are summarized in Table 5.1.

Interactions with general anaesthetic agents

Drug interactions may occur with both intravenous and inhalational agents. Although reactions due to drug incompatibility may occur with intravenous agents in *in vitro* conditions, these interactions are well-known and are easily avoided. More serious interactions between general anaesthetics may occur *in vivo*.

Due to drug incompatibility

Solutions of thiopentone sodium and methohexitone sodium are alkaline (pH 10–11). When these intravenous barbiturates are mixed with other drugs or solutions of lower pH, they may precipitate them or be precipitated by them. This drug incompatibility occurs with a wide range of compounds, some of which are used in anaesthesia (e.g. pethidine hydrochloride, propranolol hydrochloride, suxamethonium bromide). In general, thiopentone and methohexitone should not be dissolved in or mixed with oxidizing agents, acidic solutions or with drugs normally administered as sulphates, chlorides or hydrochlorides.

Other centrally acting drugs

Drugs with a significant respiratory depressant effect can modify the uptake, distribution and elimination of inhalational anaesthetic agents. However, once anaesthesia is established, all drugs which exhibit depression of CNS activity have usually been considered to have additive effects. The minimum alveolar concentration (MAC) value of halothane (which reflects the potency of this agent at steady-state conditions) is reduced by about 30% when diazepam is also administered and similar effects have been shown or may be predicted when opioid analgesics, hypnotics, tranquillizers, antidepressants and certain antihypertensive agents (e.g. clonidine) have been given. Nitrous oxide will accelerate the uptake of other inhalational agents by the 'concentration' and 'second gas' effects relating to its high diffusing capacity, but it has been demonstrated that, under steady-state conditions, MAC values of different inhalational agents are additive. However, our increasing knowledge of the varying influence of drugs used in anaesthesia on central neurotransmission (e.g. at γ-aminobutyric acid (GABA), *N*-methyl-D-aspartate (NMDA) and opioid receptors and at α_2-adrenoceptor sites) does suggest that potentiating, synergistic and perhaps antagonistic interactions could occur. Furthermore, the concomitant use of CNS stimulants (e.g. amphetamines, theophylline) could predictably increase the anaesthetic requirement.

Antiarrhythmic and antianginal agents

Organic nitrates, β-adrenoceptor antagonists and calcium-channel-blocking agents are commonly used in the management of angina; the latter two groups of drugs are also effective antihypertensive and antiarrhythmic agents. Such therapy should always be continued up to the immediate preoperative period as the risks of rebound phenomena (e.g. worsening of angina symptoms and reappearance of arrhythmias) far outweigh those due to drug interactions which may occur during anaesthesia. The percutaneous administration of glyceryl trinitrate in the management of angina is sometimes continued during anaesthesia, although the theoretical risk of potentiation of systemic hypotension or reflex tachycardia must be borne in mind.

β-Adrenoceptor antagonists

Bradycardia is frequently encountered during anaesthesia in patients receiving β-adrenoceptor antagonists, particularly when halothane (which can exhibit considerable vagomimetic activity) is being administered in relatively high concentrations. Severe bradyarrhythmias may result in hypotension; such an effect has been observed following the absorption of timolol eyedrops. Pharmacokinetic parameters may be of some import, as inhalational agents and propranolol can both reduce liver blood flow.

Calcium-channel blockers

There is now considerable evidence that volatile anaesthetic agents can themselves exert either significant calcium-channel-blocking activity or interference with the mobilization of intracellular calcium. Furthermore, verapamil has been shown in animal studies to reduce the MAC value for halothane by 25%. Additive (or synergistic) effects with these two groups of drugs are thus predictable. In consequence, a large number of studies have been undertaken, both in animals and in humans, to assess the possibility of drug interactions. It would appear that clinical concentrations of volatile anaesthetic agents and therapeutic doses of calcium-channel blockers do not produce significant unwanted effects. Nevertheless, it must be considered that the combined effect of these two groups of drugs on both cardiac output and peripheral vascular tone is more likely to lead to intraoperative hypotension. Class 1 calcium-channel blockers, such as verapamil, may also induce varying degrees of heart block and this effect is likely to be enhanced in the presence of halothane or enflurane. Furthermore, the summative effects which may be anticipated from combined therapy with β-adrenoceptor antagonists and calcium-channel blockers in the presence of these volatile agents suggests that special vigilance is necessary during anaesthesia. β-Adrenoceptor antagonists will depress the reflex responses associated with class 3 calcium-channel blockers and augment their effects by reducing the availability of calcium channels (an effect which may be mediated by the reduced intracellular synthesis of cyclic adenosine monophosphate).

The myocardial depressant effect and resultant decrease in cardiac output associated with both β-adrenoceptor antagonists and calcium-channel blockers may also modify the pharmacokinetic behaviour of inhalational agents and effectively increase their potency by secondary reflex mechanisms which facilitate cerebral blood flow.

A significant increase in the incidence of bradyarrhythmias, complete heart block and pacemaker dependence has been reported in patients undergoing cardiac surgery and involving varying anaesthetic regimes (e.g. using halothane, isoflurane, fentanyl and benzodiazepines) who were concurrently receiving the class 3 antiarrhythmic agent amiodarone. This may reflect the additive effects of drugs used in anaesthesia in combination with an antiarrhythmic agent with a long elimination half-life.

Sympathomimetic amines

Sympathomimetic amines with β-adrenergic activity may precipitate dangerous or fatal arrhythmias during inhalational anaesthesia with cyclopropane or halogenated hydrocarbons. In current clinical practice, tachyarrhythmias may be predicted due to the presence of endogenous or exogenous catecholamines during halothane anaesthesia. Some of these may be of the re-entrant type; since halothane slows the conduction of impulses, and is likely to increase the refractory period in conducting tissue it creates the conditions necessary for re-entry, namely a unidirectional block with slow retrograde condition. Halothane may also increase the automaticity of the myocardium. Increased secretion of adrenaline due to surgical stimulation, hypoxia and hypercarbia can potentiate this risk. Ventricular arrhythmias, in particular multiple ectopic beats (pulsus bigeminus) can be induced and may progress to tachycardia or even fibrillation. Injection of adrenaline is thus potentially hazardous; however, the risk of arrhythmias is unlikely if the dose of adrenaline used for haemostasis is limited to 100 μg, a concentration of 10 μg ml^{-1} (1 in 100 000) is not exceeded and due consideration is given to ventilatory parameters and to the depth of anaesthesia. The presence of lignocaine in the vasoconstrictor solution may afford some protection. Dysrhythmias are less common with the anaesthetic ethers in common use (Table 5.2).

Ketamine produces central stimulation of sympathetic activity, resulting in raised plasma catecholamine levels; both tachyarrhythmias and the development of seizures have been reported with the concomitant use of theophylline (which has similar central and peripheral effects).

Interactions with sympathomimetic amines are mainly encountered when these drugs are administered during anaesthesia. However, it is uncertain whether patients on oral sympathomimetic drugs such as ephedrine, phenylephrine and phenylpropanolamine (some of which are present in over-the-counter cold and cough remedies) are also at risk during general anaesthesia. Similarly, phenylephrine (10%) and neutral adrenaline (1%) eyedrops are sometimes used in ophthalmic practice. Small amounts of these agents are absorbed and may cause transient dysrhythmias or unexpected hypertension on occasions; in these conditions, general anaesthesia with halogenated compounds may increase their effects on the heart. A similar phenomenon may be produced by large doses of oral fenfluramine, and this drug should be discontinued a week before surgery is contemplated, if this is possible.

Cardiovascular effects may occur during anaesthesia from the prior administration of levodopa. Such effects appear to be dose-related in that large doses of levodopa tend to produce tachyarrhythmias and vasoconstriction, presumably due to the metabolite dopamine; with smaller doses, vasodilatation usually predominates.

Arrhythmias induced by sympathomimetic amines during inhalational anaesthesia can usually be prevented or controlled by β-adrenoceptor antagonists. Propranolol (1 mg i.v.) is commonly used for this purpose. The dose may be repeated

Table 5.2 Doses of submucosal adrenaline required to induce ventricular extrasystoles in the presence of inhalational agents (median effective dose (ED_{50}) at 1.25 minimum alveolar concentration (MAC)).

Inhalational agent	Dose
Halothane	2.1 μg kg^{-1}*
Isoflurane	6.7 μg kg^{-1}
Enflurane	10.9 μg kg^{-1}

* When given in a mixture with lignocaine, the ED_{50} increases to 3.7 μg kg^{-1}.
The arrhythmogenic potential of adrenaline during desflurane and sevoflurane anaesthesia is similar to isoflurane.

at 2-min intervals until a maximum of 5 mg has been administered. Propranolol may enhance the effects of the increase in vagal tone and the hypotension induced by most halogenated anaesthetics, and may cause bronchospasm (particularly in susceptible patients concurrently given histamine-releasing agents, such as tubocurarine and morphine); atenolol is a suitable alternative.

Antihypertensive agents

During general anaesthesia, hypotensive responses may be induced by a number of drug interactions. Most of these reactions are simply due to the additive effects of drugs that affect blood pressure. For instance, halothane and the intravenous barbiturates tend to lower blood pressure, and may interact with α- or β-adrenoceptor blocking agents or with other drugs that can produce vasodilatation (e.g. chlorpromazine, morphine, tubocurarine). These actions are predictable and may be desirable in normotensive patients during anaesthesia.

In hypertensive patients on drug therapy, severe hypotension may occur during general anaesthesia, or postural hypotension may be seen on recovery. Intravenous agents are particularly liable to induce such responses in treated hypertensive patients. Both thiopentone and methohexitone reduce cardiac output and often decrease blood pressure in both hypertensive and normotensive subjects. Similarly, inhalational agents (via negative inotropic or chronotropic effects or by a reduction in peripheral resistance) may lead to falls in systemic pressure which can be exaggerated in the hypertensive patient; in particular, severe and unexpected hypotension has been observed during anaesthesia in patients receiving angiotensin-converting enzyme (ACE) inhibitors. These reactions are usually predictable and can readily be explained on a physiological basis. It is well-known that the treated hypertensive patient carries a greater risk of perioperative hypotension than the normotensive subject. However, if attention is given to circulating volume requirements and appropriate dose modification of the anaesthetic agents used is made, drug interaction should not be a major problem.

Drugs that modify electrolyte balance

Drugs affecting electrolyte balance may also predispose or contribute to the occurrence of cardiac arrhythmias during inhalational anaesthesia. For instance, drugs that lower serum potassium (e.g. most diuretics, corticosteroids, carbenoxolone, insulin) may induce supraventricular or ventricular ectopic beats during inhalational anaesthesia, particularly in patients who are digitalized or have disorders of electrolyte balance. Conversely, drugs that induce hyperkalaemia (e.g. suxamethonium, potassium-sparing diuretics) tend to impair cardiac conduction and may cause sino-atrial block. Agents that lower serum calcium (e.g. calcitonin, blood transfusions or intravenous infusions containing citrates, edetates or other chelating agents) depress cardiac contractility and may predispose to cardiac arrhythmias. Additional factors unrelated to drug administration may also be involved (e.g. stimulation during anaesthesia or surgery).

Muscle relaxants

Many inhalational agents increase the neuromuscular block induced by non-depolarizing muscle relaxants. Enhancement of myoneural blockade is dependent on the nature and concentration of the anaesthetic agent; enflurane and isoflurane (and probably diethyl ether) produce a greater degree of skeletal muscle relaxation than halothane at equivalent MAC values. The mechanism of this effect is not entirely clear; it may be due to central actions, presynaptic effects or to increased sensitivity of the postsynaptic receptor or the muscle cell membrane. The variable potencies of individual inhalational agents in this context (isoflurane, desflurane or sevoflurane are more potent than halothane or enflurane) may reflect differing effects on calcium influx at the neuromuscular junction.

Volatile anaesthetics may also affect the kinetic disposition of muscle relaxants. For instance, when gradually increasing concentrations of halothane are administered neuromuscular junction sensitivity increases, but the rate of equilibration between the plasma concentration of the relaxant and the onset of paralysis will decrease. This reflects decreased perfusion to the neuromuscular junction, resulting in a reduced rate of drug delivery.

In contrast, the action of a single dose of suxamethonium is not significantly affected by general anaesthetic agents in current use, although some enhancement of its effect was observed when the now obsolete intravenous induction agent, propanidid, which shared a common metabolic pathway, was used concomitantly. The muscarinic effects of suxamethonium may be enhanced when used in combination with propofol; a lack of central vagolytic activity of the latter drug has been implicated in this interaction.

There is a considerable amount of evidence to suggest that the transition from phase I (depolarizing) to phase II (non-depolarizing) block occurs at a lower dosage of suxamethonium, when repeated doses are used by either intermittent or continuous administration, when volatile agents are being used concurrently. Isoflurane not only accelerates the onset of phase II blockade but also potentiates its intensity. Mechanisms involved in this interaction are not fully explained but may involve translocation of calcium ions at pre- and postsynaptic sites.

Enzyme induction

Many agents used in anaesthesia (e.g. thiopentone, nitrous oxide, halothane) have been shown to induce the activity of drug-metabolizing enzymes. It is thus possible that the plasma concentration and therefore the pharmacological activity of certain other drugs concurrently used (e.g. steroids, anticoagulants, anticonvulsants) could be reduced; alternatively, an increase in the production of toxic metabolites of certain agents (e.g. isoniazid) might be envisaged. The problem is complicated by the fact that the underlying disease and associated trauma may have a depressant effect on drug metabolism and lead to higher plasma concentrations of drugs administered in the postoperative period. Studies using antipyrine clearance as an index of the efficiency of drug-metabolizing enzymes have shown that short procedures are followed by increased enzyme activity, but in protracted operations activity is diminished.

In contrast, the presence of drugs with significant enzyme-inducing properties (e.g. rifampicin, phenobarbitone) may increase the likelihood of halothane hepatotoxicity due to an increased production of toxic metabolites.

Nephrotoxic agents

The use of methoxyflurane, a halogenated ether which has now been withdrawn, was not uncommonly associated with the development of impaired renal function, and was related to the increased elimination of the main metabolite, inorganic fluoride. A limited increase in the urinary excretion of fluoride ions follows the administration of enflurane and sevoflurane, and there is a slight risk of renal damage, particularly when other nephrotoxic agents (e.g. tetracyclines) are being used concomitantly.

Interactions with local anaesthetic agents

Although local anaesthetics are extensively used in current practice, undesirable or adverse drug reactions are uncommon. Nevertheless, interactions involving local anaesthetic solutions are a potential risk when they are administered to patients who are taking certain other drugs. Preparations of local anaesthetics often contain vasoconstrictors, and drug interaction can occur with either the vasoconstrictor or the local anaesthetic agent. Other constituents of local anaesthetic solutions (reducing agents, preservatives and fungicides) have not been incriminated in drug interactions.

Tricyclic antidepressants and related drugs

Endogenous noradrenaline which is released in response to sympathetic nerve stimulation is partly removed from the synaptic cleft by active transport back into the nerve terminal — this process is known as $Uptake_1$ or the amine pump (Chapter 12). Exogenous noradrenaline (and to a lesser extent, adrenaline) is removed from the circulation in a similar manner. This mechanism can be blocked by most tricyclic antidepressant drugs and their derivatives, which compete with the catecholamines for axonal transport. The pressor response to noradrenaline is potentiated four to nine times in the presence of tricyclic agents, whilst the effect of adrenaline is increased by two- to threefold. Deaths have occurred in patients receiving tricyclic antidepressants to whom local anaesthetics containing noradrenaline were administered. Such solutions are no longer commercially available in the UK. Infusion or injection of noradrenaline or other α-adrenoceptor agonists such as methoxamine or phenylephrine to patients on tricyclic antidepressants may cause a marked rise in blood pressure that can precipitate subarachnoid haemorrhage. There is some evidence that pancuronium may also sensitize tissues to adrenaline and noradrenaline by a similar mechanism, and special care should be taken when these substances or other pressor amines are administered in the presence of this muscle relaxant.

Reservations have long been expressed concerning the use of adrenaline-containing solutions of local anaesthetics in patients receiving tricyclic antidepressants. Current opinion suggests that, providing proper attention is given to dosage and technique, clinically significant drug interaction will not ensue. Similar considerations should also be given to other drugs which can compete for or inhibit Uptake_1 (e.g. phenothiazines and adrenergic neurone-blocking agents) when local anaesthetics containing vasoconstrictors are being used. Local anaesthetics containing catecholamines are perhaps more dangerous in patients with ischaemic heart disease or significant hypertension. A suitable alternative preparation is prilocaine hydrochloride (3%) and felypressin (0.03 i.u. ml^{-1}). Felypressin is a polypeptide which produces vasoconstriction but which is not dependent on the amine pump for its removal from the circulation; drug interactions with the use of this vasoconstrictor have not been reported.

Muscle relaxants and their antagonists

Local anaesthetics can enhance the effects of both depolarizing and non-depolarizing muscle relaxants on neuromuscular transmission. In high concentrations, local anaesthetics of the ester group (e.g. procaine and amethocaine) can compete with suxamethonium for plasma ChE; in these conditions, they may prevent the hydrolysis of suxamethonium and enhance depolarizing block. Conversely, the effects of local anaesthetic esters may themselves be prolonged by drugs that inhibit, compete for, or degrade ChE. Interactions of this type may occur between ester anaesthetics and neostigmine, pyridostigmine, suxamethonium, acetazolamide and cytotoxic drugs.

Many local anaesthetics may also augment non-depolarizing block, although their mechanism of action is uncertain. Local anaesthetics decrease acetylcholine release from the nerve terminal, and stabilize the postsynaptic receptor and the muscle-cell membrane. These effects can clearly contribute to and enhance non-depolarizing blockade.

Sulphonamides

Some local anaesthetics antagonize the actions of sulphonamides in both *in vivo* and *in vitro* conditions. The antibacterial effects of sulphonamides are dependent on the antagonism of *para*-aminobenzoate, which is essential for nucleic acid synthesis in certain organisms. Drugs that release *para*-aminobenzoate in tissues, such as procaine and related esters, can overcome this antagonism and prevent the bacteriostatic effects of sulphonamides. Since local anaesthetics and their metabolites are rapidly removed from the circulation, antagonism of sulphonamide-induced bacteriostasis only occurs at the site of injection. Instances of this interaction have only rarely been reported, and its significance is now mainly of historical interest. Nevertheless, local anaesthetic solutions or sprays containing procaine or amethocaine should be avoided in patients with infections that are being concurrently treated with sulphonamides or sulphonamide combinations (e.g. co-trimoxazole).

Other interactions

Clinical reports and experimental studies suggest that the cardiovascular toxicity of local anaesthetic amides is increased in the presence of calcium-channel blockers (e.g. verapamil, nifedipine); additive effects on myocardial contraction and conduction are likely. A significant failure rare of spinal anaesthesia using bupivacaine has been reported in patients with either a high alcohol intake, long-term treatment with NSAIDs (e.g. indomethacin) or both. The mechanism of such apparent drug antagonism is obscure.

Interactions of muscle relaxants and their antagonists

The effects and duration of action of depolarizing and non-depolarizing neuromuscular blocking agents may be modified by many other drugs. These can affect transmitter release, modify the enzymic hydrolysis of acetylcholine, act on the postsynaptic receptor or directly affect the voluntary muscle cell. Interactions of this type may be associated with prescribed or self-administered oral therapy, with parenteral or locally applied preparations or with agents concurrently administered in the course of anaesthesia.

General anaesthetics

Most inhalational agents will affect both the pharmacodynamic activity and the kinetic behaviour of non-depolarizing neuromuscular blocking agents. The enhanced and prolonged effects observed may be related to depression of the CNS, decreased neurotransmitter release, reduced motor endplate sensitivity or to direct effects on the muscle membrane. Furthermore, the cardiovascular effects of most volatile agents may result in decreased tissue perfusion and thus influence the rate of uptake and subsequent removal of the muscle relaxants from their site of action. Interactions involving inhalational anaesthetic agents and suxamethonium are unlikely to occur, except when the depolarizing agent is administered in repeated dosage. There is no evidence that intravenous induction agents in common use (e.g. thiopentone, propofol) interact with muscle relaxants, although the original formulation of propofol in Cremophor increased the blockade due to vecuronium.

Local anaesthetics

Most local anaesthetic agents enhance the effects of non-depolarizing agents on neuromuscular transmission. Many other drugs, including phenothiazines, antihistamines and antiarrhythmic drugs such as quinidine, procainamide and calcium-channel blockers, have local anaesthetic or membrane-stabilizing properties, and may also augment neuromuscular blockade. However, the chronic administration of certain anticonvulsants (e.g. phenytoin, carbamazepine), which themselves have a membrane-stabilizing effect, has been associated with a diminished response to certain muscle relaxants (e.g. vecuronium, atracurium); pharmacokinetic and pharmacodynamic mechanisms have both been implicated.

In addition, local anaesthetic esters may compete with suxamethonium for plasma cholinesterase and prolong depolarization blockade.

Drugs that affect electrolyte balance

Drugs that modify electrolyte balance (in particular, those that affect the plasma concentration of magnesium, calcium and potassium ions) may profoundly influence neuromuscular transmission. Magnesium salts decrease acetylcholine release and the sensitivity of the motor endplate; in consequence, the amplitude of the endplate potential is reduced. In these conditions non-depolarizing blockade is augmented and depolarization is antagonized. In general, opposite effects are produced by calcium salts and by drugs that raise plasma calcium levels (e.g. parathormone and possibly thiazide diuretics); acetylcholine release is increased and excitation–contraction coupling is enhanced. Calcium ions also stabilize the postjunctional membrane.

Drugs that increase plasma potassium (e.g. spironolactone, triamterene, amiloride) decrease the resting membrane potential of muscle and augment depolarization blockade, while drugs that induce hypokalaemia (e.g. carbenoloxone, thiazide diuretics) increase the resting potential and enhance the effects of non-depolarizing agents. Changes in plasma potassium may also modify transmitter release. In the presence of hypokalaemia the dosage of non-depolarizing agents should be reduced; conversely, the dose of suxamethonium may need to be increased.

There is much conflicting evidence related to interactions between corticosteroids and muscle relaxants. Potentiation and antagonism have both been described in association with non-depolarizing agents. The resultant effects may be dose-related or dependent on the timing of administration of the steroid. In relation to pre-existing therapy with corticosteroids, the duration of exposure to the drug or the reasons for its usage (e.g. replacement or specific therapy) may be important considerations. A number of mechanism may be involved: these include permissive effects on neurotransmission, enzyme induction (of choline acetyltransferase or ChE), structural similarities (e.g. pancuronium, vecuronium), disturbances of electrolyte balance and the development of myopathies.

Drugs that modify acid–base balance

Neuromuscular blockade can be modified by changes in acid–base balance. In particular, both respiratory acidosis and metabolic alkalosis appear to enhance and prolong non-depolarizing blockade. Any drug which induces respiratory acidosis (e.g. carbon dioxide, opioid analgesics, barbiturates) or metabolic alkalosis (e.g. thiazide diuretics and certain antacids) may therefore enhance the response to non-depolarizing agents. The effect of other alterations in acid–base balance on neuromuscular blockade is less clear.

Potentiation of the response to muscle relaxants by respiratory acidosis and metabolic alkalosis is probably due to changes in intracellular pH and potassium balance. During hypokalaemia, the resting membrane potential of excitable tissues is increased, resulting in an enhanced response to non-depolarizing agents. Although pH changes can also affect binding of muscle relaxants and receptor ionization at the motor endplate, the role of these factors is uncertain.

In vitro studies suggest that changes in acid–base balance may also affect the ionization of certain muscle relaxants in *in vivo* conditions. Many of the experimental and clinical studies concerned with the modification of neuromuscular blockade have involved the use of *d*-tubocurarine. This drug is a monoquaternary amine, but also has a basic (tertiary amine) group that attracts H^+ during acidosis. In these conditions, *d*-tubocurarine has a similar configuration to bisquaternary amines which have a greater potency and activity at the neuromuscular junction. Other non-depolarizing agents do not have these pH-dependent physicochemical properties, and changes in acid–base balance may affect their activity in a different manner.

Calcium-channel blockers

The importance of calcium ions in the presynaptic release of acetylcholine and subsequent muscle contraction has already been considered. The potentiation of neuromuscular blockade by drugs which inhibit transmembrane calcium transport and intracellular calcium mobilization may thus be anticipated. The problem is likely to be enhanced in the presence of volatile anaesthetic agents; in this context isoflurane may cause particular problems.

Drugs that inhibit plasma cholinesterase

Such drugs may interact with both main groups of muscle relaxants. Many drugs are known to affect the enzymatic hydrolysis of suxmethonium. Thus drugs which compete for or inhibit ChE, such as neostigmine, edrophonium, organophosphorus compound and local anaesthetic esters, or which interfere with the synthesis of the enzyme (certain cytotoxic agents such as cyclophosphamide and possibly thiotepa), can prolong the duration of action of suxamethonium. In the past, certain inhibitors of ChE (particularly tetrahydroaminacrine and hexafluorenium) were deliberately used to prolong the action of suxamethonium; they are no longer commercially available in the UK. Pancuronium is a moderately potent inhibitor of ChE, and may prolong the action of drugs that are normally metabolized by the enzyme. Unpredictable effects are sometimes observed when certain ganglion-blocking agents (e.g. hexamethonium, trimetaphan) are used in the presence of muscle relaxants. Competition at both junctional enzymatic sites and at the postsynaptic receptor have been reported from animal studies; trimetaphan may also inhibit ChE.

Metoclopramide and aprotinin are weak inhibitors of ChE, whilst bambuterol, a β_2-agonist, is an inactive prodrug which is converted to the active metabolite terbutaline: the carbamate groups which are split off by enzyme activity can selectively inhibit ChE. Such interactions may assume more significance in heterozygous subjects.

The effects of all non-depolarizing muscle relaxants are antagonized (reversed) by drugs which inhibit junctional acetylcholinesterase. In anaesthetic practice, neostigmine is commonly used for this purpose. Other drugs which inhibit this enzyme (e.g. pyridostigmine, organophosphorus compounds) may also modify neuromuscular blockade. It is uncertain whether the reversal of neuromuscular block is directly due to enzyme inhibition or to other properties of the drug.

In some countries, drugs that release acetylcholine from nerve terminals such as 4-aminopyridine have been used to antagonize neuromuscular blockade. Although 4-aminopyridine has some advantages over the anticholinesterase drugs (e.g. the concurrent administration of atropine is not required), it enters the CNS and may cause cerebral excitation and convulsions.

Antibiotics

Some antibiotics can induce neuromuscular blockade and may potentiate the effects of non-depolarizing agents. Occasionally, depolarization block produced by suxamethonium or decamethonium is also enhanced. This phenomenon was first observed when antibiotic sprays containing streptomycin or neomycin were applied to the peritoneum after abdominal surgery; in these conditions hypoventilation may supervene postoperatively due to the local effects of the antibiotic on the diaphragm. Similar interactions after the systemic administration of antibiotics are relatively rare, and usually involve the aminoglycosides (e.g. neomycin, streptomycin, kanamycin, gentamicin), polymyxins, colistin, tetracyclines or lincomycin and clindamycin. In these circumstances, neuromuscular block is probably dependent on several factors which may vary with different antibiotics.

Blockade induced by aminoglycoside antibiotics or tetracyclines is variably affected by anticholinesterase drugs and is more commonly antagonized by calcium salts (e.g. calcium gluconate 2–3 mg kg^{-1} min^{-1} for 5 min). The neuromuscular blockade induced by such antibiotics may be due to competition for calcium-binding sites in the nerve terminal or the prejunctional membrane (in the case of tetracyclines, localized chelation of calcium ions may be of import). By contrast, neuromuscular blockade which is induced by the polymyxins, colistin, lincomycin and clindomycin is usually unaffected by anticholinesterases and calcium salts. These interactions are usually managed by controlled ventilation until normal neuromuscular function is restored, although 4-aminopyridine is sometimes effective. Potentiation of neuromuscular blockade usually occurs when non-depolarizing agents are administered to patients on antibiotics; however, similar effects may be induced when antibacterial drugs are given to patients with myasthenia gravis.

Miscellaneous drugs

Certain immunosuppressants (e.g. azathioprine, cyclosporin) can antagonize the effects of a number of non-depolarizing neuromuscular blocking agents. Mechanisms are obscure but in the case of the cyclosporin–pancuronium interaction, the Cremophor used as a vehicle for the cyclosporin has been implicated. Occasional reports of prolongation of neuromuscular blockade and the concomitant use of a number of other drugs (benzodiazepines, lithium carbonate, H_1-antagonists and chloroquine) have also been documented.

Interactions with analgesics

Opioid analgesics

Opioid analgesics are extensively used in anaesthesia, and drug interaction between them and other agents is of particular concern to the anaesthetist. In patients receiving certain other drugs (e.g. monoamine oxidase inhibitors) dangerous interactions may occur after single doses of some opioid analgesics (e.g. pethidine). However, in most cases drug interactions with opiates are readily predictable from a knowledge of the pharmacological effects of these agents.

Other central depressants

Effective analgesic doses of opiates tend to cause sedation and invariably produce some respiratory depression. Their depressant effects on ventilation may be enhanced by other drugs that affect medullary centres such as inhalational anaesthetics, intravenous induction agents and some hypnotics and tranquillizers. Tricyclic antidepressants may also enhance the effects of opioid analgesics (an increase in the bioavailability of morphine combined with an intrinsic analgesic effect of the antidepressant are the suggested mechanisms). Similarly, the administration of more than one opiate may cause summation of this depressant effect. Conversely, the respiratory depression induced by morphine and related compounds may decrease the rate of uptake and subsequent removal of general anaesthetics given by inhalational techniques.

Monoamine oxidase inhibitors

Although monoamine oxidase inhibitors primarily interfere with the metabolism of monoamines (e.g. tyramine, dopamine) they may also affect the biotransformation of other drugs. In particular, dangerous interactions may occur between these agents and pethidine. Serious side-effects have been considered to be due to the accumulation of the principal metabolite, norpethidine; an increase in levels of 5-hydroxytryptamine within the CNS has also been postulated. Signs and symptoms include mental confusion, cerebral excitation, hyperpyrexia and either hypertension or circulatory collapse. This interaction has also been observed when pethidine has been administered to patients who have received the selective inhibitor of type B monoamine oxidase, selegiline. Although similar interactions have occasionally been reported with other opiates, they appear to be far less common. Pethidine should never be administered to patients receiving monoamine oxidase inhibitors; but buprenorphine and possibly fentanyl have been considered to be safe alternatives. Moclobemide, a reversible inhibitor of monoamine oxidase type A, may cause fewer problems in this context.

Opioid antagonists

The effects of all opioid analgesics may be modified by drugs that compete with them for opioid receptors in the CNS. Naloxone competitively antagonizes the effects of all opioid analgesics; it is a pure antagonist and has no agonist activity. By contrast, other antagonists (e.g. nalorphine, levallorphan, pentazocine) also possess some agonist activity at opioid receptors. These drugs (partial agonists) antagonize some of the effects of other opioid analgesics, but also produce central effects of their own (e.g. dysphoria, analgesia and respiratory depression) due to their intrinsic activity at other opioid receptors.

Other interactions

The effects of methadone are considerably reduced, and withdrawal symptoms enhanced, in the presence of drugs with significant enzyme-inducing properties (e.g. carbamazepine, rifampicin), and presumably this reflects increased metabolism and excretion. A decrease in the plasma concentration of tramadol, with an associated loss of analgesic efficacy, has been reported in patients who are also receiving carbamazepine. Similarly, the clearance of morphine is significantly increased with the concurrent use of oral contraceptives; it is suggested that the oestrogen component stimulates glucuronyl transferase activity.

Most opioid analgesics may delay the oral absorption of other drugs by decreasing gastric motility and slowing down the rate of gastric emptying. The urinary elimination of some analgesics (e.g. pethidine, fentanyl, phenoperidine) is increased by acids or by drugs that increase acidosis. Since these drugs are extensively metabolized, their enhanced elimination in acid urine is of little value in the treatment of drug overdosage; it is sometimes of value in the detection of drug dependence. Nausea and vomiting are common side-effects of many opioid analgesics; these effects may be modified by antiemetic drugs (e.g. chlorpromazine and the antihistamines).

Non-opioid analgesics

Non-opioid analgesics include aspirin and other NSAIDs (e.g. ibuprofen, diclofenac, naproxen) and paracetamol. These drugs, which are being increasingly used in the perioperative period and in the management of chronic pain, are the commonest group of compounds involved in drug interactions in humans.

In particular, aspirin and other salicylates have been associated with clinically significant interactions of this type. In most instances, these interactions have only been reported with large and repeated doses of such drugs; the possible effect of restricted administration or of single dosage is more difficult to evaluate.

Aspirin and related compounds may induce drug interactions by two principal mechanisms. First, aspirin-like drugs bind firmly to plasma proteins and thus can displace other drugs (e.g. warfarin anticoagulants, oral hypoglycaemic agents) from binding sites. The problem with warfarin is accentuated because aspirin itself can cause gastric bleeding due to mucosal damage, inhibit platelet aggregation and in large doses reduce the synthesis of prothrombin. The use of standard doses of aspirin should be avoided in patients receiving warfarin therapy, although low-dose aspirin (up to 75 mg daily) appears to be safe. Ketorolac is also contraindicated in the presence of anticoagulants, including low-dose heparin regimes. Paracetamol, which is virtually devoid of such effects and does not compete for protein-binding sites, is a suitable alternative.

Second, salicylates produce dose-dependent effects on tubular secretion in the kidney. Aspirin can decrease the urinary elimination of urates, and may antagonize the effects of uricosuric agents (e.g. probenecid, sulphinpyrazone) which are being administered concurrently. Furthermore, salicylates may interfere with the removal of other drugs which rely on active transport processes such as methotrexate and can potentiate their effects.

Certain NSAIDs (e.g. indomethacin) have been shown to inhibit the renal excretion of sodium and possibly antagonize the effects of other drugs used in the treatment of hypertension and heart failure (e.g. diuretics, ACE inhibitors, β-adrenoceptor antagonists). Aspirin and most other related drugs have been less commonly implicated; nevertheless, this effect is worth remembering when refractory hypertension or oedema develops during treatment with NSAIDs and appropriate adjustment of dosage may be necessary.

Drug interactions involving paracetamol appear to be extremely uncommon, although absorption may be modified by cholestyramine and metabolism is increased in the presence of anticonvulsants and oral contraceptives. However, a number of compound preparations containing paracetamol may also include either codeine or dextropropoxyphene. Both these drugs are potential respiratory depressants and such effects may be enhanced by the concurrent administration of general anaesthetics, sedatives and tranquillizers. Dextropropoxyphene poisoning is not infrequently associated with excessive consumption of alcohol. Dextropropoxyphene may prolong and enhance the effects of oral anticoagulants; interactions between this drug and the anticholinergic compound orphenadrine have also been reported.

Interactions with drugs used for premedication and sedation

Drugs which induce sleep (hypnotics) or which relieve anxiety and tension (tranquillizers) are closely related to each other and are probably the most frequently prescribed drugs in general medical practice. Benzodiazepines are commonly administered in the perioperative period. Diazepam is often used for premedication to allay anxiety prior to surgery, and temazepam may be prescribed as a hypnotic on the night before operation. In addition, intravenous benzodiazepines (e.g. diazepam, midazolam) are commonly used to induce sedation during endoscopy and minor surgical procedures. Other drugs with sedative or anticholinergic properties (e.g. antihistamine compounds, atropine or hyoscine) may also be used for premedication.

Other central depressants

Doses of tranquillizers or sedatives that relieve anxiety and tension may induce drowsiness and cause loss of concentration in susceptible subjects. These drugs should not be given to ambulant patients without warning them of the possible hazards of their administration, particularly in relation to driving. Furthermore, all such drugs may interact with other agents which have depressant effects on the

CNS (e.g. other sedatives, general anaesthetics, alcohol). Their effects may also be enhanced during the concurrent administration of antidepressant drugs, although authentic reports of this interaction are extremely rare. The effects of drugs that induce respiratory depression (e.g. intravenous barbiturates, opioid analgesics) may also be potentiated. In contrast, aminophylline and caffeine can antagonize the CNS effects induced by benzodiazepines.

Enzyme-inducing and inhibiting agents

Some drugs which may be used as hypnotics and sedatives (e.g. barbiturates, dichloralphenazone) can induce hepatic enzymes and stimulate the metabolism of other drugs such as warfarin and oral contraceptives; they are potentially capable of interactions with a wide range of other drugs.

Interactions of this type involving benzodiazepines are relatively rare, although both diazepam and chlordiazepoxide may inhibit the metabolism of phenytoin and increase its toxicity. In contrast, the H_2-receptor antagonist, cimetidine, binds to some isoforms of cytochrome P-450 and can inhibit the metabolism of diazepam and related compounds, although this interaction rarely appears to be of clinical significance. Serum levels of midazolam (and triazolam) are markedly increased in the presence of the macrolide antibiotic erythromycin. Prolonged hypnosis and amnesia have been reported in association with this drug combination; inhibitory effects on the enzyme subfamily CYP 3A by the macrolide are the likely cause (the effects of the opioid analgesic alfentanil may be enhanced and prolonged by a similar mechanism). Diltiazem and verapamil may have similar effects on the pharmacokinetic disposition of midazolam. The sedative effects of diazepam may also be increased by other drugs which reduce the clearance of the benzodiazepine (e.g. omeprazole, isoniazid, probenecid).

Other interactions involving premedicant drugs

Drugs with significant anticholinergic properties that are used for premedication (e.g. atropine, hyoscine) can induce a marked antisialagogue effect and decrease the effect of other drugs which may be administered sublingually (e.g. glyceryl trinitrate, buprenorphine). Anticholinergic drugs may also antagonize the effects of certain antiemetic agents (e.g. domperidone, metoclopramide) on the gastrointestinal tract.

Phenothiazines and butyrophenones are often used during anaesthesia, principally for their antiemetic effect. In patients who are receiving levodopa, the action of these antiemetic drugs with central antidopaminergic properties may be inhibited; conversely the mutual antagonism of these drugs and levodopa may result in an exacerbation of the extrapyramidal disorder. Metoclopramide will produce antagonistic effects at dopamine receptors within the CNS; however, it will also increase the bioavailability of levodopa by its effects on gut motility and the resultant interaction is thus unpredictable.

Phenothiazines will potentiate the sedative and analgesic properties of drugs used in anaesthesia by central mechanisms, augment the hypotensive responses of inhalational and neuromuscular blocking agents by α_1-adrenoceptor antagonist effects, and produce summative responses with anticholinergic drugs at muscarinic sites, although there are opposing effects in the extrapyramidal system. There appear to be mutual increases in the levels of both drugs, and a resultant enhancement of clinical effects, when phenothiazines are administered in the presence of either α-adrenoceptor antagonists or tricyclic antidepressants. Mechanisms involving enzyme inhibition and/or effects on liver blood flow may be involved.

Prevention of adverse drug interactions

Although adverse drug interactions cannot be entirely prevented, their incidence may be minimized by an appreciation of the factors which contribute to their occurrence. In the first place, many interactions occur with prescribed or self-administered oral therapy; it is therefore important to take a drug history before the administration of any other agent, and to be conversant with the effects of the drugs that are involved. Second, the possibility of adverse interactions rises exponentially as the number of drugs administered is increased (although only two agents are usually involved). Third, drug interactions are more likely when drug elimination is prolonged, as in hepatic or renal disease or in elderly patients. Finally, adverse interactions are more common with agents which have a relatively steep dose–response curve, or when there is little difference between the toxic and therapeutic doses of drugs.

Further reading

Aronson JK, Grahame-Smith DG. Clinical pharmacology: adverse drug interactions. *British Medical Journal* 1981; **282**: 288–291.

Attia RR, Grogono AW (eds). Drug and disease interactions. In: *Practical Anesthetic Pharmacology*. New York: Appleton Century Crofts, 1978; 243–261.

Backman JT, Olkkola KT, Aranko K *et al.* Dose of midazolam should be reduced during diltiazem and verapamil treatments. *British Journal of Clinical Pharmacology* 1994; **37**: 221–226.

Bang U, Viby-Mogensen J, Wiren JE. The effect of bambuterol on plasma cholinesterase activity and suxamethonium induced neuromuscular blockade in subjects heterozygous for abnormal plasma cholinesterase. *Acta Anaesthesiologica Scandinavica* 1990; **34**: 600–604.

Baraka A. The influence of carbon dioxide on the neuromuscular block produced by tubocurarine chloride in the human subject. *British Journal of Anaesthesia* 1964; **36**: 272–278.

Bennett JA, Eltrincham RJ. Possible dangers of anaesthesia in patients receiving fenfluramine. Results of animal studies following a case of human cardiac arrest. *Anaesthesia* 1977; **32**: 8–13.

Bevan DR, Monks PS, Calne DB. Cardiovascular reaction to anaesthesia during treatment with levodopa. *Anaesthesia* 1973; **28**: 29–31.

Blackman JG, Gauldie RW, Milne RJ. Interaction of competitive antagonists. The anti-curare action of hexamethonium and other antagonists at the skeletal neuromuscular junction. *British Journal of Pharmacology* 1975; **54**: 91–100.

Blackwell B. Monoamine oxidase inhibitor interactions with other drugs. *Journal of Clinical Psychopharmacology* 1991; **11**: 55–59.

Bowman WC, Webb SN. Neuromuscular blocking and ganglion-blocking activities of some acetylcholine antagonists in the cat. *Journal of Pharmacy and Pharmacology* 1972; **24**: 262–272.

Calvey TN. Drugs affecting administration of anaesthetics. *British Dental Journal* 1980; **149**: 185–186.

Calvey TN. Synergy and isoboles. *British Journal of Anaesthesia* 1993; **70**: 246–247.

Calvey TN, Milne LA, Williams NE et al. Effect of antacids on the plasma concentration of phenoperidine. *British Journal of Anaesthesia* 1983; **55**: 535–539.

Clive DM, Stoff JS. Renal syndromes associated with non-steroidal anti-inflammatory drugs. *New England Journal of Medicine* 1984; **310**: 563–572.

Conney AH. Pharmacological implications of microsomal enzyme induction. *Pharmacological Reviews* 1967; **19**: 317–366.

Conrad KA, Byers JM III, Finley PR, Burnham L. Lidocaine elimination. Effects of metoprolol and propranolol. *Clinical Pharmacology and Therapeutics* 1983; **33**: 133–138.

Csogor SI, Kerek SF. Enhancement of thiopentone anaesthesia by sulphafurazole. *British Journal of Anaesthesia* 1970; **42**: 988–990.

Dodson M. Drug interactions and anaesthesia. *Hospital Update* 1982; **8**: 57–68.

Durant NN, Nguyen N, Katz RL. Potentiation of neuromuscular blockade by verapamil. *Anaesthesiology* 1984; **60**: 298–303.

Eger EI II (ed.). Ventilation, circulation and uptake. In: *Anaesthetic Uptake and Action*. Baltimore: Williams and Wilkins, 1974; 122–145.

Ellis CH, Wnuck AL, De Beer EJ, Foldes FF. Modifying actions of procaine on the myoneural blocking properties of succinylcholine, decamethonium and *d*-tubocurarine in dogs and cats. *American Journal of Physiology* 1953; **174**: 277–282.

Ellis GP. The Maillard reaction. *Advances in Carbohydrate Chemistry* 1959; **14**: 63–134.

Enderby GEH. The use and abuse of trichlorethylene. *British Medical Journal* 1944; **ii**: 300–302.

Goldberg LI. Monoamine oxidase inhibitors: adverse reactions and possible mechanisms. *Journal of the American Medical Association* 1964; **190**: 456–462.

Grayson JG. Incompatibilities of multiple additives to intravenous infusion fluids. *Pharmaceutical Journal* 1971; **206**: 64–71.

Greenblatt DJ, Abernethy DR, Morse DS et al. Clinical importance of the interaction of diazepam and cimetidine. *New England Journal of Medicine* 1984; **319**: 1639–1643.

Grogono AW. Drug interactions in anaesthesia. *British Journal of Anaesthesia* 1974; **46**: 613–618.

Halsey MJ. Drug interactions in anaesthesia. *British Journal of Anaesthesia* 1987; **59**: 112–123.

Hart AP, Royster RL, Johnston WE. Cardiac conduction interactions of propranolol and verapamil with halothane in pentobarbitone anaesthetised dogs. *British Journal of Anaesthesia* 1988; **61**: 748–753.

Hirshman CA, Kreiger W, Littlejohn G et al. Ketamine-aminophylline induced decrease in seizure threshold. *Anaesthesiology* 1982; **56**: 464–467.

Humphrey JH, McClelland M. Cranial nerve palsies with herpes following general anaesthesia. *British Medical Journal* 1944; **1**: 315–316.

Ikeda K, Katoh T. Pharmacokinetics and pharmacodynamics of new volatile agents. *Current Opinion in Anaesthesiology* 1993; **6**: 639–643.

Iversen LL. The inhibition of noradrenaline uptake by drugs. *Advances in Drug Research* 1965; **2**: 5–23.

Johnston RR, Eger EI II, Wilson C. A comparative interaction of epinephrine with enflurane, isoflurane and halothane in man. *Anesthesia and Analgesia* 1976; **55**: 709–712.

Johnstone M, Nisbet HIA. Ventricular arrhythmia during halothane anaesthesia. *British Journal of Anaesthesia* 1961; **33**: 9–16.

Karis JH, Gissen AJ, Nastuk WL. The effect of volatile agents on neuromuscular transmission. *Anaesthesiology* 1967; **28**: 128–134.

Katz RL, Katz GJ. Surgical infiltration of pressor drugs and their interaction with volatile anaesthetics. *British Journal of Anaesthesia* 1966; **38**: 712–718.

Koch-Weser J, Sellers EM. Drug interactions with coumarin anticoagulants. *New England Journal of Medicine* 1972; **285**: 487–498, 547–558.

Liberman BA, Teasdale SJ. Anaesthesia and amiodarone. *Canadian Anaesthetists Society Journal* 1985; **32**: 629–638.

Lynch C. Differential depression of myocardial contractility by halothane and isoflurane *in vitro*. *Anaesthesiology* 1986; **64**: 620–631.

McConachie I, Healey TEJ. ACE inhibitors and anaesthesia. *Postgraduate Medical Journal* 1989; **65**: 273–274.

Macphee GIA, McInnes GT, Thompson GG. Verapamil potentiates carbamazepine neurotoxicity: a clinically important inhibitor interaction. *Lancet* 1986; **i**: 700–703.

Maze M, Mason DM. Verapamil decreases the MAC for halothane in dogs. *Anesthesia and Analgesia* 1983; **62**: 274P.

Mazze RI. Fluorinated anaesthetic nephrotoxicity: an update. *Canadian Anaesthetists Society Journal* 1984; **31**: S16–S22.

Merin M. Calcium channel blocking drugs and anaesthetics: is the drug interaction beneficial or detrimental? *Anaesthesiology* 1987; **66**: 1111–1113.

Mishra P, Calvey TN, Williams NE. Intraoperative bradycardia associated with timolol and pilocarpine eye-drops. *British Journal of Anaesthesia* 1983; **55**: 897–899.

Nies AS, Shand DG, Wilkinson GR. Altered hepatic blood flow and drug disposition. *Clinical Pharmacokinetics* 1976; **1**: 135–155.

Oikkola KT, Aranko K, Saarnivaara L et al. A potentially hazardous interaction between erythromycin and midazolam. *Clinical Pharmacology and Therapeutics* 1993; **53**: 298–305.

Pantuck EJ. Ecothiopate iodide eye-drops and prolonged response to suxamethonium. *British Journal of Anaesthesia* 1966; **38**: 406–407.

Perisho JA, Buechel DR, Miller RD. The effect of diazepam on minimal alveolar anaesthetic requirement in man. *Canadian Anaesthetists Society Journal* 1971; **18**: 536–540.

Pessayre D, Allemand H, Benoist C et al. Effect of surgery under anaesthesia on antipyrine clearance. *British Journal of Clinical Pharmacology* 1978; **6**: 505–514.

Pittinger CB, Eryaza Y, Adamson R. Antibiotic-induced paralysis. *Anesthesia and Analgesia* 1970; **49**: 487–501.

Riley BB. Incompatibilities in intravenous solutions. *Journal of Hospital Pharmac*y 1970; **28**: 228–240.

Robinson BJ, Lee E, Rees D *et al*. Betamethasone-induced resistance to neuromuscular blockade; a comparison of atracurium and vecuronium *in vitro*. *Anesthesia and Analgesia* 1992; **74**: 762–765.

Rolan PE. Plasma protein displacement interactions — why are they still regarded as clinically significant? *British Journal of Clinical Pharmacology* 1994; **37**: 125–128.

Sedman AJ. Cimetidine-drug interactions. *American Journal of Medicine* 1984; **76**: 109–114.

Serlin MJ, Breckenridge AM. Drug interactions with warfarin. *Drugs* 1983; **25**: 610–620.

Smith SE. Neuromuscular blocking drugs in man. In: Zaimis E (ed.) *Handbook of Experimental Pharmacology*, vol. 42, *Neuromuscular Junction*. Heidelberg: Springer-Verlag, 1976; 593–660.

Sokoll MD, Gergis SD. Antibiotics and neuromuscular function. *Anaesthesiology* 1981; **55**: 148–159.

Soni N. Mechanisms of drug interactions (Appendix III). In: Feldman S, Scurr CF, Paton W (eds) *Drugs in Anaesthesia: Mechanisms of action*. London: Edward Arnold, 1987; 408–427.

Sprotte G, Weiss KH. Drug interaction with local anaesthetics. *British Journal of Anaesthesia* 1982; **54**: 242P.

Stack CG, Rogers P, Linter SP. Monoamine oxidase inhibitors and anaesthesia — a review. *British Journal of Anaesthesia* 1988; **60**: 222–227.

Stanski DR, Ham J, Miller RD et al. Pharmacokinetics and pharmacodynamics of *d*-tubocurarine during nitrous oxide–narcotic and halothane anaesthesia in man. *Anaesthesiology* 1979; **51**: 235–241.

Stirt JA. Aminophylline is a diazepam antagonist. *Anesthesia and Analgesia* 1981; **60**: 767–768.

Stockley I. *Drug Interactions and their Mechanisms*. London: The Pharmaceutical Press, 1974; 1–78.

Stockley IH. *Drug Interactions*, 3rd edn. Oxford: Blackwell Scientific Publications, 1994; 1–932.

Stoelting RK, Longnecker DE. Influence of end-tidal halothane concentration on *d*-tubocurarine hypotension. *Anesthesia and Analgesia* 1972; **51**: 364–367.

Tempelhoff R, Modica PA, Jellish WS, Spitznagel EL. Resistance to atracurium induced neuromuscular blockade in patients with intractable seizure disorders treated with anticonvulsants. *Anesthesia and Analgesia* 1990; **71**: 665–669.

Todd JG, Nimmo WS. Effect of premedication on drug absorption and gastric emptying time. *British Journal of Anaesthesia* 1983; **55**: 1189–1192.

Trissel LA. *Handbook on Injectable Drugs*, 3rd edn. Bethesda, MD: American Society of Hospital Pharmacists, 1983.

Welling PG. Interactions affecting drug absorption. *Clinical Pharmacokinetics* 1984; **9**: 404–434.

Williams JS, Broadbent MP, Pearce AC, Jones RM. Verapamil potentiates the neuromuscular blocking effects of enflurane *in vitro*. *Anaesthesiology* 1983; **59**: A276.

Zaimis E. The neuromuscular junction — areas of uncertainty. In: Zaimis E (ed.) *Handbook of Experimental Pharmacology*, vol. 42, *Neuromuscular Junction*. Heidelberg: Springer-Verlag, 1976; 1–21.

Zink J, Sasyniuk BI, Dresel PE. Halothane–epinephrine-induced cardiac arrhythmias and the role of heart rate. *Anaesthesiology* 1975; **43**: 548–555.

Zsigmond EK, Robins G. The effects of a series of anti-cancer drugs on plasma cholinesterase activity. *Canadian Anaesthetists Society Journal* 1972; **19**: 75–82.

Chapter 6
Variability in Drug Response

There is a wide variability in the response of different patients to identical doses of the same drug. Drugs do not produce the same effects in all subjects; they may not even produce identical responses when given to the same patient on different occasions. Consequently, dose–response curves obtained in humans may only be directly applicable to individual subjects. Nevertheless, they are often used to reflect the results obtained in a sample from a relatively homogeneous population of subjects. In these conditions, a sigmoid log dose–response curve may represent the characteristic results in the population, while the interindividual variability is represented by vertical and horizontal arrows (Fig. 6.1). The vertical arrows illustrate that a range of effects may be observed in the population after the same dose of a drug; the horizontal arrows represent the range of drug dosage which may be required to produce a specific pharmacological effect in individual subjects.

Variability in the response to drugs can be considered as part of the general phenomenon of inherent or intrinsic biological variability. Physiological and pharmacological phenomena are subject to considerable interindividual variability, which is sometimes expressed by detailed description of the individual results. More commonly, the distribution and variability of individual measurements (variables) is expressed in terms of two descriptive statistics:

1 A measurement of the central tendency of the observations (the mode, the median or the mean).

2 A measurement of the variability or scatter of individual values (the frequency, the interquartile range or the standard deviation).

The precise parameter used for the expression of the central tendency and the scatter of individual results depends on the level of measurement of the data. In general, there are three levels of measurement of biological data:

1 Nominal.

2 Ordinal.

3 Continuous.

Nominal measurements

Nominal measurements depend on the classification of data or subjects into groups that are solely dependent on their names or characteristics. Thus, patients can be classified as male or female, premedicated or unpremedicated, conscious or

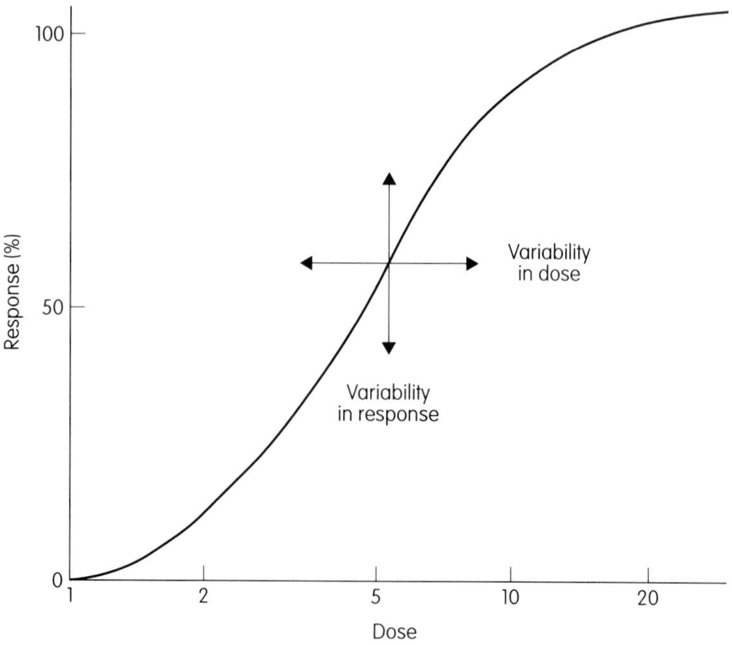

Fig. 6.1 Log dose–response curve showing the variability in dosage required to produce the same response (horizontal line), and the variability in response produced by a single dose (vertical line) in a population of subjects.

unconscious, etc. In general, quantal (all-or-none) measurements are also nominal. All measurements within a group are equivalent to each other, and there are no quantitative differences between members of the group.

The central tendency of nominal measurements is usually expressed as the most frequently occurring value, or the mode; thus, in the numerical series, 1, 2, 3, 3, 5, 5, 5, 6, 7, 9, 9, the mode is 5. The distribution of nominal measurements is expressed by the frequency of their occurrence (Table 6.1). Nominal measurements can be considered as the lowest level of description of data, and are only usually employed when their use is unavoidable.

Table 6.1 Descriptive statistics used to describe the central tendency and variability of nominal, ordinal and continuous data.

Level of measurement	Descriptive statistic	
	Central tendency	Variability
Nominal	Mode	Frequency
Ordinal	Median	Interquartile range
Continuous	Mean	Standard deviation

Ordinal measurements

Ordinal measurements depend on the ranking or order of the underlying data into a series which depends on their magnitude or relationship to each other. Individual data can be graded as lower (<) or greater (>) than other members of the series, although they cannot be given a precise quantitative value; at best, the measurements can be regarded as semiquantitative. Thus, pain scores on a visual analogue scale* and Apgar scores are ordinal measurements, since they can be placed in an order in which their relationship to each other is defined.

The central tendency of ordinal measurements is expressed as the middle or median value; for example, in 11 patients with post-operative pain scores of 1, 2, 3, 3, 5, 5, 5, 6, 7, 9, 9, the median pain score is 5. The distribution or variability of ordinal measurements can be expressed as the range (1–9), or more correctly as the interquartile range (i.e. the range which includes 25–75% of the ranked values; Table 6.1). Pain scores are not accurate quantitative values; they merely imply that a higher value represents more intense pain than a lower value. Consequently, it is incorrect to express pain scores as a mean and standard deviation (or standard error), since this implies that the scores have a quantitative value. Ordinal measurements can be considered as an intermediate level of measurement for the expression and description of data.

Continuous measurements

Continuous measurements are invariably quantitative, and the individual results have a defined magnitude and a numerical value. Consequently, there is a precisely defined and measurable difference between the individual observations or values. Quantitative measurements of drug concentrations and responses, heart rate and blood pressure are continuous data, since they have a defined value, and equal differences between individual values are comparable to each other. Continuous values are the highest level of measurement for the expression and description of biological and clinical data.

The central tendency of continuous, quantitative measurements is usually expressed as an arithmetic mean or average ($\bar{x}$):

$$\text{mean} = \frac{\Sigma x \quad \text{(the sum of their individual values)}}{n \quad \text{(the number of results or observations)}}.$$

The scatter of the individual observations about the mean (their distribution or variability) is usually described by the standard deviation (Table 6.1).

* A visual analogue scale for pain is a horizontal line which is 10 cm long; the origin of the line represents a score of 0 (no pain), while the end of the line corresponds to a score of 10 (the worst pain imaginable). Patients are asked to indicate the point on the line that corresponds best to their pain.

Standard deviation

The standard deviation (root mean square deviate) can be indirectly calculated from the expression:

$$\text{standard deviation} = \sqrt{\left(\frac{\Sigma(x-\bar{x})^2}{n-1}\right)}.$$

It is a commonly used indication of scatter or variability, and is derived from the sum of the squares of the numerical differences (deviate) between each individual value and the mean (i.e. $\Sigma\,[x_1-\bar{x}]^2+[x_2-\bar{x}]^2+[x_3-\bar{x}]^2$ etc.).

The mean deviate from the mean is given by:

$$\text{mean deviate} = \frac{\Sigma(x-\bar{x})}{n}.$$

However, the numerator of this equation ($\Sigma\,(x-\bar{x})$) will clearly be zero when the (+) and (–) signs of individual results are taken into account, since the mean is defined as the value at which the summated positive and negative deviations are equal. This problem can be eliminated by squaring the deviations about the mean before their summation, and subsequently finding their mean value; this results in an expression for the variance or mean square deviate:

$$\text{variance} = \frac{\Sigma(x-\bar{x})^2}{n}.$$

The original units for the deviation about the mean can be restored by taking the square root of the variance, resulting in an expression for the standard deviation or root mean square deviate:

$$\text{standard deviation} = \sqrt{\left(\frac{\Sigma(x-\bar{x})^2}{n}\right)}.$$

This expression can be used to estimate the standard deviation when n is > 30; however, the standard deviation is more usually based on a relatively small sample (i.e. < 30 values) which are only a small part of a much larger, unsampled population of results. In these conditions (i.e. when $n < 30$), it can be shown that a slight modification (Bessel's correction) gives a rather better estimate of the population standard deviation, using the expression:

$$\text{standard deviation} = \sqrt{\left(\frac{\Sigma(x-\bar{x})^2}{n-1}\right)}.$$

In practice, it is unnecessary to calculate each deviation from the mean (i.e. $[x_1 - \bar{x}]$, $[x_2 - \bar{x}]$, $[x_3 - \bar{x}]$, etc.), and to square and summate them, since it can be shown that $\Sigma(x - \bar{x})^2 = \Sigma x^2 - (\Sigma x)^2/n$. Consequently, the standard deviation of samples when $n < 30$ can be defined as:

$$\text{standard deviation} = \sqrt{\left(\frac{\Sigma x^2 - (\Sigma x)^2 / n}{n - 1}\right)}.$$

Most electronic calculators that are designed for statistical use can automatically calculate the mean and the standard deviation, after the individual data values have been entered.

Variance

The square of the standard deviation is known as the variance, which is defined (when $n < 30$) by the expression:

$$\text{variance} = \left(\frac{\Sigma x^2 - (\Sigma x)^2 / n}{n - 1}\right).$$

The denominator of the variance $(n - 1)$ defines its number of degrees of freedom. It is $(n - 1)$ (i.e. one less than the number of observations or results) because only $(n - 1)$ results are independent from each other; the value of the nth result is determined by the values of the remainder.

Coefficient of variation

The variability or scatter of different observations cannot be compared by their standard deviations when the means are very disparate, or when their standard deviations are calculated in different units. For example, in SI units, the weight of a group of 36 patients was 68.0 ± 20.4 kg (mean ± s.d.); when expressed in imperial units, their weight was 150 ± 45 lb. The variability of the measurements must be identical, although their standard deviations are different; clearly, the standard deviations of different groups cannot be compared unless their units of measurement are identical. This problem can be avoided by the use of the coefficient of variation, which expresses the standard deviation as a percentage of the mean:

$$\text{coefficient of variation (\%)} = \frac{\text{standard deviation}}{\text{mean}} \times 100.$$

Since the standard deviation and the mean are measured in the same units, the coefficient of variation is independent of the units of measurement. (In the above example, the coefficient of variation of body weight was 30%, whether measured in kilograms or pounds.)

Standard error of the mean

The mean ($\bar{x}$) and standard deviation (s.d.) of a relatively small sample of results are often used to provide a guide or estimate of the population mean (μ) and the population standard deviation (σ). Clearly, different samples of the entire population may provide different estimates of μ and σ. The accuracy of the sample mean ($\bar{x}$) in predicting the true value of the population mean (μ) can be estimated by the standard error of the sample mean (s.e. of the mean, or s.e.m.):

$$\text{standard error of the mean} = \frac{\text{s.d.}}{\sqrt{n}}.$$

Clearly, the larger the size of the sample, the smaller is the calculated value for the standard error of the mean.

The standard error of the mean can be used to predict the range where the population mean will be situated. When $n > 30$, there is a 95% (19/20) chance that the true population mean lies within approximately 2 standard errors of the sample mean. In the example previously discussed, a group of 36 patients had a body weight of 68.0 ± 20.4 kg (mean ± s.d.); consequently:

$$\text{mean} \pm \text{s.e.m.} = 68.0 \pm \frac{20.4}{\sqrt{36}}\,\text{kg} = 68.0 \pm 3.4\,\text{kg}.$$

Consequently, there was a probability of 95% (19/20) that the true mean of the population from which the patient sample was derived lies within the range 61.2–74.8 kg (i.e. mean ± 2 s.e.m.). In a similar manner, approximately 95% of the sample means obtained by repeated sampling of the entire population would be likely to lie within the same range. Consequently, the range from [mean – (2 × s.e.m.)] to [mean + (2 × s.e.m.)] (61.2 – 74.8 kg) represents the interval within which the population mean is likely to lie; it is called the 95% confidence interval for the population mean, while its limits are the 95% confidence limits of the mean. The s.e.m. is often incorrectly used to indicate the variability of individual values in the sample (possibly because it is always less than the standard deviation, from which it is derived). However, the variability or scatter of individual values in a population sample should always be described by the standard deviation.

The normal distribution

The variability or scatter of individual observations in a population sample can be expressed in other ways. For example, the variability in the dosage of a drug required to produce a specific pharmacological effect in 100 subjects can be expressed as a

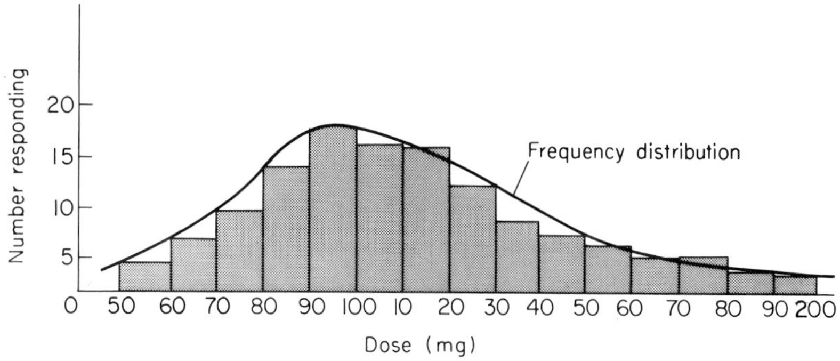

Fig. 6.2 Histogram showing the variability in dosage required to produce a specific effect. Each shaded rectangle represents the number of patients that respond to each 10 mg increment in dosage. A frequency distribution curve has been imposed on the histogram, showing that the data approximately correspond to a normal or Gaussian distribution.

histogram (Fig. 6.2); each shaded rectangle represents the number of patients who respond to each 10 mg increment in dosage (e.g. 50–60 mg, 60–70 mg, 70–80 mg, etc.). A frequency distribution curve can then be superimposed on the histogram. In the case of the data from 100 subjects, the curve is symmetrical and bell-shaped; this type of curve is known as a normal or Gaussian† distribution, and in many instances this type of frequency distribution curve provides a reasonable representation of the variability of clinical data. The peak of the normal distribution corresponds to the mean or average value; the form of the curve is determined by the degree of variability. Thus, the Gaussian curve is high and narrow when the variability and standard deviation are low, but small and wide when the variability and standard deviation are high.

In a normally distributed population, the mean (average value), the median (the central value that divides the population into two equally sized groups) and the mode (the most commonly occurring value) are identical. In addition, 68% of the values are within one standard deviation of the mean (mean ± 1 s.d.); 95% of the values are within two standard deviations of the mean (mean ± 2 s.d.). The normal distribution is the basis of many techniques of statistical analysis. Normally distributed data can be analysed by both parametric statistical tests (e.g. Student *t*-test, analysis of variance) as well as non-parametric tests (e.g. Wilcoxon signed-rank test, Mann–Whitney *U*-test, Kruskal–Wallis test, Friedman test); nevertheless, parametric tests should be used if possible, since they allow the utilization of the numerical values of quantitative data.

The normal distribution can also be plotted as a cumulative frequency distribution curve (Ogive) by calculating the proportion of patients that respond to a given dose, or to a dose below it (Fig. 6.3). In a normal distribution, 2.5% of the values are less than or equal to [mean – 2 s.d.]; 16% are less than or equal to [mean – s.d.];

† Johann Karl Friedrich Gauss (1777–1855).

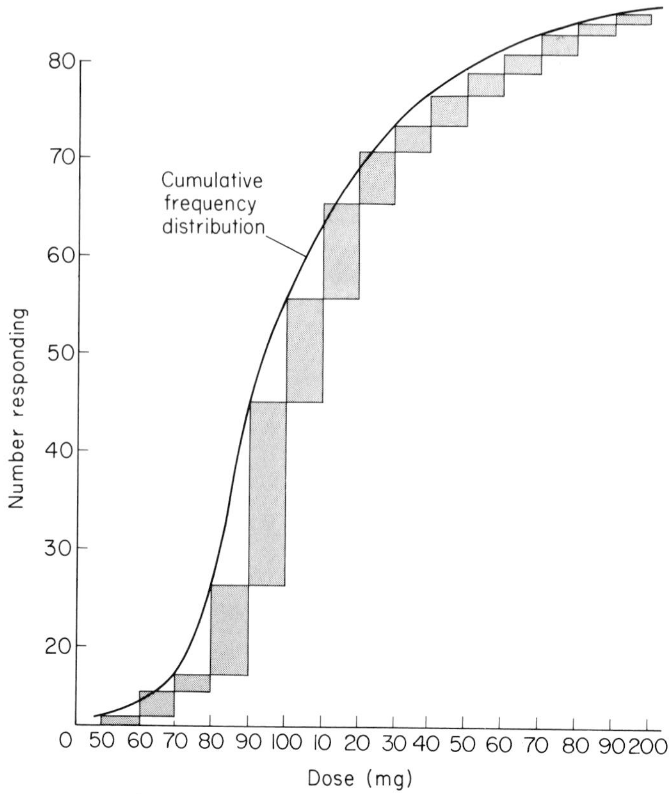

Fig. 6.3 A cumulative frequency distribution curve (Ogive) representing the summated results of Fig. 6.2.

50% are less than or equal to the mean; 84% are less than or equal to [mean + s.d.]; and 97.5% are less than or equal to [mean + 2 s.d.].

The causes of variability in drug response

Variability in the response to drugs may be related to (Table 6.2):

1 Physiological factors.

2 Pharmacological factors.

3 Pathological factors.

Physiological variability

Physiological variability in the response to drugs may occur at the extremes of age, in pregnancy, or may be related to tobacco smoking or the consumption of alcohol.

Childhood

There are marked differences in drug disposition between children and adults.

Table 6.2 Principal causes of variability in drug response.

Physiological and social
Age
Pregnancy
Tobacco
Ethyl alcohol
Pharmacological
Idiosyncracy
Supersensitivity
Tachyphylaxis
Tolerance
Hypersensitivity
Pathological
Liver disease
Renal disease
Respiratory disease
Cardiac disease
Neurological disease

In the neonatal period, absorption of drugs is slower due to a longer gastric emptying time and an increase in intestinal transit time; nevertheless, more of the drug may be absorbed because of the greater contact time with the intestinal mucosa. The gastric contents are less acidic, and some drugs (e.g. benzylpenicillin, ampicillin) will have greater overall absorption when swallowed. The vasomotor instability observed in the newborn period may result in the unreliable absorption of drugs administered by subcutaneous or intramuscular injection from tissue sites.

The distribution of drugs is influenced by a number of factors including tissue mass, fat content, blood flow, membrane permeability and the degree of protein binding. Total body water as a percentage of body weight falls from 87% in the preterm baby to 73% at 3 months, and subsequently decreases to 55% in adult patients. Consequently, doses of water-soluble drugs that are calculated by scaling down adult doses in proportion to body weight can result in lower tissue concentrations in infants and neonates. However, drug distribution is also affected by the lower body fat content and the increased permeability of the blood–brain barrier in the neonate, and lipid-soluble drugs may be relatively concentrated in the central nervous system (CNS). In addition, the decrease in plasma protein levels in the newborn leads to the increased availability of the free unbound drug, with enhanced pharmacological activity and drug metabolism. The decrease in plasma pH during neonatal life may influence the degree of drug ionization, and thus affect the membrane permeability of both acidic and basic drugs.

The rate of drug metabolism depends on both the size of the liver and the activity of hepatic microsomal enzyme systems. In the early newborn period, enzyme activity is initially immature, and may not assume the adult pattern for several months.

In older children, enzyme activity is similar to adults, although most drugs are metabolized at faster rates (probably due to the relatively greater liver volume).

Glomerular filtration rates comparable to those seen in the adult occur at about 4 months of age. In the neonatal period, the glomerular filtration rate is low (20–40% of the adult rate), and drugs removed from the body by this means (e.g. digoxin and gentamicin) are eliminated relatively slowly.

These physiological and kinetic differences may have significant practical implications. In the neonate, weight-related doses of water-soluble, polar compounds (e.g. most antibiotics) produce lower tissue concentrations than in adults, and may have decreased pharmacological effects. Dose regimes that are related to surface area are required to produce similar blood levels. However, the increased volume of distribution and the decreased renal clearance result in a longer elimination half-life, and dose intervals should therefore be prolonged. In addition, the effects of drugs on the neonatal CNS may be enhanced after their administration in labour (e.g. morphine, diazepam); this phenomenon may be due to the increased fraction of unbound drug, greater permeability of the CNS due to immaturity of the blood–brain barrier, and delayed hepatic metabolism.

For many years, it was considered that neonates were highly sensitive to doses of non-depolarizing neuromuscular blocking agents, particularly during the first 10 days of life (although they were resistant to depolarizing agents). More recent studies have not entirely confirmed these original observations. When tubocurarine is administered, neonates show an equivalent degree of neuromuscular blockade to that observed in older children and adults at lower plasma concentrations of the drug. Nevertheless, the enhanced volume of distribution of tubocurarine in the neonate, and the subsequent reduction in plasma concentrations, suggests that the initial dose requirements in terms of body weight are similar. However, since the elimination half-life of tubocurarine is longer, the interval between incremental doses should be greater. Similar studies using atracurium infusions indicate that dose requirements in the neonate (in proportion to body weight) do not differ greatly from those at other ages. Any variations may be attributed to lower body temperatures in the newborn, and their subsequent effects on drug distribution.

Abnormal responses to opioids are sometimes observed in neonates. Experimental studies in newborn animals suggest that they are relatively insensitive to morphine analgesia (although they have a marked sensitivity to its respiratory depressant effects). These changes may be related to differences in the distribution of μ_1- and μ_2-receptors in the neonatal period.

In older children in whom protein binding, hepatic microsomal enzyme activity, renal function and the permeability of the blood–brain barrier are similar to adults, differences in drug disposition are less likely. Nevertheless, drug dosage is best assessed in terms of body surface area, due to the proportional increase in body water during childhood. More frequent rates of administration, especially of the less polar compounds, may be necessary due to the relative increase in liver blood flow. Differences in pharmacodynamic activity may also be present, but are less easy to assess.

Old age

Elderly patients often respond differently to standard adult doses of drugs, and are more likely than younger patients to react adversely to drugs prescribed in hospital. Compliance with drug therapy may be unreliable, due to failing memory, confusion and poor eyesight. Nevertheless, after appropriate oral administration, drug absorption is not appreciably modified, except for substances which rely on active transport mechanisms (e.g. iron, thiamine, calcium).

In contrast to the neonate, there is a reduction in the proportion of total body water, and a relative increase in body fat. Consequently, the volume of distribution of water-soluble drugs is reduced and plasma and tissue concentrations are effectively increased. Albumin levels tend to fall with age, and the free fraction of certain drugs (e.g. phenytoin, phenylbutazone, carbenoxolone, tolbutamide) increases, thus enhancing their rate of availability to cells and tissues.

At the age of 65, hepatic blood flow may be 45% less than normal values in younger adults, and experimental evidence suggests that the activity of the microsomal enzyme systems declines to a similar extent. Consequently, the systemic bioavailability of drugs that are subject to low or high hepatic clearance is increased, with enhancement of their pharmacological effects. Similarly, glomerular filtration and tubular secretion decline with age, and the elderly patient is therefore at risk from drugs with a low therapeutic index (e.g. digoxin, gentamicin, lithium).

Enhanced effects of drugs used in anaesthetic practice should therefore be anticipated in elderly patients. Dose–response studies have shown that the dose requirements of thiopentone diminish with increasing age. Pharmacokinetic factors (e.g. decreased plasma protein binding, lowered volume of distribution and increased accumulation in fat) as well as pharmacodynamic factors play a part in this phenomenon. Similarly, the free fraction of pethidine is four times higher in elderly patients than in the young, indicating that the dose of the drug should be reduced in the aged.

In addition, changes in receptor numbers or sensitivity may account for alterations in drug responses in the elderly (e.g. the increased analgesia in elderly patients who are given opioid analgesics for postoperative pain). Altered sensitivity of the elderly to drug concentrations at receptor sites may occur with nitrazepam, warfarin and some β-adrenoceptor antagonists.

The minimum alveolar concentration (MAC) values of all inhalation anaesthetics in steady-state conditions progressively declines with advancing age, and anaesthetic requirements are significantly depressed in the elderly. Comparable data for intravenous induction agents can be superimposed on these results (Fig. 6.4); consequently, the decline in anaesthetic requirement may be due to pharmacodynamic factors

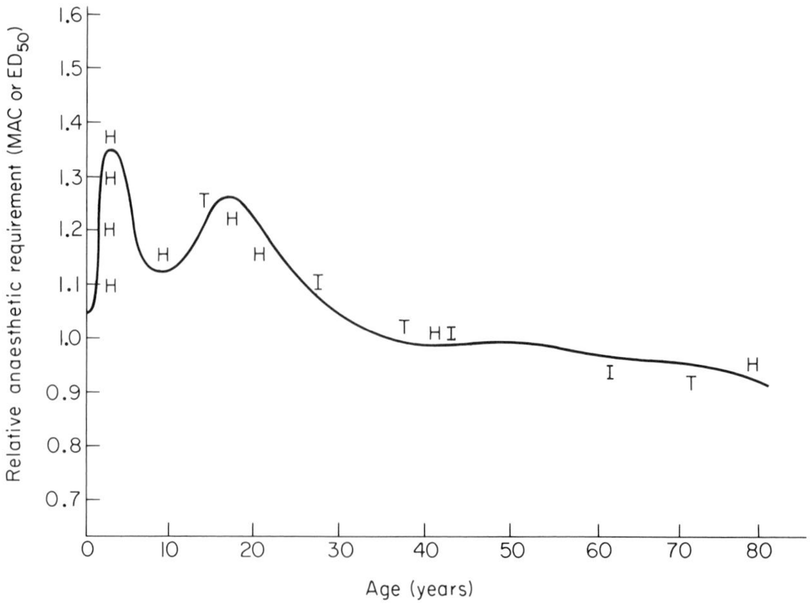

Fig. 6.4 Relative anaesthetic requirement expressed as a multiple of minimum alveolar concentration (MAC) or median effective dose (ED_{50}) for various inhalational and intravenous anaesthetic agents. Requirement normalized for established values for young healthy adults. H, Halothane; I, isoflurane; T, thiopentone.

that are based upon underlying anatomical, biochemical or functional changes associated with ageing.

Pregnancy

The absorption, distribution and elimination of drugs may alter during pregnancy. Slower gastric emptying results in the increased uptake of drugs absorbed in the stomach (e.g. diazepam) and the delayed absorption of those that are principally absorbed in the upper gastrointestinal tract (e.g. aspirin, paracetamol). Disturbances of gastrointestinal motility during pregnancy have been related to changes in the relative amounts of gastric acid and mucus secretion; increased progesterone levels during pregnancy may also cause relaxation of smooth muscle in many organs.

The placenta contains a wide range of enzymes that are concerned with the metabolism of neurotransmitters and other endogenous compounds. The decreased sensitivity to insulin which occurs in pregnancy may be due to a placental lactogen which degrades the hormone (i.e. an insulinase). Other enzymes whose activity in pregnancy is increased include alkaline phosphatase and β-glucuronidase, which is secreted by the intestinal mucosa and hydrolyses glucuronide conjugates eliminated in bile. Consequently, the effects of some drugs may be potentiated in pregnancy due to increased enterohepatic recirculation (e.g. analgesics, antibiotics).

Plasma volume and cardiac output are both increased during pregnancy (by 50% and 30% respectively, with maximum values achieved at 30–34 weeks' gestation). The clearance of many drugs (e.g. phenytoin) may be enhanced in pregnancy due to increased cardiac output, and the subsequent increase in hepatic and renal blood flow. The increase in cardiac output, associated with the modest hyperventilation which normally occurs during pregnancy, will enhance both the rate of uptake and subsequent elimination of inhalational anaesthetic agents.

Other changes in the pharmacokinetics of drugs may occur during pregnancy. Thus, the binding of many drugs (e.g. diazepam, pethidine, propranolol, theophylline) to albumin and globulins is decreased, particularly during the last trimester; it has been suggested that exogenous substances in plasma may interfere with protein binding. In the case of theophylline, decreased plasma protein binding increases the volume of distribution; since the clearance is unchanged, the terminal half-life is prolonged (Chapter 2). The pharmacokinetics of thiopentone is also modified in pregnant patients during Caesarean section. Plasma protein binding and clearance are not markedly altered, although the volume of distribution at steady state is increased; consequently, the elimination half-life of the drug is prolonged.

Smoking

Tobacco smoking results in the induction of some hepatic microsomal enzyme systems (particularly the CYP 1A2 isoform of cytochrome P-450). The rates of elimination of drugs that are metabolized by this pathway are generally greater in smokers than in non-smokers, although there is a considerable overlap. Metabolism of antipyrine, theophylline, imipramine and pentazocine is increased, while drugs such as diazepam, pethidine and warfarin are not significantly affected.

Clinical studies suggest that smokers require more opioids to obtain relief from pain, are less sedated by benzodiazepines and may obtain reduced benefit from β-blockers and nifedipine in angina. Not all these differences arise from alterations in the rate of drug metabolism, although the exact mechanism is unclear.

Ethyl alcohol

The chronic use of ethyl alcohol (ethanol) increases the capacity of the liver to metabolize this compound. At the same time pharmacodynamic tolerance occurs; higher blood concentrations are required to produce intoxication in alcohol-tolerant subjects than in normal individuals. Cross-resistance between many sedative drugs (e.g. benzodiazepines) and alcohol occurs, due to both pharmacodynamic (CNS) tolerance and more rapid metabolism. The resistance to thiopentone which is frequently encountered in chronic alcoholic patients is undoubtedly due to tolerance at a cellular level, as its duration of action is primarily determined by redistribution rather than metabolism. Changes in the availability of γ-aminobutyric acid (GABA) with possible alterations in the number and nature of GABA receptors may play a part in this phenomenon.

Similar concepts may apply to the reported tolerance of chronic alcoholics to inhalational agents, although these do not take into account the state of agitation of patients who may be on the edge of withdrawal symptoms. Nevertheless, they are only relevant in patients after prolonged prior exposure to alcohol has occurred. After the acute ingestion of alcohol, the administration of other CNS depressants may lead to supra-additive effects. The half-life of barbiturates may also be increased, presumably due to competition with alcohol for microsomal enzymes.

Pharmacological variability

Pharmacological variability in the response to drugs may be related to idiosyncracy, supersensitivity, tachyphylaxis, tolerance or hypersensitivity reactions.

Idiosyncracy

Idiosyncracy can be defined as a genetically determined abnormal reaction to a drug. It may present as extreme sensitivity to low doses, or marked insensitivity to high doses of the agent.

The term has also been used empirically to describe the side-effects (e.g. dysphoria, nausea, vomiting and other gastrointestinal tract disturbances) occurring in patients who receive certain drugs (e.g. opioids, non-steroidal anti-inflammatory drugs (NSAIDs)). These adverse effects may disappear when closely related compounds are substituted. The underlying mechanisms are unclear, but may involve hypersensitivity responses.

Important examples of idiosyncracy, i.e. genetically determined reactions to drugs, are:

1 Haemolysis after exposure to certain drugs (e.g. antimalarial agents, sulphonamides, NSAIDs), which are observed in patients with a deficiency in erythrocyte glucose-6-phosphate dehydrogenase (G6PD). The absence or deficiency of this enzyme delays the regeneration of NADPH, which protects the erythrocyte from the injurious effects of oxidative drugs. Consequently, susceptible patients may develop haemolytic anaemia and jaundice on exposure to these drugs.

2 Prolongation of the action of suxamethonium which may occur in patients with genetic variants in plasma cholinesterase. The variants show genetic polymorphism, and four separate alleles for the enzyme occur at a single locus. Consequently, there are 10 possible genotypes for plasma cholinesterase, with a wide range of enzyme activity and sensitivity to inhibition. The genetic variants of the enzyme are fully discussed in Chapter 10.

3 Toxic effects of isoniazid, hydralazine, phenelzine and certain sulphonamides in patients who are 'slow' acetylators. There is a bimodal distribution in the rate of metabolism of these drugs, since the hepatic enzyme system responsible for acetylation (*N*-acetyltransferase) shows genetic polymorphism. The toxic effects of these drugs predominantly occur in patients who are 'slow' acetylators.

4 Hereditary resistance to oral anticoagulants, which occurs in both animals and humans, due to an autosomal dominant trait. The mechanism of action is obscure. It has been suggested that a suppressant manufactured by mutant subjects has an altered reactivity with either vitamin K, its antagonists, or both. Alternatively, it has been suggested that the enzyme diaphorase (epoxide reductase), which reduces vitamin K epoxide to its active form, develops resistance to the oral anticoagulant. In addition, patients with a genetic deficiency in antithrombin III may be extremely resistant to warfarin.

5 Malignant hyperpyrexia (malignant hyperthermia), a rare but potentially fatal complication of anaesthesia. Despite its rarity, it is one of the main causes of death in anaesthetic practice. There is a strong familial susceptibility to malignant hyperthermia (which is usually inherited as an autosomal dominant condition); a similar abnormality occurs in Landrace and Pie Train pigs. The essential defect consists of a genetically determined abnormality in the Ca^{2+}-releasing channel in the sarcoplasmic reticulum of skeletal muscle (ryanodine receptor). On exposure to suxamethonium, halothane (and possibly other drugs), there is excessive Ca^{2+} release resulting in muscle contraction, rigidity and hyperthermia.

6 Acute hepatic porphyria (including acute intermittent porphyria, variegate porphyria and hereditary porphyria) which is commonly precipitated by drugs in genetically susceptible individuals. The agents commonly implicated are usually known inducers of the enzyme δ-aminolaevulinic acid (ALA) synthetase, and their administration leads to increased hepatic production and urinary excretion of porphyrins (e.g. ALA, porphobilinogen and their derivatives). Drug-induced porphyria is associated with the use of barbiturates, phenytoin, dichloralphenazone, alcohol, griseofulvin, sulphonamides, sulphonylureas, oral contraceptives and certain steroids. The use of these drugs may lead to widespread demyelination of peripheral and central pathways, resulting in sensory changes and motor paralysis.

Other genetically determined disorders associated with drug administration include defective debrisoquine oxidation, in which exaggerated hypotension after normal oral dosage may occur; increased intraocular pressure, which may be detected in some patients after the chronic administration of steroid eyedrops; and intense facial flushing which is induced by alcohol in a significant number of patients receiving chlorpropamide. Toxic reactions to gold, levamisole and procainamide have been related to specific human lymphocyte antigen (HLA) subtypes; similarly, digoxin toxicity and thromboembolism induced by oral contraceptives have been associated with specific differences in ABO blood groups.

Racial differences in drug responses also occur (although they are not usually classified as idiosyncratic reactions). Nevertheless, they often have an underlying genetic basis, which may be related to pharmacodynamic or pharmacokinetic factors, or both. For example, patients of Chinese descent may show an enhanced response to propranolol, even though its rate of clearance is greater than in Caucasians. Similarly, Scandinavians and Chileans may have a higher incidence of cholestatic jaundice induced by oral contraceptives. There is also some anecdotal evidence that the effects of thiopentone are prolonged in oriental subjects. Other studies have suggested that women may be more susceptible than men to adverse drug reactions; examples include digoxin toxicity, the development of acute dystonic reactions after metoclopramide and blood dyscrasias associated with phenylbutazone or chloramphenicol. The explanation for these differences is unclear.

Supersensitivity

Receptors play an important part in the regulation of physiological and biochemical functions, and are also subject to regulatory and homeostatic control. The continual stimulation of receptors by agonists leads to a reduction in their numbers, density and activity (down-regulation). This is exemplified by the refractory response which may follow the administration of β-adrenoceptor agonists in the treatment of bronchial asthma, and is associated with a reduction in the number of functioning β-adrenoceptors in bronchial smooth muscle. The phenomenon is partly due to the sequestration (internalization) of receptors within cells, although receptor affinity may also be modified. Adrenergic receptor density is also modified in a number of other pathological conditions (e.g. congestive cardiac failure, thyrotoxicosis).

By contrast, any decrease in catecholamine production, either following drug therapy or sympathetic denervation, increases the synthesis and numbers of adrenoceptors (up-regulation), and may also diminish the neuronal uptake of catecholamines. Similar changes in receptor density are probably produced by most neurotransmitters that act at synapses and neuroeffector junctions. In these conditions, there may be hyperreactivity or supersensitivity to the effects of drugs that act on these receptors. The phenomenon of up-regulation may explain the rebound effects which result from the sudden withdrawal of certain antihypertensive drugs (e.g. β-adrenoceptor agonists, clonidine, minoxidil) following their long-term administration, and may account for the production of tardive dyskinesia by phenothiazines and its potentiation by dopamine precursors. The increase in receptor numbers also plays an important part in the exaggerated response to vasopressors in patients on adrenergic neurone-blocking agents.

Up-regulation of receptors may be responsible for the significant hyperkalaemia which occurs after administration of suxamethonium to patients with severe burns or spinal cord injuries. In these conditions, extrajunctional receptors develop on the surface of the muscle fibre outside the motor endplate; the total number of acetylcholine receptors may increase 100 times. Consequently, the ionic changes associated with the depolarization of skeletal muscle by suxamethonium may produce significant hyperkalaemia; in extreme cases, serum potassium concentrations may be doubled.

Tachyphylaxis

Tachyphylaxis can be defined as a rapid decrease or a reduction in the response to identical doses of an agonist within a short period of time. It is sometimes used to refer to the phenomenon of acute receptor desensitization, or to the occurrence of rapid drug tolerance.

Tachyphylaxis sometimes develops after the repeated administration of suxamethonium, particularly when its elimination is compromised by enzyme abnormalities or other drugs. In these conditions, tachyphylaxis may precede the development of a second phase of non-depolarizing blockade which is difficult to antagonize (phase II blockade); it may be related to the slow dissociation of suxamethonium from the cholinergic receptor, so that receptor occupancy remains high when a second dose of the drug is given.

In current practice, tachyphylaxis is more commonly applied to the effects of drugs that act by releasing endogenous transmitters from cells or nerve endings. In these conditions, the response to repeated doses of the drug rapidly declines, presumably due to transmitter exhaustion. Tachyphylaxis is classically observed after the administration of indirectly acting sympathomimetic amines (e.g. tyramine, ephedrine, amphetamine); it may also occur with drugs that release dopamine (e.g. amantidine, tetrabenazine). In anaesthetic practice, a form of tachyphylaxis commonly occurs when trimetaphan (or other ganglion-blocking agents) is used to produce controlled hypotension during surgery.

Tolerance

Drug tolerance generally refers to the gradual decrease in the activity of drugs, which usually occurs over a period of days or weeks. It classically occurs with opioid analgesics; in these conditions, it may be related to a reduction in the number, density, or affinity of opioid receptors (i.e. down-regulation), or to modification of the synthesis or release of enkephalins or endorphins, resulting in altered responsiveness of cells in the CNS. Experimental studies suggest that some tolerance to opioids may develop within several hours, and a negative-feedback system involving endogenous opioids may be involved.

Tolerance also develops to the haemodynamic and vasodilator effects of organic nitrates during their continuous administration. Nitrate tolerance was first observed in munition workers exposed to nitroglycerine during the manufacture of explosives. Headaches and dizziness often occurred on first exposure to nitroglycerine during their initial period of employment. These symptoms rapidly abated following a few days absence from work, but frequently recurred on re-exposure ('Monday-morning headache'). Similarly, the use of intermittent regimes of drug therapy with organic nitrates avoids the gradual attenuation of their therapeutic effects, although it may expose the patient to the further risk of anginal episodes during the nitrate-free period (Chapter 15).

The basic mechanism of nitrate tolerance has recently been clarified. Organic nitrates are lipid-soluble compounds which readily penetrate smooth-muscle cells. They are metabolized intracellularly to nitric oxide, which combines with sulphydryl groups to form reactive intermediates (*S*-nitrosothiols). These compounds activate soluble guanylate cyclase, which converts guanosine triphosphate to cyclic guanosine monophosphate (cGMP); this in turn activates protein kinases, causing relaxation of vascular smooth muscle (Chapters 3 and 15). Tolerance may be due to the depletion of sulphydryl groups from vascular smooth muscle; this prevents the formation of *S*-nitrosothiols from nitric oxide. In some studies, the administration of sulphydryl donors such as *N*-acetylcysteine can delay or prevent tolerance to nitrates.

Tolerance may also occur to the effects of barbiturates (and possibly other centrally acting drugs). Increased drug metabolism, due to the autoinduction of hepatic microsomal enzymes (particularly the CYP 1A2 isoforms of cytochrome P-450) may be partly responsible.

Hypersensitivity

Hypersensitivity responses are abnormal reactions to drugs that are dependent on immunological mechanisms, and usually involve the formation of antibodies. Approximately 10% of adverse reactions to drugs are due to drug hypersensitivity, and its associated humoral responses. Most drugs are low molecular weight compounds, and many of them can act as haptens to form relatively fairly stable complexes (e.g. by conjugation with lysyl side-chains of tissue proteins).

Hypersensitivity reactions have been grouped into four main types, depending on the mechanism involved.

Type I hypersensitivity (immediate-type hypersensitivity)

Type I hypersensitivity is invariably mediated by reaginic antibodies (immunoglobulin E; IgE). Drugs combine covalently with normal plasma or tissue proteins, forming a drug–protein complex which is antigenic. The drug–protein complex gains access to antibody-forming cells (B lymphocytes and plasma cells) and induces the formation of IgE cytophilic antibodies, which become attached to mast cells in various tissues of the body (e.g. skin, bronchial and intestinal mucosa, vascular capillaries or basophil leukocytes). On subsequent exposure to the drug–protein complex, adjacent IgE molecules on the cytoplasmic membrane are bound by the hapten or antigen; consequently, type I hypersensitivity is only commonly seen with drugs that form multivalent protein complexes, or are inherently divalent due to the presence of symmetrical molecular features (e.g. most muscle relaxants). Subsequently calcium ions enter mast cells, resulting in their degranulation, and the release of pharmacological mediators (e.g. histamine, heparin, 5-hydroxytryptamine, leukotrienes, platelet-activating factor and anaphylatoxin).

Type I hypersensitivity responses are not uncommon with certain drugs (e.g. penicillin, sulphonamides, cephalosporins, phenindione), and may also follow insect stings or the oral ingestion of certain proteins. In some instances, an exaggerated 'triple response' to histamine occurs, and may result in generalized urticaria or angioneurotic oedema.

Anaphylactic shock presents as severe hypotension due to profound peripheral vasodilatation and venous pooling, usually associated with bronchiolar constriction. The blood pressure may be unrecordable and the pulse impalpable. Emergency treatment consists of the promotion of venous return, adequate oxygenation and the use of intravenous adrenaline. Glucocorticoids are of no immediate benefit, although they may be of long-term value. H_1 and H_2 histamine antagonists are of little or no use.

Type 2 hypersensitivity (cytolytic reactions)

Cytolytic reactions depend upon the reaction of circulating antibodies (either IgE or IgM) with antigens that are usually associated with blood cell membranes. In type 2 hypersensitivity, drugs combine with proteins in the cell membrane of erythrocytes, granulocytes or platelets, and induce the formation of antibodies. (Alternatively, drugs may produce conformational changes in membrane proteins, so that previously dormant antigenic sites can induce the formation of antibodies.) The immunoglobulins IgE or IgM then cross-react with the antigenic sites in the cell membrane in the presence of complement, causing cell lysis or agglutination.

Known or putative examples of type 2 hypersensitivity include: (i) haemolytic anaemia due to sulphonamides or methyldopa; (ii) agranulocytosis induced by phenothiazines, phenylbutazone or antithyroid drugs and; (iii) thrombocytopenia induced by thiazide diuretics. Nevertheless, drug-induced blood dyscrasias may be due to other mechanisms; thus, haemolytic anaemia may be related to deficiency of erythrocyte G6PD, and agranulocytosis may be due to the direct effects of cytotoxic drugs on the bone marrow.

Recent evidence suggests that 'halothane hepatitis' is also due to a type 2 hypersensitivity reaction. One of the oxidative metabolites of halothane (trifluoroacetyl chloride) can bind covalently to lysine residues on hepatic proteins. In susceptible individuals, the alkylated protein may act as an antigen, inducing the formation of antibodies which react with hepatocytes, causing cellular damage (Chapter 8).

Type 3 hypersensitivity (immune complex-mediated responses)

Immune complex-mediated hypersensitivity is due to the formation of precipitin complexes by the reaction of circulating antibodies with soluble antigens (e.g. bacterial toxins). Normally, precipitins are removed by the reticuloendothelial system, but when excess antigen is present, immune complexes are deposited in the endothelial lining of small blood vessels, glomerular membranes and the connective tissue of joints. Type 3 reactions may be the basis for pathological changes in certain systemic diseases, e.g. acute glomerulonephritis, polyarteritis nodosa and rheumatoid arthritis. Similarly, some drugs may act as haptens, induce the formation of antibodies and form circulating antigen–antibody complexes which fix complement; they are then deposited in tissues (particularly vascular endothelium) as immune complexes.

Immune complex-mediated hypersensitivity was first described as the Arthus phenomenon. A localized type of inflammatory response occurs 4–8 h after the administration of a drug or toxoid; similarly, injection of a large dose of antigen which remains in the circulation may produce an inflammatory response (serum sickness) after 7–14 days. Serum sickness presents as malaise and fever followed by arthritis or arthralgia; an urticarial rash and albuminuria may also occur. At one time it was a relatively common complication of treatment with horse serum (e.g. in the treatment of diphtheria or the prevention of tetanus). Serum sickness is an occasional complication of sulphonamide therapy, but may occur with other drugs (e.g. penicillin, streptomycin, thiouracil derivatives). It does not require previous exposure to these drugs, but depends upon the continuous production of antibodies (particularly IgG). Serum sickness usually resolves spontaneously and treatment is only rarely required.

Type 4 hypersensitivity (delayed, cell-mediated responses)

In delayed hypersensitivity antibody formation is not involved, and the reaction solely results from the combination of antigen with T-cell (killer) lymphocytes. The antigen or hapten is introduced by contact or injection, and combines covalently with receptors on the lymphocyte membrane. This results in lymphocyte mitosis and the local release of lymphokines that promote vascular leakage (e.g. lymph node permeability factor). A local inflammatory reaction usually occurs within 24–48 h, resulting in erythema, induration, blistering and exfoliation, due to the accumulation of macrophages and lymphocytes at the site of injection.

Delayed hypersensitivity is responsible for the positive response to the Mantoux reaction, and occurs in most forms of contact dermatitis, whether produced by metals (e.g. nickel or copper) or by drugs (e.g. penicillin, streptomycin, sulphonamides, chlorpromazine). It is also involved in the local reactions which are sometimes seen after prolonged contact with local anaesthetic esters and in other cutaneous reactions to drugs. For example, it is a factor in many drug rashes, erythema multiforme (the Stevens–Johnson syndrome) and in the morbilliform rashes that are sometimes induced by ampicillin and amoxycillin in patients with glandular fever or chronic lymphatic leukaemia.

Anaphylactoid reactions

Anaphylactoid responses may be difficult or impossible to distinguish clinically from anaphylactic responses; they occur through direct or non-immunological mechanisms, and are often due to the release of vasoactive substances (e.g. histamine, 5-hydroxytryptamine) from circulating basophils and mast cells after the intravenous administration of certain drugs. Many agents have been suspected or incriminated, including intravenous induction agents, neuromuscular and ganglion-blocking compounds, and certain contrast media and colloid infusions. Clinical evidence suggests that these reactions are directly related to the dose and rate of injection of the offending agent and that their effects are often transient. Anaphylactoid reactions may occur more frequently when several different drugs are administered through small infusion needles. In these conditions, physicochemical combination may result in the production of colloid aggregates which are eventually taken up by the lung, producing more serious sequelae.

Local evidence of histamine release is often observed after the intravenous administration of many opioid analgesics and neuromuscular blocking agents. Disruption and degranulation of mast cells in vessel walls may occur; these local effects are unlikely to be of any clinical consequence. Occasionally, generalized histamine release occurs, producing systemic consequences (e.g. hypotension and bronchospasm).

Both type 2 and type 3 hypersensitivity responses involve the fixation of complement and activation of the complement cascade (C3–C9), leading to opsonization of cellular debris and subsequent augmentation of the inflammatory response (Fig. 6.5). A reduction in the activity of the classical pathway (particularly affecting the function and activation of C3) has been demonstrated in patients undergoing anaesthesia and surgery.

Activation of the alternate pathway (with conversion of C3 to C3a and C3b, and the subsequent release of C5a) was associated with the use of two intravenous induction agents which are no longer available commercially in the UK (propanidid and Althesin). The resultant release of histamine and vasoactive peptides (e.g. bradykinin) had similar effects to type 1 reactions, but without previous exposure to the drug. Activation of the alternate pathway was undoubtedly due to Cremophor-EL (a polyethoxylated derivative of castor oil), which was used as a solubilizing agent with both drugs. Large polysaccharide molecules also activate the alternate pathway, and the anaphylactoid responses occasionally observed after administration of large molecular weight dextrans, hydroxyethyl starch and possibly heparin may be due to a similar mechanism.

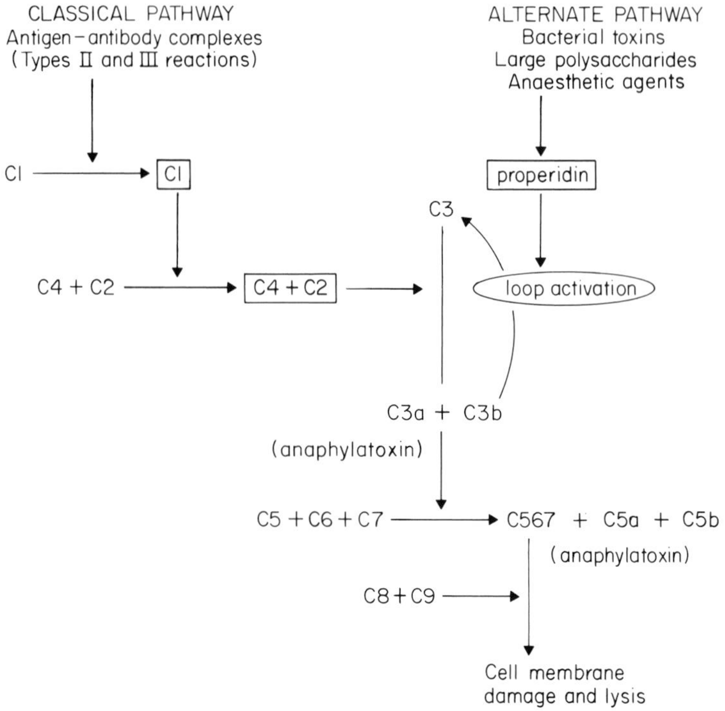

Fig. 6.5 Routes of activation of classical and alternate complement pathways. Boxes indicate activated factors.

Other responses to drugs occasionally resemble anaphylactic and anaphylactoid reactions. For example, salicylates and other NSAIDs inhibit cyclooxygenase in inflammatory cells, and may therefore increase the conversion of its substrate arachidonic acid by lipo-oxygenase to various leukotrienes. One or more of these compounds have been identified as the slow-reacting substance of anaphylaxis (SRS-A), and are important mediators of bronchospasm secondary to inflammation of the airways. Consequently, attacks of bronchoconstriction that are occasionally induced by NSAIDs may be related to the increased synthesis of leukotrienes.

Hypersensitivity responses associated with anaesthesia

Hypersensitivity responses to anaesthetic drugs are not infrequent and occasionally result in life-threatening problems. In many instances, commonly used drugs such as thiopentone, suxamethonium, alcuronium and morphine are involved and colloid infusions may have been administered. It may be particularly difficult to detect patients who are at risk from such responses, although those with a history of atopy (asthma, hayfever or eczema) or with a previous or family history of adverse reactions must be considered as vulnerable. It has been suggested that some drugs are relatively safe, e.g. etomidate, pancuronium, fentanyl and local anaesthetic amides. Pretreatment with both H_1- and H_2-receptor antagonists (e.g. chlorpheniramine and ranitidine) may confer considerable protection on susceptible patients.

Although halothane hepatitis is an extremely rare hypersensitivity response, it is usually unpredictable and can only be prevented by completely avoiding the clinical use of the drug.

Not all adverse responses to drugs in 'normal' individuals can be related to immunological mechanisms or underlying genetic disorders. In some cases, adverse responses can be considered as an extension of the pharmacological effects of the agent, or may reflect intrinsic toxicity which is primarily dependent on the chemical properties of the drug or its reactive metabolites. These effects are usually dose-dependent and can often be reproduced in animals. Adverse responses of this type have become less frequent, due to increased understanding of the structural features of drugs that contribute to their intrinsic toxicity. In addition, these toxic effects are frequently disclosed in preclinical and clinical trials.

Pathological variability

Liver disease

Liver disease can affect hepatic drug clearance by several different mechanisms. There may be alterations in hepatic blood flow (both in total flow and in the degree of intrahepatic shunting), plasma protein binding and intrinsic clearance. Severe liver disorders may also be associated with a reduction in renal blood flow.

Effects on drug disposition are complex and vary according to the type and duration of liver pathology. This is well-exemplified by studies on pancuronium kinetics in different types of liver disease. Obstructive disorders lead to decreased clearance of the muscle relaxant, presumably due to the decreased elimination of pancuronium and its metabolites in the bile; clinically, a slower recovery from neuromuscular blockade occurs. When cirrhosis predominates, the increased volume of distribution, associated with changes in plasma protein binding, results in lower plasma concentrations and decreased uptake at receptor sites. The apparent resistance to the effects of the drug is consistent with the original observations on the response to *d*-tubocurarine in liver disease.

In chronic hepatic dysfunction, dose requirements of thiopentone are decreased, and its duration of action is prolonged. These findings are consistent with decreased plasma protein binding, an increase in the unbound, diffusible fraction that is available to cross the blood–brain barrier, and a prolonged distribution half-life.

General anaesthesia will undoubtedly influence hepatic clearance, due to alterations in cardiac output and redistribution of regional blood flow. Splanchnic perfusion is invariably decreased and the elimination of drugs with a high hepatic clearance (e.g. opioid analgesics, local anaesthetics, β-adrenoceptor antagonists) will be reduced. The problem may be accentuated in the presence of pre-existing liver disease.

Renal disease

Most drugs and their metabolites are partly or wholly eliminated by the kidneys. Consequently, enhanced and prolonged responses to many drugs, with increased toxicity due to the accumulation of metabolites, are predictable in renal failure. Nomograms for the adjustment of drug dosage in renal diseases have been developed, using creatinine clearance as an indication of renal function. Elimination of acidic drugs (e.g. penicillin, NSAIDs) is further complicated by the accumulation of organic acids, which compete with them for active tubular transport processes.

Alterations in protein binding may also occur in renal failure. The binding of acidic drugs (which are normally bound to albumin) is usually decreased in plasma from uraemic patients. Basic drugs show a more variable response, although an increase in the free fraction of some drugs (e.g. diazepam, morphine, chloramphenicol) may occur. Endogenous binding inhibitors which accumulate in renal failure may also increase the unbound concentration of drugs in plasma.

It is generally considered that dosage requirements of thiopentone are reduced in renal failure. It is unclear whether this is due to an increase in the free fraction of the drug, an altered permeability of the blood–brain barrier, or to abnormal cerebral metabolism.

Renal clearance is partly responsible for the removal of opioid analgesics and their metabolites. Dose requirements are reduced in renal failure and active metabolites (e.g. morphine-6-glucuronide, norpethidine) may accumulate. Fentanyl undergoes rapid and extensive hepatic metabolism, but its metabolites have little or no activity or toxicity. Consequently, in renal failure fentanyl may have considerable advantages over other opioid analgesics.

Renal impairment may have a profound effect on the pharmacokinetics of muscle relaxants. Apparent resistance to the onset of neuromuscular blockade is sometimes observed clinically, and this may be related to altered distribution associated with changes in plasma protein binding. Renal elimination accounts for 40–50% of the clearance of pancuronium and *d*-tubocurarine, and more than 90% of gallamine clearance; the removal of these drugs diminishes proportionally with the decline in renal function. In these conditions, tubocurarine may have some advantages; when the renal elimination of tubocurarine is compromised, higher drug concentrations in the liver result in significant biliary excretion (12–40%). Reparalysis after reversal is unlikely to occur in patients with renal failure, because the clearance and elimination half-life of anticholinesterase drugs change in parallel with non-depolarizing relaxants.

In contrast, the pharmacokinetic properties of atracurium and cisatracurium are unaffected by renal failure, since both drugs are spontaneously degraded by

Hofmann elimination (a non-enzymatic process that is dependent on pH and temperature). The duration of action of single and repeated doses of these agents is not prolonged. Both atracurium and cisatracurium are partly broken down to laudanosine, and this metabolite may accumulate to a limited but unimportant extent in patients with renal failure. The elimination of mivacurium is also independent of renal function, since the drug is rapidly broken down by plasma cholinesterase. Variability in the response to suxamethonium in renal disease only occurs when there is concomitant hyperkalaemia. Vecuronium is predominantly metabolized by the liver or excreted in bile; its elimination is slightly prolonged in renal failure.

The duration of action of some other drugs may be affected in an unpredictable manner in renal disease. The duration of action of local anaesthetic blockade may be reduced in renal failure, possibly because drug removal from the site of action is facilitated by an associated increase in cardiac output. The elimination half-life of diazepam may be reduced in chronic renal failure (from approximately 97 to 37 h); protein binding is lower, but the volume of distribution of the unbound drug is decreased, although the clinical significance of this is unclear. The elimination of active metabolites (e.g. nordiazepam and temazepam) is decreased and their sedative effects are prolonged.

Respiratory disease

A variable response to a number of drugs used in anaesthesia and in other situations may occur in patients with chronic respiratory disorders. In chronic obstructive airways disease (COAD), the respiratory centre may become insensitive to carbon dioxide and rely on the hypoxic drive. Consequently, the respiratory depressant effects of opioid analgesics and intravenous induction agents may be exaggerated. Furthermore, the administration of benzodiazepines in doses used for endoscopy to these patients may cause carbon dioxide narcosis. Acid–base changes and electrolyte imbalance associated with long-standing respiratory disorders may result in variable responses to muscle relaxants. Coexisting bronchospasm may lead to further problems when drugs with potential histamine-releasing properties (e.g. morphine, tubocurarine) or which alter the autonomic balance in the bronchial musculature (e.g. propranolol, neostigmine) are administered.

Ventilation–perfusion abnormalities which occur during anaesthesia may be enhanced by pre-existing respiratory disease. The rate of induction of anaesthesia with poorly soluble agents (e.g. nitrous oxide, desflurane) may well be delayed, but is not affected when more soluble agents such as diethylether are used, as compensatory increases in alveolar concentrations of this agent can be attained. When surgical anaesthesia is achieved, hypoventilation can be a problem if spontaneous ventilation is maintained. Exaggerated effects on respiratory function occur; the activity of the accessory muscles appears to be abolished at relatively light planes of anaesthesia. Further problems relating to the uptake and elimination of inhalational agents may thus occur.

Cardiac disease

Considerable alteration in the response to drugs which may be administered to patients with pre-existing cardiovascular disease can be anticipated. Systemic disorders may present with one or more different clinicopathological patterns, such as congestive cardiac failure, fixed-output cardiac dysfunction, ischaemic heart disease, conduction defects and associated dysrhythmias and arterial hypertension.

Most general anaesthetics that are administered by intravenous or inhalational routes can induce depressant effects on different cardiovascular parameters (e.g. myocardial contractility, systemic vascular resistance, coronary blood flow, baroreceptor reflex activity, circulating catecholamine levels), and these effects can undoubtedly be enhanced in patients with diminished cardiac reserve. The resultant clinical features are complex. In some cases they can be extremely hazardous; for instance, in patients with constrictive pericarditis the myocardial depressant effects of thiopentone can induce profound hypotension and pulmonary oedema. Alternatively, a beneficial effect may be achieved, as demonstrated by the reduction in cardiac work and systemic afterload which occurs when moderate concentrations of halothane are administered to patients with congestive cardiac failure.

More specifically, pronounced differences in the distribution and elimination of drugs used in anaesthesia may occur in patients with low cardiac output states. Drugs with significant cardiac muscarinic effects (e.g. suxamethonium, halothane) can lower the sensitivity of the myocardium to circulating catecholamines and pre-existing dysrhythmias may be enhanced. Isoflurane, although a potent coronary vasodilator, may induce maldistribution of myocardial blood flow in the presence of ischaemic heart disease (the steal effect). Similar effects can be produced by desflurane and sevoflurane. Exaggerated changes in blood pressure may be observed following the induction of anaesthesia in hypertensive patients. Although such effects are usually more pronounced when the hypertension is untreated, no specific anaesthetic agent has been incriminated and the mechanism of this response remains unclear.

Neurological disease

Many neurological diseases are associated with abnormal responses to muscle relaxants. In conditions which primarily affect the neuromuscular junction (myasthenia gravis and the Eaton–Lambert syndrome), there is a markedly increased sensitivity to non-depolarizing neuromuscular blocking drugs. In these circumstances, the response to depolarizing drugs is variable. Myasthenia gravis is an autoimmune disease in which there is a quantitative reduction in acetylcholine receptors. In untreated cases, apparent resistance occurs following the administration of a single dose of suxamethonium or decamethonium, although there is an increased likelihood of the development of dual block. In patients who are receiving anticholinesterase therapy, the effects of suxamethonium will be prolonged due to inhibition of enzymatic hydrolysis. In the Eaton–Lambert syndrome, where there is a defect in acetylcholine synthesis or release, increased sensitivity to suxamethonium is usually observed. Depolarizing agents are best avoided in diseases affecting the neuromuscular junction.

Dystrophia myotonica is an inherited disorder in which the primary defect is in the muscle fibre itself. A variety of signs and symptoms are usually associated with this condition, including mental disturbances, cataracts, testicular atrophy, premature baldness and various endocrine disturbances. The underlying muscle dysfunction results in generalized muscular weakness (including those involved in respiration and deglutition) associated with prolonged contracture after stimulation. The latter is particularly noticeable as difficulty in releasing the grip after shaking hands. There is a high incidence of cardiomyopathy with abnormalities of conduction linked with this disorder, and this may reflect the underlying muscle pathology. Prolonged and generalized myotonia has been reported following the administration of suxamethonium. Excessive quantities of potassium may be released from the abnormal muscle and enhance any existing dysrhythmia. Depolarizing agents are absolutely contraindicated in this condition. The response to non-depolarizing neuromuscular blocking agents in unpredictable. Their duration of action may be normal or prolonged, and reduced doses of these drugs should be used. Undue sensitivity to the effect of respiratory depressants (e.g. general anaesthetic agents, opioid analgesics) may also be anticipated, while the administration of volatile agents such as halothane may induce cardiotoxic effects.

In a number of neurological diseases in which muscle wasting is a predominant feature (e.g. motor neurone disease, long-standing spinal injuries and the advanced stage of multiple sclerosis), there is often an increased sensitivity to the effects of suxamethonium. Degeneration of the motor endplate is followed by the up-regulation of receptors so that the whole muscle membrane responds to agonists. Potassium loss is greatly increased, and there is a possibility of dysrhythmias or cardiac arrest. In some other neurological diseases (e.g. muscular dystrophies, Friedreich's ataxia, Huntington's chorea) unpredictable responses to both depolarizing and non-depolarizing agents may occur. In Duchenne progressive muscular dystrophy, hazards associated with induction and recovery have been reported; these are likely to be due to the associated cardiomyopathy. Furthermore, the development of a hyperpyrexia-like response has been associated with the use of suxamethonium.

In those neurological disorders which involve autonomic disturbances (e.g. diabetic autonomic neuropathy, acute polyneuritis, Shy–Drager syndrome), enhanced falls in arterial pressure can be predicted following the administration of most general anaesthetic agents or other drugs with significant cardiovascular effects (e.g.

phenothiazines, tubocurarine). This is undoubtedly due to the inadequacy of compensatory baroreceptor mechanisms.

Endocrine disease

There have been suggestions that an increased response to drugs acting on the CNS, including opioid analgesics and various general anaesthetic agents, may occur in patients with myxoedema. Various factors, including a decreased efficiency of microsomal enzyme systems, alterations in drug distribution due to associated bradycardia or congestive cardiac failure, prolonged gastrointestinal transit and changes in body temperature may be involved.

Thyrotoxicosis is well-known to affect metabolism and more specific pharmacokinetic studies have shown enhancement of microsomal drug oxidation. Binding of both acidic and basic drugs to plasma proteins is decreased in hyperthyroidism. Evidence of sympathetic overactivity is an accompanying feature of uncontrolled thyrotoxicosis. A varying response to a number of drugs used during anaesthesia may thus be anticipated.

Adrenocorticosteroids exert permissive effects on catecholamines. Thus, an exaggerated response to a variety of drugs with a propensity to reduce the systemic blood pressure may occur in patients with inadequate adrenal function, and adequate replacement therapy should always be provided.

In patients with a phaeochromocytoma, drugs with the ability to release histamine (e.g. morphine, tubocurarine) or to induce dysrhythmias (e.g. halothane, enflurane) may induce exaggerated hypertensive responses or disorders of cardiac conduction. Similarly, patients with carcinoid tumours are also at risk of developing tachyarrhythmias and hypertension when drugs with histamine-provoking activity are administered.

Further reading

Abbott TR. Anaesthesia in untreated myxoedema. *British Journal of Anaesthesia* 1967; **39**: 510–514.

Armitage P, Berry G. *Statistical Methods in Medical Research*, 2nd edn. Oxford: Blackwell Scientific Publications, 1987.

Bentley JB, Borel JD, Nenad RE Jr, Gillespie TJ. Age and fentanyl pharmacokinetics. *Anesthesia and Analgesia* 1982; **61**: 968–971.

Bentley JB, Vaughan RW, Gandolfi J, Cork RC. Halothane biotransformation in obese and non-obese patients. *Anesthesiology* 1982; **57**: 94–97.

Berry G. Statistical significance and confidence intervals. *Medical Journal of Australia* 1986; **144**: 618–619.

Bradford Hill A. *A Short Textbook of Medical Statistics*, 11th edn. London Hodder and Stoughton, 1984.

Brown GW. Standard deviation, standard error: which 'standard' should we use? *American Journal of Diseases of Childhood* 1982; **136**: 937–941.

Bulpitt CJ. Confidence intervals. *Lancet* 1987; **i**: 494–497.

Bush GH, Stead AL. The use of *d*-tubocurarine in neonatal anaesthesia. *British Journal of Anaesthesia* 1962; **34**: 721–728.

Christiensen JH, Andreasen F. Individual variation in the response to thiopental. *Acta Anaesthetica Scandinavica* 1978; **22**: 303–313.

Churchill-Davidson HC, Wise RP. Neuromuscular transmission in the newborn infant. *Anesthesiology* 1963; **24**: 271–278.

Cohen EN, Brewer HW, Smith D. The metabolism and elimination of *d*-tubocurarine-H^3. *Anesthesiology* 1967; **28**: 309–317.

Crooks J, O'Malley K, Stevenson IH. Pharmacokinetics in the elderly. *Clinical Pharmacokinetics* 1976; **1**: 280–296.

Day RO, Brooks PM. Variations in response to non-steroidal anti-inflammatory drugs. *British Journal of Clinical Pharmacology* 1987; **23**: 655–658.

Dean G. *The Porphyrias — A Story of Inheritance and Environment*, 2nd edn. London: Pitman, 1971; 1–118.

Doenicke R, Grote B, Lorenz W. Blood and blood substitutes. *British Journal of Anaesthesia* 1977; **49**: 681–688.

Dundee JW, Gray TC. Resistance to *d*-tubocurarine chloride in the presence of liver damage. *Lancet* 1953; **ii**: 16–17.

Duvaldestin P, Agoston S, Henzel D *et al*. Pancuronium pharmacokinetics in patients with liver cirrhosis. *British Journal of Anaesthesia* 1978; **50**: 1131–1136.

Edwards R, Mosher VB. Alcohol abuse, anaesthesia and intensive care. *Anaesthesia* 1980; **35**: 474–489.

Eger EI II, Severinghaus JW. Effect of uneven pulmonary distribution of blood and gas on induction with inhalational anaesthetics. *Anesthesiology* 1964; **25**: 620–626.

Eichelbaum M. Drug metabolism in thyroid disease. *Clinical Pharmacokinetics* 1976; **1**: 339–350.

Evans DAP, Manley KA, McKusick VA. Genetic control of isoniazid metabolism in man. *British Medical Journal* 1960; **2**: 485–491.

Fisher DM, O'Keeffe C, Stanski DR *et al*. Pharmacokinetics and pharmacodynamics of *d*-tubocurarine in infants, children and adults. *Anesthesiology* 1982; **57**: 203–208.

Flaherty JT. Nitrate tolerance — a review of the evidence. *Drugs* 1989; **37**: 523–550.

Frederiksen MC, Ruo TI, Chow MJ, Atkinson AJ Jr. Theophylline pharmacokinetics in pregnancy. *Clinical Pharmacology and Therapeutics* 1986; **40**: 321–326.

Friis-Hansen B. Body water compartments in children. Changes during growth and related changes in body composition. *Pediatrics* 1961; **28**: 169–181.

Gardner MJ, Altman DG. *Statistics with Confidence*. London: British Medical Journal, 1989.

Gell PGH, Coombes RRA. *Clinical Aspects of Immunology*, 2nd edn. Oxford: Blackwell Scientific Publications, 1968.

Gibaldi M. Drug distribution in renal failure. *American Journal of Medicine* 1977; **62**: 471–474.

Gregory GA, Eger EI II, Munson ES. The relationship between age and halothane requirement in man. *Anesthesiology* 1969; **30**: 488–491.

Gronert GA. Malignant hyperthermia. *Anesthesiology* 1980; **53**: 395–423.

Hockings NF. Problems in prescribing for the elderly. *Hospital Update* 1981; **7**: 1201–1204.

Horowitz JD, Henry CA, Syrjanen ML *et al*. Combined use of nitroglycerin and acetylcysteine in the management of unstable angina pectoris. *Circulation* 1988; **77**: 787–794.

Hunter JM, Jones RS, Utting JE. Use of atracurium in patients with no renal function. *British Journal of Anaesthesia* 1982; **54**: 1251–1258.

Hurwitz N, Wade OL. Intensive hospital monitoring of adverse reactions to drugs. *British Medical Journal* 1969; **1**: 531–536.

James ML. Endocrine disease and anaesthesia. *Anaesthesia* 1970; **25**: 232–252.

Jusko WJ. Influence of cigarette smoking on drug metabolism in man. *Drug Metabolism Reviews* 1979; **9**: 221–226.

Kirkwood BR. *Essentials of Medical Statistics*. Oxford: Blackwell Scientific Publications, 1980.

Koch-Weser J, Greenblatt DS *et al*. Drug disposition in old age. *New England Journal of Medicine* 1982; **306**: 1081–1082.

Krauer B, Krauer F. Drug kinetics in pregnancy. *Clinical Pharmacokinetics* 1977; **2**: 167–181.

Langman MJS. Towards estimation and confidence intervals. *British Medical Journal* 1986; **292**: 716.

Lewis RE, Cruse JM, Richley JV. Effects of anaesthesia and operation on the classical pathway of complement activation. *Clinical Immunology and Immunopathology* 1982; **23**: 666–671.

Lindenbaum J, Mellow MH, Blackstone MO *et al*. Variations in biological availability of digoxin from four preparations. *New England Journal of Medicine* 1971; **285**: 1344–1347.

Mather LE, Meffin PJ. Clinical pharmacokinetics of pethidine. *Clinical Pharmacokinetics* 1978; **3**: 352–368.

Morgan DJ, Blackman GL, Paull JD *et al.* Pharmacokinetics and plasma binding of thiopental: studies at Cesarian section. *Anesthesiology* 1981; **54**: 474–480.

Muravchick S. Immediate and long-term nervous system effects of anaesthesia in elderly patients. *Clinics in Anaesthesiology* 1986; **4**: 1035–1048.

Neuberger J, Kenna JG. Halothane hepatitis: a model of immune mediated toxicity. *Clinical Science* 1987; **72**: 263–270.

Nightingale DA. Use of atracurium in neonatal anaesthesia. *British Journal of Anaesthesia* 1986; **58**: 32S–36S.

Perucca E, Crema A. Plasma protein binding of drugs in pregnancy. *Clinical Pharmacokinetics* 1982; **7**: 336–352.

Pickles H. Prescriptions, adverse reactions and the elderly. *Lancet* 1986; **ii**: 40–41.

Radford SG, Lockyer JA, Simpson PJ. Immunological aspects of adverse reactions in anaesthesia. *British Journal of Anaesthesia* 1982; **54**: 859–864.

Rylance G. Drugs in children. *British Medical Journal* 1981; **282**: 50–51.

Sauder RA, Hirshman CA. Anaesthesia for the patient with reactive airway disease. *Current Opinions in Anaesthesiology* 1989; **2**: 776–781.

Sear JW. Adverse effects of drugs given by injection. In: Taylor TH, Major E (eds). *Hazards and Complications of Anaesthesia.* Edinburgh: Churchill Livingstone, 1987; 213–236.

Sjöholm I, Kober A, Odar-Cederlöf I, Borga O. Protein binding of drugs in uremic and normal serum. The role of endogenous binding inhibitors. *Biochemical Pharmacology* 1976; **25**: 1205–1213.

Smith CL, Bush GH. Anaesthesia and progressive muscular dystrophy. *British Journal of Anaesthesia* 1985; **57**: 1113–1118.

Stevens WC, Dolan WM, Gibbons RT *et al.* Minimal alveolar concentration (MAC) of isoflurane with and without nitrous oxide in patients of various ages. *Anesthesiology* 1975; **42**: 197–200.

Tarlov AR, Brewer GJ, Carson PE, Alving AS. Primaquine sensitivity. *Archives of Internal Medicine* 1962; **109**: 209–234.

Vestal RE. Drug use in the elderly: a review of problems and special considerations. *Drugs* 1978; **16**: 358–362.

Watkins J. Intravenous therapy and immunological disasters. *Theoretical Surgery* 1986; **1**: 103–112.

West JR, Smith HW, Chasis H. Glomerular filtration rate, effective renal blood flow and maximal tubular excretory capacity in infants. *Journal of Pediatrics* 1948; **32**: 10–18.

Wilkinson GR, Shenker S. Drug disposition and liver disease. *Drug Metabolism Reviews* 1975; **4**: 139–175.

Williams RL, Mamelok RD. Hepatic diseases and drug pharmacokinetics. *Clinical Pharmacokinetics* 1980; **5**: 528–547.

Wooley PH, Griffin J, Panayi GS, Batchelor JR, Welsh KI, Gibson TJ. HLA-DR antigens and toxic reaction to sodium aurothiomalate and *d*-penicillamine in patients with rheumatoid arthritis. *New England Journal of Medicine* 1980; **303**: 300–302.

Zhang A-Z, Pasternak GW. Opiates and enkephalins: a common binding site mediates their analgesic action in rats. *Life Sciences* 1981; **29**: 843–847.

Zhou H-H, Koshakji RP, Silberstein DJ, Wilkinson GP. Racial differences in drug response: altered sensitivity to and clearance of propranolol in men of Chinese descent as compared with American Whites. *New England Journal of Medicine* 1989; **320**: 565–570.

Chapter 7
Intravenous Anaesthetic Agents

Intravenous anaesthetic agents are usually defined as drugs which induce loss of consciousness in one arm–brain circulation time (normally 10–20 s), when given in appropriate dosage. In the late 19th century and the early years of the 20th century many drugs were administered intravenously in an attempt to produce rapid unconsciousness; these included several opiates, chloral hydrate, bromethol, infusions of chloroform and ether and various intravenous preparations of the available barbiturate derivatives (e.g. amylobarbitone, butobarbitone, pentobarbitone). Unfortunately, problems with the delayed onset and prolonged duration of anaesthesia, as well as the toxic effects of the individual drugs, were frequently encountered.

In the early 1930s, a milestone in anaesthetic practice was achieved with the introduction of barbiturates with a rapid onset of hypnotic activity and an extremely short duration of action. In 1932, hexobarbitone was introduced by Weese and Scharpff in Germany; its rapid onset of action was responsible for its acceptance as an induction agent. It was soon superseded by thiopentone, which was independently studied by Lundy and Waters in the USA. The potential hazards of thiopentone (particularly when used alone in large doses) were not fully appreciated until the disaster at Pearl Harbor in 1941. In subsequent years thiopentone became widely accepted as an intravenous induction agent; however, many thiobarbiturates have essentially similar properties, and in some respects it is remarkable that the drug has stood the test of time. Methohexitone, which became generally available in the UK in 1959, is the only other barbiturate derivative in current use.

In 1941 Hans Selye reported on the ability of certain steroids to produce reversible sleep in animals. The development of many such drugs was precluded because of their hormonal effects; nevertheless, several steroids have been used as anaesthetic agents. In the late 1950s hydroxydione was introduced into anaesthetic practice; it had a marked hypnotic potency but no hormonal actions. Due to the poor solubility of the drug, administration was dependent on its continuous infusion in a large volume of saline, and the onset of action was delayed. A polymerized and more concentrated preparation of the drug was subsequently introduced; unfortunately this led to the frequent occurrence of thrombophlebitis, and the use of hydroxydione was discontinued.

More recently, Althesin (a combination of the steroids alphaxolone and alphadolone) was used as an intravenous anaesthetic agent. Despite its many advantages, the occurrence of anaphylactic or anaphylactoid phenomena (particularly bronchospasm and severe hypotension) led to the withdrawal of the drug in 1984. These phenomena were probably related to the polyethoxylated castor oil (Cremophor EL) which was used in Althesin to increase the solubility of the steroids. Minaxolone, a water-soluble steroid, has also been used in humans as an induction agent. Its use was associated with a significant incidence of excitatory effects; in addition it was shown to induce neoplasia in experimental animals and development was subsequently discontinued.

No steroid anaesthetics are currently available in the UK. However, 5β-pregnanolone, a steroid compound originally studied but rejected because of its aqueous insolubility, has more recently been reformulated as an emulsion and evaluated in clinical studies in humans. Induction with this agent appeared to be reliable and pain on injection was not a feature. Haemodynamic changes were minimal and excitatory effects were not significant.

A number of derivatives of eugenol have also been used as intravenous anaesthetics. Eugenol is chemically related to phenoxyacetic acid and is one of the main constituents of oil of cloves. The eugenol derivative propanidid was used as an occasional induction agent for approximately 20 years, but was withdrawn in 1983. Propanidid is an ester which is poorly soluble in water; preparations of the drug also contained Cremophor EL, and occasionally produced bronchospasm and profound hypotension during induction. In addition, propanidid caused various excitatory effects (e.g. hiccup, abnormal muscle movements, respiratory stimulation and convulsions).

Other drugs which have been used as intravenous anaesthetic agents are structurally related to cyclohexamine. One analogue, phencyclidine, was used in the 1950s as an induction agent; however, it was soon discarded because of severe psychotomimetic reactions. The related compound ketamine was introduced in 1970; although it does not produce loss of consciousness in one arm–brain circulation time, it is usually classified as an intravenous anaesthetic agent. In spite of several disadvantages, the drug has a definite, albeit limited, place in anasthetic practice.

In contrast, etomidate is an imidazole ester with hypnotic activity but little or no analgesic effects. Although etomidate has a high margin of safety, it has several disadvantages which have restricted its use as an anaesthetic agent.

Propofol is a chemically inert phenolic derivative with anaesthetic properties. The clinical use of propofol in its original Cremophor EL formulation was first described in 1977. It was reformulated as an aqueous emulsion which has been generally available since 1985. The rapid and symptom-free recovery associated with the use of this drug has undoubtedly contributed to its current popularity. It is widely used as an induction agent (particularly in day-case procedures) and for maintenance of anaesthesia by infusion techniques.

All intravenous anaesthetics must be administered in aqueous solution or as an oil or emulsion which is readily miscible with plasma. In addition, they must be partially non-ionized and lipid-soluble in plasma at pH 7.4 in order to cross the blood–brain barrier and produce rapid loss of consciousness. These conflicting physicochemical requirements are usually resolved by the use of alkaline solutions or by the administration of lipid-soluble drugs in water-miscible oils and emulsions. In consequence bases, buffers or solubilizing agents are frequently added to solutions of anaesthetic agents.

In this chapter, the following drugs are considered as anaesthetic agents:

1 Barbiturates (thiopentone and methohexitone).

2 Etomidate.

3 Propofol.

4 Ketamine.

Although other drugs (e.g. benzodiazepines, opioids, neuroleptic agents) are sometimes used to induce anaesthesia, they do not produce rapid loss of consciousness in therapeutic doses and are not usually considered as intravenous anaesthetics.

Barbiturates

Barbiturates are derivatives of barbituric acid, which was first prepared in 1863 as a condensation product of urea and malonic acid.

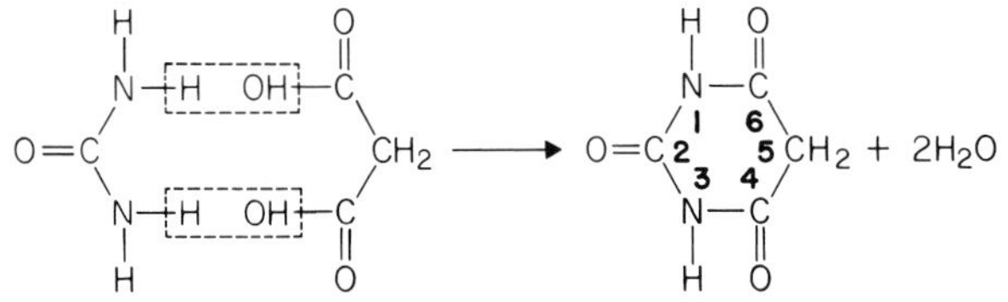

Although barbituric acid itself is inert, the substitution of both hydrogen atoms at the C5 position by organic groups produces compounds with hypnotic activity. These compounds are referred to as oxybarbiturates. An analogous series of compounds can be regarded as substitution products of thiobarbituric acid.

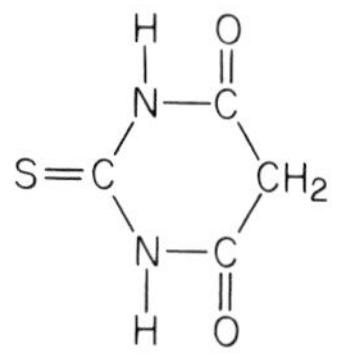

In general thiobarbiturates (e.g. thiopentone) have a greater lipid solubility than their oxybarbiturate analogues (e.g. pentobarbitone) and thus cross the blood–brain barrier more rapidly. Most of the barbiturates which have been used as sedatives, hypnotics or anticonvulsants contain two alkyl groups with 2–5 carbon atoms at the C5 position of the ring. Within certain limits, an increase in the length of these alkyl groups enhances hypnotic potency and activity. Substitution by extremely long alkyl groups decreases hypnotic activity and may be associated with convulsant properties. Similarly, *N*-methylation of the N1 or N3 nitrogen atom produces compounds which can have excitatory or convulsant side-effects (e.g. methohexitone and methylphenobarbitone). Conversely, substitution by aromatic or heterocyclic groups at C5 is often associated with anticonvulsant effects (e.g. phenobarbitone).

Barbiturates are not readily soluble in water (except in alkaline solutions). In aqueous conditions their solubility is dependent on isomerism from the keto to the enol form (tautomerism), and their presence in solution as weak acids:

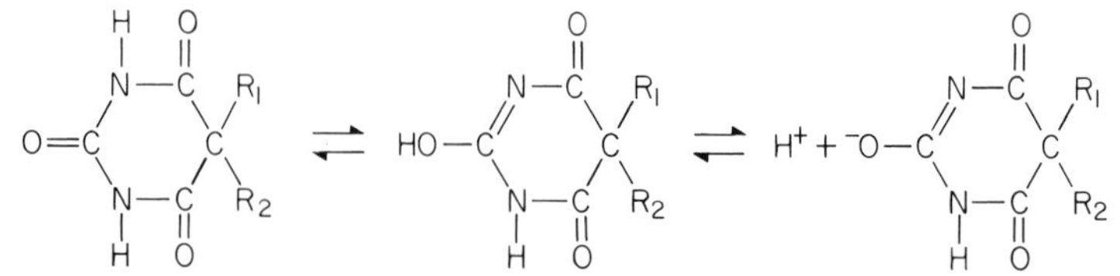

Isomerism from the keto to the enol form is pH-dependent, and readily occurs in alkaline solutions. The water solubility of sodium salts of barbituric acids relies upon the presence of the enol form and its subsequent ionization in alkaline solution:

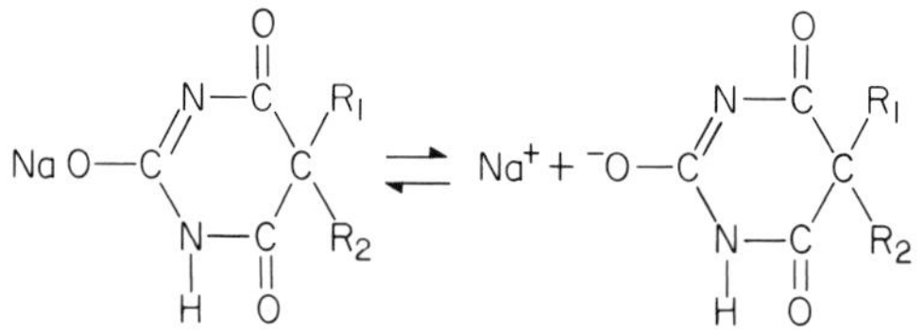

The dissociation constants of most barbiturates range from 7.3 to 8.0; consequently, in *in vivo* conditions the degree of ionization of different drugs is relatively constant.

In contrast, there are marked differences between the various barbiturates with regard to lipid solubility, plasma protein binding and the extent of drug metabolism. In general, thiobarbiturates have a high lipid solubility, are extensively bound to plasma proteins (usually 60–90%) and are completely metabolized by liver enzymes. Some oxybarbiturates (e.g. cyclobarbitone and pentobarbitone) are 20 times less lipid-soluble, moderately bound to plasma proteins (i.e. 30–50%) and are mainly eliminated by hepatic metabolism. Other oxybarbiturates (e.g. barbitone and phenobarbitone) are approximately 200 times less lipid-soluble, only slightly bound to plasma proteins (i.e. less than 20%) and are almost entirely excreted unchanged in the urine. In consequence, barbitone and phenobarbitone have a relatively long terminal half-life.

Although barbiturates have depressant effects on cellular function in many tissues and organs, the central nervous system (CNS) is particularly sensitive to their effects. Early neurophysiological studies suggested that the responses to barbiturates were dependent on the suppression of the midbrain reticular formation (the reticular activating system). Thus, barbiturates modified sensory and auditory cortical evoked responses, and depressed the electroencephalogram (EEG) and arousal response to reticular stimulation. These effects were generally considered to be due to the modification of synaptic activity.

It was subsequently shown that excitatory neurotransmission (and excitatory postsynaptic potentials) were depressed by barbiturates while inhibitory transmission was unaltered or enhanced. These effects were initially believed to be related to actions on cellular metabolism; thus barbiturates decrease cerebral oxygen consumption and mitochondrial respiration, increase glycogen and phosphate levels, reduce acetylcholine release, and depress dopamine, noradrenaline and 5-hydroxytryptamine turnover in certain areas of the brain. It is now considered that these changes represent indirect and secondary effects of barbiturates on the CNS.

In the past 15 years it has been demonstrated that barbiturates have significant effects on γ-aminobutyric acid (GABA)-dependent chloride channels in the brain. GABA is probably the main inhibitory neurotransmitter in the CNS, and is believed to mediate both presynaptic and postsynaptic inhibition at 20–40% of all synapses. In the presence of GABA, chloride channels in neuronal membranes open, allowing chloride ions to diffuse into the neurone; this results in hyperpolarization and decreased neuronal excitability (i.e. inhibition).

Two subtypes of the GABA receptor, designated $GABA_A$ and $GABA_B$, are now recognized. $GABA_A$ receptors are sited in a macromolecular complex which includes specific interaction sites for benzodiazepines, barbiturates and steroid anaesthetic agents, as well as for several categories of convulsants. Barbiturates appear to act by increasing the duration of GABA-dependent chloride channel opening. This effect is thought to be principally mediated via β subunits of the $GABA_A$ receptor, in contrast to benzodiazepines, which increase the frequency of channel opening and have a greater affinity for α subunits of the receptor. Barbiturates also inhibit the binding of radiolabelled picrotoxin analogues at sites related to chloride channels, and the chronic administration of phenobarbitone increases GABA levels in all regions of the CNS. These neurochemical phenomena may well account for many of the electrophysiological effects of barbiturates on the brain.

However, recent experimental evidence using a patch clamp method and the planar lipid bilayer technique (in which a single membrane protein is isolated and fused into an artificial lipid membrane) have demonstrated that barbiturates can have direct effects on sodium channels. A reduction of voltage-dependent activation, with a decreased frequency and duration of channel opening times, has been observed in the presence of clinically relevant concentrations of barbiturates. It would also appear that barbiturates may have differential effects on the several potassium channel subtypes. K^+ channel activation and blockade (resulting in hyperpolarization and depolarization respectively) have been demonstrated in different species and at varying neuronal sites. It could thus be inferred that the hypnotic effects (and excitatory side-effects) of barbiturates may depend upon an integration of the responses of the various ion channels at differing sites within the CNS. However, as both intravenous barbiturates in common use (thiopentone and methohexitone) are chiral compounds (Chapter 4), the receptor affinity and pharmacodynamic effects of the different enantiomers may also be of considerable import in this context.

Barbiturates have been widely used as sedatives and hypnotics for many years and proprietary preparations of amylobarbitone, butobarbitone and quinalbarbitone are still available in the UK. Although they are currently classified as controlled drugs, they are sometimes used to induce sleep. In some patients with long-standing and intractable insomnia, they may produce more predictable and reliable effects than the benzodiazepines. Nevertheless, there are many disadvantages associated with their use. Like other hypnotic drugs, they impair judgement and increase reaction time; ambulant patients should always be warned of their hazards in relation to driving, working at heights and operating dangerous machinery. All barbiturates may impair psychomotor performance or produce hangover effects on the day after administration. In addition, hypnotic doses may affect respiration; accidental or deliberate barbiturate overdosage is classically associated with severe respiratory depression. Barbiturates can act with other central depressants, including ethyl alcohol, and are particularly dangerous in patients with pulmonary disease (e.g. chronic bronchitis and asthma). They induce hepatic enzymes concerned with drug metabolism, and may affect the breakdown of other drugs (e.g. oral anticoagulants, tricyclic antidepressants, anticonvulsants and oral contraceptives). They may also precipitate acute porphyria in genetically susceptible patients. The elimination of barbiturates may be compromised in hepatic and renal impairment and in patients over 60 years old. In general they are poorly tolerated by elderly patients and drowsiness, disorientation and ataxia may result in slurred speech, falls and fractures, poor memory and acute confusional states. This increased susceptibility is partly due to pharmacokinetic factors (i.e. decreased hepatic oxidative drug metabolism) and partly to enhanced sensitivity at neuronal sites in the CNS.

Continuous or long-term barbiturate administration commonly causes drug tolerance, due to hepatic enzyme induction (pharmacokinetic tolerance) as well as due to increased neuronal sensitivity (pharmacodynamic tolerance). Barbiturates may antagonize the effects of analgesics, and may induce physical and psychological dependence. Consequently, barbiturate abuse is not uncommon.

In addition to their use as hypnotics, some barbiturates (particularly phenobarbitone and primidone) are used as anticonvulsant drugs. Only two barbiturates (thiopentone and methohexitone) are currently used as anaesthetic agents.

Thiopentone

Thiopentone (5-ethyl-5′-(1-methylbutyl)-2-thiobarbituric acid; Fig. 7.1) is the sulphur analogue of the oxybarbiturate pentobarbitone. The sodium salt is a pale yellow powder with a bitter taste and is readily soluble in water. The solution commonly used to induce anaesthesia (2.5% w/v) has a pH of 10.5.

Thiopentone

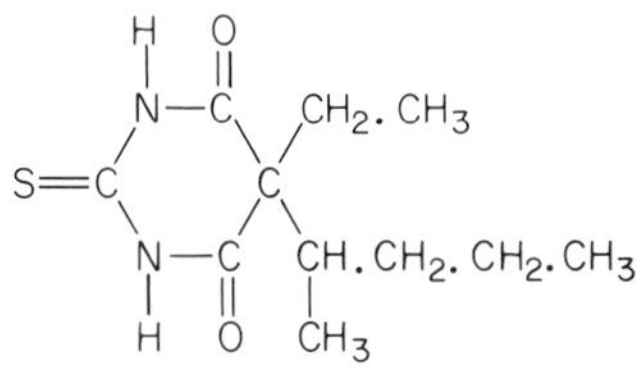

Methohexitone

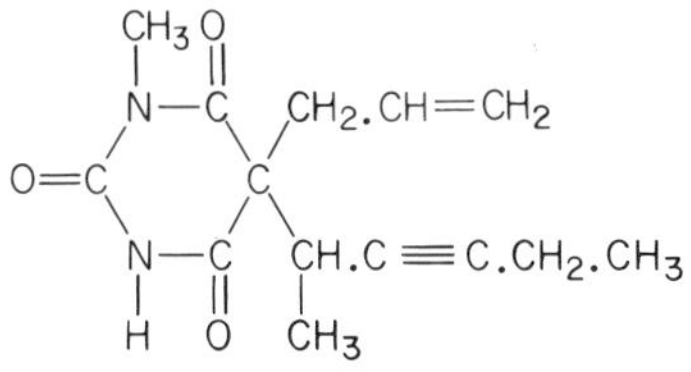

Etomidate

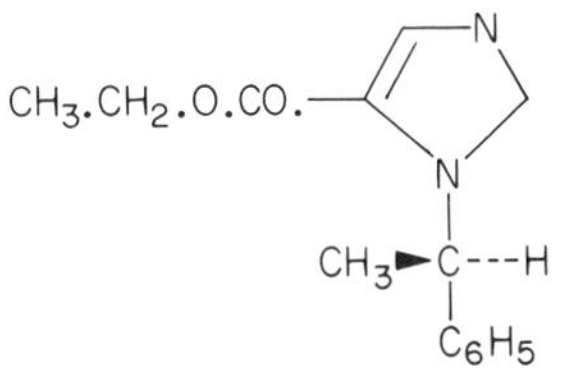

Propofol

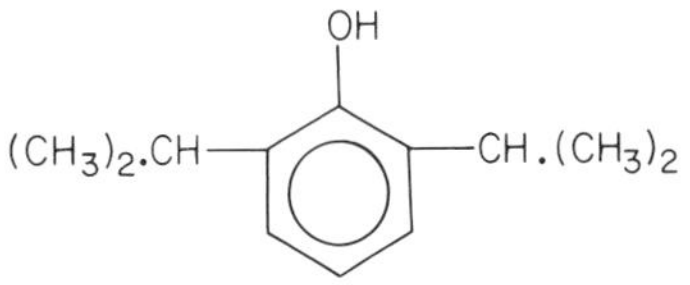

Ketamine

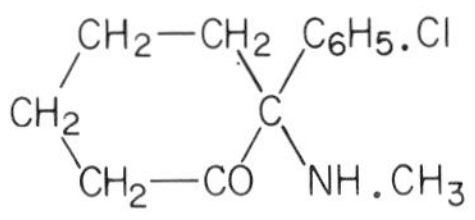

Fig. 7.1 Chemical structure of intravenous anaesthetics.

There are two reasons for this:

1 All salts of weak acids form alkaline solutions when dissolved in water. In these conditions, sodium thiopentone ($pK_a = 7.6$) ionizes and the thiopentone anion can attract H^+, forming an undissociated weak acid. Thus, the resulting solution is alkaline:

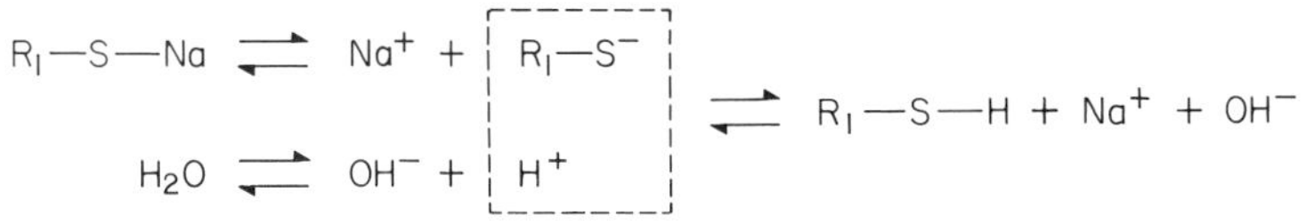

Nevertheless the extent to which this occurs is limited, due to the small concentration of H^+ in solution. At pH 10.5, about 99.9% of thiopentone is still present in the ionized form R_1—S^-. The solubility of the non-ionized form R_1—S—H in water is extremely low and in concentrations above 0.003% (30 μg ml^{-1}) it readily precipitates from solution.

2 Commercial preparations of thiopentone sodium contain 6 parts of sodium carbonate to 100 parts of barbiturate (by weight). Sodium carbonate produces free hydroxyl ions in solution, and is added to prevent the precipitation of the insoluble free acid (R_1—S—H) by atmospheric carbon dioxide. Solutions of thiopentone sodium may remain stable at room temperature for up to 2 weeks (and for longer at 4°C) but should be immediately discarded if they become cloudy. They are not normally used more than 48 h after their preparation.

Due to their alkaline pH, 2.5% solutions of thiopentone are usually bacteriostatic, but may be incompatible with many basic drugs. In general, thiopentone should not be mixed with oxidizing agents, acidic solutions or drugs normally administered as sulphates, chlorides or hydrochlorides.

Effects on the central nervous system

The effects of thiopentone on the CNS are closely related to the dose and rate of administration of the drug. After a normal induction dose of thiopentone (3–5 mg kg^{-1}), the rapid loss of consciousness is principally due to two factors. In the first place, brain tissue is extremely vascular and normally receives about 25% of the cardiac output. Second, thiopentone is highly lipid-soluble (oil/water solubility coefficient = 500–700) and more than 90% of the drug in the cerebral capillaries immediately crosses the blood–brain barrier. At pH 7.4, 39% of the drug is ionized (pK_a = 7.6) and approximately 80% is bound to plasma albumin. However, these factors do not significantly restrict the transfer of thiopentone to the brain. The initial loss of consciousness is usually smooth and excitatory side-effects are rare. The onset of sleep is often preceded by one or more deep breaths and may be associated with rapid eye movements and associated EEG changes. Characteristically, the EEG shows a variable amplitude and high frequency pattern (predominantly at 20–30 Hz); this is usually replaced by slow-wave activity as anaesthesia deepens. The high-frequency response may be due to the selective depression of inhibitory neurones in the reticular formation. It may correspond to the second (excitement) stage of anaesthesia described by Guedel and could account for an enhanced reflex response to surgical stimulation, increased vagal activity and laryngospasm and hyperalgesia (a decreased threshold for the appreciation of a painful stimulus). These effects may be shown to occur when small doses of thiopentone are administered or they may be observed clinically during recovery from barbiturate anaesthesia.

As anaesthesia deepens due to the increased cerebral uptake of thiopentone, cortical responsiveness declines and EEG waveforms of low voltage become predominant. As the dose of thiopentone is increased, effects on the brainstem are produced. Respiratory depression is due to a direct action on the respiratory centre and its pontine connections; the sensitivity to carbon dioxide is decreased in proportion to the depth of anaesthesia. Consequently, $Paco_2$ increases, pH falls and apnoea may occur. In deep barbiturate anaesthesia, hypoxic drive mediated by the aortic and carotid chemoreceptors may play an important part in the maintenance of respiration. Fetal respiration is particularly sensitive to thiopentone. In contrast to the opiates, barbiturates predominantly affect the depth rather than the rate of respiration. In clinical practice the respiratory effects of thiopentone may be considerably modified by the degree of surgical stimulation and by the concomitant use of other central depressant drugs. Patients with impaired cardiovascular and respiratory function may be particularly sensitive to the effects of thiopentone.

A phenomenon described as acute tolerance may occur with thiopentone. After the administration of different doses, the plasma concentration at the time of recovery is directly related to the dose (i.e. CNS sensitivity declines as the dose of thiopentone is increased). The earlier return of consciousness has also been related to the increased rate of injection of a given dose of the drug. It is unclear whether this phenomenon truly reflects an alteration in CNS sensitivity to thiopentone (i.e. a pharmacodynamic effect), or may be explained by distribution disequilibrium (hysteresis; a pharmacokinetic effect). Indeed, the concept of acute tolerance to thiopentone has recently been challenged.

Thiopentone and other barbiturates also decrease cerebral metabolism and reduce oxygen consumption (see p. 213). Cerebral blood flow, cerebral blood volume and cerebrospinal fluid pressure also fall during barbiturate anaesthesia, possibly due to the decreased production of carbon dioxide. Consequently, thiopentone is sometimes used for cerebral resuscitation or to reduce raised intracranial pressure. These effects may be modified by any changes in systemic $Paco_2$ produced by respiratory depression, which will have opposing effects on cerebrovascular tone and pressure.

Effects on the cardiovascular system

In healthy patients, the plasma concentration of thiopentone associated with surgical anaesthesia causes minimal cardiovascular depression. Nevertheless, normal induction doses cause a variable degree of hypotension. Particular problems may occur in hypovolaemic states, in patients with cardiovascular disease (including hypertension) or in patients who are concurrently receiving drugs which affect the sympathetic nervous system (e.g. vasodilators and β-adrenoceptor antagonists). In these conditions, the ability of the cardiovascular system to compensate for the haemodynamic effects of thiopentone is impaired and dose requirements are reduced. The reduction in blood pressure produced by thiopentone is primarily due to decreased stroke volume and cardiac output; indeed, there may be a compensatory reflex increase in systemic vascular resistance.

The changes in cardiac output may be due to several factors. In the first place, the vasomotor centre and the hypothalamic nuclei controlling the force of cardiac contraction may be depressed by thiopentone. In addition, ganglionic transmission and the contractility of vascular smooth muscle may be impaired, causing venodilatation and the peripheral pooling of blood. High doses may directly depress cardiac contractility, probably due to the local anaesthetic (membrane-stabilizing) effects of thiopentone.

Renal effects

During thiopentone anaesthesia glomerular filtration rate, renal plasma flow and electrolyte and water excretion are decreased. These effects may be partly due to the reduction in renal blood flow produced by thiopentone, but are mainly related to the increased release of antidiuretic hormone (ADH) from the posterior lobe of the pituitary gland. Secretion of ADH is dependent on the activity of the hypothalamic nuclei and the integrity of the hypophyseal tract. Suppression of inhibitory pathways affecting hypothalamic nuclei (particularly the supraoptic nucleus) increases the secretion of ADH. Consequently, urine output during thiopentone anaesthesia is approximately 0.1 ml min^{-1} (about 10% of normal). In uraemic patients a decrease in the protein binding of thiopentone may occur and cause potentiation of its effects.

Hepatic effects

There is little or no definite evidence that normal induction doses of thiopentone cause any impairment of hepatic function. Nevertheless, respiratory depression (producing hypoxia and hypercarbia), as well as some systemic and hepatic diseases, may adversely affect liver blood flow and hepatocellular function; this may explain the occasional association of thiopentone with toxic jaundice and abnormal liver function tests. In common with other barbiturates, thiopentone may induce hepatic enzymes, increasing the activity of the mixed-function oxidase system (cytochrome P-450) in the smooth endoplasmic reticulum. Enzyme activity may be increased following anaesthesia with thiopentone (although other agents, such as nitrous oxide and halothane, have also been shown to stimulate enzyme activity). Thiopentone may also precipitate acute intermittent porphyria, and its use (as well as all other barbiturates) is absolutely contraindicated in this condition (p. 220).

In chronic hepatic dysfunction, the effects of thiopentone may be prolonged and slower recovery of consciousness may be anticipated. In liver disease the protein binding of thiopentone may be modified by a reduction in albumin synthesis.

Pharmacokinetics

The rapid onset of action of thiopentone is due to the immediate uptake of non-ionized and non-protein-bound drug by the brain. At pH 7.4, 75–80% of thiopentone is bound to plasma albumin, and 61% of the non-protein-bound fraction is non-ionized. As a result, alterations in extracellular pH and protein binding may affect the uptake of thiopentone by the brain. In experimental conditions, the plasma concentration of thiopentone at pH 6.8 is reduced by 40%, presumably due to the enhanced uptake of the non-ionized drug by the tissues. Similarly, alkalosis (e.g. hyperventilation) may increase the concentration and proportion of ionized thiopentone in plasma and diminish the effects of a given dose. In addition, protein-binding sites on plasma albumin may be occupied by other drugs (e.g. probenecid and iodine-containing contrast media): their prior administration may enhance the effects of thiopentone. In *in vitro* conditions high concentrations of many non-steroidal anti-inflammatory drugs (e.g. indomethacin, phenylbutazone and aspirin) displace thiopentone from albumin; the clinical significance of this phenomenon is a matter of conjecture.

High concentrations of thiopentone are present in the brain and other well-perfused tissues within 1 min of intravenous administration. The rapid emergence from sleep after single-dose thiopentone anaesthesia is due to redistribution from the brain to less vascular regions (particularly muscle and skin). These tissues become saturated with thiopentone within 15–30 min; as thiopentone is taken up, the plasma concentration rapidly falls and the drug diffuses out of the brain. In contrast, the fat depots, which have a poor blood supply, may require several hours to take up significant amounts of thiopentone and reach saturation. The concentration of thiopentone in blood, skeletal muscle and fat at various times after its administration is consistent with a physiological pharmacokinetic model with a central blood pool and six tissue compartments (Chapter 2). The model supports the concept that thiopentone is primarily removed from the brain by lean body tissues (e.g. muscle) and that subcutaneous fat only plays a small part in the termination of its anaesthetic effects.

After intravenous administration of thiopentone there is a triexponential decline in the plasma concentration of the drug. The initial rapid disposition phase (half-life = 2–4 min) presumably reflects the distribution of the drug to well-perfused organs (e.g. brain and hepatorenal tissues); this is followed by a slower disposition phase (half-life = 45–60 min) due to the uptake of thiopentone by muscle and skin. Finally, the elimination of the drug from the body is reflected by the terminal decline in plasma concentration (half-life = 5–10 h). The volume of distribution of thiopentone at steady state is slightly greater than body water (1–4 l kg^{-1}), whilst its clearance is approximately 10–20% of liver blood flow (i.e. 1–5 ml min^{-1} kg^{-1}). The low hepatic extraction ratio of thiopentone is consistent with capacity-limited elimination by the liver and will be sensitive to changes in plasma protein binding.

The clearance of thiopentone is greater in infants and children than in adults; it is significantly decreased in obese patients and in elderly subjects.

Since thiopentone is highly lipid-soluble, it is extensively metabolized by the liver (and possibly by other tissues). Only trace amounts are eliminated in the urine (normally less than 1% of the dose). Although metabolism only plays a limited part in recovery from the effects of thiopentone, it is entirely responsible for the eventual elimination of the drug from the body. Drug metabolism is relatively slow (6–15% h^{-1}) and is mainly due to ω-oxidation of thiopentone to the inactive metabolite thiopentone carboxylic acid (ω-oxidation refers to the oxidation of the terminal methyl group on the 1-methylbutyl side-chain to the corresponding carboxylic acid). To some extent, thiopentone is also metabolized by (ω-1) oxidation to hydroxythiopentone, and by desulphuration to its oxybarbiturate analogue pentobarbitone. This compound has a longer half-life than thiopentone (20–50 h) and is itself metabolized to inactive products (e.g. pentobarbitone carboxylic acid, hydroxypentobarbitone). When large doses of thiopentone are used in cerebral resuscitation, thiopentone metabolism becomes non-linear (zero-order) due to saturation of hepatic enzyme systems. In these conditions significant concentrations of thiopentone are present in plasma and may contribute to delayed recovery.

Unwanted effects

Thiopentone is undoubtedly a safe and reliable intravenous induction agent, as long as certain precautions are observed. Facilities for artificial ventilation and oxygenation must always be available. Deep thiopentone anaesthesia can reduce smooth-muscle tone in the gut and depress reflex laryngeal activity, and the risk of aspiration of gastric contents must always be recognized. In particular, the usual recommended dose (4–5 mg kg^{-1}) may need to be considerably reduced in elderly, debilitated and hypovolaemic patients.

In subjects with acute intermittent porphyria and porphyria variegata, thiopentone increases the synthesis of cytochrome P-450 from haem, and thus induces (derepresses) the enzyme ALA synthetase. This enzyme plays a crucial role in porphyrin synthesis by the liver and other tissues. Increased synthesis of porphobilinogen and other porphyrins may cause progressive demyelination and neuropathy, voluntary muscle weakness and paralysis, abdominal pain or psychiatric sequelae. The urine usually contains porphobilinogen and uroporphyrin and may turn red when allowed to stand in daylight for several hours. Some types of porphyria (e.g. erythropoietic, cutanea tarda) are not adversely affected by thiopentone; even in acute intermittent porphyria, barbiturates do not always induce an attack. Nevertheless, the precipitation of acute porphyria may be fatal and barbiturates should be excluded in all types of porphyria.

Thiopentone may induce transient urticarial or erythematous rashes (and occasionally other cutaneous reactions). Urticarial responses are usually related to histamine release from mast cells and may be associated with raised plasma histamine concentrations. This may be related to the dose and speed of injection. True hypersensitivity or anaphylactic responses (i.e. reactions involving immunoglobulins or T lymphocytes) are very rare, with a suggested incidence of 1 in 14 000 to 1 in 20 000. They usually present as bronchospasm, hypotension, generalized oedema or peripheral vascular collapse and may be associated with a significant mortality.

The relatively slow elimination of thiopentone (terminal half-life = 5–10 h) necessitates care and supervision during the prolonged recovery. Patients should be advised not to drive or operate machinery for 24 h after anaesthesia and to avoid alcohol and sedative drugs.

Although intravenous thiopentone is usually painless, inadvertent extravascular administration can cause significant adverse effects. Subcutaneous or perivenous injection may produce local complications ranging from slight pain to extensive tissue necrosis. They are far less frequent with dilute thiopentone (2.5%) than with more concentrated solutions (e.g. 5%, which was widely used at one time). These effects are probably due to local tissue irritation produced by precipitation of insoluble non-ionized thiopentone acid at the pH of extracellular fluid. They are unlikely to be primarily related to the pH of solutions of thiopentone since they are less frequently observed when the slightly more alkaline solution of methohexitone (1%) is used. Dispersal of thiopentone by local injection of hyaluronidase and topically applied demulcents may be useful in the treatment of local complications.

Intra-arterial injection of thiopentone causes immediate, severe and agonizing shooting pain which is usually followed by signs of arterial spasm, with blanching of the limb, increasing cyanosis and disappearance of a pulse. The onset of unconsciousness may be delayed. When more dilute solutions are used the incidence and severity of the sequelae are reduced but gangrene may develop in untreated cases.

The precise explanation for these complications is unclear. Arterial injection is rapidly followed by the precipitation of insoluble thiopentone acid crystals (which have a maximum solubility of 0.003% or 30 $\mu g\ ml^{-1}$ at pH 7.4); these are transported in a progressively narrowing arterial vasculature (where there is no opportunity for dilution) and aggregate in small arterioles. Initial vascular spasm may be due to the local release of noradrenaline from the arterial or arteriolar wall. This is followed by an intense chemical endarteritis which rapidly involves the endothelium and periendothelial tissues. In addition, blood vessels may be occluded by crystals of thiopentone and by erythrocyte and platelet aggregation resulting in arterial thrombosis and gangrene. The important factor in the pathogenesis of the condition is the injection of thiopentone into the arterial tree where the drug is neutralized but is not subsequently diluted. Although crystal formation may occur immediately after intravenous injection due to the alteration in pH, it is of little or no importance as the drug is rapidly diluted within 1–2 s by the collateral venous return.

Table 7.1 Pharmacological properties of intravenous anaesthetic agents.

	Onset of action	Recovery	Cardiovascular effects	Other effects
Thiopentone	Rapid	Relatively rapid; complete recovery delayed	BP ↓ CO ↓	Extravascular complications Arterial thrombosis Laryngospasm and bronchospasm Enzyme induction ↑ ↓ Intracranial pressure
Methohexitone	Rapid	Rapid	BP ↓ CO ↓ HR ↑	Pain on injection Excitatory effects Abnormal muscle movement Cough and hiccup
Etomidate	Rapid	Moderately rapid	Minimal	Pain on injection Excitatory effects Adrenocortical suppression
Propofol	Rapid	Rapid	BP ↓ CO ↓	Pain on injection Delayed recovery after prolonged administration
Ketamine	Slow	Slow	BP ↑ CO ↑ HR ↑	Analgesia ↑ Intracranial pressure Psychotomimetic effects

BP, Blood pressure; CO, cardiac output; HR, heart rate.

Table 7.2 Pharmacokinetics and metabolism of intravenous anaesthetic agents.

	Terminal half-life (min)	Clearance (ml min^{-1} kg^{-1})	Apparent volume of distribution (l kg^{-1})	Metabolites
Thiopentone	300–600	1.4–5.7	1.0–4.0	Thiopentone carboxylic acid Hydroxythiopentone Pentobarbitone
Methohexitone	90–250	10.0–13.0	1.2–2.2	Hydroxymethohexitone Hydroxymethohexitone glucuronide
Etomidate	60–90	10.0–24.3	2.2–4.3	Ethyl alcohol 1-(α-methylbenzyl)-imidazole-5-carboxylic acid
Propofol	300–700	21.4–28.6	3.3–5.7	2,6-Diisopropylphenol glucuronide 2,6-Diisopropylquinol glucuronide
Ketamine	150–200	17.1–20.0	2.9–3.1	Norketamine Hydroxynorketamine Hydroxyketamine glucuronide Hydroxynorketamine glucuronide

After intra-arterial injection of thiopentone, immediate treatment is necessary. If the needle is still *in situ* in the artery, injection of a vasodilator (e.g. papaverine or procaine, 80–120 mg, or possibly a calcium-channel blocker) is required. Temporary sympathetic blockade by continuous axillary block or repeated stellate ganglion block will open up the collateral circulation, and heparin is often useful.

The pharmacological properties and pharmacokinetics of thiopentone are summarized in Tables 7.1 and 7.2.

Methohexitone

Methohexitone is 1-methyl-5-allyl-5′-(1-methyl-2-pentynyl)-2-barbituric acid (Fig. 7.1). There are four possible optically active isomers of the compound; a racemic mixture of two of these stereoisomers (α-*d*-methohexitone and α-*l*-methohexitone) is used for clinical anaesthesia. The sodium salts of both these enantiomorphs are white powders which are readily soluble in water. Commercial preparations of methohexitone also contain 6 parts of sodium carbonate to 100 parts of barbiturate and the drug is usually prepared as a 1% solution with a pH of approximately 11. Aqueous solutions of methohexitone, when maintained at room temperature, have a shelf-life of at least 6 weeks; if other media (e.g. dextrose or saline) are used for the continuous infusion of methohexitone, solutions may become unstable within 24 h. Solutions of methohexitone are usually bacteriostatic due to their alkaline pH, and are often incompatible with solutions of many basic drugs.

Methohexitone is approximately three times as potent as thiopentone (usual induction dose 1–2 mg kg^{-1}), but has a similar profile of pharmacological activity. The rapid onset of action of methohexitone is due to its high lipid solubility (oil : water solubility is approximately 300) and the extensive blood supply to the brain, which normally receives 25% of the cardiac output. The short duration of unconsciousness reflects the redistribution of the drug to less well-perfused organs and tissues, such as muscle and subcutaneous fat. In most respects (e.g. its effects on the CNS, the cardiovascular system, renal and hepatic function, as well as the propensity to induce hepatic enzymes, acute intermittent porphyria and undesirable systemic reactions) methohexitone is similar to thiopentone (Table 7.1). Nevertheless, there are several important differences between the two drugs.

1 There is less danger of tissue damage and vascular complications when methohexitone is injected subcutaneously or intra-arterially. This appears to be directly related to the lower concentration of methohexitone in solutions of the drug. As discussed previously, complications produced by thiopentone in this context are commoner and more serious when concentrated solutions of the drug are injected. Furthermore, experimental studies suggest that high concentrations of methohexitone (e.g. 5%) injected intra-arterially produce similar effects to thiopentone. Thus the dilution of the drug would appear to be the main factor limiting these complications; other properties of barbiturates appear to be of little importance. Paradoxically, localized pain on injection of 1% methohexitone into small veins occurs more frequently than with 2.5% thiopentone; the explanation for this is unknown.

2 Methohexitone (and other barbiturates that are methylated at the N1 position of the oxybarbiturate ring, e.g. methylphenobarbitone) may cause excitatory side-effects. Although these occasionally occur with thiopentone, they are more frequently associated with the use of methohexitone. Involuntary muscle movements, tremor, hypertonus, coughing and hiccuping may be observed in up to 80% of patients. Their incidence is dependent on the dose and rate of administration of the drug and may be modified by appropriate premedication.

Methohexitone can precipitate convulsive activity in patients with an abnormal EEG or a history of focal epilepsy (and has been used for this specific purpose during neurosurgery). Nevertheless, the use of methohexitone in patients with convulsive disorders is controversial, and some authorities consider that the drug can be used safely in patients with a history of epilepsy.

3 Methohexitone may induce tachycardia and is considered to produce less hypotension than thiopentone; some anaesthetists have considered that it may have advantages over thiopentone for induction of anaesthesia in patients in shock.

4 Complete recovery from anaesthesia is significantly quicker after methohexitone than after equivalent doses of thiopentone. Similarly, when given by intermittent injection or infusion, methohexitone is less likely to cumulate. These differences are related to the different pharmacokinetic properties of the two drugs (Table 7.2). After the intravenous injection of a single dose of methohexitone, there may be a biexponential or triexponential decline in the plasma concentration of the drug. The initial rapid distribution phase (half-life = 5–6 min) is due to the distribution of the drug to well-perfused tissues; this may be followed by a slower distribution phase (half-life = 60 min), which presumably indicates the uptake of the drug by less well-perfused tissues, such as muscle and subcutaneous fat. Finally, the elimination of methohexitone from the body is reflected by the terminal decline in plasma concentration (half-life = 1.5–4 h).

5 Methohexitone has been associated with a greater incidence of hypersensitivity responses than thiopentone. However, in contrast to the latter drug, most patients have exhibited periorbital and facial oedema and no deaths have been reported.

The elimination half-life is considerably less than thiopentone. This difference is principally due to the more rapid clearance of methohexitone by the liver as the apparent volumes of distribution are essentially similar. The clearance of methohexitone is approximately 50% of liver blood flow, and the relatively high extraction ratio is consistent with flow-limited hepatic elimination. Thus the clearance of methohexitone may be modified by changes in hepatic blood flow, but is unaffected by changes in protein binding or alterations in hepatic enzyme activity. Both thiopentone and methohexitone are approximately 80% bound to plasma proteins (mainly albumin) at physiological pH values.

Methohexitone is metabolized by (ω-1) oxidation to hydroxymethohexitone, which may also have some hypnotic activity. Hydroxymethohexitone may be eliminated in urine as the glucuronide metabolite. Only trace amounts of the unchanged drug methohexitone can be recovered from bile and urine.

Uses of intravenous barbiturates

Thiopentone is still widely used as an induction agent in anaesthesia. Methohexitone is commonly used in dental outpatient anaesthesia, but its role in day-case surgery has declined since the advent of propofol. Both drugs (particularly methohexitone) have been used by continuous infusion techniques to supplement nitrous oxide anaesthesia. Pharmacokinetic models can be used to determine the dose and the required infusion rate.

When facilities for controlled ventilation are available, thiopentone may be the drug of choice for the treatment of status epilepticus. In this context, it has a more rapid onset of action than diazepam, which can be a considerable advantage. In addition, the drug can be extremely useful in the management of status epilepticus which does not respond to conventional anticonvulsant therapy, particularly when controlled ventilation under neuromuscular blockade is practicable.

Thiopentone and other barbiturates have been used to protect the brain from the effects of hypoxia after stroke and head injury. The haemodynamic effects of the barbiturates may tend to reduce cerebral blood flow. However, the depression of cerebral metabolism reduces brain oedema and intracranial pressure, so that cerebral perfusion actually improves. For such therapeutic procedures, meticulous care of the airway and monitoring of cardiovascular parameters and, when possible, the intracranial pressure are indicated. In the UK, the use of barbiturates for cerebral resuscitation is controversial.

Etomidate

Etomidate (R-(+)-1-(α-methylbenzyl)-imidazole-5-ethylcarboxylate sulphate) is an imidazole derivative and an ester (Fig. 7.1). Although the sulphate salt is freely soluble in water, proprietary preparations of the drug usually contain propylene glycol (35% v/v). This improves the stability of the solution and reduces its local irritant effects. Etomidate is usually prepared and administered as a 0.2% solution (2 mg ml^{-1}). Normal induction doses (0.3 mg kg^{-1}) produce immediate loss of consciousness; the duration of action is dose-dependent and the drug shows little or no tendency to cumulate even with repeated dosage. The mode of action on neuronal membranes and/or neurotransmitters within the CNS has not been clearly defined.

The most significant advantage of etomidate is its relatively high safety margin. There is a 30-fold difference between the anaesthetic dose and the lethal dose, which compares favourably with the five- to 10-fold difference for the intravenous barbiturates. In particular, etomidate has little or no effect on the cardiovascular system. It usually causes a slight fall in peripheral resistance and blood pressure; blood flow in most organs is generally unchanged or slightly increased. Myocardial contractility, oxygen consumption and coronary blood flow are usually unaffected. Etomidate reduces cerebral blood flow and intracranial pressure, and hypnotic doses cause respiratory depression (as assessed by changes in ventilation produced by alterations in inspired $P\text{CO}_2$).

Both anaphylactic and anaphylactoid reactions are uncommon. Occasionally histamine release from mast cells causes skin rashes during the induction of anaesthesia. Severe reactions (e.g. generalized erythema, hypotension, bronchospasm) appear to be commoner when etomidate is used with other drugs. Indeed, some authorities consider that etomidate is the safest induction agent in this context and may be the drug of choice in patients where a hypersensitivity response could be anticipated.

Following the intravenous administration of etomidate, there is usually a biexponential decline in the plasma concentration of the drug. The initial fall in concentration (half-life = 2–5 min) reflects the distribution of the drug to well-perfused tissues. The subsequent slower decline in plasma concentration is due to the elimination of the drug from the body (terminal half-life = 68–75 min). The apparent volume of distribution of etomidate is slightly greater than total body water, and its clearance is 50–80% of liver blood flow (Table 7.2). The relatively high extraction ratio is consistent with flow-limited hepatic clearance (although it is uncertain whether the liver is the only organ concerned with the metabolism of etomidate). Etomidate is bound to albumin to a significant extent (70–80%) and the effects of the drug may be enhanced in the elderly and in hypoalbuminaemic states.

Etomidate is mainly eliminated from the body by metabolism; only trace amounts (1–2% of the dose) are detected in urine and bile. The drug is principally metabolized by ester hydrolysis to ethyl alcohol and its corresponding carboxylic acid metabolite (1-(α-methylbenzyl)-imidazole-5-carboxylic acid). The metabolism of etomidate appears to be mainly dependent on non-specific hepatic esterases, although the drug may also be hydrolysed by plasma cholinesterase. Etomidate can also inhibit plasma cholinesterase by competing with other substrates for the enzyme.

In spite of its advantages, several undesirable effects have restricted the use of etomidate in anaesthetic practice. Etomidate may cause pain on injection in 25–50% of patients. Similarly, etomidate may cause haemolysis (although this appears to be clinically insignificant). Both these problems have been related to the solvent (propylene glycol). Furthermore, etomidate commonly causes excitatory side-effects, particularly spontaneous movements and hypertonicity of voluntary muscle. These phenomena can be modified by suitable premedication or the prior administration of fentanyl or alfentanil. Postoperative nausea and vomiting are also more commonly associated with etomidate than with other induction agents.

Prolonged administration of etomidate by intravenous infusion may result in suppression of adrenocortical function. Etomidate can impair the synthesis of both glucocorticoids and mineralocorticoids by the adrenal cortex. This effect is mediated by high-affinity binding of etomidate to cytochrome P-450 isoforms, resulting in inhibition of the synthesis of 11-hydroxylated, biologically active corticosteroids. Experimental studies also indicate that a continuous infusion of etomidate will cause an increase in levels of the enzyme δ-aminolaevulinic acid (ALA) synthetase. The use of etomidate should therefore be avoided in patients with acute intermittent porphyria.

Propofol

Propofol (2,6-diisopropylphenol; Fig. 7.1) is a chemically inert phenolic compound with anaesthetic properties. It has a high lipid solubility, but is almost insoluble in water; the original preparation contained the solubilizing agent Cremophor EL (polyethoxylated castor oil). This formulation was assessed in a number of preliminary clinical studies but was discarded due to the anaphylactoid potential of Cremophor EL. In the current preparation, propofol is available as a 1% (10 mg ml^{-1}) isotonic emulsion, which contains soya bean oil and purified egg phosphatide.

The normal induction dose of propofol (1.5–2.5 mg kg^{-1}) produces loss of consciousness due to the immediate uptake of the lipid-soluble drug by the CNS. Within several minutes of intravenous administration, the plasma concentration of propofol decreases due to the distribution of the drug throughout the body and its uptake by peripheral tissues. As the plasma concentration falls, propofol diffuses from the CNS into the systemic circulation; when bolus doses of the drug are used to induce anesthesia, there is a rapid recovery of full consciousness and awareness. Postoperative nausea and vomiting appear to be extremely uncommon, particularly when propofol is used as the sole anaesthetic agent. These advantageous properties have undoubtedly contributed to the current popularity of propofol as an induction agent for short procedures and day-case surgery (Table 7.1).

The safety margin of propofol is generally considered to be lower than that of etomidate but greater than the intravenous barbiturates, both with regard to undesirable side-effects and to hypersensitivity responses. Propofol frequently causes a significant reduction in systemic blood pressure, which may fall to 70–80% of the preoperative level. Hypotension is related to the dose and rate of injection and is usually maximal within 5–10 min. The reduction in blood pressure is principally due to a decrease in systemic vascular resistance and is not usually accompanied by tachycardia. Indeed, it has been suggested that, in this context, propofol may act as a calcium-channel blocker or by promoting the release of nitric oxide. Cardiac output may fall, and recent studies indicate that propofol may depress cardiac output in a manner comparable to that of thiopentone. Respiratory side-effects (e.g. cough, laryngospasm) during induction are rarely encountered and propofol is frequently the induction agent of choice for the insertion of the laryngeal mask airway (LMA). Respiratory depression may be observed; apnoea is usually transient, but may be more prolonged when doses at the higher end of the recommended range are used, or when other respiratory depressants are used concomitantly. However excitatory side-effects, including myoclonus, opisthotonos and convulsions, are sometimes associated with the administration of propofol and current data suggest that the use of this drug is contraindicated in epileptic patients. The high placental transfer of propofol and associated neonatal depression preclude its use in obstetric anaesthesia.

There is no evidence to suggest that propofol has any significant effects on renal or hepatic function. Propofol does not induce enzymes involved in drug metabolism or porphyrin synthesis. However, experimental studies suggest that propofol (in common with many inhalation anaesthetic agents) can depress the chemotactic activity of leukocytes.

Pain on injection commonly occurs when propofol is injected into small veins on the dorsum of the hand or wrist. Pain may manifest at more proximal sites (e.g. upper arm and shoulder) during injection. The mechanism is obscure; the pain is transitory and thrombophlebitic sequelae are extremely rare. The incidence of pain is lessened if large veins in the antecubital fossa are used for administration or if a small dose of lignocaine (5–10 mg) is added to the propofol.

Current evidence suggests that the principal mode of action of propofol in the CNS is to produce a reduction in sodium-channel opening times in neuronal membranes (c.f. barbiturates, p. 213). Effects on inhibitory neurotransmitters (e.g. GABA, glycine) are less clear. Experimental studies indicate that propofol does not directly affect the GABA–chloride receptor complex. Furthermore, the anaesthetic effects of propofol are not modified by the benzodiazepine antagonist flumazenil. Recent studies have implied that the excitatory side-effects of propofol (and methohexitone) may be related to antagonism of glycine receptors at subcortical levels, although propofol may have permissive effects at other sites in the CNS which involve this inhibitory neurotransmitter.

Propofol is extensively bound to plasma proteins; after anaesthetic doses approximately 97–98% is bound to albumin. After intravenous injection the plasma concentration of propofol usually declines in a biexponential or triexponential manner. The initial fall in concentration is extremely rapid (half-life 1–3 min), reflecting the almost immediate distribution of the lipid-soluble drug from plasma to tissue. Indeed, most of the drug removed from the blood in the first 2 h is due to tissue uptake. Estimated values for pharmacokinetic constants after injection of propofol are extremely variable. In early studies it was suggested that the terminal half-life of propofol was 1–5 h and that the total apparent volume of distribution of the drug was approximately 10 times greater than total body water. The clearance of propofol was more than liver blood flow, indicating that there might be significant extrahepatic metabolism of the drug. This observation was confirmed when significant amounts of a glucuronide metabolite were recovered from the urine of a patient during the anhepatic phase of liver transplantation.

Prolonged blood sampling suggests that the half-life of propofol is about 60 h and that its clearance is less than hepatic blood flow (i.e. approximately 1000 ml min^{-1}). These studies suggest that the elimination of propofol is extensively dependent on hepatic metabolism and may be sensitive to changes in liver blood flow (but not to protein binding or enzyme activity). Propofol is mainly metabolized to the glucuronide conjugates of 2.6-diisopropylphenol and 2.6-diisopropylquinol which are subsequently eliminated in urine.

The main advantage of propofol in clinical practice is that rapid recovery of consciousness and full awareness occurs when bolus doses are used to induce anaesthesia; similarly, significant cumulation does not occur after infusion or repeated administration of the drug. Nevertheless, a number of studies suggest that the drug has a relatively long half-life, and prolonged infusions and multiple doses should be used with caution.

Unexpected deaths in children under long-term sedation with propofol in an intensive care unit have been reported. Increasing metabolic acidosis, bradycardia and progressive myocardial failure were the presenting symptoms. The drug itself and the lipid content of the solvent have both been implicated, but the aetiology is obscure.

The pharmacological properties and pharmacokinetics of propofol are summarized in Tables 7.1 and 7.2.

Ketamine

Ketamine ((2-chlorphenyl)-2-(methylamino)-cyclohexanone hydrochloride; Fig. 7.1) is chemically related to cyclohexamine and phencyclidine. Although it does not usually produce loss of consciousness in one arm–brain circulation time, it is commonly classified as an induction agent. Ketamine hydrochloride is freely soluble in water, forming an acidic solution (pH = 3.5–5.5). Three different concentrations (10, 50 and 100 mg ml^{-1}) are available for intravenous injection (dose = 1–4.5 mg kg^{-1}) or intramuscular administration (dose = 5–10 mg kg^{-1}). Ketamine is a racemic mixture of two enantiomers; the S(+) enantiomer is 3.4 times more potent than the R(–) isomer.

Ketamine differs from other intravenous agents in that it is almost devoid of hypnotic properties but produces a state of dissociative anaesthesia in which dose-related anterograde amnesia and profound analgesia are present. The drug has a relatively slow onset of action compared with other intravenous anaesthetics; up to 90 s may elapse after injection before any CNS effect is observed. This delay can be as much as 8 min after intramuscular injection. It can be difficult to determine the precise time of the onset of action and patients may gaze into the distance for several minutes without closing their eyes. Hypertonus and spontaneous involuntary muscle movements, including tonic–clonic activity of the limbs, may occur during induction. Muscular relaxation is often poor and the tone of the jaw muscle may be increased, causing obstruction of the airway. Respiratory activity is little affected (although respiratory rate may slightly increase), and the response to alterations in $Paco_2$ is normal. Coughing and laryngospasm are extremely rare: indeed, experimental studies suggest that ketamine antagonizes the effects of histamine, acetylcholine and 5-hydroxytryptamine on bronchial smooth muscle. The drug is safe for use in asthmatic patients. Although most reflex responses are not affected by ketamine, some depression of laryngeal reflexes may occur, which precludes its use for operations on the upper airway.

In contrast to most other anaesthetic agents, ketamine invariably produces tachycardia, increases cardiac output and raises plasma noradrenaline concentrations. Both systolic and diastolic blood pressure (as well as pulmonary vascular resistance and arterial pressure) are usually increased by 20–40%. These changes usually occur within 5 min and last for 10–20 min. Nevertheless, cardiac arrhythmias are uncommon and ketamine may produce an increase in peripheral blood flow. The effects of ketamine on the cardiovascular system may be partly due to its direct action on neuronal pathways in the CNS. However, experimental evidence indicates that the positive inotropic effects of ketamine are mediated by indirect activation of cardiac β-adrenoceptors (by inhibition of noradrenaline reuptake at these sites) and that ketamine appears to have a depressant effect on denervated cardiac muscle. Ketamine causes an increase in cerebral blood flow, oxygen consumption and intracranial pressure.

The duration of action of ketamine (like that of most intravenous agents) is dependent on the dose of the drug. Normal intravenous doses act for 10–20 min, although the precise duration of action may be difficult to assess. Nausea and vomiting are not infrequent in the postoperative period. In addition, there is a significant possibility of emergence phenomena, ranging from vivid dreams and visual images to hallucinations and delirium which may continue for 24 h after administration. Psychotomimetic sequelae may be extremely unpleasant, and it has been suggested that they are due to the misperception or misinterpretation of sensory information (particularly visual or auditory stimuli). Emergence phenomena may be considerably modified by the use of appropriate premedication with opiates, benzodiazepines or droperidol (which itself may give rise to psychotomimetic side-effects when used alone). Such problems tend to be more common in women but are rarer in children, particularly when their postoperative recovery is undisturbed.

The effect of ketamine on the CNS is associated with characteristic changes in the electrocardiogram (ECG). The α-rhythm is usually depressed and is replaced by θ- and δ-wave activity. These changes may persist for the duration of analgesia. Electrophysiological studies suggest that ketamine mainly affects thalamocortical projection pathways and has only minimal effects on the reticular activating system, the limbic system and most thalamic nuclei. Analgesia may be due to effects on afferent pathways in the spinoreticular tracts that are concerned with the perception of pain or to the binding of the drug by opioid receptors (particularly δ-receptors). More recent evidence suggests that ketamine and other phencyclidine analogues specifically antagonize glutamate (an excitatory neurotransmitter) at *N*-methyl-D-aspartate (NMDA) receptor sites in the CNS. Antagonism between ketamine and NMDA is non-competitive, indicating that the drug may produce indirect changes at receptor sites (e.g. it may produce conformational changes in ion channels that are normally activated by glutamate and other excitatory amino acids). In the CNS, glutamate is known to be released at corticostriate nerve endings and plays an important role as a central neurotransmitter.

Ketamine is approximately 45% non-ionized at pH 7.4. After intravenous administration the drug is rapidly distributed in tissues and readily crosses the blood–brain barrier (and placental barrier). Plasma concentrations usually decrease in a biexponential manner; the initial rapid fall in plasma concentration (half-life = 10–20 min) is followed by a slower decline (half-life 150–200 min) which is due to the elimination of ketamine, principally by hepatic metabolism. The apparent volume of distribution is two to three times greater than body water, and the clearance is approximately equal to liver blood flow. The relatively high extraction ratio is consistent with 'flow-limited' hepatic clearance and drugs which reduce liver blood flow (e.g. inhalational agents, β-adrenoceptor antagonists, cimetidine) can decrease the clearance of ketamine and prolong its terminal half-life. After intramuscular administration, ketamine is rapidly absorbed and maximum plasma concentrations are invariably present within 30 min.

The elimination of ketamine depends on the mixed-function oxidase system associated with the smooth endoplasmic reticulum. Its main metabolite, norketamine, has some hypnotic activity but is generally less potent than ketamine. Both ketamine and norketamine may be further metabolized to hydroxylated derivatives. These are subsequently conjugated and eliminated as glucuronides (Table 7.2).

Ketamine has only a limited place in anaesthetic practice, due to its undesirable effects on the CNS and the cardiovascular system. It is usually avoided in patients with cardiac impairment, trauma, or a history of psychotic illness. Nevertheless, the drug has a definite role in certain situations. In paediatric practice, it is a useful agent when venepuncture is difficult or poorly tolerated or when repeated anaesthesia is necessary. Thus it may be used to provide anaesthesia for cardiac catheterization, burns dressings and other minor procedures (e.g. radiotherapy, bone marrow biopsy). The use of ketamine by oral and rectal routes for sedation and premedication in small children has also been described. In these situations, ketamine appears to have a low bioavailability and to undergo significant first-pass metabolism.

In adults, the indications for its use are more controversial and less well-defined. It may be of value for repeated burns dressings, in the poor-risk elderly patient and in certain emergency situations (e.g. on-site procedures following road traffic accidents). Ketamine has also been administered by intrathecal and extradural routes for the treatment of postoperative or intractable pain.

Adverse reactions to intravenous anaesthetic agents

Since the first conclusive case of an adverse reaction associated with the use of thiopentone was reported in 1952, there has been a progressive increase in the apparent incidence of hypersensitivity reactions to intravenous anaesthetic agents. This coincided with the introduction and use of a number of non-barbiturate induction agents. In recent years two of these agents (propanidid and Althesin) have been withdrawn because of their association with such adverse effects. Both these drugs contained the solubilizing agent Cremophor EL (polyethoxylated castor oil), which is a mixture of fatty acids with a molecular weight of approximately 3200, and is also present in some vitamin preparations and antifungal drugs. Although early studies suggested that Cremophor EL had no immunogenic or anaphylactoid potential, subsequent evidence indicated that it played an important role in the occurrence of adverse reactions to intravenous anaesthetics. Alternatively, its surfactant properties may have enhanced the immunogenic potential of propanidid and alphaxolone (the active steroid in Althesin).

The incidence of anaphylactoid and hypersensitivity responses during anaesthesia has recently been estimated as 1 in 6000 (but neuromuscular blocking agents may have been involved in 80% of the cases); the reported incidence of such responses associated with the intravenous induction agents in current use is summarized in Table 7.3. The severity of hypersensitivity responses is difficult to assess and, although adverse reactions to thiopentone appear to be relatively uncommon, approximately 10 deaths have been recorded in this context. On the other hand, it is probable that many incidences are not reported (particularly those in which serious sequelae do not occur).

However, in a number of instances, some undesirable effects (e.g. hypotension) may be due to the direct actions of the anaesthetic agent on the myocardium or on vascular smooth muscle, or an enhanced vasovagal response to venepuncture. In addition, mechanical problems with the airway, related to kinked or misplaced

Table 7.3 Incidence of hypersensitivity responses associated with current preparations of intravenous induction agents.

Agent	Incidence
Thiopentone	1 in 14 000–1 in 20 000
Methohexitone	1 in 1600–1 in 7000
Propofol	1 in 80 000–1 in 100 000
Etomidate	1 in 50 000–1 in 450 000
Ketamine	2 cases

endotracheal tubes, may present as apparent bronchospasm. Anaesthetic techniques invariably involve some polypharmacy and the role of other drugs (e.g. muscle relaxants, colloid infusions) may be difficult to determine. Furthermore, the outcome of a hypersensitivity response may obviously depend upon the early recognition of the problem and the ability to institute immediate therapeutic measures.

The clinical features of anaphylactoid and hypersensitivity reactions to intravenous anaesthetics may include bronchospasm, hypotension, peripheral vascular collapse, erythema, urticaria, oedema and abdominal pain. The clinical course of the reaction is variable; localized or generalized vasodilatation may occur within seconds of the injection, and can be rapidly followed by bronchospasm and cyanosis. The pulse may be impalpable and the blood pressure unrecordable (although the ECG usually shows an increase in heart rate). Localized or generalized oedema may subsequently develop. Occasionally, reactions to intravenous anaesthetics have a slower onset (over 10–90 min); their clinical manifestations are often relatively benign and their cause may not be recognized.

Many of the presenting symptoms resemble the pharmacological effects of histamine in humans, or may be produced by other mediators. These include bradykinin, 5-hydroxytryptamine, leukotrienes, prostaglandins and heparin. The mechanisms involved may be of four types:

1 A type I hypersensitivity reaction, which depends upon previous exposure and sensitization to the induction agent and the formation of immunoglobulin E (IgE) reaginic antibodies. The antibodies become bound to mast cells and basophils; subsequent exposure to the agent results in an antigen–antibody reaction on the mast cell membrane and the disruption of its cytoplasmic granules, which release histamine and other vasoactive amines.

2 Occasionally a type II (cytotoxic) hypersensitivity response has been reported. In this mechanism, IgG or IgM antibodies bind to an antigen on the cell surface. The antigen–antibody reaction then activates the classical complement pathway, which results in the consumption of C4 and C3, leading to a cascade of activation of the remaining complement proteins (C5–9) and cell lysis and some production of C3a (anaphylotoxin). This reaction has been identified following a hypersensitivity response to propofol.

3 An anaphylactoid response which does not require prior exposure to the drug. This involves an alternate complement pathway, which involves a larger proportion of C3 being converted into the anaphylotoxins C3a and C5a. Many of the reactions of Althesin involved this mechanism.

4 A direct action of the drug on circulating basophils and mast cells resulting in the release of histamine which appears to be related to the dose and speed of injection. This mechanism usually accounts for the erythema and unexpected hypotension which is not infrequently observed after the induction of anaesthesia, and may also occur with other agents used (e.g. analgesics, muscle relaxants). Previous exposure to the drug is not a feature and the systemic manifestations are usually mild. This reaction may also be regarded as an anaphylactoid response, but could be considered as a direct pharmacological effect of the drug concerned.

Treatment

The diagnosis should be firmly established and airway obstruction must be excluded. Bronchospasm is the most life-threatening of the symptoms and treatment must primarily be aimed at preventing severe hypoxia. Endotracheal intubation and positive-pressure ventilation with 100% oxygen are usually required. Intravenous adrenaline (1 in 10 000, i.e. 100 μg ml^{-1}) is the first-line drug of choice. In addition to its bronchodilator effect, adrenaline may prevent further release of histamine and improve peripheral vascular tone. In the most severe clinical circumstances, and with full cardiovascular monitoring facilities available, adrenaline may be administered by slow intravenous injection in aliquots of 3–5 ml (300–500 μg) and repeated at 5-min intervals until a satisfactory therapeutic response is achieved. If bronchospasm is less profound, smaller doses of adrenaline (i.e. 50–100 μg) may be effective. The development of glottic or subglottic oedema due to extravasation of fluid into the pharyngeal and laryngeal tissues may further compromise the airway. An H_1-receptor antagonist should be administered for the prophylaxis and treatment of this complication (and for the development of urticaria); chlorpheniramine (10 mg intravenously) is the drug of choice in this context.

Hydrocortisone hemisuccinate (up to 200 mg intravenously) should also be given; although the maximum response does not occur for 1–3 h, bronchospasm and hypotension may persist. The use of intravenous aminophylline or nebulized salbutamol may also be considered in cases of refractory bronchospasm. Crystalloid or, preferably, colloid infusions should be used as plasma expanders; 1–2 l of the circulating volume may have extravasated into the tissues.

Prevention of reactions

1 The rate of injection and the dose of the induction agent should be carefully considered. The severity of many reactions is reduced by the slow administration of moderate doses of intravenous agents.
2 Patients with a history of allergy or atopy may be especially sensitive to type I hypersensitivity responses (particularly when there is evidence of increased IgE concentrations). The repeated exposure of these patients to induction agents known to produce such reactions is particularly hazardous. Alternative drugs or techniques (e.g. local or regional anaesthesia) should be considered.
3 When general anaesthesia is required in such patients, premedication with an H_1 antagonist (e.g. chlorpheniramine), an H_2 antagonist (e.g. ranitidine), which may have complementary beneficial effects against the cardiovascular manifestations of histamine, and a steroid is indicated.

4 It can be extremely important, for both therapeutic and medicolegal purposes, to distinguish between true hypersensitivity reactions and similar clinical manifestations associated with the enhanced pharmacological effects of the drugs involved, pharmacodynamic interactions or mechanical problems involving the airway. Plasma histamine levels can be measured by radioimmunoassay on blood samples taken after the event. Plasma levels of tryptase, a proteolytic enzyme released from mast cell granules (but not basophils) following activation, may be elevated for approximately 6 h following a hypersensitivity response. Enhanced levels of the main metabolite of histamine, *N*-methylhistamine, may be detected in urinary samples and also aid in diagnosis. More specific investigations at a later stage may be useful to identify the responsible drug; these include intradermal skin testing, estimations of IgE antibodies and possibly radioallergosorbent tests (RAST) for specific antibodies.

Total intravenous anaesthesia

Total intravenous anaesthesia (TIVA) is usually applied to techniques in which all anaesthetic agents are given intravenously during major surgical procedures. Thus intravenous anaesthetics are used to induce hypnosis, opioids are given to prevent intraoperative pain and neuromuscular blockade is induced during controlled ventilation with oxygen-enriched air. In recent years there has been considerable interest in TIVA, due to environmental considerations and the introduction of drugs with suitable pharmacokinetic properties (e.g. propofol, alfentanil and atracurium). The use of continuous infusion techniques has considerable practical advantages, including minimal cardiovascular depression, rapid recovery and the avoidance of hazards of exposure to inhalational agents. Unfortunately, they are relatively expensive since they usually depend on the accurate and controlled infusion of drugs with a short duration of action and a rapid recovery. In addition they require precise pharmacokinetic data that have been previously collated from a defined patient population, as well as the determination and assessment of the various factors that are liable to influence the behaviour of drugs in the body. Thus the concurrent administration of other drugs as well as cardiovascular, renal and hepatic impairment may affect the disposition and the activity of many intravenous agents. Present evidence suggests that there is considerable interindividual variability in the metabolism and elimination of anaesthetic drugs, at least some of which may be determined by genetic factors. Awareness and intraoperative dreaming are also problems of concern with TIVA. In spite of the obvious ecological advantages of this technique, a greater knowledge of potential drug interactions and more accurate methods of assessment of cerebral function are required before TIVA becomes a generally accepted practice.

Further reading

Aveling W, Sear JW, Fitch W *et al.* Early clinical evaluation of minaxolone: a new intravenous anaesthetic agent. *Lancet* 1979; **ii**: 71–73.

Avery AF, Evans A. Reactions to Althesin. *British Journal of Anaesthesia* 1973; **45**: 301–303.

Bevan JC. Propofol related convulsions. *Canadian Journal of Anaesthesia* 1993; **40**: 805–809.

Breimer DD. Pharmacokinetics of methohexitone following intravenous infusion in humans. *British Journal of Anaesthesia* 1976; **48**: 643–649.

Briggs LP, Clarke RSJ, Dundee JW *et al.* Use of di-isopropylphenol as main agent for short procedures. *British Journal of Anaesthesia* 1981; **53**: 1197–1202.

Christiensen JH, Andreasen F, Janssen JA. Influence of age and sex on the pharmacokinetics of propofol. *British Journal of Anaesthesia* 1981; **53**: 1189–1196.

Christiensen JH, Andreasen F, Janssen JA. Pharmacokinetics and pharmacodynamics of thiopentone — a comparison between young and elderly patients. *Anaesthesia* 1982; **37**: 398–404.

Clarke RSJ, Dundee JW, Barron DW *et al.* Clinical studies of induction agents. XXVI: The relative potencies of thiopentone, methohexitone and propanidid. *British Journal of Anaesthesia* 1968; **40**: 593–601.

Clarke RSJ, Dundee JW, Carson JW. A new steroid anaesthetic — Althesin. *Proceedings of the Royal Society of Medicine* 1973; **66**: 1027–1029.

Collins CGS. Effects of the anaesthetic 2,6-diisopropylphenol on synaptic transmission in the rat olfactory cortex slice. *British Journal of Pharmacology* 1988; **95**: 939–949.

Cook DJ, Carton EG, Housmans PR. Mechanism of the positive inotropic effect of ketamine in isolated ferret ventricular papillary muscle. *Anaesthesiology* 1991; **74**: 880–888.

Doenicke A. Etomidate, a new intravenous hypnotic. *Acta Anaesthesiologica Belgica* 1974; **25**: 307–315.

Doenicke J, Kugler J, Penzel G *et al.* Hirnfunktion und Toleranzbreiten ach Etomidate einem neuen barbituratfreien i.v. applizierbaren Hypnoticum. *Der Anaesthetist* 1973; **22**: 357–366.

Dolin SR, Smith MB, Soar J, Morris PJ. Does glycine antagonism underly the excitatory side-effects of methohexitone and propofol? *British Journal of Anaesthesia* 1992; **68**: 523–526.

Domino EF, Chodoff P, Corrsen G. Pharmacological effects of CI 581, a new dissociative anaesthetic in man. *Clinical Pharmacology and Therapeutics* 1965; **6**: 279–290.

Dundee JW, Barron JW. The barbiturates. *British Journal of Anaesthesia* 1962; **34**: 240–246.

Dundee JW, Clarke RSJ. Propofol. *European Journal of Anaesthesiology* 1989; **6**: 5–22.

Dundee JW, Knox JWD, Black GW *et al.* Ketamine as an induction agent in anaesthetics. *Lancet* 1970; **i**: 1370–1371.

Dundee JW, McIlroy PDA. The history of the barbiturates. *Anaesthesia* 1982; **37**: 726–734.

Dundee JW, Moore J. Thiopentone and methohexital. A comparison as main anaesthetic agents for a standard operation. *Anaesthesia* 1961; **16**: 50–60.

Dundee JW, Price HL, Dripps RD. Acute tolerance to thiopentone in man. *Anaesthesia* 1956; **28**: 344–352.

Dundee JW, Wyant GM. *Intravenous Anaesthesia.* Edinburgh: Churchill Livingstone, 1988; 1–358.

Edwards R, Ellis FR. Clinical significance of thiopentone binding to haemoglobin and plasma protein. *British Journal of Anaesthesia* 1973; **45**: 891–893.

Firestone LL, Quinlan JJ, Homanics GE. The role of gamma-amino butyric acid type-A receptor subtypes in the pharmacology of general anaesthesia. *Current Opinion in Anaesthesiology* 1995; **8**: 311–314.

Fisher M. Treatment of acute anaphylaxis. *British Medical Journal* 1995; **311**: 731–733.

Frenkel C, Duch DS, Urban BW. Effects of IV anaesthetics on human brain sodium channels. *British Journal of Anaesthesia* 1993; **71**: 15–24.

Gjessing J. Ketamine (CI-581) in clinical anaesthesia. *Acta Anaesthesiologica Scandinavica* 1968; **12**: 15–21.

Horton JN. Adverse reaction to Althesin. *Anaesthesia* 1973; **28**: 182–183.

Hudson RJ, Stanski DR, Burch PG. Pharmacokinetics of methohexital and thiopental in surgical patients. *Anaesthesiology* 1983; **59**: 215–219.

Jarman R, Abel AL. Intravenous anaesthesia with pentothal sodium. *Lancet* 1936; **230**: 422–423.

Jessop E, Grounds RM, Morgan M, Lumley J. Comparison of infusions of propofol and methohexitone to provide light general anaesthesia during surgery with regional blockade. *British Journal of Anaesthesia* 1985; **57**: 1173–1177.

Johnston R, Noseworthy TW, Anderson B *et al.* Propofol versus thiopentone for outpatient anaesthesia. *Anaesthesiology* 1987; **67**: 431–433.

Knell PJW. Total intravenous anaesthesia by an intermittent technique. Use of methohexitone, ketamine and a muscle relaxant. *Anaesthesia* 1983; **38**: 586–587.

Langrehr D. Dissoziative anasthesie durch Ketamine. *Actuelle Chirurgie* 1969; **4**: 71–78.

Laroche D, Vergnaud MC, Sillard B *et al.* Biochemical markers of anaphylactoid reactions to drugs. Comparison of plasma histamine and tryptase. *Anesthesiology* 1991; **75**: 945–949.

Lindgren L. Anaesthetic activity and side effects of propofol. *Current Opinion in Anaesthesiology* 1994; **7**: 321–325.

Logan MR, Duggan JE, Levack ID, Spence AA. Single-shot iv anaesthesia for out-patient dental anaesthesia. Comparison of 2,6-diisopropylphenol and methohexitone. *British Journal of Anaesthesia* 1987; **59**: 179–183.

Lundy JS. Intravenous anesthesia: preliminary report of the use of two new thiobarbiturates. *Proceedings of Staff Meetings of the Mayo Clinic* 1935; **10**: 534–543.

Lundy JS, Tovell RM. Some of the newer local and general anesthetic agents. Methods of their administration. *Northwest Medicine (Seattle)* 1934; **33**: 308–311.

Mackenzie N, Grant IS. Comparison of the new emulsion formulation of propofol with methohexitone and thiopentone for induction of anaesthesia in day cases. *British Journal of Anaesthesia* 1985; **57**: 725–731.

Major E, Verniquet AJW, Waddell TK *et al.* A study of three doses of ICI 35868 for induction and maintenance of anaesthesia. *British Journal of Anaesthesia* 1981; **53**: 267–272.

Miller E, Munch JC, Crossley FS, Hartnung WH. Thiobarbiturates. *Journal of the American Chemical Society* 1936; **58**: 1090–1091.

Morgan M. Total intravenous anaesthesia. *Anaesthesia* 1983; **38** (suppl.): 1–72.

Morgan M, Lunn JN. Experiences with propofol. *Anaesthesia* 1988; **43** (suppl.): 1–121.

Nebauer AE, Doenicke A, Hoernecke R *et al.* Does etomidate cause haemolysis? *British Journal of Anaesthesia* 1992; **69**: 58–60.

Parke TJ, Stevens JE, Rice ASC *et al.* Metabolic acidosis and fatal myocardial failure after propofol infusion in children: five case reports. *British Medical Journal* 1992; **305**: 613–615.

Paul DR, Logan MR, Wildsmith JW. Which intravenous induction agent for day case surgery? A comparison of propofol, thiopentone, methohexitone andetomidate. *Anaesthesia* 1988; **43**: 362–364.

Petros AJ, Bogle RG, Pearson JD. Propofol stimulates nitric oxide release from porcine aortic endothelial cells. *British Journal of Pharmacology* 1993; **109**: 6–7.

Powell H, Morgan M, Sear JW. Pregnanolone: a new steroid intravenous anaesthetic: dose finding study. *Anaesthesia* 1992; **47**: 287–290.

Sanders LD, Isaac PA, Yeomans WA *et al.* Propofol-induced anaesthesia. Double-blind comparison of recovery after anaesthesia induced by propofol or thiopentone. *Anaesthesia* 1989; **44**: 200–204.

Schuermans V, Dom J, Dony J *et al.* Multinational evaluation of etomidate for anaesthesia induction. Conclusions and consequences. *Anaesthetist* 1978; **27**: 52–59.

Selye H. Anesthetic effect of steroid hormones. *Proceedings of the Society for Experimental Biology and Medicine* 1941; **46**: 116–121.

Selye H. Studies concerning the correlation between anesthetic potency, hormonal activity and chemical structure among steroid compounds. *Anesthesia and Analgesia* 1942; **21**: 41–47.

Servin F, Desmonts JM, Haberer JP *et al.* Pharmacokinetics and protein-binding of propofol in patients with cirrhosis. *Anesthesiology* 1988; **69**: 887–891.

Stanski DR. Intravenous barbiturates. *Anaesthesia* 1981; **36**: 548–549.

Stoelting VK. Use of a new intravenous oxygen barbiturate 25398 for intravenous anesthesia. *Anesthesia and Analgesia* 1957; **36**: 49–51.

Trotter C, Serpell MG. Neurological sequelae in children after prolonged propofol infusion. *Anaesthesia* 1992; **47**: 340–342.

Valtonen M, Iisalo E, Kanto J, Rosenberg P. Propofol as an induction agent in children: pain on injection and pharmacokinetics. *Acta Anaesthesiologica Scandinavica* 1989; **33**: 152–155.

Veroli P, O'Reilly B, Bertrand F *et al.* Extrahepatic metabolism of propofol in man during the anhepatic phase of orthoptic liver transplantation. *British Journal of Anaesthesia* 1992; **68**: 183–186.

Wann KT. Neuronal sodium and potassium channels: structure and function. *British Journal of Anaesthesia* 1993; **71**: 2–14.

Weese H, Scharpff W. Evipan, ein neuartiges Einschlafmittel. *Deutsche Medizinische Wochenschrift* 1932; **58**: 1205–1207.

White PF, Ham J, Way WL, Trevor AJ. Pharmacology of ketamine isomers in surgical patients. *Anesthesiology* 1980; **52**: 231–239.

Whitwam JG. Methohexitone. *British Journal of Anaesthesia* 1976; **48**: 617–619.

Wyant GM, Barr JS. Further comparative studies of sodium methohexital. *Canadian Anaesthetists Society Journal* 1960; **7**: 127–135.

Wyant GM, Chang CA. Sodium methohexital: a clinical study. *Canadian Anaesthetists Society Journal* 1959; **6**: 40–50.

Chapter 8
Inhalational Anaesthetic Agents

Although the introduction of inhalational anaesthetics revolutionized operative surgery, their general acceptance by the medical profession was relatively slow. The effects of nitrous oxide on sensation and voluntary power were described by Joseph Priestley as early as 1772; nevertheless, the gas was not generally used as an analgesic or an inhalational anaesthetic until well into the 19th century. Diethyl ether and chloroform, which were initially used in the 1840s, were more rapidly accepted. There were few significant further advances until 1934, when trichlorethylene and cyclopropane were introduced into anaesthetic practice. Some 20 years later halothane was synthesized, and its general acceptance has been followed by the introduction of other fluorinated anaesthetics, e.g. methoxyflurane, enflurane, isoflurane, desflurane and sevoflurane.

General anaesthesia normally consists of a state of reversible insensibility associated with loss of consciousness, absence of pain and some degree of muscle relaxation. In the early days of anaesthesia, these effects were produced by administration of a single anaesthetic agent. By contrast, during the past 40 years balanced techniques have been widely used, in which several different drugs have produced these effects. By these methods, the hazards of general anaesthesia are greatly reduced and postoperative recovery of vital functions is extremely rapid.

Drugs that are classified as inhalational anaesthetics primarily produce loss of consciousness; however, they may also produce significant analgesia (e.g. nitrous oxide) or muscle relaxation (e.g. isoflurane). They are stored at ambient temperatures either as liquified gases under pressure, or as volatile liquids.

Mode of action

The molecular basis of inhalational anaesthesia is unknown. Consequently, the mode of action of individual agents is uncertain. All inhalational anaesthetics have a relatively rapid onset of action, and their effects are readily reversible. It therefore seems improbable that the molecular basis of anaesthesia depends on the formation of stable, covalent chemical bonds in the central nervous system (CNS). Inhalational anaesthesia is more likely to be related to the physical properties of individual agents, or to reversible, low-energy intermolecular forces (e.g. van der Waals forces, dipole–dipole interactions or ionic and hydrogen bonds).

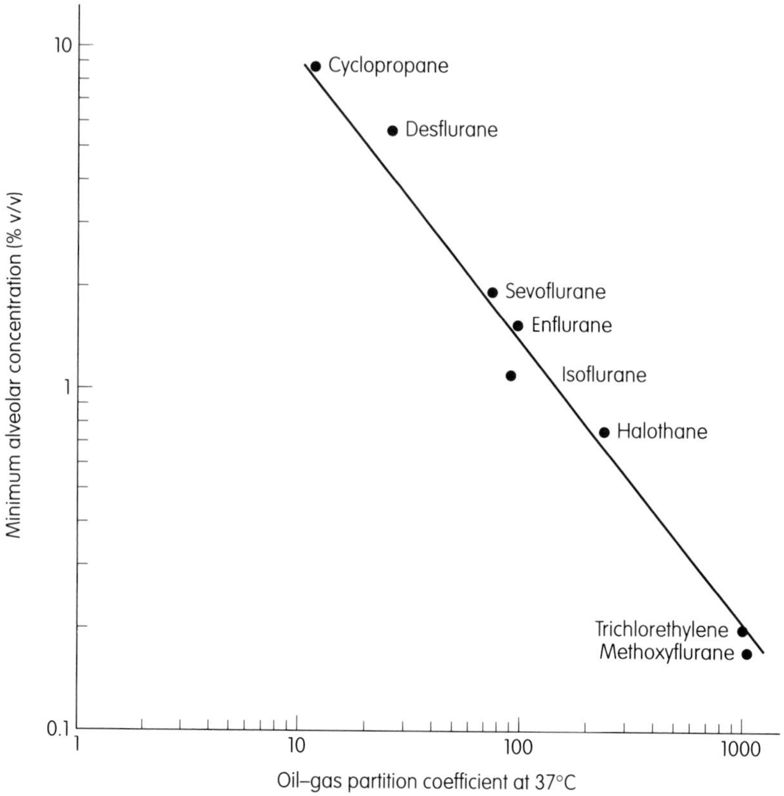

Fig. 8.1 Relation between the oil–gas partition coefficient at 37°C and the minimum alveolar concentration (% v/v) of different anaesthetic agents.

In general, different inhalational anaesthetics have certain physicochemical properties in common. Almost all these agents are simple aliphatic hydrocarbons or ethers with 1–4 carbon atoms, and have boiling points less than 90°C. They have varying degrees of lipid solubility; the anaesthetic potencies of different agents are additive, and closely related to their lipid solubility. In addition, their effects may be modified or reversed by the application of pressure. Many simple chemical agents can behave as inhalational anaesthetics in appropriate circumstances, including some gases, hydrocarbons, halogenated hydrocarbons, ethers, halogenated ethers and organic solvents. Most of these agents cannot be used clinically, due to their side-effects or toxicity. Some agents only produce anaesthetic effects at high partial pressures [e.g. nitrogen, which requires a pressure of approximately 3000 kPa (30 atm)]. Consequently, in humans, the anaesthetic effects of nitrogen gas are only evident during scuba diving or similar activities.

Previous theories of anaesthesia

Early theories of anaesthesia were based on the relation between anaesthetic potency and the physical properties of individual agents. In 1899–1901, Meyer and Overton independently showed that the potency of many anaesthetics and hypnotics was closely related to their solubility in olive oil (relative to their aqueous solubility). Since that time, many hypotheses have been based on the correlation between anaesthetic potency and lipid solubility, as assessed by the oil–gas partition coefficient at 37°C (Fig. 8.1). In subsequent work, Ferguson expressed the thermodynamic activity (or molal free energy) of anaesthetics in terms of their vapour pressure. Alternatively, it was suggested that individual molecules form hydrates or clathrates, i.e. that they are enclosed within a cage-like structure of water molecules as hydrated compounds which are oriented and stabilized by hydrogen bonds. The involvement of structural proteins within the clathrate could result in conformational changes and thus interfere with the function of cellular membranes. Current evidence suggests that the correlation between hydrate dissociation and anaesthetic potency is incomplete and unsatisfactory, and these concepts are only of historical interest.

The Meyer–Overton theory, and the general acceptance of the correlation between anaesthetic potency and lipid solubility, identified neuronal membranes as a likely site of anaesthetic action in the CNS.

Structure of neuronal membranes

In the CNS and other tissues, the limiting membrane of most cells is approximately 10 nm wide and consists of a bimolecular layer of phospholipid with intercalated molecules of protein (Fig. 1.1). Some protein molecules are situated on the internal or external aspects of the membrane; others (integral proteins) are contained within and may traverse the lipid membrane. Some integral proteins form a ring surrounding fine pores or channels, approximately 0.5 nm in diameter. The opening and closing of these channels results in ionic changes that govern neuronal activity. The phospholipid components can migrate within the neuronal membrane, and are responsible for the permeability barrier that limits the diffusion of most polar compounds. The phospholipids immediately surrounding integral membrane proteins (boundary lipids) are particularly important in the modification of the activity of enzymes and ion channels, and may influence the conformational changes that are associated with enzyme or receptor function.

Consequently, if inhalational agents produce anaesthesia by acting on neuronal membranes, they may primarily affect either the phospholipid or the protein components of the membrane.

Actions on membrane phospholipids

The correlation between the oil : gas partition coefficient and anaesthetic potency suggests that inhalational anaesthetics mainly produce their effects by actions at non-polar hydrophobic sites on the lipid or protein components of neuronal membranes. Inhalational anaesthetics may initially dissolve in membrane phospholipids and change their physical properties (e.g. their fluidity, volume, surface tension or lateral surface pressure), and thus modify the degree of order or disorder within the membrane. Alterations in the physical properties of lipids (particularly boundary lipids) may have secondary effects on associated integral membrane proteins (e.g. receptors, enzymes, ion channels), resulting in conformational changes and the subsequent modification of their activity. These changes may reduce or prevent the release of neurotransmitters, or increase the volume and width of neuronal membranes, so that ion channels do not function effectively. According to these concepts, phospholipids can be considered as the primary targets of anaesthetic action, while integral membrane proteins are the secondary targets. Nevertheless, it seems unlikely that alterations in the physical properties of membrane phospholipids are primarily responsible for anaesthesia, since the changes produced are relatively small and insignificant.

A related theory suggests that inhalational anaesthetics affect non-polar sites in an inert manner, and physically modify the relationships between pressure and volume within the neuronal membrane. This theory is based on the phenomenon of the pressure reversal of anaesthesia; numerous studies with luminous bacteria, tadpoles and mice have shown that anaesthesia can be modified or reversed when external environmental pressures are increased. A similar phenomenon occurs during Althesin anaesthesia in hyperbaric conditions in humans. In the 1970s, these observations were explained by the critical volume hypothesis, which proposed that anaesthetics and pressure act at the same site, and by means of a common mechanism. According to this hypothesis, anaesthesia occurs when the volume of the hydrophobic regions in neuronal membranes expands beyond a certain critical amount; when this volume is restored by changes in temperature or pressure, anaesthesia is reversed. Subsequent modifications of this hypothesis have been proposed, e.g. the mean excess volume hypothesis and the multisite expansion hypothesis, which suggested that anaesthesia (and the pressure reversal of anaesthesia) were produced by actions at more than one type of molecular site and varied with different agents. Consequently, each anaesthetic agent produces its own pattern of CNS depression and activation.

These hypotheses, which are mainly or solely based on the phenomenon of pressure reversal of anaesthesia, are not now generally accepted. Recent experimental evidence suggests that pressure reversal is highly specific and selective, and may be due to effects on pressure-sensitive glycine channels, which play an important role in mediating inhibitory tone in the CNS. It therefore seems unlikely that anaesthesia and pressure act by means of a common mechanism. The pressure reversal of anaesthesia may be related to the high-pressure neurological syndrome; this condition (which is characterized by tremor, convulsions and periods of microsleep) occurs in many experimental animals and humans at pressures above 3000 kPa (30 atm).

In addition, most recent experimental evidence suggests that phospholipids in neuronal membranes may not be the primary target or site of action of inhalational anaesthetics. In particular, structural and dynamic studies in *in vitro* conditions suggest that the concentrations of inhalational agents that are present during clinical anaesthesia have little or no effect on pure lipid bilayers. Significant effects on lipid membranes are only produced by much higher concentrations of anaesthetics.

Actions on membrane proteins

Until recently, membrane proteins were not considered to be likely primary targets of inhalational anaesthetics, since their well-constrained structure seemed unlikely to be modified in an identical manner by different anaesthetic molecules. Nevertheless, there is now considerable evidence that inhalational agents may directly interact with neuronal membrane proteins in the CNS, producing conformational changes in their structure which directly affect the function of ion channels, receptors or enzymes. Inhalational anaesthetics may combine with integral proteins at hydrophobic sites that are exposed to boundary lipids; alternatively, they may combine with membrane proteins on the internal or external aspects of the lipid bilayer (Fig. 1.1).

In recent years, preparations of purified and soluble proteins have been used to study the effects of inhalational anaesthetics on ion channels, receptors and enzymes in a lipid-free environment. Many soluble proteins and enzyme systems are unresponsive or resistant to clinical concentrations of inhalational anaesthetics; these include glycolytic enzymes, glutamate receptors and most voltage-gated ion channels and active transport systems. The phosphatidyl-inositol system, cyclic nucleotides and regulatory G proteins are also relatively resistant to inhalational agents. Other proteins (e.g. haemoglobin, albumin) are bound by inhalational agents, and appear to undergo reversible conformational changes without any alteration in their physiological roles.

In contrast, the functional properties of other proteins are selectively modified by clinical concentrations of inhalational anaesthetic agents. These proteins include some receptors and their associated ion channels (e.g. γ-aminobutyric $acid_A$ ($GABA_A$) and nicotinic acetylcholine receptors) as well as certain enzymes (e.g. protein kinase C). For instance, in adrenal chromaffin cells, low concentrations of halothane inhibit cholinoceptor depolarization by carbachol, resulting in decreased Ca^{2+} entry and catecholamine secretion. Isoflurane has similar inhibitory effects on acetylcholine-induced chloride currents in certain molluscs (e.g. the pond snail, *Lymnaea stagnalis*). In this species, inhalational anaesthetics also selectively activate a potassium current ($I_{K(An)}$) in certain identified ganglion cells, resulting in hyperpolarization and inexcitability of the neuronal membrane. Inhalational anaesthetics have also been shown to interact competitively with a soluble purified lipid-free enzyme (luciferase) in bacteria and fireflies; there is a close correlation between the concentrations that induce anaesthesia in humans and those that inhibit firefly luciferase. Consequently, the relationship between anaesthetic potency and lipid solubility (the Meyer–Overton law) can be interpreted in terms of interaction with proteins, as well as solution in lipids. The anaesthetic potency of a homologous series of alcohols initially increases with their chain length, but eventually becomes constant at a certain molecular weight (the cut-off phenomenon); a similar phenomenon occurs with the binding and inhibition of firefly luciferase. The cut-off phenomenon may reflect the binding of alcohols by a hydrophobic site of limited capacity on the interior or exterior of the neuronal membrane, where it is exposed to an aqueous environment.

Other studies with the stereoisomers of isoflurane suggest that inhalational anaesthetics directly interact with proteins in the cell membrane. Enantiomeric forms of inhalational anaesthetics appear to have similar properties in the relatively achiral environment of lipid bilayers; in contrast, they may have different effects on protein targets (i.e. receptors, enzymes and ion channels), which consist of chiral amino acids (L-amino acids) with stereoselective properties (Chapter 4). Recent studies with the enantiomers of isoflurane suggest that their effects are moderately stereoselective. Thus, the potency of S(+)-isoflurane in experimental animals (as assessed by anaesthetic sleep times) is significantly greater than its R(–) enantiomer. In addition, in isolated neurones of the pond snail (*Lymnaea stagnalis*), the two stereoisomers inhibit acetylcholine-induced currents to a different extent: S(+)-isoflurane is approximately twice as potent as its R(–) enantiomer in the inhibition of inward, acetylcholine-activated chloride currents at some nicotinic cholinoceptors. The pond snail also contains certain identified neurones in which a potassium current ($I_{K(An)}$) can be reversibly activated by small concentrations of inhalational anaesthetics, as well as by synaptic transmission. Activation of $I_{K(An)}$ by inhalational agents hyperpolarizes the neurone to below its threshold value, and thus inhibits the generation of action potentials and normal neuronal activity. This process is also stereoselective; thus, S(+)-isoflurane is approximately twice as effective as its R(–) enantiomer in the activation of $I_{K(An)}$ in identified neurones in the pond snail. Unfortunately, the relationship of $I_{K(An)}$ to inhalational anaesthesia in humans is obscure.

Clinical studies have also attempted to define the possible role of receptor or ion channel proteins in the production of inhalation anaesthesia. In these studies, the effects of receptor agonists or antagonists on anaesthetic potency has been assessed (as measured by induced changes in the minimum alveolar concentration (MAC) values of individual inhalational agents). Alterations in the MAC values of inhalational agents suggest that the receptor or ion channel protein may play a part in the production of anaesthesia. For example, α_2-adrenoceptor agonists such as clonidine, azepexole and dexmedetomidine reduce the MAC values of most inhalational agents (Table 8.1), and may be used to partially replace them. These effects can be reversed or prevented by α_2-adrenoceptor antagonists (e.g.

Table 8.1 Some factors that affect the minimum alveolar concentration (MAC) of inhalational anaesthetics.

	Effect on MAC
Physiological and metabolic factors	
Age	↑ in infancy and childhood ↓ in maturity and old age
Pregnancy	↓
Circadian rhythms	↑ during metabolic activity
Hyperthermia (> 40°C)	↑
Hypothermia (< 30°C)	↓↓
Hypotension	↓
Hyperthyroidism	↑
Hypothyroidism	↓
Pharmacological factors	
Catecholamines	
↑	↑
↓	↓
α_2-Adrenoceptor agonists	↓
Sedatives and tranquillizers	↓↓
Opioid analgesics	
Acute dosage	↓
Chronic dosage	↑
Amphetamines	
Acute dosage	↑↑↑
Chronic dosage	↓
Ethyl alcohol	
Acute dosage	↓
Chronic dosage	↑
Lithium	↓

↑ or ↓, 0–30% change; ↑↑ or ↓↓, 30–60% change; ↑↑↑, more than 60% change.

tolazoline, yohimbine), suggesting that these receptors may play an important role in the induction of anaesthesia. Nevertheless, reductions in anaesthetic potency do not necessarily indicate the direct involvement of receptor systems in the CNS; for example, decreases in MAC values induced by opioid analgesics may be due to a direct reduction in afferent input rather than other effects on inhalational anaesthesia.

In conclusion, recent studies suggest that inhalational anaesthetic agents may be relatively selective in their effects on the CNS, and directly affect one or more unidentified proteins in the neuronal membrane, producing conformational changes in their structure. These changes directly affect the functional activity of certain receptors, enzymes or ion channels, resulting in hyperpolarization and inexcitability. Clinical concentrations of inhalational agents appear mainly to affect ligand-gated ion channels in the CNS, resulting in the postsynaptic inhibition of neuronal activity.

Site of action

Analysis of evoked cortical responses during anaesthesia shows that inhalational agents can affect the conduction of impulses at many sites between the peripheral nervous system and the cerebral cortex. Nervous conduction in the main afferent pathways is modified, although there are also effects on the reticular activating system, the basal ganglia, the cerebellum, medullary centres and motor pathways in the spinal cord. Consequently, the neurological manifestations of anaesthesia appear to be due to multiple actions at different sites in the CNS, depending on the agent that is used; they are unlikely to be solely dependent on the selective depression of afferent pathways. There is some experimental evidence that cortical cells are more sensitive to inhalational anaesthetics than the reticular activating system (despite the many synaptic relays in the reticular formation). Indeed, monosynaptic transmission may be more sensitive to depression by inhalational anaesthetic agents.

Potency

Inhalational anaesthetics vary greatly in potency (i.e. the alveolar concentration that is required to produce a given anaesthetic effect). Nitrous oxide is a relatively non-potent anaesthetic, and even concentrations of 80% in oxygen are usually insufficient to maintain anaesthesia. By contrast, concentrations of 15% cyclopropane, 5–10% diethylether or desflurane, or 1–4% of halothane, enflurane, isoflurane or sevoflurane will produce general anaesthesia. These differences in the potency of inhalational anaesthetics are primarily related to their lipid solubility (the Meyer–Overton relationship). The potency of inhalational anaesthetics is traditionally expressed in terms of their MAC, i.e. the minimum concentrations at steady state that produces no reaction to a surgical stimulus (skin incision) in 50% of subjects at atmospheric pressure. When the MAC (% v/v) of different inhalational agents is plotted against their lipid solubility (as expressed by their oil : gas partition coefficients at 37°C), a linear relationship is obtained (Fig. 8.1).

The relationship between anaesthetic potency and lipid solubility was established independently by Meyer and Overton in 1899–1901; they showed that the potency of many anaesthetics and hypnotics was closely related to their solubility in olive oil (relative to their aqueous solubility). Olive oil is a variable, inconsistent mixture of many naturally occurring lipids; it is now known that the solubility of inhalational anaesthetics in purified solvents of rather greater polarity (e.g. octanol, lecithin) provides a better correlation with potency, and may be more representative of the site of action of inhalational anaesthetics. In addition, these results suggest that ideal anaesthetic agents are amphipathic, and have both hydrophobic (non-polar) and hydrophilic (polar) properties.

The MAC of inhalational anaesthetic agents is affected by many physiological and pharmacological factors (Table 8.1). In addition, when two different inhalational anaesthetics are administered simultaneously, their activities (when expressed as MAC values) are additive. Thus, 50% of the MAC of nitrous oxide and 50% of the MAC of enflurane has an equal effect to the MAC of nitrous oxide, enflurane or any other inhalational agent. In practice, there may be slight deviations from exact additivity (e.g. with combinations of nitrous oxide and isoflurane). These deviations are generally considered to reflect patient variability.

The concept of MAC values has recently been extended to cover other responses to surgical stimuli, intubation and awareness during the recovery period.

Onset of action

General anaesthesia occurs when the concentration of inhalational agents in the CNS (as reflected by their partial pressure or tension) is sufficiently great to induce loss of consciousness. The uptake and elimination of volatile anaesthetics can be considered as a series of exponential processes. During the induction of anaesthesia by the inhalation of a constant concentration of an anaesthetic agent, a series of diffusion gradients is established. These diffusion gradients occur:

1 Between the concentration of inspired gas or vapour and its tension in pulmonary alveoli.

2 Between the alveolar tension and the pulmonary capillary blood tension.

3 Between the pulmonary capillary blood tension and the cerebral blood tension.

4 Between the cerebral blood tension and the tension of the anaesthetic in the cells and tissues in the CNS.

In practice, the rapidity of action is mainly dependent on the rate at which the alveolar tension increases and approaches the inspired gas or vapour tension (Fig. 8.2). A rapid rise in alveolar tension produces a large diffusion gradient between the alveoli and the pulmonary capillary blood; consequently, the tension in pulmonary capillary blood also rises rapidly and drives the other diffusion gradients. When equilibrium is achieved, the partial pressure of anaesthetic in the alveoli is approximately equal to its tension in the brain.

These changes are reversed during recovery from inhalational anaesthesia. The inspired gas tension falls to zero and a series of diffusion gradients is established between the partial pressure of anaesthetic in the CNS and the exhaled vapour. The speed of recovery is mainly dependent on the rapidity with which the alveolar tension decreases, and thus produces a large diffusion gradient between pulmonary capillary blood and the alveoli. Consequently, factors that affect the onset of action of inhalational anaesthetics also affect recovery to an equal and opposite extent.

Blood–gas partition coefficient

The potency of inhalational anaesthetic agents, when expressed as their minimum alveolar concentrations, is closely related to their lipid solubility, as reflected by

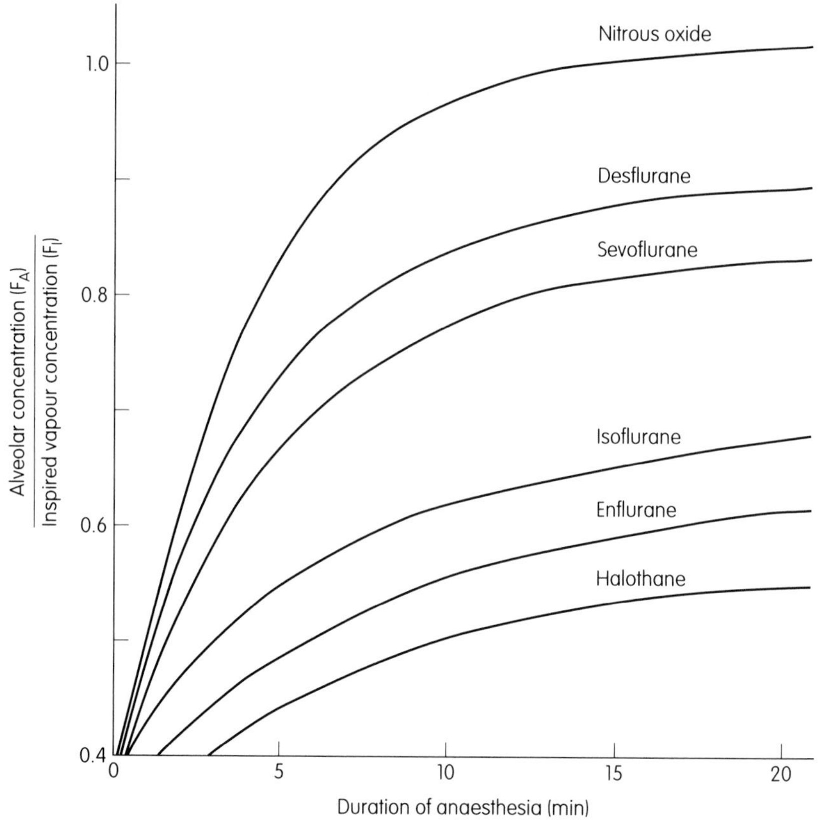

Fig. 8.2 Relation between the duration of anaesthesia and the rate of approach of alveolar concentration (F_A) to the inspired gas or vapour concentration (F_I). Inhalational anaesthetics that are less soluble in blood show a rapid rise in alveolar concentration, so that the ratio F_A/F_I approaches unity.

their oil : gas partition coefficients (Fig. 8.1). In contrast, the rate of onset of anaesthetic action is mainly determined by a different physical property, i.e. their solubility in blood. This is expressed numerically as the blood : gas partition coefficient at 37°C, and defined as the ratio of the amount of anaesthetic in blood and gas at 37°C, when the two phases are of equal volume and in equilibrium (i.e. at equal partial pressures). The blood : gas partition coefficient ranges in value from 0.45 (desflurane) to 12.0 (diethylether and methoxyflurane), and is numerically equal to the Ostwald solubility coefficient (λ) in blood at 37°C.

Inhalational anaesthetics with a low blood : gas partition coefficient are poorly soluble in blood and have a rapid onset of action; on induction of anaesthesia their alveolar concentration rapidly increases and approaches the inspired gas or vapour concentration (Fig. 8.2), and diffusion into pulmonary capillaries causes a rapid rise in their partial pressure in blood. Consequently, diffusion into the CNS occurs quickly and the onset of anaesthesia is rapid. In contrast, agents with a high blood : gas partition coefficient are more soluble in blood and have a slower onset of action. Although they are extensively removed from the alveoli due to solution in pulmonary capillary blood, their partial pressure in the alveoli and the vascular system remains relatively low (Fig. 8.2). The onset of anaesthesia is therefore slower, since the diffusion gradient between cerebral blood and the CNS is relatively small. Changes in the composition of blood (e.g. changes in free fatty acids, albumin and haemoglobin) may also affect the blood : gas partition coefficient. All inhalational anaesthetics in current use in the UK have a low blood : gas partition coefficient, are poorly soluble in blood and have a rapid onset of action.

Other factors also affect the speed of induction of isoflurane and desflurane anaesthesia; for example, both drugs have a pungent, ethereal smell and may cause irritation of the upper airway, which can delay the onset of anaesthesia. Similar principles generally govern the changes that occur during recovery from inhalational anaesthesia. During halothane anaesthesia, substantial amounts (about 25%) of the drug are metabolized; the formation of sedative metabolites (e.g. bromide ions) may contribute to postanaesthetic drowsiness, particularly after prolonged procedures. In these conditions, complete recovery from isoflurane anaesthesia is much more rapid.

Pulmonary ventilation

In non-rebreathing systems, hyperventilation increases the rate of rise in alveolar tension of inhalational anaesthetics, resulting in the more rapid onset of anaesthesia by enhancing the diffusion gradient between cerebral blood and the CNS. Conversely, any reduction in pulmonary ventilation decreases the rate of rise in alveolar tension during inhalation of the anaesthetic. The effects of changes in ventilation are most obvious when anaesthesia is induced with a soluble agent (i.e. an agent with a high blood : gas partition coefficient), and all the anaesthetic that enters the lung is taken up by pulmonary capillary blood. In these conditions, doubling alveolar ventilation doubles anaesthetic uptake.

The functional residual capacity (FRC) of the lung also affects the alveolar tension of inhalational anaesthetics, since it acts as a buffer between the inspired concentration of a gas or vapour and its alveolar concentration. A reduction in the FRC increases the rate at which the alveolar concentration rises; conversely, an increase in FRC significantly slows the rate of rise in alveolar tension. Abnormal ventilation : perfusion ratios may also alter alveolar partial pressure and anaesthetic uptake, either by increasing end-tidal anaesthetic concentrations (dead-space effect) or by reducing arterial transfer (shunting effect).

Inspired concentration

Any increase in the inspired gas or vapour tension raises alveolar partial pressures and produces more rapid onset of anaesthesia. During induction, higher concentrations than those required for maintenance may be used to accelerate the onset of anaesthesia. This principle is demonstrated by the use of the single-breath technique for the induction of anaesthesia. After maximum expiration, the subject breathes a mixture containing either 2% isoflurane (or 4% halothane) and holds it in the lungs for as long as possible, followed by normal tidal breathing. Consciousness is usually lost within 1–2 min.

Concentration effect

The relation between the inspired gas tension and its alveolar partial pressure is complex; with some anaesthetics (e.g. nitrous oxide) any increase in inspired gas tension causes a disproportionate increase in alveolar partial pressure and its rate of approximation to the inhaled concentration (the concentration effect). In practice, the concentration effect is only observed with nitrous oxide, since this is the only agent in current use that is administered in sufficiently high volumes and rapidly taken up by the lungs. In an adult subject breathing an inspired concentration of 60% nitrous oxide, the uptake in the first few minutes is usually more than 1 l min^{-1}.

Second gas effect

When two inhalational anaesthetics are given simultaneously, the uptake of large volumes of one agent may increase the alveolar tension of the other, thus accelerating the induction of anaesthesia. For example, when a constant concentration of halothane is inspired, the rise in its alveolar concentration is accelerated by the concurrent administration of nitrous oxide. The second gas effect is usually considered to be due to the rapid uptake of nitrous oxide, resulting in the concentration of halothane within a smaller volume, thus increasing its alveolar tension. Consequently, the uptake of halothane and the onset of anaesthesia is accelerated. In practice, the second gas effect is only seen when nitrous oxide is one of the inhalational anaesthetics.

Both the concentration effect and the second gas effect may have minor effects in accelerating the onset of anaesthesia during the first few minutes of inhalation.

Cardiac output

Changes in cardiac output affect pulmonary blood flow and alter the diffusion gradients of inhalational agents between the alveoli, pulmonary capillaries and tissues during the induction of anaesthesia. A high cardiac output increases the diffusion gradient and anaesthetic uptake, and slows the rate of rise in alveolar concentrations; a low cardiac output (either due to drugs or pathological conditions) reduces the diffusion gradient and anaesthetic uptake and may accelerate the rise in alveolar tension. These effects are most marked when soluble anaesthetic agents with a high blood : gas partition coefficient are used. Similarly, during the course of anaesthesia the diffusion gradient across the pulmonary epithelium is reduced as the partial pressure of the anaesthetic in systemic venous blood rises. When complete equilibration occurs (i.e. when the tension in the alveoli and pulmonary capillary blood are equal), diffusion ceases and no anaesthetic uptake occurs. In practice, complete equilibration takes a considerable time and may never occur, since most anaesthetics are partly removed from the body by metabolism and excretion. Consequently, inhalational anaesthesia can be regarded as a state of partial equilibrium.

Anaesthetic circuit

The inspired gas or vapour tension, and the alveolar partial pressure, may be altered by the absorption of inhalational agents by various components of the anaesthetic circuit. All halogenated anaesthetics are partly soluble in rubber, and some may react with soda lime; consequently, the concentration leaving the vaporizer and the inspired concentration may be different. The release of inhalational agents from rubber may also influence the course of subsequent anaesthesia. Although saturation of inhalational agents in components of the circuit never occurs (even after several weeks), significant gradients may be present at the beginning and the end of anaesthesia.

In circle breathing systems, some halogenated anaesthetics may also be taken up or react with soda lime or baralyme, especially when the absorbent is dry and warm. In these conditions, the use of halogenated anaesthetics containing the difluoromethyl (—CHF_2) group (e.g. enflurane, isoflurane and desflurane) may result in the formation of carbon monoxide, and the conversion of haemoglobin to carboxyhaemoglobin. This reaction does not occur in the presence of moisture, or if the soda lime (or baralyme) is normally (6–19%) hydrated.

The effect of ventilation on the uptake of inhalational agents is also influenced by anaesthetic systems and circuitry. In non-rebreathing systems, anaesthetic uptake is primarily dependent upon ventilation, since the inspired concentration is set by the vaporizer. By contrast, in a circle system the inspired concentration depends upon the expired concentration, as well as the anaesthetic in the fresh gas supply. When anaesthetic uptake is low (e.g. due to hypoventilation) higher concentrations are expired; nevertheless, more anaesthetic is still added to the system, thus increasing the inspiratory concentration, the alveolar–arterial gradient, and anaesthetic uptake. Consequently, in circle systems ventilation may have little effect on the rate of anaesthetic uptake. In contrast, the effect of changes in cardiac output on alveolar concentration is greater in circle systems, since the uptake of anaesthetics by the blood has a greater effect on the residual concentration in the circuit.

Effects of chronic exposure

In recent years, there has been considerable interest in the effects of chronic occupational exposure to small concentrations of inhalational anaesthetics. Hospital staff working in operating theatres are continually exposed to trace amounts of inhalational anaesthetics, and small concentrations of volatile agents or their metabolites can be detected in plasma, urine and exhaled air for several days after exposure. The hazards of chronic occupational exposure are poorly defined or unknown, although a number of epidemiological studies have attempted to assess the possible risks in female anaesthetists. In one study, it was suggested that there was a slightly increased incidence of spontaneous abortion, but little or no other evidence of significant toxic effects. In subsequent work, a 10-year prospective study of all women doctors aged 40 years or less was carried out between 1977 and 1986; it was concluded that there was no obvious association between the miscarriage rate and medical specialty, the hours spent in the operating theatre or the use of scavenging systems. There is no significant evidence that the administration of general anaesthetics during pregnancy increases the risk of fetal malformations.

In other studies, abnormal liver function tests have been observed in anaesthetists chronically exposed to low concentrations of halogenated anaesthetics; in some instances, this was associated with hepatitis which resolved when exposure to inhalational agents ceased.

In addition, continuous exposure to nitrous oxide for 2–24 h may cause megaloblastic changes in the bone marrow; exposure for 4–6 days may result in agranulocytosis. Other evidence suggests that high concentrations can interfere with DNA synthesis; in both experimental animals and humans, nitrous oxide converts cobalt in vitamin B_{12} from the monovalent form (cob[I]alamin) to the oxidized divalent form (cob[II]alamin). Since the vitamin is the cofactor of methionine synthase, activity of the enzyme is inhibited, resulting in the impaired synthesis of methionine, tetrahydrofolate and DNA (p. 261).

Nevertheless, there is very little convincing evidence that exposure to nitrous oxide in early pregnancy (either as a patient or as a hospital employee) results in any adverse effects; in addition, efficient scavenging systems reduce the concentration in operating theatres to approximately 5–10% of the levels known to affect methionine synthesis. However, it may be considered prudent to avoid exposure to nitrous oxide during the first 6 weeks of pregnancy, when this is possible.

Although the hazards of trace concentrations of inhalational anaesthetics appear to be extremely small, large numbers of hospital staff are chronically exposed to these agents. Consequently, in recent years there has been considerable interest in the development and introduction of efficient monitoring and scavenging systems in operating theatres. Despite their high cost, the use of these systems is probably justifiable, since they will minimize the hazards of exposure to inhalational anaesthetics in the operating theatre. Similarly, the use of low-flow anaesthesia will tend to reduce occupational exposure to inhalational agents.

Metabolism of inhalational anaesthetics

Since the 1960s, it has been generally recognized that most inhalational anaesthetics are metabolized to a variable extent. All of the halogenated anaesthetics in current use contain more than one carbon–halogen bond (i.e. C–F, C–Cl, or C–Br), which differ in their chemical stability and reactivity and in their susceptibility to drug metabolism. In general, C–F bonds are highly stable, and resistant to metabolic breakdown, since fluoride ions are stronger bases than other halide ions; chemical stability declines in the order C–F > C–Cl > C–Br > C–I. Thus, the trifluoromethyl group (CF_3) in halothane, isoflurane, desflurane and sevoflurane is particularly stable, and is not significantly metabolized. In contrast, when one or more chlorine atoms are attached to a terminal carbon atom (e.g. in chloroform, trichlorethylene and methoxyflurane), metabolism is extensive.

When inhalational anaesthetics are metabolized, the carbon–halogen bonds are usually broken down by oxidative enzymes, resulting in the release of reactive metabolites and halogen ions (e.g. F^-, Br^- or Cl^-), which may cause renal or hepatic damage. For example, when methoxyflurane was used as an inhalational agent, it was extensively metabolized to fluoride ions, which could cause reversible nephropathy at plasma concentrations above 40 $\mu mol\ l^{-1}$. Similarly, the metabolism of halothane results in the release of bromide ions, which may cause significant postoperative sedation after prolonged anaesthetic procedures.

Inhalational anaesthetics are mainly metabolized by the cytochrome P-450 enzyme system in the liver. In humans and other mammals, this system consists of a superfamily of haemoproteins associated with the endoplasmic reticulum; they have different but overlapping substrate specificities, and metabolize drugs at different rates. The cytochrome P-450 enzymes are the terminal oxidases of the mixed-function oxidase system (Chapter 1). Recent work suggests that one of the isoforms of cytochrome P-450 (the isoform 2E1) may be specifically responsible for the defluorination of many common inhalational anaesthetics, including enflurane, isoflurane, desflurane and sevoflurane. The rate of defluorination of anaesthetics by cytochrome P-450 2E1 in human liver, as assessed by fluoride production, occurs in the order methoxyflurane > sevoflurane > enflurane > isoflurane > desflurane. Cytochrome P-450 2E1 is also expressed in renal tubules, where it may play some part in the defluorination of anaesthetics. Methoxyflurane, but not the fluorinated agents in current use, is partially metabolized by other enzyme isoforms in liver and kidney (e.g. 1A2, 2C9/10, and 2D6), as well as by some other tissues. Enzyme induction with ethanol or isoniazid (but not barbiturates or phenytoin) increases the rate of defluorination by cytochrome P-450 2E1; the enzyme isoform may also be induced by fasting, obesity, diabetes, ketones and isopropyl alcohol. In experimental animals, cytochrome P-450 2E1 is responsible for the metabolic activation of numerous toxins and chemicals (including carbon tetrachloride, many alcohols and nitrosamines, aniline, benzene, acetone and paracetamol). In addition, it may be responsible for the activation of many suspected carcinogens (e.g. vinyl chloride, ethyl carbamate and benzene). The human isoform 2E1 specifically hydroxylates chlorzoxazone, and is specifically inhibited by disulfiram and methoxypsoralen.

Halothane may be metabolized in a different manner. Approximately 15–25% of the drug is normally metabolized to oxidative products (trifluoroacetic acid, bromide and chloride ions) by one or more cytochrome P-450 isoforms. Thus, in normal conditions, little or no defluorination of halothane occurs. In contrast, in hypoxia cytochrome P-450 mediates the reductive metabolism of halothane, resulting in the formation of fluoride and other reductive metabolites, which are excreted in a conjugated form in urine. Consequently, halothane metabolism depends on cellular oxygen availability in the liver. In normal conditions, little or no defluorination of halothane takes place; by contrast, during hepatic hypoxia, significant amounts of fluoride may be produced by reductive metabolism.

Present evidence suggests that halothane hepatitis is primarily related to the oxidative metabolism of the drug. Some of the classical enzyme-inducing agents, such as the barbiturates and phenytoin, may not induce the isoforms of cytochrome P-450 that are primarily concerned with the metabolism of inhalational anaesthetics. Consequently, different enzyme-inducing agents may have variable effects on the disposition of these agents. In addition, some inhalational anaesthetics may directly induce certain hepatic enzyme isoforms. The effects produced by exposure during a single anaesthetic procedure are unclear; hepatic microsomal enzymes may be induced after minor surgery in humans, although this may be related to the stress of surgery rather than to general anaesthesia. In practice, maintenance and recovery from general anaesthesia are usually unaffected by enzyme-inducing agents, since the elimination of most agents is dependent on respiration rather than metabolism.

In general, the toxic effects of inhalational anaesthetics appear to be related to their metabolism. Anaesthetic agents that are significantly metabolized by hepatic enzyme systems (e.g. methoxyflurane and halothane) are particularly associated with hepatic or renal toxicity. Consequently, the simultaneous use of enzyme-inducing agents may enhance the metabolism and toxicity of some anaesthetic agents (particularly methoxyflurane). In addition, the solubility of anaesthetic agents and their metabolites in blood and tissues may also have an important influence on their toxicity. In recent years, these problems have been minimized by the introduction of inhalational agents which are only metabolized to a limited extent, and are not significantly affected by most enzyme-inducing agents (e.g. enflurane, isoflurane, sevoflurane and desflurane). All these inhalational anaesthetics are relatively potent, and have low blood and tissue solubilities, which will tend to limit their accumulation in tissues. Consequently, the toxic hazards associated with the metabolism of inhalational anaesthetics are progressively declining as newer fluorinated agents are introduced into clinical practice.

Properties of individual anaesthetic agents

Although the general effects of inhalational anaesthetics on the brain are similar, some of them possess unique properties or individual toxic effects that may limit or modify their clinical use. For this reason, the properties of different inhalational anaesthetics are described separately. The physical properties of inhalational agents are summarized in Table 8.2, their biological properties are described in Table 8.3, and their structural formulae are given in Fig. 8.3.

Nitrous oxide

In 1772, Joseph Priestley prepared nitrous oxide and described its subjective and objective effects; approximately 20 years later Humphrey Davy suggested that its analgesic properties might be useful in the management of pain during operative surgery. Nevertheless, its potential advantages as an analgesic and anaesthetic agent were ignored for many years. In 1844, Horace Wells, an American dentist, first used nitrous oxide to facilitate dental extraction. Unfortunately, the

Table 8.2 Physical properties of inhalational anaesthetics in current use in the UK.

Physical properties	Nitrous oxide	Halothane	Enflurane	Isoflurane	Desflurane	Sevoflurane
Boiling point at atmospheric pressure (°C)	−88	50.2	56.5	48.5	23.5	58.5
Vapour pressure at 20°C (kPa)	5200	32.1	23.3	32.5	89.2	22.7
MAC in oxygen (% v/v)	104	0.75	1.63	1.17	6.6	1.80
MAC in 70% nitrous oxide (% v/v)	36	0.26	0.57	0.41	2.3	0.62
Oil : gas partition coefficient	1.4	224	98	98	29	80
Blood : gas partition coefficient	0.47	2.4	1.8	1.4	0.45	0.65

MAC, minimum alveolar concentration.

Table 8.3 Biological properties of inhalational anaesthetics in current use in the UK.

Properties	Nitrous oxide	Halothane	Enflurane
Onset/offset of action	Extremely rapid	Less rapid	Rapid
Analgesic properties	Marked	Poor	Moderate
Effect on respiration	Non-irritant Respiratory rate ↑ Tidal volume ↓ $Pa\text{CO}_2$ normal Enters air spaces	Non-irritant Respiratory rate ↑ Tidal volume ↓↓ $Pa\text{CO}_2$ ↑ (less depressant)	Non-irritant Respiratory rate ↑ Tidal volume ↓↓ $Pa\text{CO}_2$ ↑↑ (most depressant)
Effect on cardiovascular system	Little or no effect Cardiac sensitivity to catecholamines ↑/↓	Heart rate ↓↓ Blood pressure ↓↓ Cardiac output ↓↓ Peripheral resistance ↓ Cardiac sensitivity to catecholamines ↑↑↑	Heart rate ↑ Blood pressure ↓↓ Cardiac output ↓ Peripheral resistance ↓ Cardiac sensitivity to catecholamines ↑
Effects on electroencephalogram	None	Decreased voltage Burst suppression	Changes similar to grand mal or focal seizure activity + muscle twitching
Cerebral blood flow	↑	↑↑↑	↑
Potentiation of non-depolarizing neuromuscular blockade	None	Moderate	Marked
Effect on uterus	None	Slight relaxation	Slight relaxation
Metabolism (%)	Minimal	15–25	2
Fluoride production	None	Minimal	Significant
Toxicity and hypersensitivity reactions	Inactivation of vitamin B_{12} Neutropenia	Hepatic damage (rare)	Hepatic damage (extremely rare) Renal toxicity ?

↑ or ↓, Minimal change; ↑↑ or ↓↓, moderate change; ↑↑↑, marked change; ↑/↓, no change.

clinical demonstration of its effects was unsuccessful, and its use fell into disrepute. The low potency of nitrous oxide, and the necessity for adequate oxygenation during anaesthesia, were only recognized in the 1870s. Since then, the gas has been frequently used as an adjuvant, and as a vehicle for the administration of more potent agents during inhalational anaesthesia. It is also used to provide analgesia, particularly in obstetric practice, as an equal mixture of nitrous oxide and oxygen (50% : 50%, v/v; Entonox).

Physical and chemical properties

At ambient temperatures and pressures, nitrous oxide is a colourless and odourless

Isoflurane	Desflurane	Sevoflurane
Rapid	Extremely rapid	Extremely rapid
Moderate	Moderate	Moderate
Slightly irritant Respiratory rate ↑ Tidal volume ↓↓ $Pa{CO_2}$ ↑	Pungent and irritant Respiratory rate ↑ Tidal volume ↓↓ $Pa{CO_2}$ ↑	Non-irritant Respiratory rate ↑ Tidal volume ↓↓ $Pa{CO_2}$ ↑
Heart rate ↑↑ Blood pressure ↓↓ Cardiac output ↓ Peripheral resistance ↓↓ Cardiac sensitivity to catecholamines ↑ Coronary steal ?	Heart rate ↑ Blood pressure ↓↓ Cardiac output ↓ Peripheral resistance ↓↓ Cardiac sensitivity to catecholamines ↑ Coronary steal ?	Heart rate ↑/↓ Blood pressure ↓↓ Cardiac output ↓ (slight) Peripheral resistance ↓ Cardiac sensitivity to catecholamines ↑ Coronary steal ?
Decreased voltage Burst suppression	Decreased voltage Burst suppression	Decreased voltage Burst suppression
↑	↑	↑
Marked	Marked	Marked
Slight relaxation	Slight relaxation	Slight relaxation
0.2	0.02	3
Minimal	Minimal	Significant
None	None	Renal toxicity?

gas which boils at –88°C, and is heavier than air (specific gravity = 1.54). Although it is non-flammable, it strongly supports combustion. It is usually prepared by heating ammonium nitrate at 250°C; if the reaction temperature is poorly controlled, higher oxides of nitrogen are formed. The contamination of nitrous oxide by these impurities may have fatal effects in anaesthetized patients. After preparation, the compressed gas is cooled to –40°C, and stored as a liquid under pressure in steel cylinders (5000 kPa; 50 atm).

Nitrous oxide is a relatively insoluble agent, with a low blood : gas partition coefficient (0.47). It has a lower lipid solubility than other anaesthetics, and its oil : gas solubility coefficient is only 1.4.

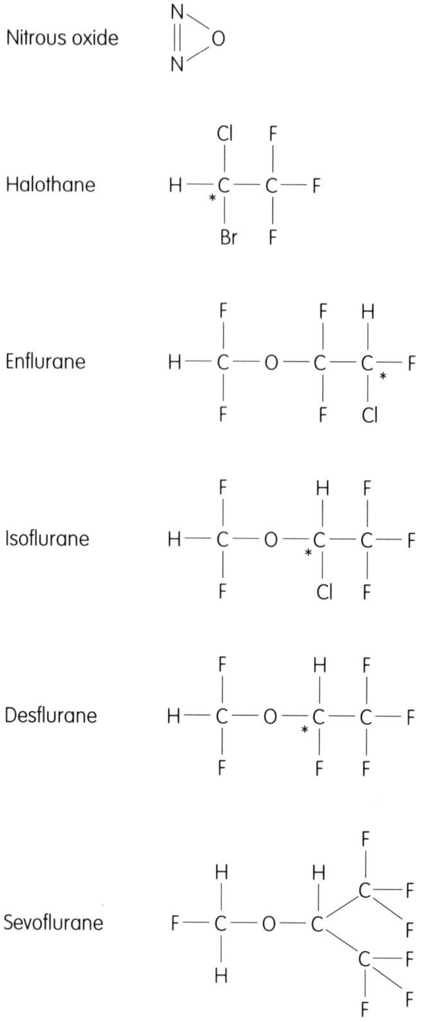

Fig. 8.3 The structural formulae of common inhalational anaesthetic agents. The presence of chiral carbon atoms is shown by an asterisk.

Induction and recovery

Both induction and recovery from anaesthesia are extremely rapid, and its alveolar concentration rapidly approaches the inspired gas concentration (Fig. 8.2). During induction, nitrous oxide may cause exhilaration and euphoria. In the 19th century, it became generally known as laughing gas (since subjects who inhaled it became jovial and boisterous). Unpremedicated patients solely anaesthetized with nitrous oxide and oxygen may also experience bizarre dreams during surgery.

Although nitrous oxide has a low blood solubility, it is 15–25 times more soluble than oxygen or nitrogen, and diffuses across membranes some 15 times more rapidly than oxygen, and 25 times more rapidly than nitrogen. Consequently, nitrous oxide diffuses across the alveolar epithelium into pulmonary capillaries more rapidly than oxygen, and the alveolar oxygen tension may therefore temporarily increase during induction. Reverse changes may occur during recovery from anaesthesia, due to the rapid diffusion of nitrous oxide from pulmonary capillary blood into the alveoli, and may cause temporary hypoxia (diffusion hypoxia). Nitrous oxide diffuses through tissues more readily than other anaesthetics; in the average adult, the percutaneous diffusion rate is about 10 ml min^{-1}.

Since nitrous oxide is more diffusible than oxygen or nitrogen, it enters enclosed air-containing spaces more rapidly than oxygen or nitrogen can leave. These spaces include the cuff of an endotracheal tube, the bowel, pneumothoraces and air emboli; nitrous oxide will increase their volume by an amount that is related to its alveolar concentration. During prolonged intra-abdominal procedures, distension of the gut may adversely affect operating conditions and make wound closure more difficult. Similarly, administration of 75% nitrous oxide doubles the size of a pneumothorax in 10 min, and triples it in 30–45 min. Nitrous oxide may also cause pressure changes in some non-compliant spaces, e.g. the middle ear, nasal sinuses and the eye.

Potency

Nitrous oxide is not a potent anaesthetic (although it is a good analgesic); due to its low lipid solubility, its MAC is 104% v/v at atmospheric pressure.* The low potency of nitrous oxide restricts its use as an inhalational anaesthetic, and when the inspired concentration of nitrous oxide is more than 70%, arterial and tissue hypoxia may occur. A mixture of nitrous oxide and oxygen (usually 65% : 35%) is widely used as a carrier gas for more potent inhalational agents, or is combined with other drugs (e.g. intravenous anaesthetics and opioid analgesics).

Analgesia

Nitrous oxide is a powerful analgesic; inhalation of 20–50% mixtures in oxygen may have similar effects to standard doses of morphine or pethidine. A mixture of nitrous oxide and oxygen containing equal volumes of both gases (Entonox) is widely used in obstetric practice to relieve pain during childbirth. It is also used in minor surgical procedures (e.g. the dressing of small burns and superficial wounds). The explanation for the analgesic effects of nitrous oxide is obscure; it may involve actions at opioid receptors, since the analgesia is partially antagonized by naloxone.

* The MAC of nitrous oxide can be determined by hyperbaric techniques, or by the additive potencies, when expressed as MAC values, of individual inhalational agents; thus, 0.5 MAC halothane + 0.5 MAC nitrous oxide is equivalent to 1.0 MAC of either agent.

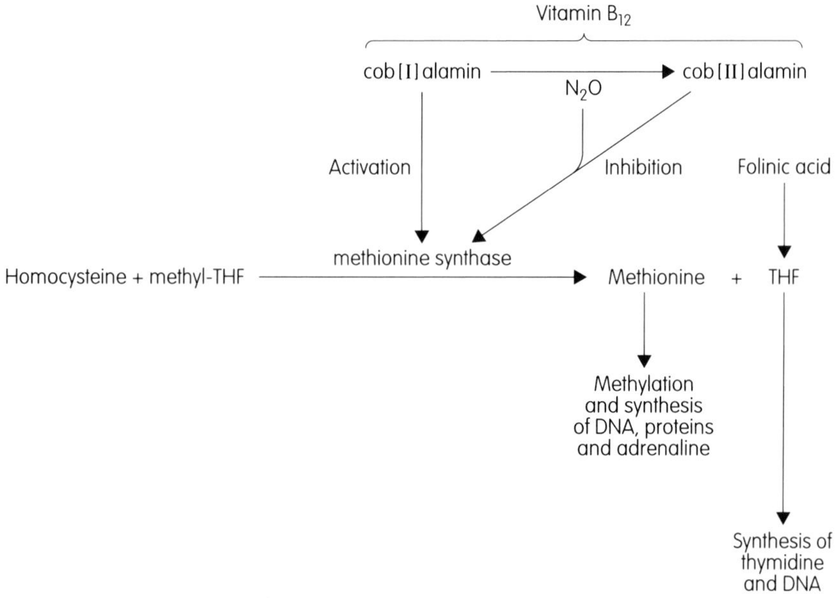

Fig. 8.4 Metabolic pathways that are affected by nitrous oxide. An active form of vitamin B_{12} (cob[I]alamin) is the cofactor of methionine synthase and activates the enzyme. Nitrous oxide oxidizes the cobalt ion in vitamin B_{12} from this active monovalent form to an inactive divalent form (cob[II]alamin). The resultant inhibition of methionine synthase impairs the synthesis of methionine and tetrahydrofolate (THF) and has subsequent effects on DNA and protein synthesis.

Respiratory effects

In anaesthetic concentrations, nitrous oxide tends to increase the respiratory rate; this compensates for any decrease in tidal volume, so that alveolar ventilation and $Paco_2$ are maintained at normal levels. In the presence of nitrous oxide, the increases in $Paco_2$ produced by the more potent fluorinated anaesthetics are minimized. Nevertheless, nitrous oxide depresses the ventilatory response to increased $Paco_2$ or hypoxaemia in a similar manner to other anaesthetic agents. Nitrous oxide anaesthesia is associated with a reduction in FRC, an increased incidence of atelectasis and a reduced Pao_2 during the postoperative period. It also depresses mucociliary function, and has a depressant effect on neutrophil motility.

Cardiovascular effects

Although nitrous oxide has mild myocardial depressant effects, and slightly reduces myocardial contractility, it also increases sympathetic activity by its central effects. In most patients, the increase in sympathetic activity counteracts the direct myocardial depressant effects, and may also offset the depressant effects of other inhalational agents. Consequently, administration of 70% nitrous oxide usually has no significant effect on haemodynamic performance, even in patients undergoing coronary artery surgery. In the absence of excitement, heart rate is generally unaffected by nitrous oxide, but systemic vascular resistance may slightly increase, due to sympathetic stimulation. Extrasystoles or ectopic rhythms are only rarely induced and there is no evidence that sensitivity to endogenous or exogenous catecholamines is modified. Thus, nitrous oxide is not contraindicated in patients with serious cardiac disease.

Nitrous oxide increases cerebral blood flow, and may also potentiate similar responses to halogenated inhalational agents. Consequently, it is sometimes avoided in subjects with serious intracranial pathology. In other patients, these effects are relatively minor and of little practical importance.

Metabolism and toxic effects

There is no evidence that significant amounts of nitrous oxide are metabolized in humans; in this respect, the anaesthetic may differ from most other inhalational agents. Extremely small amounts may be converted to nitrogen during the oxidation of vitamin B_{12}, and some may also be reduced to nitrogen by intestinal bacteria.

Administration of nitrous oxide may interfere with the synthesis of methionine, deoxythymidine and DNA (Fig. 8.4). Nitrous oxide oxidizes the cobalt ion in the vitamin B_{12} molecule from the monovalent form (cob[I]alamin) to the divalent form (cob[II]alamin). Since vitamin B_{12} is the cofactor of methionine synthase, oxidation of vitamin B_{12} results in inhibition of the enzyme. The inhibition of methionine synthase results in impaired synthesis of methionine and tetrahydrofolate, with subsequent effects on deoxythymidine, thymidine and DNA synthesis (Fig. 8.4). Methionine synthase is also directly inactivated by nitrous oxide, possibly due to the production of free radicals.

The effects of nitrous oxide on vitamin B_{12} metabolism and methionine synthase occur rapidly; in rats exposed to 50% nitrous oxide, thymidine synthesis is impaired within 1 h. In humans, exposure to nitrous oxide for 2–24 h may cause impairment of deoxythymidine synthesis and megaloblastic changes in the bone marrow; their severity appears to be related to the duration of anaesthesia. More prolonged exposure to nitrous oxide (e.g. for 4–6 days) results in agranulocytosis, although some patients are relatively resistant. These effects are accompanied by a rise in serum folate, and decreased serum methionine concentrations.

After exposure to nitrous oxide has ceased, the marrow gradually returns to normal within approximately 1 week. Recovery can be accelerated by folinic acid; this acts as an alternative source of tetrahydrofolate, and restores normal thymidine synthesis within several hours (Fig. 8.4). Administration of methionine, even in large dosages, is less effective. Although vitamin B_{12} may assist recovery, the time required for the formation of new methionine synthase (2–3 days) appears to be the main rate-limiting factor. Intermittent or repeated exposure to nitrous oxide within a short period may not allow sufficient time for enzyme activity to recover.

Nitrous oxide has little or no effect on vitamin B_{12} or methionine synthase at inhaled concentrations of 450 p.p.m. or less, regardless of the duration of exposure. Hospital staff working in unscavenged operating theatres are exposed to concentrations between 200 and 400 p.p.m., and have normal serum methionine levels; concentrations in a scavenged operating theatre are approximately 50 p.p.m. In these conditions, the possible hazards of occupational exposure to nitrous oxide are relatively slight. In contrast, prolonged exposure to nitrous oxide in heavily contaminated and unscavenged environments (e.g. dental surgeries) can produce neurological syndromes resembling subacute combined degeneration of the spinal cord; their occurrence presumably reflects the chronic deficiency in vitamin B_{12} induced by nitrous oxide.

In experimental animals, nitrous oxide is a mild teratogen when administered in concentrations of 50% or more for several days. These effects can be prevented by pretreatment with folinic acid, suggesting their relationship to impaired DNA synthesis. There is very little convincing evidence that exposure to nitrous oxide in early pregnancy (either as a patient or as a hospital employee) results in any adverse effects, in spite of the very large numbers of women that have been exposed over many years. Nevertheless, it may be considered prudent to avoid exposure to nitrous oxide during the first 6 weeks of pregnancy (or to cover the anaesthetic with folinic acid), when this is possible.

Halothane

Halothane is a fluorinated hydrocarbon synthesized by Charles Suckling between 1950 and 1955; its pharmacology was subsequently investigated by James Raventós, and its anaesthetic effects in humans were first described by Michael Johnstone in 1958. At the time, it was a notable advance in inhalational anaesthesia, and was the volatile agent of choice for at least 20 years. During the past decade, its clinical use in the UK has markedly declined, mainly due to the extremely rare complication of halothane hepatitis, and the introduction and availability of other fluorinated anaesthetics. Nevertheless, halothane is probably still the most commonly used inhalational anaesthetic in the world.

Physical and chemical properties

Halothane (2-bromo-2-chloro-1,1,1-trifluoroethane) is a volatile, colourless liquid, which boils at 50.2°C, and is unstable in the presence of light. Decomposition is usually prevented by storage in amber-coloured bottles containing thymol (0.01%), in order to prevent the liberation of free bromine. In the conditions and concentrations used in anaesthesia, it is non-flammable and non-explosive. Halothane has a relatively low blood : gas partition coefficient (2.4); consequently, both induction and recovery are relatively rapid and the level of anaesthesia is easily controlled. The oil–gas partition coefficient of halothane at 37°C is 224, and its MAC value in oxygen is 0.75% v/v; consequently, it is a relatively lipid-soluble and potent anaesthetic. Concentrations of 2–4% are usually required for induction, and 0.5–1.5% for the maintenance of anaesthesia. It has poor analgesic properties; indeed, in certain circumstances, it may have antanalgesic effects and lower the pain threshold.

Halothane is a chiral drug and can exist in two distinct, optically active forms, which may have different biological properties (Chapter 4). The drug used clinically is a racemic mixture of the two enantiomeric forms.

Respiratory effects

Halothane is a respiratory depressant, and typically increases respiratory rate, but decreases tidal volume and minute ventilation volume. $P\text{aco}_2$ may be increased. In small concentrations (< 1 MAC) these effects are relatively slight, although the ventilatory response to hypercarbia and hypoxia is usually partially suppressed, due to inhibitory effects on peripheral vascular chemoreceptors. At higher concentrations (1–2 MAC) respiratory depression is more pronounced, due to the additional inhibition of neuronal pathways in the brainstem. In general, the degree of respiratory depression is partially reversed by sensory or surgical stimulation.

Bronchial and bronchiolar smooth-muscle tone are also reduced, due to a decrease in cholinergic tone. Histamine-induced bronchoconstriction is suppressed, and the drug may be useful in asthmatic patients.

Halothane does not irritate the respiratory tract or increase salivary, laryngeal or bronchial secretions. In the concentrations used to induce anaesthesia, it depresses pharyngeal and laryngeal reflexes, and has complex effects on mucus production and mucociliary flow rates.

Cardiovascular effects

Halothane anaesthesia has important effects on the heart and the circulation. In the heart, vagal tone is increased, the automaticity of the sino-atrial node is depressed, and atrioventricular conduction is delayed, producing sinus bradycardia or an atrioventricular junctional rhythm. Myocardial contractility and cardiac output are also decreased, although these parameters may return to normal during prolonged anaesthesia. In addition, halothane slightly reduces cardiac afterload, increases the myocardial oxygen supply-to-demand ratio and enhances the myocardial tolerance of ischaemia. Consequently, intraoperative ST depression is less common than with other fluorinated agents. Myocardial depression induced by halothane is potentiated by β-adrenoceptor blockade and calcium antagonists, and is the main explanation for the reduction in blood pressure during anaesthesia. The actions of halothane on the myocardium have been compared with the effects of calcium antagonists (particularly verapamil).

During halothane anaesthesia, the peripheral circulation is also affected, and there is a slight overall reduction in systemic vascular resistance (about 5% at 1 MAC). The precise effects on peripheral resistance and regional blood flow vary in different vascular beds. Cutaneous and cerebral blood flow are increased, due to a fall in peripheral resistance; pulmonary blood flow is also slightly increased, and the vasoconstrictor response to hypoxia is inhibited. In contrast, splanchnic, hepatic and renal blood flow are reduced. There is usually little or no direct effect on coronary blood flow. The basis of these actions is unclear; they may be related to effects on central sympathetic pathways and baroreceptors, blockade of cholinergic receptors in autonomic ganglia, or to direct effects on vascular smooth muscle. The autoregulation of blood flow in various organs is also impaired; consequently, alterations in cerebral blood flow may reflect any changes in cardiac output. Halothane also modifies the responsiveness of the cerebral circulation to changes in $P\mathrm{aco}_2$; thus, hypocarbia may not reverse the increase in cerebral blood flow. During halothane anaesthesia, there is a fall in the plasma concentration of most endogenous catecholamines (including dopamine, noradrenaline and adrenaline). It is possible that these hormonal changes may partially mediate the effects of halothane on the circulation. The effects of halothane on the heart and the peripheral circulation tend to reduce systemic blood pressure, to an extent that is directly related to the inhaled concentration; consequently, the anaesthetic can be used to produce controlled hypotension.

Halothane sensitizes the myocardium to catecholamines, and cardiac arrhythmias may occur during halothane anaesthesia. Simple and relatively innocuous arrhythmias (e.g. bradycardia and atrioventricular junctional rhythms) are fairly common; alternatively, bigeminal rhythm or multifocal ventricular extrasystoles may occur, and can progress to ventricular tachycardia or fibrillation. There are many well-recognized precipitating factors, including hypokalaemia, hypocalcaemia, acidosis, alkalosis and sudden hypertensive responses; in addition, changes in the concentration of circulating catecholamines may induce cardiac arrhythmias. Increased endogenous secretion of adrenaline (which may be due to endotracheal intubation, hypoxia, hypercarbia or the presence of a phaeochromocytoma) or drugs with β-adrenergic actions or sympathomimetic effects can precipitate arrhythmias during halothane anaesthesia. A particular hazard is presented by injected or infused adrenaline, and its use should be avoided, if possible, during halothane anaesthesia. If adrenaline is required to produce local haemostasis during surgery, concentrations of 1 : 100 000 (10 μg ml^{-1}) or less should be used, and no more than 100 μg should be given within a 10-min period (in an adult). The dose may be doubled if administered with 0.5% lignocaine. In contrast to catecholamines, vasoconstrictor polypeptides such as felypressin do not affect the excitability of the heart, or increase the risk of arrhythmias during halothane anaesthesia.

Arrhythmias induced during halothane anaesthesia often resolve spontaneously when precipitating factors (e.g. hypokalaemia or hypercarbia) are treated. Specific therapy may be indicated in the management of life-threatening arrhythmias; its efficacy will be greatly enhanced by the institution of general supportive measures. Adrenaline-induced ventricular arrhythmias are usually treated with a β-adrenoceptor antagonist such as propranolol, or intravenous lignocaine. Metoprolol and atenolol are relatively cardioselective (β_1) adrenoceptor antagonists, and are more acceptable alternatives in patients in whom the use of propranolol may be inadvisable (e.g. in asthma or diabetes).

Halothane (and other fluorinated anaesthetics, particularly enflurane) may interact with calcium-channel antagonists (e.g. verapamil, diltiazem); consequently, combinations of these drugs may have adverse effects on the cardiovascular system (Chapter 5). In patients with reasonable ventricular function, significant haemodynamic effects may only occur when high doses of inhalational agents are used (> 1.5 MAC) in the presence of calcium-channel antagonists. Hypotension is commonly seen, due to reductions in systemic vascular resistance and myocardial contractility; atrioventricular block or sinus arrest may also occur (particularly with verapamil). By contrast, in patients with poor ventricular function (and during open-chest surgery) myocardial depression may occur with small doses of calcium antagonists; the presence of β-adrenergic blockade may further enhance cardiac depression.

Other effects

Halothane, like other volatile agents, has a depressant effect on the activity of many types of smooth muscle (e.g. vascular, gastrointestinal, vesical and uterine muscle), as well as skeletal and cardiac muscle. In the uterus, equipotent concentrations of halothane, enflurane and isoflurane produce the same degree of muscle relaxation. Although they are generally considered to be unsuitable as sole anaesthetic agents in obstetric practice, low concentrations (e.g. 0.5 MAC) are commonly used to prevent awareness during Caesarean section.

Halothane augments the effects of non-depolarizing muscle relaxants in a dose-dependent manner (but to a lesser extent than the fluorinated ethers). The explanation for the potentiation of neuromuscular blockade is obscure, although both central and peripheral factors may be involved. Halogenated anaesthetics depress the central nervous system, inhibit the presynaptic release of acetylcholine, and may desensitize postsynaptic acetylcholine receptors. In these conditions, smaller amounts of non-depolarizing agents are required to produce adequate muscle relaxation, and their duration of action may be prolonged. These effects are greatest with tubocurarine and pancuronium, and are usually less marked with atracurium and vecuronium.

When halothane is eliminated, the potentiation of neuromuscular blockade is rapidly reversed.

Metabolism

Approximately 25% of halothane is normally metabolized by one or more cytochrome P-450 isoforms to trifluoroacetic acid, chloride ions and bromide ions. These metabolites are slowly excreted in urine; bromide ions may be detected in the body for several weeks after prolonged anaesthesia, and their concentration may be high enough to cause significant postoperative sedation. In oxidative conditions, there is little or no defluorination of halothane, and fluoride ions are not formed. In contrast, in hypoxic conditions, reductive metabolism of halothane occurs, resulting in the formation of fluoride and other reduced metabolites, which are excreted in a conjugated form in urine. Consequently, halothane metabolism depends on cellular oxygen availability in the liver. In normal conditions, little or no defluorination of halothane takes place; by contrast, during hepatic hypoxia, significant amounts of fluoride may be produced by reductive metabolism. Most of the evidence suggests that halothane hepatitis is primarily related to the oxidative metabolism of the drug.

Hepatotoxicity (halothane hepatitis)

Administration or exposure to halogenated hydrocarbons (e.g. carbon tetrachloride and methylene dichloride) is classically associated with hepatocellular damage. During the past 35 years, the extensive use of halothane has also been associated with severe hepatic damage.

Postoperative jaundice and death after exposure to halothane were reported soon after the introduction of the drug, and the condition was compared with chloroform poisoning. Since then, it has become clear that severe hepatic necrosis is a definite but extremely uncommon complication of halothane anaesthesia; indeed, the condition is so rare that it cannot always be differentiated from viral hepatitis, or other causes of perioperative jaundice.

Administration of halothane affects the liver in two different ways. In the first place, the drug can cause mild and transient liver damage in approximately 25% of patients within 3 days of administration; there are characteristic changes in liver function tests (particularly in aminotransferase enzymes) but minimal clinical signs or abnormalities. This relatively common and mild type of hepatic dysfunction may be related to slight hypoxia, particularly in the centrilobular region of hepatic lobules, and is sometimes associated with the reductive metabolism of halothane.

In contrast, halothane occasionally causes severe fulminant hepatic necrosis with a high mortality rate (typically 50–80%); the condition usually occurs within 5 days of exposure to the drug, and is accompanied by a large increase in amino-transferase levels. The duration of exposure is not usually critical, and many cases occur after relatively short operative procedures. The overall incidence of hepatic necrosis is approximately 1 in 10 000 (range: 1 in 7000 to 1 in 35 000); it is more common, and has a higher mortality, after repeated exposure to halothane, suggesting that the condition may have an immunological basis.

In the past, experimental models of halothane hepatitis have been developed, in an attempt to study the cause of the severe hepatic necrosis. These paradigms include the polychlorinated biphenyls (PCB)–halothane model; the halothane–hypoxia model; and the triiodothyronine model. There is no evidence that any of these experimental models are similar to halothane hepatitis in humans, and their validity is extremely questionable. More recent studies have been concerned with the immunological mechanisms that may be involved in halothane hepatotoxicity. One of the oxidative metabolites of halothane, trifluoroacetyl chloride, is covalently bound to lysine residues on hepatic proteins, including isoforms of cytochrome P-450 itself. In susceptible individuals, the alkylated protein may act as an antigen, inducing the formation of antibodies that react with liver cells. By means of enzyme-linked immunosorbent assay (ELISA), serum antibodies to trifluoroacetyl-lysine residues can be detected in about 70% of patients with hepatic failure after exposure to halothane; they are not detected in patients with other forms of liver disease, or in those who have had uneventful halothane anaesthesia. The presence of the antibodies is specific to halothane-induced hepatitis, and titres usually persist for 1–5 years. Only an extremely small minority of individuals are sensitive to the antigen; the reasons for this are unclear.

A number of risk factors for halothane hepatitis are recognized; these include multiple exposures (with a maximum susceptibility of 28 days between exposures); obesity (particularly in females); and middle age (although a number of cases have been reported in children). The condition is twice as common in females, and there is sometimes an association with hepatic enzyme-inducing agents. In practical terms, it is generally recommended that anaesthetists should: (i) take a careful anaesthetic history; (ii) avoid repeated exposure to halothane within a period of at least 3 months; and (iii) avoid the use of halothane in patients with a history of jaundice or pyrexia after previous exposure. Nevertheless, the safety period of 3 months is completely arbitrary; if the condition has an immunological basis, any repeated exposure to halothane may increase the risk of hepatotoxicity in susceptible patients. Significant antibody titres may be present for up to 5 years, and cases of hepatotoxicity have been reported after a similar interval between exposures. In addition, some postoperative pyrexia is not uncommon after surgery, and many patients may be excluded from subsequent halothane anaesthesia by the adoption of this criterion. It is almost impossible to eliminate the risk of halothane hepatitis entirely, except by avoiding the use of the drug; the possibility of its occurrence has undoubtedly been the major factor in the decline in the use of halothane in the UK during the past decade.

Other fluorinated anaesthetics (particularly enflurane, isoflurane and desflurane) are less extensively metabolized than halothane; consequently, they are less likely to produce significant amounts of hepatic metabolites that can act as haptens and induce the formation of antibodies. Occasional cases of jaundice and hepatotoxicity have been reported after enflurane anaesthesia, although they are extremely rare; it has been estimated that postoperative hepatic dysfunction will be produced by enflurane in 1–2 million anaesthetics. Current evidence suggests that isoflurane, desflurane and sevoflurane anaesthesia are not associated with hepatotoxicity. Nevertheless, metabolites of enflurane are covalently bound to liver proteins, and can react with antibodies from patients with halothane hepatitis. In addition, isoflurane is metabolized to trifluoroacetyl derivatives, which may be the important haptenic group in halothane hepatitis (although antibodies have not been detected in patients after isoflurane anaesthesia). It is clear that several fluorinated anaesthetics can produce metabolites that are covalently bound by hepatic proteins, and that cross-sensitization between different anaesthetic agents could occur. Nevertheless, since halothane is more extensively metabolized than other agents, it is likely to produce the highest concentrations of haptenic determinants, immunoreactive proteins and hepatotoxic antibodies.

Enflurane

Enflurane is a fluorinated ethyl methyl ether, which was synthesized by R.C. Terrell in 1963. During the past 15 years, it has been widely used as an acceptable alternative to halothane; at the present time, enflurane and its structural isomer isoflurane are by far the most popular volatile agents in the UK and most developed countries.

Physical and chemical properties

Enflurane (2-chloro-1,1,2-trifluoroethyl difluoromethyl ether) is a volatile, colourless liquid which boils at 56.5°C, and has a relatively pleasant smell. Enflurane has a low blood : gas partition coefficient (1.8), induction and recovery are rapid, and the level of anaesthesia is easily controlled. Its oil : gas partition coefficient at 37°C is 98, and its MAC value in oxygen is 1.63% v/v; consequently, it is less lipid-soluble and less potent than halothane. Concentrations of up to 5% are required for induction, and 1–2% for the maintenance of anaesthesia. Enflurane has analgesic properties when administered in subanaesthetic concentrations (about 0.8%) and may be used effectively during labour and for burns dressings. Continuous administration of subanaesthetic doses can cause excessive drowsiness.

Enflurane is a structural isomer of isoflurane (Chapter 4), and is also a chiral drug; it contains a single asymmetric carbon atom, and is used clinically as an equal mixture of two enantiomeric forms.

Respiratory effects

Enflurane depresses respiration more than other fluorinated anaesthetics in current use. Although the respiratory rate rises, both tidal volume and the minute respiratory volume are decreased. In spontaneously breathing subjects, $Pa\text{CO}_2$ increases, and the ventilatory response to carbon dioxide is diminished. In addition, the respiratory responses to hypoxia and hypoxic pulmonary vasoconstriction are depressed. Respiratory depression is usually reduced or diminished by surgical stimulation.

Enflurane does not irritate the respiratory tract, and typically produces bronchodilation (although to a lesser extent than halothane). It does not usually induce bronchospasm or laryngospasm, and causes a reversible increase in mucus production.

Cardiovascular effects

Enflurane characteristically depresses many cardiovascular parameters (e.g. cardiac output, myocardial contractility and blood pressure), but increases heart rate. There is usually a slight decrease in systemic vascular resistance. Relatively small changes in the inhaled concentration of enflurane may have a marked effect on cardiac function, and enflurane has a narrower margin of safety than most other fluorinated agents in current use.

During light enflurane anaesthesia (0.5 MAC), stroke volume and cardiac output are usually well-maintained, but the blood pressure decreases slightly (due to a fall in systemic vascular resistance). Heart rate is generally unaffected. Higher concentrations of enflurane (1.5 MAC) significantly depress cardiac contractility; stroke volume falls to about 50% of control values, although heart rate usually increases. Consequently there is a moderate reduction in cardiac output, which is usually less than the decrease in stroke volume or contractility. Nevertheless, during deep enflurane anaesthesia (1.5 MAC) cardiac output is approximately 70% of its preoperative value. In these conditions, the negative inotropic effects of enflurane may be enhanced by β-adrenoceptor antagonists and some calcium-channel antagonists (e.g. verapamil and diltiazem); it is generally considered that enflurane modifies the movement of Ca^{2+} across cardiac cellular membranes.

Enflurane anaesthesia is occasionally associated with cardiac arrhythmias, although it is less likely than halothane to sensitize the heart to the effects of adrenaline and other catecholamines. Enflurane anaesthesia alone causes little or no change in atrioventricular conduction; however, in the presence of some calcium and β-adrenoceptor antagonists, increases in conduction time may occur and induce cardiac arrhythmias (particularly atrioventricular junctional escape rhythms). In practice, during enflurane anaesthesia arrhythmias are unlikely to occur after the subcutaneous injection or local application of adrenaline; enflurane is clearly preferable to halothane in any situation that is associated with the presence of excessive concentrations of catecholamines. The difference between the anaesthetics appears to be related to their chemical structure. Halothane is a halogenated hydrocarbon while enflurane is a fluorinated ether; the anaesthetic ethers are classically associated with a high degree of cardiovascular stability.

During enflurane anaesthesia, peripheral vascular resistance is usually reduced by approximately 25%, regardless of the depth of anaesthesia. The reduction in vascular resistance, and the associated myocardial depression, cause a marked fall in systemic arterial blood pressure. When compared with halothane, less myocardial depression may be required to produce a given fall in blood pressure; consequently, enflurane may be a more acceptable agent for the induction of controlled hypotension. Coronary vascular resistance is slightly decreased by enflurane; in contrast, resistance in the splanchnic vessels may be increased (thus reducing renal and mesenteric blood flow). Enflurane anaesthesia usually increases cerebral blood flow; autoregulation is also impaired or abolished, so that changes in cerebral perfusion may be produced by alterations in systemic blood pressure. These changes are potentiated by hypercarbia and antagonized by hypocarbia.

Central nervous system effects

Inhalation of high concentrations of enflurane (approximately 3% v/v) produces abnormal electroencephalogram (EEG) activity, particularly when $P\text{aco}_2$ tensions are decreased by hyperventilation. In children, paroxysms of generalized electrical activity that resemble grand mal epilepsy may be induced. In adults, changes indicative of focal seizure activity are more commonly observed. Abnormal EEG activity may be reduced or abolished by decreasing the concentration of enflurane and increasing the $P\text{aco}_2$ tension, but may persist for days or weeks after anaesthesia. Occasionally, EEG changes are associated with peripheral effects such as fasciculation, twitching or tonic–clonic movements of the face and limbs; permanent neurological disturbances or sequelae have not been reported. Although there is no evidence that these phenomena are commoner in epileptic patients, the use of enflurane is best avoided in subjects with convulsive disorders.

Other effects

Enflurane causes relaxation of voluntary muscle and enhances the effects of non-depolarizing muscle relaxants. It is more potent than halothane, but approximately equipotent with isoflurane, desflurane and sevoflurane. The phenomenon is due to the central effects of enflurane, as well as its peripheral actions on voluntary muscle; potentiation of muscle relaxants rapidly disappears when the anaesthetic is discontinued. It is generally considered that the dosage of non-depolarizing agents should be modified when enflurane is used (particularly in high concentrations).

Enflurane also causes relaxation of uterine smooth muscle; nevertheless, it is commonly used in low concentrations to prevent awareness during Caesarean section. Similar effects are produced on the ocular muscles, and there may be a significant fall in intraocular tension (about 30–40%). In this respect, enflurane is slightly less potent than halothane or isoflurane.

Metabolism and toxicity

Enflurane is mainly eliminated unchanged; only 2% of the inhaled drug is metabolized by the liver. The main metabolites of the drug are carbon dioxide, difluoromethoxy-difluoroacetic acid and inorganic fluoride and chloride ions. Enflurane is metabolized by a specific isoform of cytochrome P-450 (CYP 2E1), which is induced by isoniazid, alcohol and similar compounds, as well as fasting, obesity and diabetes. Other enzyme-inducing or enzyme-inhibiting agents do not affect CYP 2E1, and do not appear to modify the metabolism of enflurane.

Enflurane is partly metabolized by CYP 2E1 to fluoride ions; high plasma fluoride concentrations ($> 40\ \mu mol\ l^{-1}$) are known to cause reversible nephropathy and antidiuretic hormone (ADH)-resistant polyuria. After enflurane anaesthesia, peak plasma fluoride concentrations are commonly observed within 4–8 h, and are usually less than $20\ \mu mol\ l^{-1}$. Since enflurane is relatively insoluble and is rapidly eliminated from the body, plasma fluoride concentrations usually decline within 1–2 h; however, they may not return to baseline levels for several days. After prolonged enflurane anaesthesia, there may be some reduction in ADH sensitivity that lasts for several hours. Although the possibility of permanent renal damage is extremely small, enflurane is probably best avoided in patients with pre-existing renal disease, particularly when prolonged anaesthesia is contemplated.

Toxic or hypersensitivity reactions to enflurane that affect the liver are extremely uncommon, and prolonged anaesthesia only causes minimal changes in hepatic function. Occasional cases of jaundice and hepatotoxicity have been reported after enflurane anaesthesia, although they are exceptionally rare; it has been estimated that postoperative hepatic dysfunction will be produced by enflurane in 1–2 million anaesthetics. Nevertheless, metabolites of enflurane are covalently bound to liver proteins, and can react with antibodies from patients with halothane hepatitis; it therefore seems possible that cross-sensitization between halothane and enflurane may take place.

Isoflurane

In some respects, isoflurane is similar to its structural isomer enflurane; in other ways, its properties are quite different. Isoflurane is a fluorinated ethyl methyl ether, which was synthesized by R.C. Terrell during the 1960s. It is now commonly used as an inhalational anaesthetic agent.

Physical and chemical properties

Isoflurane (1-chloro-2,2,2-trifluoroethyl difluoromethyl ether) is a volatile colourless liquid which boils at 48.5°C and is not flammable at normal anaesthetic concentrations. It is extremely stable at ambient temperatures, and does not decompose in the presence of light or react with soda lime. Isoflurane is relatively insoluble, and has a lower blood : gas partition coefficient than halothane or enflurane (1.4). Consequently, the induction of anaesthesia is usually rapid and the level of anaesthesia is easily controlled. Unfortunately, isoflurane has a slightly unpleasant odour, which may cause problems (e.g. breath-holding) during the inhalational induction of anaesthesia. Its oil–gas partition coefficient at 37°C is 98, and its MAC value in oxygen is 1.17% v/v; consequently, it is less lipid-soluble and less potent than halothane, but more potent than enflurane (Table 8.2). Inhaled concentrations of approximately 4% are required for induction, and 1–1.5% for the maintenance of anaesthesia. Isoflurane, like enflurane, has analgesic properties when administered in subanaesthetic concentrations (e.g. 0.5%); it has been used to provide analgesia during labour, and for burns dressings. The continuous administration of subanaesthetic doses may cause drowsiness.

Isoflurane is a structural isomer of enflurane, and is also a chiral drug. It is administered clinically as a mixture of two enantiomeric forms which have similar physical and chemical properties, but have different biological effects (Chapter 4).

Respiratory effects

During spontaneous ventilation, isoflurane causes dose-dependent respiratory depression (to a lesser extent than enflurane but greater than halothane). Consequently, the respiratory rate rises, tidal volume decreases and the minute volume is reduced. In spontaneously breathing subjects, $P\text{aco}_2$ increases, and the ventilatory response to carbon dioxide is diminished. Respiratory responses to hypoxia and hypoxic pulmonary vasoconstriction are depressed to approximately the same extent as halothane. Respiratory depression is usually reduced or diminished by surgical stimulation.

Isoflurane has a slightly pungent and ethereal odour; it irritates the upper airway, but does not cause bronchoconstriction in normal humans. The incidence of postoperative pulmonary complications is similar to halothane. Isoflurane has mild bronchodilator effects, and causes a reversible depression in mucus production.

Cardiovascular effects

Isoflurane has little direct effect on the heart (in contrast to halothane and enlurane).

Anaesthetic concentrations (i.e. 1–1.5 MAC) only cause a slight fall in myocardial contractility and stroke volume. Cardiac output is usually maintained or even increased, due to baroreceptor reflex activity. Isoflurane causes peripheral vasodilatation, lowers blood pressure, but has only slight depressant effects on baroreceptors; consequently, reflex sympathetic activity is increased. There is a variable rise in pulse rate, which usually maintains cardiac output above preoperative levels. In patients under 40, there may be considerable tachycardia (i.e. more than 100 beats min^{-1}); in older subjects, baroreceptor reflexes are more depressed, and little or no change in pulse rate may occur. In these conditions, cardiac output may fall.

In general, isoflurane does not affect atrioventricular conduction or cardiac rhythm (although it may prolong the increased conduction time produced by β-adrenergic blockade or calcium-channel antagonists). In addition, isoflurane does not significantly sensitize the heart to adrenaline or other catecholamines. Nevertheless, thiopentone may reduce the arrhythmic threshold during isoflurane anaesthesia.

Isoflurane decreases peripheral resistance and is a potent vasodilator (particularly at higher concentrations). In many vascular beds, it maintains or increases blood flow (e.g. in the hepatic arterial circulation and coronary blood vessels), and therefore allows better tissue oxygenation. In the cerebral circulation, low concentrations of isoflurane (< 1 MAC) do not increase cerebral blood flow or intracranial pressure, although significant vasodilatation may occur at higher concentrations. There is little or no impairment of cerebral autoregulation or carbon dioxide responsiveness, and isoflurane is commonly used as an inhalational agent in neurosurgical practice.

The use of isoflurane in patients with coronary arterial disease is controversial. Isoflurane is a potent coronary vasodilator, and it has been suggested that the drug may cause the redistribution of blood in the coronary circulation (coronary steal), and thus induce myocardial ischaemia. In this phenomenon, blood is diverted from a myocardial area with restricted or inadequate perfusion to an area with relatively normal perfusion and autoregulation by dilatation of the coronary vasculature. Clinical studies in patients prior to coronary artery bypass grafting suggest that isoflurane may decrease blood flow through the great cardiac vein, and thus reduce regional perfusion of the myocardium. Similarly, studies in experimental animals with stenosis of the left anterior descending coronary artery suggest that isoflurane reduces blood flow through the stenosed segment, but increases perfusion in the unconstricted vasculature (the coronary steal phenomenon). Nevertheless, isoflurane appears to have little or no effect on the overall incidence of ischaemic episodes or mortality associated with bypass surgery.

Clearly, other important factors may modify myocardial blood flow and thus affect the incidence of intraoperative ischaemia. The occurrence of hypotension and tachycardia may induce myocardial ischaemia (particularly if the ratio of mean blood pressure to heart rate falls to less than 1.0). These effects are not uncommon during isoflurane anaesthesia, due to peripheral vasodilatation and the reflex increase in heart rate. Consequently, isoflurane is generally avoided in patients with severe coronary artery disease, particularly when associated with left ventricular failure. In susceptible patients, it is clearly important that blood pressure is maintained, and that tachycardia is avoided.

Other effects

Isoflurane causes relaxation of voluntary muscle, and enhances the effects of non-depolarizing muscle relaxants. In this respect, it is more potent than halothane, but approximately equipotent with enflurane, desflurane and sevoflurane. The phenomenon is due to the central effects of isoflurane, as well as its peripheral actions on voluntary muscle; the potentiation rapidly disappears when the anaesthetic is discontinued. In general, the dosage of non-depolarizing agents should be modified when isoflurane is used.

Isoflurane depresses cortical EEG activity, and does not induce abnormal electrical activity or convulsions. It also causes relaxation of uterine smooth muscle; nevertheless, it can be used in low concentrations to prevent awareness during Caesarean section. In this situation, it has approximately the same potency as halothane and enflurane.

Metabolism and toxicity

Isoflurane is mainly eliminated unchanged; approximately 0.2% of the dose is metabolized by a specific isoform of cytochrome P-450 (CYP 2E1). The main metabolites of isoflurane are trifluoroacetic acid, fluoride ions and small amounts of other fluorinated compounds. None of the breakdown products of isoflurane have been related to anaesthetic toxicity. Peak inorganic fluoride levels are approximately 5 μmol l^{-1}; they never appear to be high enough to cause renal damage (even in the presence of hepatic enzyme-inducing agents). Peak concentrations of fluoride occur at the time of anaesthesia (reflecting the low tissue solubility of isoflurane).

Desflurane

Although desflurane was synthesized in the 1960s, it has only recently been introduced into anaesthetic practice in the UK. Initially, there was little interest in desflurane, since the drug was difficult and dangerous to prepare, and had a lower anaesthetic potency than other related compounds. In addition, it was recognized that desflurane was extremely volatile, and so could not be administered by conventional anaesthetic vaporizers. Clinical studies of its suitability as an inhalational anaesthetic agent only began in 1987; in recent years, it has been recognized that it allows rather more precise control of anaesthesia than many other agents. Desflurane is closely related chemically to isoflurane and only differs in the replacement of a chloride atom by fluorine.

Physical and chemical properties

Desflurane (1-fluoro-2,2,2-trifluoroethyl difluoromethyl ether) is an extremely volatile colourless liquid which boils at 23.5°C. Its vapour pressure at 20°C is 669 mmHg (89.2 kPa), and a heated and pressurized vaporizer is required for its administration. It is non-flammable and extremely stable at ambient temperatures, and does not decompose in the presence of light, or react with soda lime or baralyme. Desflurane is relatively insoluble, and has a lower blood : gas partition coefficient than any other inhalational anaesthetic (0.45). Tissue : blood partition coefficients are also lower than the values for other volatile agents. Consequently, induction and recovery from anaesthesia should be more rapid than with other inhalational agents, and the level of anaesthesia should be easier to control. Its oil–gas partition coefficient at 37°C is 29, and its MAC value in oxygen is 6.6% v/v; consequently, it is less lipid-soluble and less potent than other fluorinated inhalational agents. Inhaled concentrations of 6–9% are required for induction, and 3–5% for the maintenance of anaesthesia. When administered in subanaesthetic concentrations, desflurane has analgesic properties.

Desflurane is closely related chemically to isoflurane; the only difference is the replacement of the single chlorine atom in isoflurane by a fluorine atom. Consequently, desflurane has 6 fluorine atoms per molecule. It is also a chiral drug, and can exist in two enantiomeric forms, which may have different biological properties (Chapter 4). When desflurane is used clinically, it is administered as an equal mixture of two stereoisomers.

Respiratory effects

Desflurane is a respiratory depressant, and has similar effects on respiration as other inhalational anaesthetics. In this respect, it is rather less potent than isoflurane or enflurane. There is a rise in the respiratory rate, and a decrease in tidal volume and minute volume; in spontaneously breathing subjects, $Paco_2$ increases, and the ventilatory response to carbon dioxide is depressed. Respiratory depression is usually reduced or diminished by surgical stimulation. Desflurane has a pungent, ethereal odour, to a greater extent than isoflurane or other inhalational agents; this often causes irritation of the airway and limits the rate of induction of inhalational anaesthesia. Consequently, desflurane frequently causes increased salivation, breath-holding, coughing or laryngospasm, and may increase the incidence of hypoxaemia during induction. It is generally accepted that desflurane should not be used to induce inhalational anaesthesia in children.

Cardiovascular effects

The effects of desflurane on the heart and the circulation are generally similar to isoflurane. Desflurane decreases blood pressure by peripheral vasodilatation and reflexly increases heart rate, so that cardiac output is usually maintained at preanaesthetic values. The rise in heart rate is associated with increased secretion of catecholamines. In general, there is little or no direct effect on the heart; occasionally cardiac contractility is depressed during anaesthesia, and may produce cardiovascular collapse. Desflurane does not usually affect atrioventricular conduction or cardiac rhythm, or sensitize the heart to adrenaline or other catecholamines.

Desflurane is a potent peripheral vasodilator, and lowers blood pressure by decreasing systemic vascular resistance. Consequently, blood flow in most peripheral blood vessels is maintained or increased (e.g. in the splanchnic and renal circulation). Cerebral vascular resistance is decreased, and cerebral blood flow may increase (depending on the concurrent effects on systemic blood pressure). Desflurane also increases coronary blood flow, and may induce the coronary steal phenomenon.

Other effects

Desflurane causes relaxation of voluntary muscle, and enhances the effects of non-depolarizing muscle relaxants. It is more potent than halothane, but approximately equipotent with the other fluorinated ethers. The relaxation of voluntary muscle is due to both the central and the peripheral effects of desflurane; the potentiation rapidly disappears when the anaesthetic is discontinued. Desflurane also causes relaxation of uterine smooth muscle, and has approximately the same potency as halothane, enflurane and isoflurane.

Metabolism and toxicity

Desflurane contains six relatively stable C—F bonds, and only minute amounts (approximately 0.02%) are metabolized in humans. After inhalation of desflurane, there are small but significant increases in serum and urine trifluoroacetate levels (although concentrations are only 10–20% of those observed after exposure to isoflurane. There are also slight but insignificant increases in inorganic and organic fluorides. The limited metabolism of desflurane is entirely mediated by an isoform of cytochrome P-450 (CYP 2E1). Enzyme induction with ethanol (or possibly phenobarbitone) increases the formation of fluoride.

Since desflurane is almost entirely eliminated unchanged, its ability to produce hepatic or renal toxicity is extremely limited. Indeed, there is no evidence that desflurane is associated with any cellular or organ toxicity. In experimental animals treated with enzyme-inducing agents, repeated and prolonged desflurane anaesthesia does not produce any significant histological or histochemical changes.

Sevoflurane

Although sevoflurane was synthesized in the 1970s, its introduction into anaesthetic practice was delayed, due to the occurrence of possible toxic effects in experimental animals. In recent years it has been widely used as an inhalational agent in Japan, and has recently been introduced into clinical use in the UK.

Physical and chemical properties

Sevoflurane (1-trifluoromethyl-2,2,2-trifluoroethyl monofluoromethyl ether) is a volatile colourless liquid which boils at 58.5°C; its vapour pressure at 20°C is 170 mmHg (22.7 kPa). It is non-flammable in air and relatively stable at ambient temperatures. It is partially hydrolysed on prolonged contact with water, or on exposure to strong bases, including soda lime and baralyme. The breakdown of sevoflurane by soda lime and baralyme is temperature dependent, and results in the formation of two breakdown products; one of these compounds (compound A, an olefin) has lethal effects in experimental animals and may have nephrotoxic effects in humans. Increased concentrations of these compounds are produced by low-flow anaesthesia. Sevoflurane is relatively insoluble, and has a low blood : gas partition coefficient (0.65); it is slightly more soluble than nitrous oxide or desflurane. Since its tissue : blood partition coefficients are also low, induction and recovery from anaesthesia are rapid, and the level of anaesthesia is easily controlled. Sevoflurane is less soluble than isoflurane in the plastic and rubber components of anaesthetic circuitry, which is an advantage in low-flow systems. Its oil–gas partition coefficient at 37°C is 80, and its MAC value in oxygen is 1.80% v/v; consequently, it is less lipid-soluble and less potent than halothane or isoflurane, but more potent than desflurane. Inhaled concentrations of 4–6% are required for induction, and 1–3% for the maintenance of anaesthesia. When administered in subanaesthetic concentrations, sevoflurane has analgesic properties.

Sevoflurane is a chemical analogue of isoflurane, and contains seven fluorine atoms per molecule. Unlike halothane, enflurane, isoflurane and desflurane, it is an achiral compound and has no optical activity.

Respiratory effects

Sevoflurane is a respiratory depressant, and has similar effects as other inhalational anaesthetics. It produces a rise in the respiratory rate, with a decrease in the tidal volume and minute volume; in spontaneously breathing subjects, $Pa\text{CO}_2$ increases, and the ventilatory response to increases in carbon dioxide is depressed. Respiratory depression is usually reduced or diminished by surgical stimulation. Sevoflurane has little or no odour or pungency, and does not irritate the airway. In Japan, sevoflurane has been widely used to induce inhalational anaesthesia in children.

Cardiovascular effects

Sevoflurane decreases blood pressure, mainly by reducing peripheral resistance. Heart rate is generally stable, and tachycardia does not usually occur. Cardiac output is usually maintained at preoperative levels. In general, sevoflurane has little or no direct effect on the heart, although cardiac contractility is occasionally depressed. Cardiac rhythm and atrioventricular conduction are usually unaffected; since sevoflurane is a fluorinated ether, it does not sensitize the heart to adrenaline or other catecholamines.

Sevoflurane primarily lowers blood pressure by decreasing systemic vascular resistance. Blood flow in most peripheral vessels is maintained or increased (e.g. in the splanchnic and renal circulation). Cerebral vascular resistance is decreased, and cerebral blood flow may increase. Sevoflurane also increases coronary blood flow, and may induce the coronary steal phenomenon.

Other effects

Sevoflurane causes relaxation of voluntary muscle, and enhances the effects of non-depolarizing muscle relaxants. It is approximately equipotent with other fluorinated ethers but more potent than halothane. Sevoflurane also causes relaxation of uterine muscle.

Metabolism and toxicity

Sevoflurane is more extensively metabolized than other fluorinated ethers, and approximately 3% of the inhaled anaesthetic is converted to inorganic and organic fluorides by the liver. The metabolism of sevoflurane is entirely dependent on a specific isoform of the mixed-function oxidase system (cytochrome P-450 2E1). Enzyme induction with ethanol, and possibly phenobarbitone, increases the formation of fluorides. Significant plasma fluoride concentrations (i.e. approximately 20 μmol l^{-1}) may occur during anaesthesia. Sevoflurane is also metabolized to hexafluoro-isopropanol, which is partly eliminated as a glucuronide conjugate with a relatively long half-life (about 55 h).

Cyclopropane

Cyclopropane is a colourless and odourless gas, which was synthesized in 1882, and introduced into anaesthetic practice in 1934. It is stored in metal cylinders, as a liquid under pressure (500 kPa; 5 atm). Like nitrous oxide, it has a low blood : gas partition coefficient (0.5), and both induction and recovery are extremely rapid. Respiratory depression may be more marked than with other inhalational agents, and hypercarbia is likely to occur in the absence of controlled ventilation. Cyclopropane does not irritate the respiratory tract, although laryngospasm or bronchospasm may occur (particularly in asthmatic subjects), due to an increase in the tone of bronchial muscle. During anaesthesia, there is usually a slight but generalized increase in sympathetic tone, producing a small rise in blood pressure. Cyclopropane is a potent muscle relaxant, and may potentiate the effects of non-depolarizing agents. Little is known of its metabolism in humans, although experimental evidence suggests that it is partly metabolized to carbon dioxide; no significant toxic effects are produced by its use.

Unfortunately, cyclopropane anaesthesia is associated with two significant hazards. First, cardiac excitability is increased and a variety of arrhythmias may occur, particularly during the induction of anaesthesia. In these conditions, ventricular ectopic beats or ventricular tachycardia may precipitate ventricular fibrillation. Similar arrhythmias are more likely to be induced by β-adrenoceptor agonists, by factors that increase endogenous adrenaline levels (such as hypercarbia), or by anticholinergic drugs. During cyclopropane anaesthesia, the use of sympathomimetic amines is extremely hazardous. Second, cyclopropane is explosive and inflammable in the concentrations required to produce anaesthesia. For these reasons, cyclopropane is rarely, if ever, used in current anaesthetic practice, and is mainly of historical interest.

Diethylether

Diethylether was introduced by William Morton in 1846, and was the first inhalational anaesthetic to be used successfully during surgical operations. It is a volatile inflammable liquid, which is extremely soluble in blood (blood : gas partition coefficient = 12.0). Thus, both induction and recovery are relatively slow, and it may take many hours to be entirely eliminated from the body. Diethylether tends to increase sympathetic tone so that respiratory rate, blood pressure and heart rate are maintained or slightly increased during anaesthesia. (In contrast, in the denervated heart diethylether has a depressant effect.) There is marked irritation of the respiratory tract, with an increase in secretions, and premedication with atropine or a similar drug is usually essential. Diethylether enhances the action of non-depolarizing agents and causes some relaxation of uterine muscle.

Little is known of the metabolism of diethylether in humans, although its administration is not associated with any significant toxicity. In experimental animals, about 6% of an administered dose is metabolized to a number of compounds including ethanol, acetaldehyde and acetic acid. One of the main advantages of diethylether is the absence of any deleterious effects on the cardiovascular system. There is no tendency to arrhythmias or increased sensitivity to catecholamines. However, postoperative nausea and vomiting are frequent side-effects.

The main disadvantages of diethylether are its slow onset and recovery, its irritant effect on the respiratory tract and its inflammability. Nevertheless, the drug was widely used until the advent of halothane in 1958. In recent years, its use has greatly declined and it is rarely, if ever, employed in current anaesthetic practice. Diethylether is still occasionally used in intensive care in the management of severe asthma. In this situation it causes bronchorrhoea, which increases the effectiveness of bronchial lavage in asthmatic patients.

Further reading

Albrecht RF, Miletich DJ. Speculations on the molecular nature of anesthesia. *General Pharmacology* 1988; **19**: 339–346.

Atlee JL III, Hamann SR, Brownlee SW, Kreigh C. Conscious state comparisons of the effects of the inhalational anesthetics and diltiazem, nifedipine, or verapamil on specialized atrioventricular conduction times in spontaneously beating dog hearts. *Anesthesiology* 1988; **68**: 519–528.

Benjamin SB, Goodman ZD, Ishak KG, Zimmerman HJ, Irey NS. The morphologic spectrum of halothane-induced hepatic injury: analysis of 77 cases. *Hepatology* 1985; **5**: 1163–1171.

Brett RS, Dilger JP, Yland KF. Isoflurane causes 'flickering' of the acetylcholine receptor channel: observations using the patch clamp. *Anesthesiology* 1988; **69**: 161–170.

Brown BR Jr, Gandolfi AJ. Adverse effects of volatile anaesthetics. *British Journal of Anaesthesia* 1987; **59**: 14–23.

Buffington CW. Hemodynamic determinants of ischemic myocardial dysfunction in the presence of coronary stenosis in dogs. *Anesthesiology* 1985; **63**: 651–662.

Carpenter RL, Eger EI II, Johnson BH, Unadkat JD, Sheiner LB. Pharmacokinetics of inhaled anesthetics in humans: measurements during and after the simultaneous administration of enflurane, halothane, isoflurane, methoxyflurane, and nitrous oxide. *Anesthesia and Analgesia* 1986; **65**: 575–582.

Cheng S-Z, Brunner EA. A hypothetical model on the mechanism of anesthesia. *Medical Hypotheses* 1987; **23**: 1–9.

Christ DD, Kenna JG, Kammerer W, Satoh H, Pohl LR. Enflurane metabolism produces covalently bound liver adducts recognised by antibodies from patients with halothane hepatitis. *Anesthesiology* 1988; **69**: 833–838.

Conway CM. Gaseous homeostasis and the circle system. Factors influencing anaesthetic gas exchange. *British Journal of Anaesthesia* 1986; **58**: 1167–1180.

Daniels S, Smith EB. Effects of general anaesthetics on ligand-gated ion channels. *British Journal of Anaesthesia* 1993; **71**: 59–64.

Eger EI II (ed.) *Anesthetic Uptake and Action*. Baltimore: Williams and Wilkins, 1974.

Eger EI II. New inhaled anesthetics. *Anesthesiology* 1994; **80**: 906–922.

Eger EI II, Saidman LJ, Bandstater B. Minimum alveolar concentration: a standard of anesthetic potency. *Anesthesiology* 1965; **26**: 756–763.

Eger EI II, Smith NT, Stoelting RK, Cullen DJ, Kadis L, Whitcher CE. Cardiovascular effects of halothane in man. *Anesthesiology* 1970; **32**: 396–409.

Eger EI II, Smuckler EA, Ferrell LD, Goldsmith CH, Johnson BH. Is enflurane hepatotoxic? *Anesthesia and Analgesia* 1986; **65**: 21–30.

Epstein RM, Rackow H, Salanitre E, Wolf GL. Influence of the concentration effect on the uptake of anaesthetic mixtures: the second gas effect. *Anesthesiology* 1964; **25**: 364–371.

Firestone L. General anaesthetics. *International Anesthesiology Clinics* 1988; **26**: 248–253.

Fogdall RP, Miller RD. Neuromuscular effects of enflurane, alone and combined with *d*-tubocurarine, pancuronium, and succinylcholine in man. *Anesthesiology* 1975; **42**: 173–178.

Forrest JB, Chambers C. Effects of volatile anaesthetics on tracheai mucociliary transport. *Canadian Anaesthetists Society Journal* 1983; **30**: S76–S77.

Franks NP, Lieb WR. What is the molecular nature of the general anaesthetic target sites? *Trends in Pharmacological Sciences* 1987; **8**: 169–174.

Franks NP, Lieb WR. Stereospecific effects of inhalational general anesthetic optical isomers on nerve ion channels. *Science* 1991; **254**: 427–430.

Franks NP, Lieb WR. Selective actions of volatile general anaesthetics at molecular and cellular levels. *British Journal of Anaesthesia* 1993; **71**: 65–76.

Franks NP, Lieb WR. Molecular and cellular mechanisms of general anaesthesia. *Nature* 1994; **367**: 607–614.

Frost EAM. Inhalation anaesthetic agents in neurosurgery. *British Journal of Anaesthesia* 1984; **56**: 47S–56S.

Gelman S, Fowler KC, Smith LR. Regional blood flow during isoflurane and halothane anesthesia. *Anesthesia and Analgesia* 1984; **63**: 557–565.

Gillman MA. Analgesia (sub-anesthetic) nitrous oxide interacts with endogenous opioid system: a review of the evidence. *Life Sciences* 1986; **39**: 1209–1221.

Halsey MJ. A reassessment of the molecular structure–functional relationships of the inhaled general anaesthetics. *British Journal of Anaesthesia* 1984; **56**: 9S–25S.

Halsey MJ. Anaesthetic mechanisms. *British Journal of Hospital Medicine* 1986; **36**: 445–447.

Halsey MJ. Drug interactions in anaesthesia. *British Journal of Anaesthesia* 1987; **59**: 112–123.

Halsey MJ, Wardley-Smith B, Green CJ. Pressure reversal of general anaesthesia — a multisite expansion hypothesis. *British Journal of Anaesthesia* 1978; **50**: 1091–1096.

Hansen TD, Warner DS, Todd MM, Vust LJ. Effects of nitrous oxide and volatile anaesthetics on cerebral blood flow. *British Journal of Anaesthesia* 1989; **63**: 290–295.

Hayashi Y, Maze M. $Alpha_2$ adrenoceptor agonists and anaesthesia. *British Journal of Anaesthesia* 1993; **71**: 108–118.

Hayashi Y, Sumikawa K, Tashiro C, Yamatodani A, Yoshiya I. Arrhythmogenic threshold of epinephrine during sevoflurane, enflurane, and isoflurane anaesthesia in dogs. *Anesthesiology* 1988; **69**: 145–147.

Haydon DA, Hendry BM, Levinson SR. The molecular mechanisms of anaesthesia. *Nature* 1977; **268**: 356–358.

Jones RM. Clinical comparison of inhalation anaesthetic agents. *British Journal of Anaesthesia* 1984; **56**: 57S–69S.

Jones RM, Cashman JN, Eger EI II, Damask MC, Johnson BH. Kinetics and potency of desflurane (I-653) in volunteers. *Anesthesia and Analgesia* 1990; **70**: 3–7.

Kapur PA, Matarazzo DA, Fung DM, Sullivan KB. The cardiovascular and adrenergic actions of verapamil or diltiazem in combination with propranolol during halothane anesthesia in the dog. *Anesthesiology* 1987; **66**: 122–129.

Keane PE, Biziere K. Minireview. The effects of general anaesthesics on GABAergic synaptic transmission. *Life Sciences* 1987; **41**: 1437–1448.

Kenna JG, Neuberger J, Williams R. An enzyme-linked immunosorbent assay for detection of antibodies against halothane-altered hepatocyte antigens. *Journal of Immunological Methods* 1984; **75**: 3–14.

Kenna JG, Neuberger J, Williams R. Specific antibodies to halothane-induced liver antigens in halothane-associated hepatitis. *British Journal of Anaesthesia* 1987; **59**: 1286–1290.

Kenna JG, Satoh H, Christ DD, Pohl LR. Metabolic basis for a drug hypersensitivity: antibodies in sera from patients with halothane hepatitis recognize liver neoantigens that contain the trifluoroacetyl group derived from halothane. *Journal of Pharmacology and Experimental Therapeutics* 1988; **245**: 1103–1109.

Khambatta HJ, Sonntag H, Larsen R, Stephan H, Stone G, Kettler D. Global and regional myocardial blood flow and metabolism during equipotent halothane and isoflurane anesthesia in patients with coronary artery disease. *Anesthesia and Analgesia* 1988; **67**: 936–942.

Krnjević K. Cellular mechanisms of anesthesia. *Annals of the New York Academy of Sciences* 1991; **625**: 1–16.

Landers DF, Becker GL, Wong KC. Calcium, calmodulin, and anesthesiology. *Anesthesia and Analgesia* 1989; **69**: 110–112.

Mapleson WW. Effect of age on MAC in humans: a meta-analysis. *British Journal of Anaesthesia* 1996; **76**: 179–185.

Mazze RI. Metabolism of the inhaled anaesthetics: implications of enzyme induction. *British Journal of Anaesthesia* 1984; **56**: 27S–41S.

Merin RG. Calcium channel blocking drugs and anesthetics: is the drug interaction beneficial or detrimental? *Anesthesiology* 1987; **66**: 111–112.

Merrell WJ, Gordon L, Wood AJJ, Shay S, Jackson EK, Wood M. The effect of halothane on morphine disposition: relative contributions of the liver and kidney to morphine glucuronidation in the dog. *Anesthesiology* 1990; **72**: 308–314.

Meyer HH. Zur Theorie der Alkoholnarkose. I. Mitt. Welche Eigenschaft der Anästhetika bedingt ihre narkotische Wirkung? *Archiv für Experimentelle Pathologie und Pharmakologie (Naunyn-Schmiedeberg)* 1899; **42**: 109–118.

Miletich DJ, Ivankovitch AD, Albrecht RF, Reimann CR, Rosenberg R, McKissic ED. Absence of autoregulation of cerebral blood flow during halothane and enflurane anaesthesia. *Anesthesia and Analgesia* 1976; **55**: 100–105.

Mitchell MM, Prakesh O, Rulf ENR, van Daele MERM, Cahalan MK, Roelandt JRTC. Nitrous oxide does not induce myocardial ischemia in patients with ischemic heart disease and poor ventricular function. *Anesthesiology* 1989; **71**: 526–534.

Moody EJ, Suzdak PD, Paul SM, Skolnick P. Modulation of the benzodiazepine/gamma-aminobutyric acid receptor chloride channel complex by inhalation anesthetics. *Journal of Neurochemistry* 1988; **51**: 1386–1393.

Munson ES, Embro WJ. Enflurane, isoflurane, and halothane and isolated human uterine muscle. *Anesthesiology* 1977; **46**: 11–14.

Neigh JL, Garman JK, Harp JR. The electroencephalographic pattern during anesthesia with enflurane. *Anesthesiology* 1971; **35**: 482–487.

Neuberger J, Williams R. Halothane anaesthesia and liver damage. *British Medical Journal* 1984; **289**: 1136–1139.

Nunn JF. Clinical aspects of the interaction between nitrous oxide and vitamin B_{12}. *British Journal of Anaesthesia* 1987; **59**: 3–13.

Nunn JF, Chanarin I, Tanner AG, Owen ERTC. Megaloblastic bone marrow changes after repeated nitrous oxide anaesthesia. *British Journal of Anaesthesia* 1986; **58**: 1469–1470.

Overton CE. *Studien über die Narkose: zugleich ein Beitrag zur allgemeinen Pharmakologie*. Jena: Gustav Fischer, 1901.

Plummer JL, Wanwimolruk S, Jenner MA, Hall P de la M, Cousins MJ. Effects of cimetidine and ranitidine on halothane metabolism and hepatotoxicity in an animal model. *Drug Metabolism and Disposition* 1984; **12**: 106–110.

Pocock G, Richards CD. Excitatory and inhibitory synaptic mechanisms in anaesthesia. *British Journal of Anaesthesia* 1993; **71**: 134–147.

Priebe HJ. Isoflurane and coronary hemodynamics. *Anesthesiology* 1989; **71**: 960–976.

Priebe HJ, Skarvan K. Cardiovascular and electrophysiologic interactions between diltiazem and isoflurane in the dog. *Anesthesiology* 1987; **66**: 114–121.

Quasha AL, Eger EI II, Tinker JH. Determination and applications of MAC. *Anesthesiology* 1980; **53**: 315–334.

Rasmussen H. The calcium messenger system — Part I. *New England Journal of Medicine* 1986; **314**: 1094–1101.

Rasmussen H. The calcium messenger system — Part II. *New England Journal of Medicine* 1986; **314**: 1164–1170.

Reilly CS, Wood AJJ, Koshakji RP, Wood M. The effect of halothane on drug disposition: contribution of changes in intrinsic drug metabolising capacity and hepatic blood flow. *Anesthesiology* 1985; **63**: 70–76.

Reiz S, Bălfors E, Sorenson MG, Ariola S Jr, Friedman A, Truedsson H. Isoflurane — a powerful coronary vasodilator in patients with coronary artery disease. *Anesthesiology* 1983; **59**: 91–97.

Ruffle JM, Snider MT, Rosenberger JL, Latta WB. Rapid induction of halothane anaesthesia in man. *British Journal of Anaesthesia* 1985; **57**: 607–611.

Rupp SM, Miller RD, Gencarelli PJ. Vecuronium-induced neuromuscular blockade during enflurane, isoflurane, and halothane anesthesia in humans. *Anesthesiology* 1984; **60**: 102–105.

Sahlman L, Henriksson B-A, Martner J, Ricksten S-E. Effect of halothane, enflurane, and isoflurane on coronary vascular tone, myocardial performance, and oxygen consumption during controlled changes in aortic and left atrial pressure. *Anesthesiology* 1988; **68**: 1–10.

Segal I, Vickery RG, Walton JK, Doze VA, Maze M. Dexmedetomidine diminishes halothane anesthetic requirements in rats through a postsynaptic alpha$_2$ adrenergic receptor. *Anesthesiology* 1988; **69**: 818–823.

Shackleton S, Harrington JM. The pollution controversy. In: Lunn JN (ed.) *Epidemiology in Anaesthesia*. London: Arnold, 1986; 93–122.

Slogoff S, Keats AS. Randomized trial of primary anesthetic agents on outcome of coronary artery bypass operations. *Anesthesiology* 1989; **70**: 179–188.

Stoetling RK, Blitt CD, Cohen PJ, Merin RG. Hepatic dysfunction after isoflurane anesthesia. *Anesthesia and Analgesia* 1987; **66**: 147–153.

Stoetling RK, Eger EI II. An additional explanation for the second gas effect: a concentrating effect. *Anesthesiology* 1969; **30**: 273–277.

Targ AG, Yasuda N, Eger EI II. Solubility of I-653, sevoflurane, isoflurane, and halothane in plastics and rubber composing a conventional anesthetic circuit. *Anesthesia and Analgesia* 1989; **69**: 218–225.

Targ AG, Yasuda N, Eger EI II, Huang G, Vernice GG, Terrell RC. Halogenation and anesthetic potency. *Anesthesia and Analgesia* 1989; **68**: 599–602.

Terrell RC. Physical and chemical properties of anaesthetic agents. *British Journal of Anaesthesia* 1984; **56**: 3S–7S.

Trudell JR. A unitary theory of anesthesia based on lateral phase separations in nerve membranes. *Anesthesiology* 1977; **46**: 5–10.

Ueda I, Kamaya H. Molecular mechanisms of anesthesia. *Anesthesia and Analgesia* 1984; **63**: 929–945.

Weiskopf RB. New inhaled anesthetics. *Current Opinion in Anesthesiology* 1989; **2**: 421–424.

White DC. A review of nitrous oxide. In: Atkinson RS, Adams AP (eds) *Recent Advances in Anaesthesia and Analgesia*, vol. 16. Edinburgh: Churchill Livingstone, 1989; 19–42.

Williams R. Halothane and the liver — a medical review. In: *Halothane and the Liver: The Problem Revisited. Proceedings of a Symposium, 1986*. Bristol: Sir Humphrey Davy Department of Anaesthesia, 1986; 12–21.

Chapter 9
Local Anaesthetic Agents

Local anaesthetic agents can be defined as drugs which are used clinically to produce reversible inhibition of the excitation–conduction process in peripheral nerve fibres and nerve endings, and thus produce the loss of sensation in a circumscribed area of the body. In the UK, only a small number of drugs are commonly used to induce local anaesthesia (prilocaine, lignocaine and bupivacaine). Nevertheless, many other agents that are primarily used for other purposes have similar actions, which are often referred to as local anaesthetic (membrane-stabilizing) properties. These drugs include:

1 Anticonvulsants (e.g. phenytoin, carbamazepine).
2 Phenothiazines (e.g. chlorpromazine).
3 Antihistamines (H_1 histamine antagonists; e.g. cyclizine).
4 Barbiturates (e.g. pentobarbitone).
5 Opioid analgesics (e.g. pethidine).
6 Antiarrhythmic drugs (e.g. quinidine, disopyramide).
7 β-Adrenoceptor antagonists (e.g. propranolol).

Similarly, local anaesthetic drugs are commonly used as antiarrhythmic agents, and have occasionally been used as anticonvulsants.

In addition, a number of naturally occurring biotoxins reversibly inhibit the conduction of impulses in peripheral nerves and nerve endings. Thus, one variety of the Japanese puffer fish (*Spheroides spengleri*) contains the poison tetrodotoxin; it is also present in the octopus, salamanders, newts and amphibia, and is probably derived from microorganisms that synthesize the toxin. (During his voyages of discovery in the South Seas, Captain James Cook tasted puffer fish and subsequently suffered from tetrodotoxin poisoning.) An unrelated series of toxins (the saxitoxins) is produced by the dinoflagellates (i.e. flagellated unicellular organisms which contaminate shellfish). Both tetrodotoxin and saxitoxin are extremely potent local anaesthetics; unfortunately, they are relatively polar compounds and do not readily penetrate perineuronal tissues.

Structure and function of nerve fibres

Peripheral nerves consist of the dendrites and axons of sensory and/or motor neurones, which are bound together and surrounded by connective tissue. Layers of longitudinally arranged collagen surround individual nerve fibres (the endoneurium) or groups of nerve fibres (the perineurium); an outer connective tissue sheath (the epineurium) surrounds the nerve trunk and carries its blood vessels and lymphatics. Each nerve fibre is connected with a central cell body or perikaryon from which it receives its metabolic and nutritional requirements, and is surrounded by a sheath of Schwann-cell cytoplasm. Unmyelinated fibres are usually enclosed in groups by the sheath of a single Schwann cell (which may be up to 0.5 mm long); at junctions, the cytoplasm of adjacent Schwann cells is in contact. In contrast, each myelinated fibre is enclosed by the cytoplasm of a single Schwann cell, with its phospholipid cell membrane wound spirally around the axon to form the myelin sheath (Fig. 9.1). Between individual Schwann cells the myelin sheath is absent; the resultant junctions are known as the nodes of Ranvier. The internodal distance is related to the size of the Schwann cells and the diameter of the nerve fibres. In large myelinated nerves, the internodal distance may be 1–2 mm.

Nerve fibres consist of a central core (the axoplasm) which is enclosed by a limiting cell membrane (the axolemma or axonal membrane). The axoplasm contains mitochondria, microtubules and neurofilaments, which are required for normal neuronal nutrition and metabolism. In contrast, the axonal membrane is a characteristic phospholipid membrane (p. 1), containing integral proteins which play an important functional role as ion channels.

Various techniques have been used to study the electrophysiology of neuronal conduction and its modification by drugs. These methods include measurement of changes in potential by intracellular microelectrodes, the use of fluorescent probes and the analysis of voltage clamp recordings, in which the membrane potential is changed in small steps, and separate phases of ionic flow are studied.

In the inactive state, there is a difference in potential of approximately 80 mV across the neuronal membrane (i.e. the inside is electronegative relative to the outside). This potential difference (the resting potential) mainly reflects the selective permeability of the neuronal membrane to potassium ions, and can be regarded as a potassium diffusion potential. In nerve fibres, as in many other cells, an ionic pump

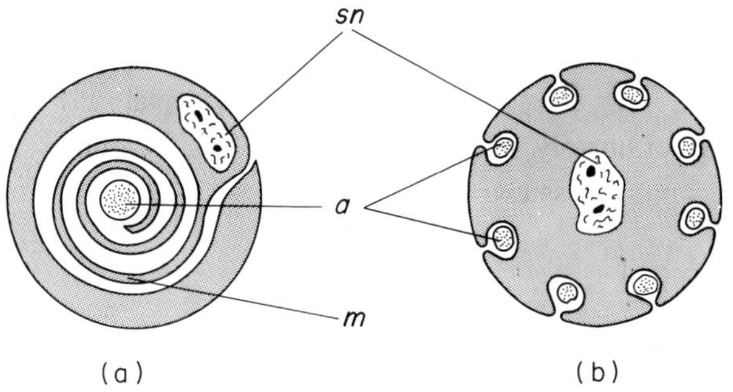

Fig. 9.1 Diagram showing transverse section of (a) myelinated nerve fibres and (b) unmyelinated nerve fibres. sn, Schwann cell nucleus; a, axon; m, myelin sheath.

(the enzyme Na^+/K^+ ATPase) maintains a high internal potassium concentration and a high external sodium concentration. The intracellular concentration of potassium (K_i^+) is normally 25–30 times greater than in extracellular fluid (K_o^+). In the resting state, the neuronal membrane is effectively impermeable to sodium ions (Fig. 9.2); consequently, sodium ions play little or no part in the production of the resting membrane potential. In contrast, the membrane is relatively permeable to potassium ions, and there is a tendency for potassium ions to diffuse from the axon. This propensity is opposed by the anionic charge on intracellular proteins, which tends to prevent potassium diffusion, and the balance between these two forces represents the resting membrane potential (–80 mV). Consequently, the resting membrane potential is closely related to the intracellular/extracellular concentration ratio of potassium ions (K_i^+/K_o^+). The neurone acts as a potassium electrode, and the resting potential can be modified by alterations in extracellular potassium concentration.

During neuronal activity, characteristic changes occur in the transmembrane potential. Initially, there is a slow phase of depolarization as the cell becomes progressively less negative. When the threshold potential is reached, there is rapid and transient depolarization to approximately +25 mV, followed by a return to the resting value (repolarization). These changes in transmembrane potential are referred to as the action potential, and occur within 1–2 ms; they are due to changes in the ionic permeability of the axonal membrane to Na^+. The property of electrical excitability (i.e. the ability to generate an action potential) depends on the presence of voltage-sensitive sodium channels in the axonal membrane. During excitation, the neurone slowly depolarizes until the threshold potential is reached at approximately –50 mV. At this point, sodium permeability rapidly

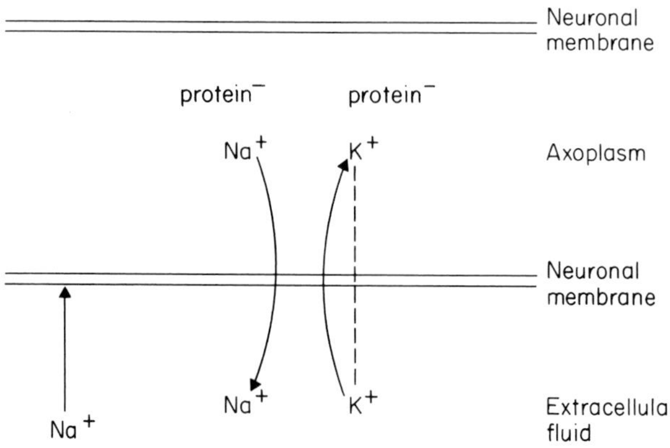

Fig. 9.2 The origin of the resting membrane potential. The sodium pump (i.e. the enzyme Na^+/K^+ ATPase) maintains a high internal potassium concentration and a high external sodium concentration. In the resting state, the membrane is effectively impermeable to sodium ions, although potassium ions can diffuse from the axoplasm to extracellular fluid. The tendency for potassium ions to leave the fibre is opposed by the ionic charges on intracellular protein, giving rise to the resting membrane potential.

increases due to the opening of voltage-dependent ion channels, and sodium ions rapidly diffuse across the axonal membrane (Fig. 9.3). This causes a transient reversal of the membrane potential to approximately +25 mV. Na^+ diffusion ceases since the transmembrane potential is equal to the equilibrium potential, and the channels close spontaneously (inactivation). At the same time, potassium permeability increases due to the opening of K^+ channels in the axonal membrane. Potassium ions diffuse across the axonal membrane into extracellular fluid, resulting in repolarization and the restoration of the resting membrane potential. During the refractory period these changes are reversed (i.e. sodium ions are transferred from the axoplasm to extracellular fluid, and potassium ions are concentrated by the neurone). Re-establishment of the ionic gradient depends on active transport by the enzyme Na^+/K^+ ATPase (the sodium pump), and requires the expenditure of cellular energy.

Calcium ions are present in the neuronal membrane (and other cellular membranes), and can interact with negatively charged phosphate groups associated with the heads of phospholipids. These hydrophilic groups are present at the internal and external aspects of the membrane (Chapter 1); interaction with calcium ions alters the charge distribution in the membrane, impedes sodium conductance and may modify the action of local anaesthetics. In experimental conditions, the threshold potential required for sodium channel opening is reduced when the local concentration of Ca^{2+} is increased (although the resting potential is unaltered).

The activation and depolarization of unmyelinated fibres produce a local flow of current in the neuronal membrane which decreases the transmembrane potential of the adjacent nerve. Voltage-sensitive sodium channels are activated and impulses are propagated along the nerve fibre. Retrograde conduction cannot occur, due to the inactivation of sodium channels in the wake of the impulse.

In myelinated fibres, current flows from one node of Ranvier to another; since the internodal distance may be 1–2 mm, conduction in myelinated fibres (saltatory conduction) is much more rapid (approximately 120 m s^{-1}).

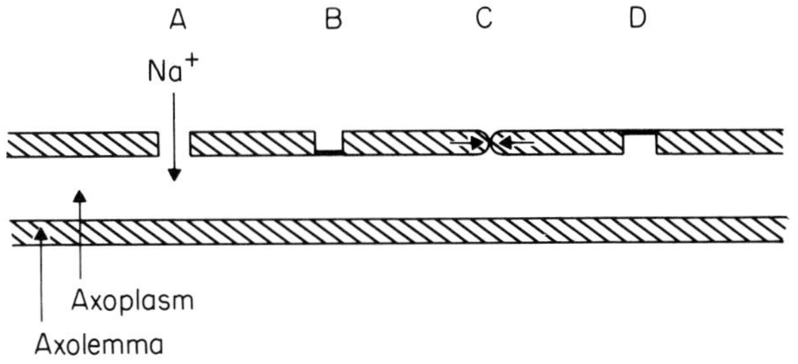

Fig. 9.3 Site of action of local anaesthetic agents. A, The influx of Na^+ through unblocked channels produces neuronal depolarization. B, Na^+ channels blocked by the cationic forms of local anaesthetic esters or amides. C, Na^+ channels blocked by the uncharged forms of local anaesthetics, due to membrane expansion. D, Na^+ channels blocked by the naturally occurring poison tetrodotoxin.

History of local anaesthetics

The alkaloid cocaine is the only naturally occurring local anaesthetic, and was the first of these drugs to be used clinically. It is derived from a shrub (*Erythroxylon coca*) that grows in the foothills of the Andes, and for many centuries its leaves were chewed by Peruvian Indians in order to obtain cocaine. The drug was particularly valued for its mood-elevating and stimulant properties, and its numbing effects on the buccal mucosa were well-known. Pure cocaine was first isolated in 1860 by Niemann, who confirmed its effects on sensation; its pharmacological actions were studied by Von Anrep between 1870 and 1880. The drug was first introduced into clinical practice by Freud and Köller in 1884. Sigmund Freud used cocaine in an attempt to treat a morphine-dependent colleague, but converted him into a cocaine addict; he also took cocaine himself for a period of 10 years (while he was writing *The Interpretation of Dreams*). Karl Köller initially used cocaine to produce corneal anaesthesia in experimental animals, and rapidly appreciated its potential advantages. He introduced it into ophthalmological practice as a surface anaesthetic, and its use for infiltration, conduction and spinal anaesthesia soon followed.

Unfortunately, its potential for producing drug dependence was not initially appreciated. Nevertheless, by 1890 its dangers were well-recognized, and a search began for newer and safer drugs. The first synthetic local anaesthetic, the *para*-aminobenzoate (PABA) ester procaine, was introduced by Einhorn in 1905. Many other synthetic local anaesthetic esters were subsequently investigated; most of these have now been discarded, and are solely of historical interest. However amethocaine is still widely used to produce topical anaesthesia.

An important milestone occurred in 1943 when lignocaine was synthesized by Lofgren, and subsequently introduced into anaesthetic practice. This aminoacylamide was the prototype of a new group of local anaesthetic drugs. Since the advent of lignocaine, other amide anaesthetics have been introduced (e.g. mepivacaine, bupivacaine and prilocaine). Etidocaine is also an extremely potent amide anaesthetic (although it is not available for clinical use in the UK). In recent years, some amide local anaesthetics have been developed as single stereoisomers (e.g. ropivacaine and s-bupivacaine), and their use may have significant clinical advantages. Some local anaesthetics (e.g. lignocaine and bupivacaine) have also been used experimentally as liposomal preparations,* in order to prolong the duration of local anaesthesia and reduce systemic toxicity.

Local anaesthetic preparations

Most local anaesthetics are bases that are almost insoluble in water. Consequently,

* Liposomes are vesicles with a diameter of 50 nm–10 μm; they consist of an aqueous phase surrounded by a phospholipid bilayer. Drugs can be incorporated in either the lipid or the aqueous phase.

their hydrochloride salts, which are extremely water soluble, are usually dissolved in modified isotonic Ringer's solution. Dilute preparations of local anaesthetics are usually acid (pH range = 4.0–5.5), and contain a reducing agent (e.g. sodium metabisulphite) to enhance the stability of added vasoconstrictors (which may oxidize in solution). These preparations also normally contain a preservative and a fungicide. The preservative helps to maintain the stability of the local anaesthetic solution, while the fungicide (usually a small concentration of thymol) prevents the growth of contaminating fungi. Solutions of local anaesthetics are extremely stable and usually have an effective shelf-life of more than 2 years.

Most local anaesthetics also produce some degree of vasodilatation, and they may be rapidly absorbed after local injection. Consequently, vasoconstrictors are frequently added to local anaesthetic solutions, in order to enhance their potency and prolong their duration of action by localizing them in tissues. In addition, vasoconstrictors decrease the systemic toxicity and increase the safety margin of local anaesthetics by reducing their rate of absorption (which is mainly dependent on local blood flow). In these conditions, the effectiveness of vasoconstrictors is extremely variable. In most infiltration procedures and in conduction blockade, vasoconstrictors usually prolong and enhance local anaesthesia; on the other hand, they may have little effect on the duration of extradural or intrathecal blockade (particularly when induced by etidocaine or bupivacaine).

Adrenaline is the most commonly used vasoconstrictor; it is added to local anaesthetic solutions in concentrations ranging from 1 in 80 000 (12.5 $\mu g\ ml^{-1}$) to 1 in 300 000 (3.3 $\mu g\ ml^{-1}$). Preparations containing noradrenaline (1 in 80 000) have been used, but are best avoided due to their pressor effects (which are particularly hazardous in patients with ischaemic heart disease or who are on tricyclic antidepressant drugs). The vasoconstrictor felypressin is added to some local anaesthetics (i.e. prilocaine) in a concentration of 0.03 i.u. ml^{-1}. Felypressin is a non-catecholamine vasoconstrictor that is chemically related to vasopressin, the posterior pituitary hormone. It is a synthetic octapeptide that only affects peripheral blood vessels; it has no action on the heart. Although it produces less marked vasoconstriction than adrenaline, it may be useful in patients with ischaemic heart disease, or when the use of catecholamines is undesirable. Other drugs (e.g. phenylephrine) have also been used as vasoconstrictors; however, adrenaline is more effective than phenylephrine or noradrenaline in decreasing the rate of absorption of most local anaesthetics.

Chemical and physicochemical properties

All local anaesthetics have certain chemical and physicochemical properties in common. Chemically, they consist of a lipophilic aromatic group (R_1), an intermediate ester (—CO·O—) or amide (—NH·CO—) chain, and a hydrophilic secondary or tertiary amine group (R_2). The intermediate chain is an important determinant of

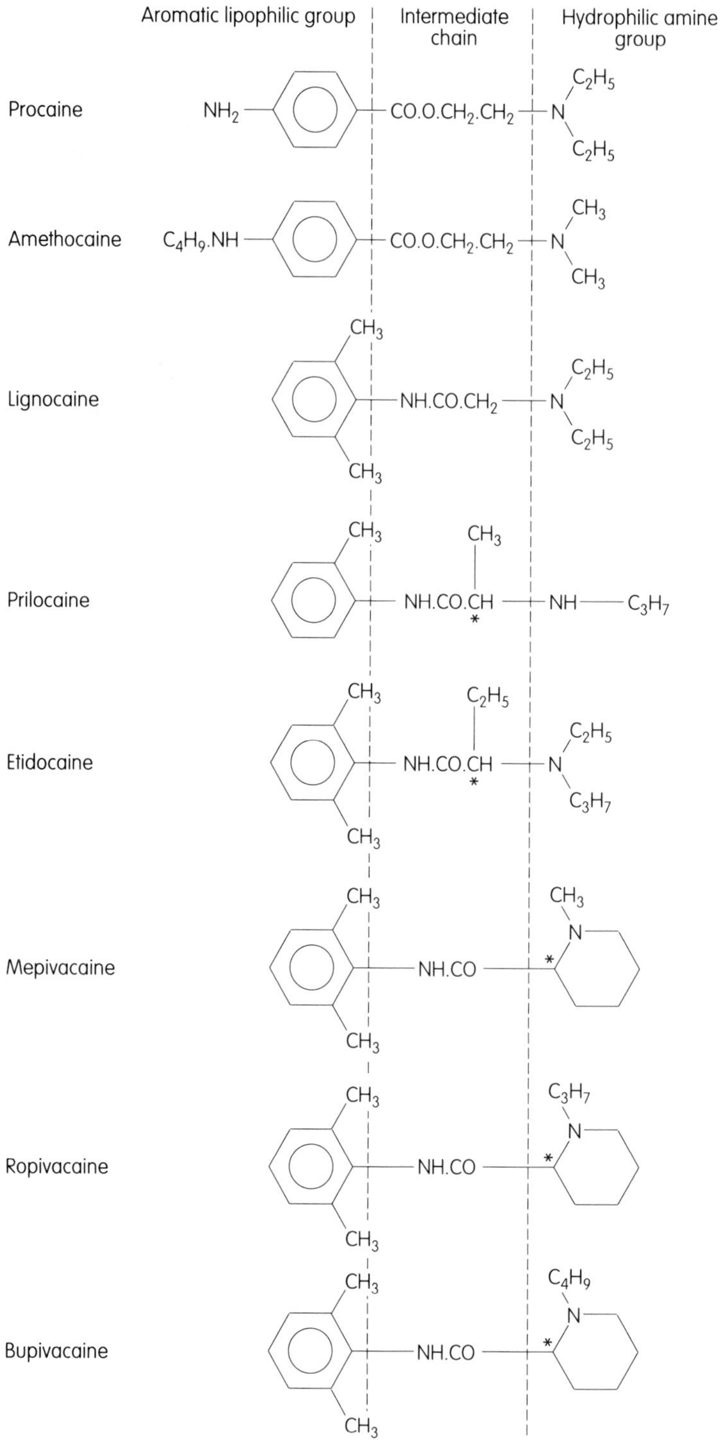

Fig. 9.4 The chemical structure of local anaesthetic agents. Chiral carbon atoms (asymmetric centres) are represented by an asterisk. Prilocaine, mepivacaine, bupivacaine and etidocaine are normally administered as racemic mixtures of R and S stereoisomers; ropivacaine is given as an S(–) enantiomer.

the duration of action; it also allows local anaesthetics to be classified as esters or amides (Fig. 9.4).

Ester local anaesthetics include:

1 Cocaine.
2 Procaine.
3 Chloroprocaine.
4 Amethocaine.

Amide local anaesthetics are:

1 Lignocaine.
2 Prilocaine.
3 Mepivacaine.
4 Bupivacaine.
5 Ropivacaine.
6 Etidocaine.

There are important practical differences between these two groups of local anaesthetics. Esters are relatively unstable in solution, and are rapidly hydrolysed in the body by plasma cholinesterase, as well as some other esterases. PABA is usually one of the main hydrolytic products, and is sometimes associated with allergic reactions. By contrast, amides are relatively stable in solution, and are slowly broken down by amidases in the liver. In addition, hypersensitivity reactions to amide local anaesthetics are almost unknown. In current practice, esters are rarely used to produce local anaesthesia.

Modification of the chemical structure of local anaesthetics may have a profound effect on their physicochemical characteristics. In particular, anaesthetic properties may be modified by changes in: (i) lipid solubility; (ii) plasma and tissue protein binding; and (iii) the dissociation constant (pK_a value). Values for these constants in ester and amide local anaesthetics are shown in Table 9.1.

In general, there is a close correlation between lipid solubility and anaesthetic potency (particularly in *in vitro* conditions). This relationship presumably reflects the ability of different anaesthetics to penetrate perineural tissues and the neuronal membrane, and reach their site of action in the axoplasm. For instance, in most clinical situations bupivacaine is approximately four times as potent as lignocaine, due to their differences in lipid solubility (Table 9.1).

Plasma and tissue protein binding primarily affect the duration of action of local anaesthetics. For example, procaine (which is not extensively bound to plasma or tissue proteins) has a short duration of action in most clinical situations; by contrast, amethocaine, bupivacaine, ropivacaine and etidocaine are extensively bound and have prolonged effects. Lignocaine, mepivacaine and prilocaine are moderately bound to plasma and tissue proteins, and have an intermediate duration of action (Table 9.1).

The dissociation constant (pK_a value) of local anaesthetics is the most important factor affecting their rapidity and onset of action. In order to produce their effects,

Table 9.1 Physicochemical properties and pharmacological effects of local anaesthetic agents.

	pK_a value (25°C)	Relative lipid solubility	Relative potency	Protein binding (%)	Onset of action	Duration of action	Clinical use	Properties
Procaine	8.9	1	1	6	Slow	Short	Limited Vascular spasm Diagnostic procedures	Vasodilatation Allergenic
Amethocaine	8.5	200	8	75	Slow	Long	Topical anaesthesia Spinal anaesthesia	Systemic toxicity
Lignocaine	7.7	150	2	65	Fast	Moderate	Infiltration anaesthesia Peripheral nerve blockade Extradural blockade IVRA	Versatile Moderate vasodilatation
Prilocaine	7.7	50	2	55	Fast	Moderate	Infiltration anaesthesia Peripheral nerve blockade IVRA	Methaemoglobinaemia Low sytemic toxicity
Etidocaine	7.7	5000	6	96	Fast	Long	Infiltration anaesthesia Peripheral nerve blockade Extradural blockade	Profound motor blockade
Mepivacaine	7.6	50	2	78	Fast	Moderate	Infiltration anaesthesia Peripheral nerve blockade	Similar to lignocaine
Ropivacaine	8.1	400	6	94	Moderate	Long	Infiltration anaesthesia Peripheral nerve blockade Extradural anaesthesia	Separation of sensory and motor blockade Reduced motor blockade
Bupivacaine	8.1	1000	8	95	Moderate	Long	Infiltration anaesthesia Peripheral nerve blockade Extradural and spinal anaesthesia	Separation of sensory and motor blockade

IVRA, Intravenous regional anaesthesia.

local anaesthetics must diffuse across the nerve sheath and the neuronal membrane in the form of the non-ionized and uncharged free base. The dissociation constant (pK_a value) represents the pH at which the concentration of the non-ionized base (B) and the ionized base (BH^+) are equal. It can be used to calculate the proportion of the non-ionized base (B) that is present in extracellular fluid at different pH values, using the equation:

$$pK_a - pH = \log_{10} \frac{[BH^+]}{[B]}.$$

For example, lignocaine and prilocaine have a pK_a value of approximately 7.7; at pH 7.4, 33% is present in solution as the non-ionized base B, and is available to diffuse across the nerve sheath. In contrast, bupivacaine and ropivacaine have a pK_a value of 8.1; at pH 7.4, only 17% of these drugs is present in solution as the non-ionized base B, and is available for diffusion. In general, high pK_a values are associated with a slower onset of blockade, since less of the drug is present as the non-ionized base. Conversely, lower pK_a values are consistent with a more rapid onset of anaesthesia, since more of the drug is present as the non-ionized base at physiological pH values. These considerations may explain the slower onset of action of procaine, amethocaine, ropivacaine and bupivacaine, and the more rapid effects of lignocaine, prilocaine, mepivacaine and etidocaine (Table 9.1). Nevertheless, the rapidity of onset and latency of action of local anaesthetics can also be modified by unrelated factors (e.g. the dose and the resultant concentration of the drug in tissues).

Most ester local anaesthetics (e.g. procaine, chloroprocaine, amethocaine), as well as lignocaine, are achiral compounds; in contrast, most of the amides are chiral drugs. Many chiral local anaesthetics (i.e. prilocaine, mepivacaine, bupivacaine and etidocaine) are commonly administered clinically as a racemic mixture of two stereoisomers. More recently, ropivacaine has been developed and used as an s(–) enantiomer, and bupivacaine may soon be available as a single isomer preparation (s(–)-bupivacaine). Although individual enantiomers of chiral compounds have approximately equal local anaesthetic activity, the s-enantiomers may have important advantages in other respects. For example, they may produce enhanced vasoconstriction and thus prolong local anaesthetic activity; they may reduce the intensity and duration of motor blockade and may be associated with a reduced risk of cardiotoxicity. There are also differences in their metabolism and pharmacokinetics (Chapter 4).

Mode of action

Most local anaesthetic agents are tertiary amine bases (B) that are administered as water-soluble hydrochlorides (B·HCl). After injection, the tertiary amine base is liberated by the relatively alkaline pH of tissue fluid:

$$B{\cdot}HCl + HCO_3^- \rightleftharpoons B + H_2CO_3 + Cl^-.$$

Consequently, in tissue fluid the local anaesthetic is present in both a non-ionized (B) and an ionized (BH^+) form; their relative proportions will depend on the pH of the solution and the pK_a of the individual compound, as determined by the modified Henderson–Hasselbalch equation:

$$pK_a - pH = \log_{10} \frac{[BH^+]}{[B]}.$$

The non-ionized base B then diffuses through the nerve sheath, perineuronal tissues and the neuronal membrane to reach the axoplasm, where it partially ionizes:

$$B + H^+ \rightleftharpoons BH^+.$$

In the ionized form BH^+, the local anaesthetic enters the sodium channel from the axoplasm (i.e. from the interior of the nerve fibre); it either occludes the channel, or combines with a receptor that results in channel closure (Fig. 9.3). Indeed, the sodium channel itself may be the receptor for local anaesthetics, or there may be multiple binding sites for drugs in the sodium channel. The diffusion of drugs through open ion channels is required for local anaesthetics to reach their site of action; consequently, in experimental conditions nerve blockade may be related to, and intensified by, neuronal excitation or activity (use-dependent blockade or phasic blockade), rather than to resting blockade (tonic blockade).

Thus, although the presence of the diffusible base is essential to reach its site of action in the axoplasm, the anaesthetic primarily acts in an ionized, cationic form. The most convincing evidence to support this explanation has been obtained from experiments in which lignocaine and its *N*-ethylated quaternary derivative have been applied to the inside and outside of the neuronal membrane. Lignocaine produces local anaesthesia when applied to the inside or the outside of the axonal membrane; in contrast, its quaternary derivative is only effective when applied to the axoplasmic aspect of the membrane, implying the presence of a site of action that is only accessible from the axoplasm.

Although local anaesthetics primarily reduce sodium entry and thus prevent depolarization, they may also affect other ionic channels (e.g. potassium channels). Nevertheless, they do not modify the resting potential of the neurone (except in extremely high concentrations). Similarly, they do not alter the threshold potential required for impulse propagation, although the rates of depolarization and repolarization are decreased, the refractory period is prolonged, and conduction velocity is diminished. Similar effects may be produced in other excitable tissues; for instance, in cardiac muscle, the rate of depolarization of ventricular muscle (phase 0) is reduced (Chapter 15). In addition, local anaesthetics may modify the effects of calcium ions on the charge distribution and excitability of neuronal membranes.

All local anaesthetics do not act in the manner described above. Certain agents (e.g. benzocaine, benzyl alcohol, *n*-butanol) are only present in the body as uncharged tertiary bases, and must therefore act in a different way. They are believed to cause conduction blockade by membrane expansion (i.e. by causing swelling of the lipoprotein matrix of the sodium channel). To some extent, other local anaesthetics (which are partly present in the axolemma and the axoplasm as the uncharged, tertiary base) may act in this manner.

In clinical practice local anaesthesia may be influenced by the local availability of the free base (B), since this is the form of the drug that readily diffuses through connective tissue and crosses the neuronal membrane. Thus, local anaesthetics are relatively inactive when injected into tissues with an acid pH (e.g. pyogenic abcesses). This is presumably due to the reduced availability of the free base for diffusion, and to the more rapid removal of the drug due to increased vascularity. Conversely, carbonated solutions have been used to improve the speed of onset and the quality of conduction blockade. In isolated preparations, carbon dioxide rapidly diffuses across the neuronal membrane and decreases the axoplasmic pH. This enhances the conversion of the local anaesthetic to the active cationic form, and the gradient for the diffusion of the free base from the extracellular fluid to the axoplasm is also increased. In these conditions, the speed of onset and the depth of local anaesthesia should be enhanced (due to the presence of a greater proportion of the free base at its site of action). It is debatable whether these advantages are present in clinical practice, since injected carbonic acid and carbon dioxide are rapidly buffered by intracellular proteins. In addition, carbonated solutions are unstable, the local anaesthetic may be precipitated, and any added vasoconstrictor is more easily hydrolysed. Consequently, carbonated solutions of local anaesthetics are not widely used in current practice. Other agents (e.g. sodium bicarbonate, various dextrans) have also been added to local anaesthetic solutions, in an attempt to increase the intensity and duration of action (presumably by modifying the proportion of the free base that is present in solution).

During conduction blockade, different modalities may be affected to an unequal extent by local anaesthetics. The sensation of pain usually disappears before touch and pressure, while motor fibres may remain functional although sensory pathways are blocked. These differences may be related to the diameter of the nerve fibres mediating different sensations; smaller diameter fibres may differ in their susceptibility to the effects of local anaesthetics. Unmyelinated fibres have a relatively large surface area (due to the absence of a myelin sheath). In contrast, myelinated fibres have a relatively small surface area, and are only susceptible to nerve blockade at the nodes of Ranvier. In addition, sequential blockade of two to three nodes of Ranvier may be required to interrupt neuronal transmission. Since the internodal distance is related to nerve fibre diameter, the larger diameter myelinated fibres are less susceptible than smaller fibres, which in turn are less susceptible than unmyelinated fibres. Consequently pain (which is partly mediated by unmyelinated

C fibres) is commonly blocked before touch and pressure (mediated by Aβ and Aγ fibres), which in turn are blocked before proprioception and motor function (which are dependent on Aα fibres). Nevertheless, these considerations do not adequately explain several clinical observations. For instance, myelinated fibres of the Aδ group (which conduct the sensation of fast or first pain) may be blocked before some non-myelinated C fibres. This phenomenon may reflect the anatomical distribution of nerve fibres and their accessibility to drugs.

Physicochemical factors may also account for the differential effects of local anaesthetics on sensory and motor function. For instance, low concentrations of bupivacaine and ropivacaine may readily affect unmyelinated C fibres, due to their high lipid solubility; in contrast, they may not rapidly diffuse across myelinated Aα fibres and cause motor blockade (due to their relatively high pK_a value). Consequently, these drugs may possess the optimal physicochemical characteristics required to cause differential sensory and motor blockade.

Pharmacokinetics

Significant absorption of local anaesthetics occurs from their site of injection. For each individual drug, the amount of local anaesthetic absorbed and the peak plasma concentration will be dependent on the dose, and may also be modified by the presence or absence of a vasoconstrictor (particularly during infiltration or conduction anaesthesia). The site of injection is also important; for example, higher blood levels are attained after intercostal and caudal blockade than with lumbar epidural or brachial plexus blockade. Thus, for every 100 mg lignocaine injected in an adult, the peak venous plasma concentration ranges from 1.5 $\mu g\ ml^{-1}$ (intercostal blockade), 1.2 $\mu g\ ml^{-1}$ (caudal and paracervical blockade), 1.0 $\mu g\ ml^{-1}$ (epidural blockade), 0.6 $\mu g\ ml^{-1}$ (brachial plexus blockade) to 0.4 $\mu g\ ml^{-1}$ (intrathecal blockade). This range of concentrations is mainly due to differences in vascularity, although other factors (e.g. uptake by tissue lipids) may also be involved. In these conditions, adherence to dose limits for local anaesthetics may obscure potential differences in systemic toxicity, depending on the site of injection. Clearly, identical doses of local anaesthetics may be more toxic in certain injection sites than in others. Many local anaesthetics are also well-absorbed from mucous membranes.

The rate of uptake is closely related to the surface area available for absorption (e.g. it is extremely rapid when topical local anaesthetic sprays are applied to the tracheobronchial tract). In addition, the inherent effects of drugs on vascular smooth-muscle tone may affect their rate of absorption. Thus, cocaine prevents the neuronal uptake of catecholamines ($Uptake_1$) and inhibits the enzyme monoamine oxidase; this produces vasoconstriction and delays drug absorption. Most other local anaesthetics tend to have a biphasic action on vascular smooth muscle; in the concentrations present clinically, they may all produce some degree of vasodilation (usually in the order procaine > prilocaine > lignocaine > mepivacaine > bupivacaine >

ropivacaine). This may affect the rate of absorption of individual drugs. In general, the S-isomers of prilocaine, mepivacaine and bupivacaine may produce more vasoconstriction (i.e. less vasodilatation) than the R-enantiomers; consequently, the S-forms of chiral local anaesthetics may have a longer duration of action than their antipodes. Procaine, chloroprocaine and related esters are potent vasodilators, and are readily absorbed after injection; they are also rapidly broken down in tissues and plasma by esterase enzymes (particularly cholinesterase). The inactivation of procaine by enzymes in many vascular mucous membranes accounts for its relative lack of surface anaesthetic activity.

After absorption from the site of injection, the plasma concentration of local anaesthetics depends on their rate of distribution in tissues and their elimination from the body. The prolonged absorption of local anaesthetics may preclude or obscure the accurate determination of their pharmacokinetics. After intravenous injection, the plasma concentration of all local anaesthetics usually declines in a biexponential manner. There is an initial rapid distribution phase (half-life = 1–3 min), associated with their rapid uptake by highly perfused organs (e.g. lung, liver and kidney, as well as skeletal muscle). Subsequently, there is a slower decline in plasma concentration; this phase represents the removal of the local anaesthetic by metabolism and excretion. The terminal half-life of most ester anaesthetics is relatively short (approximately 10 min), due to their rapid hydrolysis by plasma cholinesterase. In contrast, the elimination half-life of amides ranges from 100 min (lignocaine) to 160 min (bupivacaine). Their volume of distribution is rather greater than total body water, while their plasma clearance is comparable with liver blood flow (Table 9.2). Pathological conditions may alter the pharmacokinetics of local anaesthetics. In particular, cardiovascular disease and hepatic cirrhosis may decrease the clearance and volume of distribution of local anaesthetics, with variable effects on the terminal half-life. In neonates, the clearance of local anaesthetics is decreased and their half-life is prolonged. In addition, a number of drugs (e.g. halothane, propranolol) can decrease the clearance of amide local anaesthetics.

The binding of local anaesthetics by plasma proteins may also affect their pharmacokinetic behaviour and pharmacodynamic effects. In general, ester local anaesthetics are not significantly bound by plasma proteins (i.e. 5–10% or less). In contrast, amide local anaesthetics are mainly bound by α_1-acid glycoprotein, in the order bupivacaine > ropivacaine > mepivacaine > lignocaine > prilocaine. The extent of plasma protein binding ranges from 55 to 95%; it is usually reversible, and does not appear to limit or restrict the uptake of local anaesthetics by most tissues and organs. Plasma protein binding is significantly influenced by physiological and pathological changes in the concentration of α_1-acid glycoprotein (which may occur in infancy, pregnancy, old age, myocardial infarction, renal failure, malignant disease and after operative surgery). In these conditions, plasma protein binding is increased, the free (unbound) concentration of drugs is reduced, and the

Table 9.2 Pharmacokinetics and metabolism of local anaesthetics.

	Terminal half-life (min)	Clearance ($l\ min^{-1}$)	Apparent volume of distribution (l)	Metabolites
Cocaine	Uncertain	Uncertain	Uncertain	Norcocaine Ecgonine Benzoylated derivatives
Procaine	Uncertain	Uncertain	Uncertain	*para*-Aminobenzoate Diethylaminoethanol
Amethocaine	Uncertain	Uncertain	Uncertain	Butyl-aminobenzoate Dimethylaminoethanol
Lignocaine	100	1.0	91	Monoethylglycine-xylidide *N*-ethylglycine 2,6-Xylidine 4-Hydroxy-2,6-xylidine
Prilocaine	100	2.4	191	*o*-Toluidine *N*-propylamine
Etidocaine	160	1.1	134	Numerous unidentified metabolites
Mepivacaine	115	0.8	84	3-Hydroxymepivacaine 4-Hydroxymepivacaine
Ropivacaine	120	0.8	60	Pipecolic acid Pipecolylxylidide
Bupivacaine	160	0.6	73	Pipecolic acid Pipecolylxylidide

total plasma concentration of local anaesthetics may not be related to their effective concentration.

The protein binding of local anaesthetics may also affect placental transfer. In general, highly protein-bound drugs have a low umbilical vein : maternal blood (UV : M) concentration ratio. Thus, the UV : M ratio for bupivacaine is approximately 0.2; for lignocaine and prilocaine, the UV : M ratio is 0.5. These values do not necessarily reflect the relative safety of the local anaesthetics in pregnancy and labour (since they do not take account of differential α_1-acid glycoprotein binding in maternal and fetal blood). Nevertheless, it is generally accepted that the placental transfer of bupivacaine is less than lignocaine and prilocaine, and that this may have possible advantages in pregnancy and labour.

Metabolism and elimination

The metabolism of local anaesthetics is determined by their chemical structure. Esters and amides are metabolized in different ways by different tissues.

Ester local anaesthetics are broken down by plasma cholinesterase (and also by other esterase enzymes in certain tissues). Only small amounts of the unchanged drugs are eliminated in urine. For example, procaine is extensively hydrolysed to PABA and diethylaminoethanol (which is further metabolized by alcohol dehydrogenase to diethylglycine). Most other ester local anaesthetics (e.g. chloroprocaine and amethocaine) are metabolized in an essentially similar manner. In contrast, cocaine is relatively resistant to hydrolysis by plasma cholinesterase. It is extensively metabolized in the liver, and only trace amounts (approximately 1% of the dose) are excreted unchanged. Studies using radiolabelled cocaine suggest that the drug is converted to several metabolites (i.e. norcocaine, ecgonine and their benzoylated analogues), and that some of them may be responsible for the stimulant effects of cocaine on the central nervous system (CNS).

In contrast to most ester anaesthetics, the amides are extensively metabolized by hepatic enzymes (mainly by amidases that are associated with the cytoplasm and the smooth endoplasmic reticulum). Lignocaine is almost entirely metabolized by the liver; its clearance is approximately 70–80% of normal liver blood flow, and after oral administration only trace amounts gain access to the systemic circulation (i.e. it has an extremely high first-pass effect). It is initially dealkylated to monoethylglycine-xylidide and acetaldehyde. Monoethylglycine-xylidide is mainly hydrolysed to *N*-ethylglycine and 2,6-xylidine; the latter compound is hydroxylated to 4-hydroxy-2,6-xylidine, which is the main metabolite of lignocaine eliminated in urine (accounting for approximately 70% of the dose). Some of the metabolites of lignocaine have local anaesthetic activity, while others appear to have convulsive properties. Monoethylglycine-xylidide has antiemetic and antiarrhythmic properties, and may potentiate convulsions produced by lignocaine. Glycine-xylidide (a minor metabolite of lignocaine) has local anaesthetic effects and may depress the CNS; it has a relatively long half-life and may take several days to be eliminated from the body.

Prilocaine is more rapidly metabolized than other amide anaesthetics; although it is mainly metabolized by the liver, it may also be broken down by the kidney and the lung. Its principal metabolites are *o*-toluidine and *N*-propylamine. *o*-Toluidine is probably responsible for the methaemoglobinaemia and cyanosis which sometimes occur approximately 5–6 h after large doses of prilocaine. It usually resolves spontaneously, but may be treated with reducing agents (e.g. ascorbic acid or methylene blue). Prilocaine is administered clinically as a chiral mixture of two stereoisomers, which are metabolized by the liver at different rates. R-(−)-prilocaine is more rapidly metabolized than S-(+)-prilocaine, and may produce higher plasma concentrations of *o*-toluidine with enhanced methaemoglobinaemia. Nevertheless, since the clearance of prilocaine is limited by liver blood flow, these differences do not significantly affect the plasma concentration or the pharmacokinetics of the drug.

Mepivacaine is rapidly metabolized in the liver. At least three hydroxylated metabolites are formed; most of the drug is excreted in urine as 3-hydroxy-mepivacaine or 4-hydroxy-mepivacaine.

Bupivacaine has a relatively low hepatic clearance, and is only slowly metabolized by the liver. In humans, the main metabolite is probably pipecolic acid (a product of hydrolysis of bupivacaine); only 5% of the dose is eliminated in urine as a dealkylated metabolite (pipecolylxylidide).

The hepatic clearance of ropivacaine is also relatively low; the drug is primarily metabolized to pipecolic acid and derivatives of xylidine.

Pharmacological effects of local anaesthetics

Cardiovascular effects

Cocaine causes tachycardia and arrhythmias by both central and peripheral effects. In the CNS, it increases neuronal activity in sympathetic centres in the hypothalamus and the medulla; peripherally, it enhances the effects of endogenous catecholamines and produces sympathomimetic effects. Both these actions are due to its effects on $Uptake_1$ (the amine pump), which is responsible for the removal of catecholamines from extracellular fluid by central and peripheral nerve endings. Thus, inhibition of $Uptake_1$ by cocaine increases the central and peripheral effects of adrenaline and noradrenaline. In contrast, the membrane-stabilizing effects of other local anaesthetics have led to their development and use as antiarrhythmic agents.

Most local anaesthetics affect sodium channels in myocardial and junctional tissues (as well as in peripheral nerves). Bupivacaine may also affect calcium and potassium channels in cardiac muscle. Consequently, local anaesthetics decrease the maximum rate of increase of phase 0 of the cardiac action potential (V_{max}) in a dose-dependent manner. The slowing of conduction of the cardiac action potential prolongs the PR and the QRS intervals of the electrocardiogram. The excitability of atrial and ventricular muscle cells is decreased, and the refractory period of conducting tissue is prolonged. In the past, procaine was used as an antiarrhythmic agent. Its short duration of action led to the development of its analogue procainamide (which is not significantly broken down by plasma cholinesterase); at one time, this drug was widely used in the management of both ventricular arrhythmias and supraventricular tachycardias (Chapter 14).

In recent years, lignocaine has become the standard agent for the suppression of ventricular arrhythmias associated with myocardial infarction or cardiac surgery. In general, lignocaine does not affect atrial muscle fibres; it may act preferentially on ischaemic myocardium, prolong the effective refractory period of junctional tissues, and be more effective when the extracellular potassium concentration is high.

Lignocaine has a terminal half-life of approximately 1.6 h; thus, after constant intravenous infusion of the drug there is a latent period (approximately 7–8 h) before a steady state is reached. Consequently, lignocaine is usually administered as a loading dose (75–100 mg intravenously (i.v.) or 300 mg intramuscularly) and a constant infusion of 2–4 mg min^{-1} is then maintained. Drowsiness and numbness are frequently observed at high rates of infusion, and the metabolism of the drug is reduced in heart failure.

High doses of local anaesthetics are associated with significant cardiotoxicity, due to direct effects on cardiac conduction as well as indirect effects on medullary centres. Myocardial contractility and conduction in junctional tissues are depressed, with widening of the QRS complex and distortion of the ST segment. High concentrations of some local anaesthetics (particularly bupivacaine) may predispose to the development of re-entrant arrhythmias, which may be potentiated by hypoxia, acidosis and hyperkalaemia. In the past, cardiotoxicity (and several deaths) have occurred when bupivacaine was used during intravenous regional anaesthesia (Bier's block). Similarly, a number of maternal deaths were reported in the USA, which were associated with the accidental intravenous administration of bupivacaine during extradural anaesthesia for Caesarean section. In these conditions, ventricular arrhythmias and cardiac arrest are believed to reflect the effects of bupivacaine on calcium and/or potassium channels (as well as sodium channels). Recent evidence suggests that the use of local anaesthetic enantiomers with the S-configuration reduce the possibility of cardiac depression and cardiotoxicity (as compared with the R-isomers); consequently, ropivacaine (an S-stereoisomer) and S-bupivacaine (levobupivacaine) may have considerable advantages compared to racemic bupivacaine. The development and use of local anaesthetics with the S-configuration may considerably decrease the risks of cardiotoxicity.

Peripheral vascular effects

Cocaine possesses inherent vasoconstrictor activity, since it inhibits the uptake of adrenaline and noradrenaline by peripheral sympathetic nerve endings. Other commonly used local anaesthetics may produce variable effects on vascular smooth muscle. Exposure of isolated blood vessels to local anaesthetics frequently produces an increase in tone. Intravascular injection of most amides produces a biphasic effect on vascular smooth muscle; extremely low concentrations enhance its activity and increase peripheral resistance, while higher concentrations cause vasodilatation. This may be due to changes in the Ca^{2+} concentration of the vessel wall. In the doses commonly used to produce local anaesthesia, vasodilatation usually occurs in the order procaine > chloroprocaine > prilocaine > lignocaine > mepivacaine > bupivacaine > ropivacaine. In experimental conditions, the S-enantiomers of chiral local anaesthetics produce enhanced vasoconstriction (when compared with the R-isomers), and may have a longer duration of action. It is not clear whether these differences are also present in humans.

Procaine is an extremely effective vasodilator, and has been used in the management of vascular spasm associated with inadvertent intra-arterial injections, trauma and surgery.

Central nervous system

Local anaesthetics and their metabolites are weak bases, and cross the blood–brain barrier relatively easily. They may produce biphasic effects on the CNS. Although small doses of lignocaine (2–4 mg kg^{-1}) have anticonvulsant effects, and have been used in the treatment of status epilepticus, signs of CNS excitation usually follow the absorption of significant amounts of the drug. Increasing plasma concentrations of local anaesthetics are associated with numbness of the tongue and mouth, lightheadedness, visual disturbances, slurring of speech, muscular twitching and tremors, restlessness and irrational conversation. At concentrations of 2 μg ml^{-1} (bupivacaine) or 9 μg ml^{-1} (lignocaine), grand mal convulsions may occur. The threshold for convulsions is influenced by the presence of other drugs that affect the CNS, and by acidosis and hypoxia. Some local anaesthetics (e.g. procaine) are relatively free from convulsant activity. The excitatory effects of local anaesthetics are probably due to the selective depression of inhibitory cortical neurones, and may be followed by signs of cortical and medullary depression (e.g. unconsciousness, coma and apnoea).

Unwanted effects of local anaesthetics

Due to absolute or relative overdosage

Severe and occasionally fatal CNS and cardiovascular system toxicity may occur with gross overdosage of local anaesthetic agents (or when large doses inadvertently reach the vascular system). As long as the injection is not too rapid, the early signs of CNS toxicity described above may be recognized before more serious effects occur.

Convulsions should be treated by maintaining adequate ventilation and controlled by anticonvulsant drugs, e.g. diazepam (10–20 mg i.v., repeated if necessary). Although it has a relatively slow onset of action, it is unlikely to potentiate the phase of CNS depression. Alternatively, thiopentone (150–250 mg i.v.) may be used; it has an immediate onset but a relatively short duration of action. If convulsions are prolonged, the use of a muscle relaxant and mechanical ventilation may be required.

Profound hypotension and bradyarrhythmias may occur due to depression of the cardiovascular system. Intravenous atropine (1.2–1.8 mg) and colloid or crystalloid infusions as plasma expanders may be necessary. Fetal bradycardia and other signs of fetal distress may occur after paracervical block for analgesia in labour, due to the rapid absorption of local anaesthetics from this site.

Accidental injection of large volumes of local anaesthetic into the cerebrospinal fluid (CSF) during epidural or paravertebral block can produce total spinal anaesthesia. This presents as complete respiratory paralysis (due to motor and medullary involvement) and hypotension, due to autonomic blockade. Treatment includes mechanical ventilation and circulatory support, and the use of a vasopressor may be indicated.

As part of the therapeutic effect

If multiple intercostal blocks are performed, respiratory insufficiency may occur, due to unavoidable paralysis of some motor fibres. During spinal anaesthesia, a variable degree of hypotension is not uncommon, due to autonomic blockade; extradural analgesia during labour may potentiate the effects of hypotension due to inferior vena caval compression. Prophylactic measures usually minimize these complications, but symptomatic treatment may be required.

Due to the added vasoconstrictor

Most of these effects are undoubtedly due to accidental intravascular injection. Cardiac arrhythmias and hypertensive responses are predictable side-effects when sympathomimetic amines are used, although the local anaesthetic itself may exert some protective effect on the heart. In general, the use of sympathomimetic vasoconstrictors should be restricted in susceptible patients, e.g. those with a known history of cardiovascular disease, or who are taking drugs that inhibit Uptake_1, such as tricyclic antidepressants. It has been shown that concentrations of adrenaline greater than 1 in 200 000 do not further enhance local anaesthetic effects when most amide-type drugs are used to produce conduction blockade. Sympathomimetic amines with predominant α-adrenoceptor effects, such as noradrenaline and phenylephrine, have theoretical advantages as vasoconstrictors; in practice they appear to be less effective than adrenaline. Felypressin does not cause arrhythmias, although some elevation of blood pressure may occur.

Vasoconstrictor agents must not be given with local anaesthetics when anaesthesia is produced in digital extremities or in areas with a terminal vascular supply, as the intense ischaemia produced may lead to gangrene. Similarly, these solutions must never be given intravenously.

Specific effects

Allergic responses to most currently used local anaesthetics are extremely rare. Skin reactions following repeated handling of ester-type drugs have been most frequently reported; occasionally, anaphylactic responses have occurred. The metabolite PABA probably acts as a hapten and induces the antibody response. Allergic reactions associated with the amide group are even less common; cross-sensitization between amide and ester local anaesthetics is almost unknown. Some reactions may occur when multidose ampoules are used (possibly due to the added preservative).

Sulphonamides produce bacteriostatic effects by preventing the incorporation of PABA into the folic acid nucleus, thus inhibiting the growth and multiplication of bacteria. Procaine and related esters are hydrolysed to PABA, and thus may antagonize the effects of sulphonamides; the concurrent use of ester local anaesthetics and sulphonamides or preparations containing sulphonamides (e.g. co-trimoxazole) is therefore undesirable.

Methaemoglobinaemia formation may occur when high doses of prilocaine are given (e.g. more than 600 mg extradurally), probably due to the accumulation of its main metabolite *o*-toluidine (and various hydroxylated derivatives). The fetus is at special risk, since its erythrocytes are deficient in methaemoglobin reductase (the enzyme that reduces methaemoglobin to haemoglobin). When necessary, methylene blue (5 mg kg^{-1}) is an immediate and effective antidote in the mother and the child.

Clinical uses of local anaesthetics

Topical anaesthesia

Local anaesthetics may be applied to the skin, the eye, the ear, the nose and the mouth, as well as other mucous membranes (particularly in the tracheobronchial tree and the genitourinary tract). In general, cocaine, amethocaine, lignocaine and prilocaine are the most useful and effective local anaesthetics for this purpose. When used to produce topical anaesthesia, they usually have a rapid onset of action (5–10 min) and a moderate duration of action (30–60 min). The powerful vasoconstrictor properties of cocaine make it a useful agent when both the reduction of bleeding and local anaesthesia are required. Its main indication in current practice is to provide surface anaesthesia for intranasal procedures. Aqueous solutions containing 4–20% cocaine are commonly used for this purpose; adrenaline (1 in 1000) is sometimes added. Cocaine is occasionally used to produce corneal anaesthesia; its desiccating effect is a marked disadvantage and may lead to corneal ulceration. It has largely been replaced in this field by other drugs (e.g. amethocaine, which is an excellent topical anaesthetic).

Various preparations of lignocaine are available as aqueous solutions (4%) or in water-miscible bases as gels, ointments, creams and sprays (2–10%). These may be used as eyedrops, or to provide anaesthesia of the tracheobronchial tract prior to endotracheal intubation or bronchoscopic examination. They may also be used to produce anaesthesia of the urethra during diagnostic urological procedures, in order to eliminate the need for general anaesthesia. Sprays may be applied to mucosal surfaces to provide anaesthesia for suturing of episiotomy wounds or minor lacerations. Significant absorption may occur from the more vascular areas, and fatalities have occurred after the topical application of local anaesthetics to mucosal surfaces.

Benzocaine (a non-ionized ester) is incorporated into eardrops used for the relief of pain in otitis media, and into various ointments, creams, gels and sprays used for the symptomatic relief of muscle strains, pruritus and painful fissures.

Absorption of local anaesthetics through intact skin is usually slow and unreliable, and high concentrations (e.g. 20% benzocaine or 40% lignocaine) are required. In recent years, a eutectic mixture of local anaesthetics (EMLA) has been widely used to produce surface anaesthesia of the skin (particularly in paediatric practice). The crystalline tertiary bases of lignocaine and prilocaine melt to form an oil at temperatures greater than 16°C (a eutectic mixture). In these conditions, the droplet concentration of the local anaesthetics in an oil-in-water emulsion is high enough (approximately 80%) to produce effective surface anaesthesia. The eutectic mixture contains equal proportions (25 mg ml^{-1}) of the tertiary bases of lignocaine and prilocaine, and is used as an emulsion which can be applied as a cream to the skin. The preparation may cause transient skin blanching and erythema. An occlusive dressing is necessary to ensure cutaneous contact and at least 60 min is usually required to demonstrate significant surface analgesia.

Infiltration anaesthesia

Infiltration techniques are frequently employed in dentistry and to provide anaesthesia for minor surgical procedures. Amide compounds with a moderate duration of action (lignocaine, prilocaine or mepivacaine) are commonly used. The site of action is at the unmyelinated nerve endings; with all these agents, the onset of action is almost immediate after submucosal or subcutaneous injection, and provides satisfactory operating conditions in over 90% of cases.

The duration of local anaesthesia is variable. Procaine has a short duration of action (15–30 min), while lignocaine, mepivacaine and prilocaine have a moderate duration of action (usually 70–140 min). Bupivacaine and ropivacaine have the longest duration of action (approximately 200 min). The addition of adrenaline (1 in 200 000; 5 μg ml^{-1}) will increase the quality and prolong the duration of anaesthesia. Nevertheless, there is no significant difference in the duration of effect when lignocaine (1%) and bupivacaine (0.25%) containing adrenaline are used to produce infiltration anaesthesia. Residual anaesthesia persists longer after intradermal injection (4–7 h) than after submucosal injection (1–3 h), presumably due to differences in vascular absorption.

Conduction anaesthesia

Conduction anaesthesia can be considered as the minor nerve blockade of a moderately accessible single nerve entity (e.g. ulnar, radial or intercostal nerves) or as the major blockade of deeper nerves or nerve trunks with a wide dermatomal distribution (e.g. sciatic nerve or brachial plexus).

In current practice, amides are invariably used to produce conduction anaesthesia. Solutions containing vasoconstrictors are commonly administered in these techniques, and for each individual agent the duration of anaesthesia will be chiefly determined by the total dose of the drug, rather than the volume or the concentration used. When amide local anaesthetics are used to produce minor nerve blockade, they have a relatively rapid onset of action (3–6 min).

The duration of local anaesthesia is more variable; lignocaine, mepivacaine and prilocaine have a moderate duration of action (1–2 h), while bupivacaine, ropivacaine and etidocaine produce local anaesthesia for 2–6 h. The duration of action is prolonged by increasing the dose of the local anaesthetic, or by the addition of a vasoconstrictor. Thus, the duration of action of lignocaine during minor nerve blockade is usually increased from 1–2 to 4–5 h by the addition of adrenaline (1 in 200 000). Mixtures of local anaesthetic drugs (e.g. prilocaine and bupivacaine, or lignocaine and bupivacaine) are commonly used to combine a rapid onset with a prolonged duration of action.

In major nerve blockade, the onset of action is more variable, mainly due to anatomical factors which can delay or restrict the access of the local anaesthetic to its site of action. During brachial plexus or sciatic nerve blockade, solutions of local anaesthetics may be placed outside the fascial planes or connective tissues that surround the nerve trunks. Consequently, local anaesthetic bases must diffuse across extensive connective tissue barriers as well as the myelin sheaths of nerve trunks; they may be also taken up by the surrounding adipose tissue and by muscle. In general, lignocaine, mepivacaine and prilocaine have a more rapid onset of action (approximately 14 min) than bupivacaine (23 min). Analgesia persists for 3–4 h with lignocaine, prilocaine and mepivacaine, but up to 10 h with bupivacaine and ropivacaine. Etidocaine has a shorter onset time (9 min) but a similar duration of action to bupivacaine; however, the differential blockade of motor fibres may tend to limit its use. Persistent paraesthesia after nerve blockade is probably due to mechanical trauma, rather than a pharmacological effect.

Procaine is an ideal diagnostic agent, due to its relatively short duration of action (15–45 min) and its localizing effects (which are due to poor diffusion properties). In the treatment of chronic pain it can be used to block somatic or autonomic fibres; the efficiency of permanent neurolytic blockade can then be more easily assessed.

Extradural anaesthesia

The deposition of local anaesthetic solutions in the area between the dura mater and the periosteum lining the vertebral canal is widely used as part of a balanced anaesthesia technique, and to provide analgesia in the postoperative period and during labour. Extradural anaesthetics are commonly administered in the thoracolumbar region of the spinal cord. The epidural space is filled with adipose tissue, lymphatics and blood vessels (mainly the peridural venous plexus). After injection, local anaesthetic solutions spread widely in all directions, and produce analgesia by blocking conduction at the intradural spinal nerve roots. Local anaesthetics diffuse through the dural root sleeves, immediately proximal to the dorsal root ganglion. In this region, the dura is extremely thin, and is continuous with the epineurium of the spinal nerves. Numerous arachnoid villi are also present; some of them partly or completely protrude through fenestrations in the dura into the extradural space, and local anaesthetics may only need to diffuse across the thin arachnoid membrane. After extradural injection, high concentrations of local anaesthetics are invariably present in the intradural nerve roots, and the dermatomal spread of analgesia is consistent with conduction blockade at this site. Spread into the paravertebral spaces may also occur in younger subjects, and there may be some uptake of local anaesthetics by the spinal cord. Indeed, there is some evidence that the effect of local anaesthetics on the spinal cord may persist for some time after the spinal nerve roots have recovered from blockade.

In general terms, extradural anaesthesia may be considered as multiple minor nerve blockade. The onset of action is slightly longer (presumably due to the greater distance for diffusion), but the duration of action is equal to ulnar or intercostal nerve blockade. The quality and extent of the blockade are determined by the volume and concentration, as well as the total dose of the local anaesthetic. Raised volumes increase the spread of the solution in the extradural space and the extent of blockade; higher concentrations reduce onset time and increase the intensity of anaesthesia and motor blockade. Higher total doses increase the duration of blockade. Other important factors are the site of injection, the speed of administration and the position of the patient. A lateral posture encourages the development of sensory and motor blockade on the dependent side.

The spread of local anaesthetic solution may be more extensive in parturient women, since the peridural venous plexus is distended due to compression of the inferior vena cava, and the volume of the potential space is reduced. Consequently, the dose of local anaesthetic required to produce extradural blockade in pregnancy is usually reduced. Similarly, enhanced effects may be seen in arteriosclerotic patients and the elderly, due to the impairment of vascular absorption from the extradural space.

Extradural blockade above the lower thoracic region (T10) may be associated with significant hypotension (i.e. a reduction in systolic blood pressure of > 30 mmHg), due to the blockade of sympathetic vasoconstrictor pathways in the spinal cord and autonomic ganglia. Vascular dilatation in splanchnic blood vessels results in the pooling of blood in capacitance vessels and a substantial reduction in venous return. Hypotension can be prevented or minimized by preloading with crystalloid or colloid solutions, or treated with ephedrine (10–15 mg i.v.).

In the UK, bupivacaine (0.25–0.5%) is the only drug that is commonly used to produce extradural anaesthesia. Although it has a slow onset of action (20–30 min), it usually provides analgesia for several hours, and its high lipid solubility and significant protein binding delay its absorption into the systemic circulation. Similarly, only small amounts of the drug cross the placenta and reach the fetal circulation. Dose requirements vary between 1 and 3 ml for each segment blocked; lower concentrations (0.25%) provide analgesia with minimal motor blockade, while higher concentrations (0.5%) have a longer duration of action with a moderate degree of motor blockade (Table 9.3). Adrenaline (1 in 200 000–1 in 300 000; 3.3–5 μg ml^{-1}) is sometimes added; although the duration of blockade is unaffected, peak plasma concentrations of bupivacaine are reduced and its presence may give an early indication of inadvertent intravascular injection. Other drugs, for instance opioids (fentanyl, morphine, diamorphine), α_2-agonists (clonidine, dexmedetomidine) or benzodiazepines (midazolam), are sometimes given by extradural administration with local anaesthetics.

Bupivacaine is currently administered as a racemic mixture of two enantiomers (Chapter 4). In the near future, two related single-isomer preparations may also be used to produce extradural anaesthesia. Ropivacaine is the s(–) enantiomer of the propyl derivative of bupivacaine, and is less cardiotoxic than racemic bupivacaine. After extradural administration, sensory blockade produced by equivalent concentrations of the drugs is similar, although motor blockade produced by ropivacaine is slower in onset, less intense and shorter than racemic bupivacaine.

Table 9.3 The preparations, dosage and effects of bupivacaine used to produce extradural analgesia and subarachnoid anaesthesia in adults.

Concentration	Specific gravity*	Normal dose range: Dose (mg)	Normal dose range: Volume (ml)	Onset of action (min)	Duration of action (min)	Clinical effects
Lumbar extradural administration						
0.25% in water	1.003	15–38	6–15	15–25	60–120	Analgesia Normal muscle tone
0.5% in water	1.006	30–75	6–15	15–20	120–180	Analgesia Mild or moderate muscle relaxation
Caudal administration						
0.5% in water	1.006	100–150	20–30	10–20	120–180	Analgesia Moderate to complete muscle relaxation
Lumbar subarachnoid administration						
0.25% in water	1.003	5–8	2–3	20–25	120–180	Spinal anaesthesia Mild muscle relaxation
0.5% in water	1.006	10–15	2–3	10–20	140–200	Spinal anaesthesia Moderate muscle relaxation
0.5% in 8% dextrose	1.026	10–15	2–3	10–15	120–180	Spinal anaesthesia Moderate muscle relaxation

* The median specific gravity of cerebrospinal fluid = 1.007 at 20°C.

Consequently, ropivacaine provides better separation of sensory and motor blockade than bupivacaine (and also has a shorter half-life and more rapid clearance; Table 9.2). s(–)-bupivacaine (levobupivacaine) may soon be available as a single isomer; it is also less cardiotoxic and has a longer duration of action than the racemic mixture. When used extradurally, it may have the same advantages as ropivacaine.

When lignocaine or mepivacaine is given by extradural administration, tachyphylaxis (i.e. the development of rapid drug tolerance) may occur. It is less commonly observed with bupivacaine. When tachyphylaxis occurs, identical doses of local anaesthetics produce progressively decreasing degrees of blockade, so that an increase in the dose is required to maintain the same degree of blockade. The phenomenon may be related to the local changes in pH produced by the introduction of significant volumes of relatively acid local anaesthetic solutions (pH 4–5) into the extradural space. Since the volume and buffering capacity of extradural tissues are limited, local anaesthetic solutions may decrease its effective pH and thus reduce the relative concentration of free base that is available for diffusion into intradural spinal nerve roots. In these conditions, there may be a progressive decrease in the extent and duration of sensory blockade and analgesia. This explanation may not be entirely correct, since tachyphylaxis appears to increase as the interval between successive doses of the local anaesthetic is progressively extended.

Caudal blockade is a form of extradural anaesthesia, and is commonly used to produce blockade of the lower lumbar and sacral nerve roots. The nerves of the cauda equina descending in the sacral canal are blocked by local anaesthetics inserted through a needle in the sacral hiatus, producing sacral or perineal anaesthesia. The anaesthetic agent does not need to traverse a dural sleeve or the dura (which ends at the lower border of S2). Below this level, the sacral canal contains an abundant venous plexus (as well as sacral nerves, the filum terminale and fat).

Bupivacaine (0.5%; 20–30 ml) is usually used to produce caudal blockade (e.g. to provide supplementary analgesia after haemorrhoidectomy and perineal surgery in adults). The slow onset of blockade and the significant failure rate are probably due to considerable vascular absorption into the sacral venous plexus and internal vertebral venous plexus, and the wide distribution of the drug through the various sacral foramina. The extent of blockade may be affected by the position of the patient and the dose and speed of injection.

Spinal anaesthesia

The introduction of local anaesthetic solutions directly into the CSF produces spinal anaesthesia. The central attachments of ventral and dorsal nerve roots are unmyelinated. When local anaesthetic solutions are introduced into the subarachnoid space, their tertiary bases are rapidly taken up by the nerve roots, dorsal root ganglia and the spinal cord. Consequently, the potency of local anaesthetics after spinal subarachnoid injection is 10–15 times greater than after extradural administration, and motor blockade is more pronounced (Table 9.3). In addition, the onset of anaesthesia is more rapid, since local anaesthetics do not need to penetrate extensive tissue or diffusion barriers in order to reach their site of action. Due to the smaller doses of local anaesthetics that are used, the duration of spinal anaesthesia is usually shorter than extradural anaesthesia. The quality and extent of blockade are related to the dose of local anaesthetic administered, the speed of injection, the position of the patient and the specific gravity of the solution injected (when compared with the specific gravity of CSF, i.e. 1.007).

An increase in the dose of local anaesthetic usually improves the quality and intensity of anaesthesia, prolongs its duration and may increase its spread. The effect of the position of the patient depends on the specific gravity (baricity) of the solution injected. Hypobaric solutions (e.g. 0.25% or 0.5% bupivacaine in water; specific gravity = 1.003–1.006) tend to rise in the CSF. Their spread could depend on the position of the patient, and their effects tend to be unpredictable. Although their duration of action is usually longer than hyperbaric solutions, the blockade is frequently of variable quality. Isobaric solutions of local anaesthetics are also used; these solutions are more physiological, and their spread in the CSF does not depend on posture. Unfortunately, their effects are also less predictable.

Hyperbaric solutions of local anaesthetics are frequently used to produce subarachnoid spinal blockade. The spread of these solutions in the CSF is affected by gravity and by posture. When hyperbaric solutions are injected in the mid lumbar region (L2–3 or L3–4) and the patient is placed supine, blockade usually spreads to the mid thoracic level (T4–7); if the patient is injected in (and remains in) the sitting position, blockade only extends to T7–10. When injected at L4–5 and the patient remains sitting, a saddle blockade is produced, which can be used for perineal surgery. The spread of hyperbaric solutions in the CSF is also affected by age, height, spinal curvature and the volume and capacity of the subarachnoid space. Thus, compression of the inferior vena cava (e.g. in pregnancy or by intra-abdominal tumours) distends the vertebral venous plexus and decreases the volume of the subarachnoid space. In these conditions, the spread of the local anaesthetic and the degree of analgesia are increased.

In the UK 'heavy' bupivacaine (0.5% bupivacaine in 8% dextrose; specific gravity = 1.026) is the only hyperbaric solution that is commonly used to produce subarachnoid blockade. Moderate doses (10–15 mg, i.e. 2–3 ml) have an onset of action of 10–15 min, and a duration of action of approximately 2–3 h (Table 9.3); smaller doses (and hyperbaric lignocaine) have a shorter duration of action. The addition of vasoconstrictors (e.g. adrenaline; 1 in 200 000) causes a slight prolongation of blockade. Bupivacaine (and dextrose) are not metabolized in the CSF, but are taken up by the spinal cord or absorbed by branches of the spinal arteries, which form a vascular network in the pia mater.

Subarachnoid spinal anaesthesia above the lower thoracic region (T10) may cause significant hypotension, due to the blockade of sympathetic vasoconstrictor pathways in the spinal cord and autonomic ganglia. Vascular dilatation in splanchnic blood vessels results in the pooling of blood in capacitance vessels and a substantial reduction in venous return. Hypotension can be prevented or minimized by preloading with crystalloid or colloid solutions, or treated with ephedrine (10–15 mg i.v.).

Different sensory modalities do not have the same sensitivity to spinal subarachnoid blockade; consequently, the area of analgesia is usually greater than the area of anaesthesia. Similarly, the level of motor blockade is approximately two dermatomes lower than the level of sensory blockade. In the future, the introduction of ropivacaine and levobupivacaine may reduce the intensity and duration of motor blockade associated with spinal subarachnoid anaesthesia.

Neurological complications of spinal anaesthesia are relatively uncommon, and are usually related to CSF leakage, mechanical trauma, the introduction of infection or pre-existing pathology. However, the incidence of arachnoiditis and cauda equina syndromes is probably commoner when high concentrations of local anaesthetics are used.

Intravenous local anaesthesia

Procaine (1% in saline) has been used by intravenous infusion as a supplement to general anaesthesia, to produce analgesia for burns dressings and to relieve postoperative pain. Its action is rather unpredictable and side-effects are not uncommon. It is rarely, if ever, used for this purpose in current anaesthetic practice.

In contrast, intravenous regional anaesthesia (IVRA) is a useful method of providing analgesia for minor surgical procedures. It was first described by August Bier in 1908, but only became widely used approximately 30 years ago. In this technique, a local anaesthetic agent is slowly injected (over 2–3 min) into the vein of a limb that has been previously exsanguinated by an Esmarch bandage and occluded by an orthopaedic tourniquet, which is inflated to 100 mmHg above systolic blood pressure. The occurrence of paraesthesia and the onset of analgesia are almost immediate, and complete sensory blockade usually develops within 10 min. The quality and duration of analgesia are dependent on the dose of local anaesthetic administered, the efficiency of exsanguination, the period of ischaemia prior to injection and the site of injection. It may also be influenced by the effects of local acidosis, and vasodilatation due to carbon dioxide accumulation. The site of action is probably the unmyelinated nerve terminals, which drugs must reach by retrograde spread in the vascular bed. Nerve conduction is not usually affected, although motor paralysis and muscle relaxation usually occur within 15–20 min, due to the presynaptic and postsynaptic effects of the local anaesthetic at the neuromuscular junction.

Most of the commonly used agents produce effective local anaesthesia; the period of residual analgesia (30–350 min) is related to the drug used. Application of the tourniquet produces some discomfort or pain after 20–30 min, which can be partly avoided by the use of a double-tourniquet technique. Nevertheless, IVRA is not usually used for procedures that last longer than an hour; although nerve damage is extremely rare, it is usually associated with prolonged tourniquet times.

Local anaesthetics that are significantly bound to plasma or tissue protein (e.g. bupivacaine, ropivacaine and etidocaine) should not be used to produce IVRA; the use of bupivacaine, in particular, has been associated with several deaths during IVRA, due to cardiac complications.

Lignocaine or prilocaine (200 mg, i.e. 40 ml of a 0.5% solution) is commonly used for regional anaesthesia in the arm. Larger doses are required for the lower limb, and the results are less satisfactory. Systemic toxicity is usually associated with the accidental or inadvertent deflation of the tournique; plasma concentrations of lignocaine or prilocaine are unlikely to be significant if the tourniquet is released more than 15–20 min after injection. Nevertheless, minor symptoms of local anaesthetic toxicity (e.g. paraesthesia and tinnitus) are not uncommon after tourniquet release.

Other uses

Cocaine is sometimes used in analgesic mixtures that are administered orally (e.g. for the relief of intractable pain associated with terminal malignant disease). Gastric sedation may be related to its local anaesthetic effects, and euphoria may be produced. However, the occurrence of excitatory side-effects (as well as the world shortage of cocaine) has tended to restrict its use for this purpose. Procaine forms less soluble conjugates with some other drugs (e.g. penicillin), producing slow-release preparations; procaine may also reduce the pain of injection. Similarly, lignocaine is sometimes used with intramuscular injections of irritant drugs (e.g. amoxycillin) in order to decrease the pain of injection.

Finally dibucaine (nupercaine; cinchocaine) selectively inhibits normal (typical) plasma cholinesterase; in contrast, atypical variants of the enzyme are resistant to inhibition. Consequently, dibucaine is used to study genetic polymorphism in this condition.

Further reading

Aberg G. Toxicological and local anaesthetic effects of active isomers of two local anaesthetic compounds. *Acta Pharmacologic et Toxicologica* 1972; **31**: 273–286.

Adriani J, Campbell B. Fatalities following topical application of local anaesthetics to mucous membranes. *Journal of the American Medical Association* 1956; **162**: 1527–1530.

Adriani J, Dalili H. Penetration of local anesthetic through epithelial barriers. *Anesthesia and Analgesia* 1971; **50**: 834–841.

Adriani J, Zepernick R, Arens J, Authement E. The comparative potency and effectiveness of topical anesthetics in man. *Clinical Pharmacology and Therapeutics* 1964; **5**: 49–62.

Alahuhta S, Rasanan J, Jouppila P *et al*. The effects of epidural ropivacaine and bupivacaine for Cesarean section on utero-placental and fetal circulation. *Anesthesiology* 1995; **83**: 23–32.

Albert J, Lofström B. Bilateral ulnar nerve blocks for the evaluation of local anesthetic agents. III. Tests with a new agent, prilocaine, and with lidocaine in solutions with and without epinephrine. *Acta Anaesthesiologica Scandinavica* 1965; **9**: 203–211.

Aps C, Reynolds F. An intradermal study of the local anaesthetic and vascular effects of the isomers of bupivacaine. *British Journal of Clinical Pharmacology* 1978; **6**: 63–68.

Arthur GR, Feldman HS, Covino BG. Comparative pharmacokinetics of bupivacaine and ropivacaine, a new amide local anesthetic. *Anesthesia and Analgesia* 1988; **67**: 1053–1058.

Atkinson DI, Modell J, Moya F. Intravenous regional analgesia. *Anesthesia and Analgesia* 1965; **44**: 313–317.

Bassett AL, Wit AL. Recent advances in electrophysiology of antiarrhythmic drugs. *Progress in Drug Research* 1973; **17**: 33–58.

Bell HM, Slater EM, Harris WH. Regional anesthesia with intravenous lidocaine. *Journal of the American Medical Association* 1963; **186**: 544–549.

Bigger JT Jr. Arrhythmias and antiarrhythmic drugs. *Advances in Internal Medicine* 1972; **18**: 251–281.

Blair MR. Cardiovascular pharmacology of local anaesthetics. *British Journal of Anaesthesia* 1975; **47**: 247–252.

Blaschke TF. Protein binding and kinetics of drugs in liver diseases. *Clinical Pharmacokinetics* 1977; **2**: 32–44.

Boakes AJ, Laurence DR, Lovel KW, O'Neil R, Verrill PJ. Adverse reactions to local anaesthetic vasoconstrictor preparations: a study of the cardiovascular responses to xylestesin and hostacain-with-noradrenaline. *British Dental Journal* 1972; **133**: 137–140.

Boyes RN. A review of the metabolism of amide local anaesthetic agents. *British Journal of Anaesthesia* 1975; **47**: 225–230.

Braid DP, Scott DB. The systemic absorption of local analgesic drugs. *British Journal of Anaesthesia* 1965; **37**: 394–404.

Braun H. Ueber einige neue örtliche Anaesthetica (Stovain, Alypin, Novocain). *Deutsche Medizinische Wochenschrift* 1905; **31**: 1667–1671.

Brockway M, Bannister J, McKeown D, Wildsmith JAW. Double-blind comparison of extradural bupivacaine and ropivacaine. *British Journal of Anaesthesia* 1990; **64**: 388.

Bromage PR. Physiology and pharmacology of epidural analgesia. *Anesthesiology* 1967; **28**: 592–622.

Bromage PR. Mechanism of action of extradural analgesia. *British Journal of Anesthesia* 1975; **47**: 199–212.

Bromage PR, Gertel M. An evaluation of two new local anaesthetics for major conduction blockade. *Canadian Anaesthetists Society Journal* 1970; **17**: 557–564.

Cahalan MD, Almers W. Interactions between quaternary lidocaine, the sodium channel gates and tetrodotoxin. *Biophysical Journal* 1979; **27**: 57–74.

Calvey TN. Drugs affecting administration of anaesthetics. *British Dental Journal* 1980; **149**: 185–186.

Catchlove RFH. The influence of CO_2 and pH on local anesthetic action. *Journal of Pharmacology and Experimental Therapeutics* 1972; **181**: 298–309.

Chambers WA, Littlewood DG, Logan MR, Scott DB. Effect of added epinephrine on spinal anesthesia with lidocaine. *Anesthesia and Analgesia* 1981; **60**: 417–420.

Covino BG. Pharmacokinetics of local anaesthetic drugs. In: Prys-Roberts C, Hug CC (eds) *Pharmacokinetics of Anaesthesia*. Oxford: Blackwell Scientific Publications, 1984; 270–292.

Covino BG. Pharmacology of local anaesthetic agents. *British Journal of Anaesthesia* 1986; **58**: 701–716.

Crawford OB. Comparative evaluation in peridural anaesthesia of lidocaine, mepivacaine and L-67, a new local anesthetic agent. *Anesthesiology* 1964; **25**: 321–329.

Critchley LAH, Short TG, Gin T. Hypotension during subarachnoid anaesthesia: haemodynamic analysis of three treatments. *British Journal of Anaesthesia* 1994; **72**: 151–155.

Duncan L, Wildsmith JAW. Liposomal local anaesthetics. *British Journal of Anaesthesia* 1995; **75**: 260–261.

Eccles JC. *The Understanding of the Brain*. New York: McGraw-Hill, 1973.

Ehrenstrom Reiz GM, Reiz SL. EMLA — a eutectic mixture of local anaesthetics for topical anaesthesia. *Acta Anaesthesiologica Scandinavica* 1982; **26**: 596–598.

Finucane BT. Ropivacaine — a worthy replacement for bupivacaine? *Canadian Journal of Anaesthesia* 1990; **37**: 722–725.

Foldes FF, Davidson GM, Duncalf D, Kunabara S. The intravenous toxicity of local anesthetic agents in man. *Clinical Pharmacology and Therapeutics* 1965; **6**: 328–335.

Franz DN, Perry RS. Mechanisms for differential block among single myelinated and non-myelinated axons by procaine. *Journal of Physiology* 1974; **236**: 193–201.

Frazier DT, Narahashi T, Yamada M. The site of action and active form of local anesthetics. II. Experiments with quaternary compounds. *Journal of Pharmacology and Experimental Therapeutics* 1970; **171**: 45–51.

Gissen AJ, Covino BG, Gregus J. Differential sensitivity of mammalian nerves to local anesthetic drugs. *Anesthesiology* 1980; **53**: 467–474.

Griffin RP, Reynolds F. Extradural anaesthesia for Caesarean section: a double-blind comparison of 0.5% ropivacaine with 0.5% bupivacaine. *British Journal of Anaesthesia* 1995; **74**: 512–516.

Gristwood R, Bardsley H, Baker H, Dickens J. Reduced cardiotoxicity of levobupivacaine compared with racemic bupivacaine (Marcaine): new clinical evidence. *Expert Opinion on Investigative Drugs* 1994; **3**: 1209–1212.

Hallen B, Carlsson P, Uppfeldt A. Clinical study of a lignocaine–prilocaine cream to relieve the pain of venepuncture. *British Journal of Anaesthesia* 1985; **57**: 326–328.

Heath M. Deaths after intravenous regional anaesthesia. *British Medical Journal* 1982; **285**: 913.

Hickey R, Hoffman J, Ramamurthy S. A comparison of ropivacaine 0.5% and bupivacaine 0.5% for brachial plexus block. *Anesthesiology* 1991; **74**: 639–642.

Hille B. The common mode of action of three agents that decrease the transient charge in sodium permeability in nerves. *Nature* 1966; **210**: 1220–1222.

Hille B. *Ionic Channels of Excitable Membranes*. Sunderland, Massachussetts: Sinauer Associates, 1984.

Hodgkin AL. *The Conduction of the Nervous Impulse*. Liverpool: Liverpool University Press, 1964.

Huxley AF. Ion movements during nerve activity. *Annals of the New York Academy of Sciences* 1959; **81**: 221–246.

Huxley AF, Stampfli R. Evidence for saltatory conduction in peripheral myelinated nerve fibres. *Journal of Physiology* 1949; **108**: 315–339.

Karalliedde L. Animal toxins. *British Journal of Anaesthesia* 1995; **74**: 319–327.

Knapp RB. Drug distribution following intravenous regional analgesia. *Journal of the American Medical Association* 1967; **199**: 760–762.

Lafont ND, Boogaerts JG, Legros FJ. Use of liposome-associated bupivacaine for the management of a chronic pain syndrome. *Anesthesia and Analgesia* 1994; **6**: 818.

Lawson RA, Smart NG, Gudgeon AC, Morton NS. Evaluation of an amethocaine gel preparation for percutaneous analgesia before venous cannulation in children. *British Journal of Anaesthesia* 1995; **75**: 282–285.

Lubens HM, Ausdenmoore RW, Shafer AD, Reece RM. Anesthetic patch for painful procedures such as minor operations. *American Diseases of Children* 1974; **128**: 192–194.

McClure JH. Ropivacaine. *British Journal of Anaesthesia* 1995; **76**: 300–307.

McCrae AF, Wildsmith JAW. Prevention and treatment of hypotension during central neural block. *British Journal of Anaesthesia* 1993; **70**: 672–800.

McCrae AF, Jozwiak H, McClure JH. Comparison of ropivacaine and bupivacaine in extradural analgesia for the relief of pain in labour. *British Journal of Anaesthesia* 1995; **74**: 261–265.

Maunuksela E-L, Korpela R. Double-blind evaluation of a lignocaine–prilocaine cream (EMLA) in children. *British Journal of Anaesthesia* 1986; **58**: 1242–1245.

Mihaly GW, Moore RG, Thomas J, Triggs EJ, Thomas D, Shanks CH. The pharmacokinetics of the anilide type local anesthetics in neonates: I. Lignocaine. *European Journal of Clinical Pharmacology* 1978; **13**: 143–152.

Molodecka J, Stenhouse C, Jones JM, Tomlinson A. Comparison of percutaneous anaesthesia for venous cannulation after topical application of either amethocaine or EMLA cream. *British Journal of Anaesthesia* 1994; **72**: 174–176.

Moore DC. Local anesthetic drugs: tissue and systemic toxicity. *Acta Anaesthesiologica Scandinavica* 1981; **4**: 283–300.

Moore DC, Bridenbaugh LD, Bagdi PA, Bridenbaugh PO, Stander H. The present status of spinal (subarachnoid) and epidural (peridural) block: a comparison of the two technics. *Anesthesia and Analgesia* 1968; **47**: 40–49.

Moore DC, Bridenbaugh LD, Bridenbaugh PO, Tucker GT. Bupivacaine hydrochloride: laboratory and clinical studies. *Anesthesiology* 1970; **32**: 78–83.

Morrison LMM, Emanuelsson BM, McClure JH *et al.* Efficacy and kinetics of extradural ropivacaine: comparison with bupivacaine. *British Journal of Anaesthesia* 1994; **72**: 164–169.

Narahashi T, Yamada M, Frazier DT. Cationic forms of local anesthetics block action potentials from inside the nerve membrane. *Nature* 1969; **223**: 748–749.

Nation RL, Triggs EJ, Selig M. Lignocaine kinetics in cardiac patients and aged subjects. *British Journal of Clinical Pharmacology* 1977; **4**: 439–448.

Nishimura N, Morioka T, Sato S, Kuba T. Effects of local anesthetic agents on the peripheral vascular system. *Anesthesia and Analgesia* 1965; **44**: 135–139.

Ochs HR, Carstens G, Greenblatt DJ. Reduction in lidocaine clearance during continuous infusion and by co-administration of propranolol. *New England Journal of Medicine* 1980; **303**: 373–377.

Piafsky KM. Disease-induced changes in the plasma binding of basic drugs. *Clinical Pharmacokinetics* 1980; **5**: 246–262.

Piafsky KM, Knoppert D. Binding of local anesthetics to 1-acid glycoprotein. *Clinical Research* 1978; **26**: 836A.

Reisner LS, Hochman BN, Plumer MH. Persistent neurologic deficit and adhesive arachnoiditis following intrathecal 2-chloroprocaine injection. *Anesthesia and Analgesia* 1980; **59**: 452–454.

Reiz S, Nath S. Cardiotoxicity of local anaesthetic agents. *British Journal of Anaesthesia* 1986; **58**: 736–746.

Reynolds F. Adverse effects of local anaesthetics. *British Journal of Anaesthesia* 1987; **59**: 78–95.

Ritchie JM. Mechanism of action of local anesthetic agents and biotoxins. *British Journal of Anaesthesia* 1975; **47**: 191–198.

Ritchie JM, Ritchie B, Greengard P. The active structure of local anesthetics. *Journal of Pharmacology and Experimental Therapeutics* 1965; **150**: 152–159.

Ritchie JM, Ritchie B, Greengard P. The effect of the nerve sheath on the action of local anesthetics. *Journal of Pharmacology and Experimental Therapeutics* 1965; **150**: 160–164.

Scott DB. Toxic effects of local anaesthetic agents on the central nervous system. *British Journal of Anaesthesia* 1986; **58**: 732–735.

Scott DB, Jebson PJR, Braid DP, Ortengren B, Frisch P. Factors affecting plasma levels of lignocaine and prilocaine. *British Journal of Anaesthesia* 1972; **44**: 1040–1049.

Scott DB, McClure JH, Giasi RM, Seo J, Covino BG. Effect of concentration of local anaesthetic drugs in extradural block. *British Journal of Anaesthesia* 1980; **52**: 1033–1037.

Strichartz GR (ed.) *Local Anesthetics. Handbook of Experimental Pharmacology*, vol. 81. Heidelberg: Springer-Verlag, 1987; pp. 1–19.

Strong JM, Mayfield DE, Atkinson AJ, Burris BC, Raymon F, Webster LT. Pharmacological activity, metabolism, and pharmacokinetics of glycinexylidide. *Clinical Pharmacology and Therapeutics* 1975; **17**: 184–194.

Swerdlow M, Jones R. The duration of action of bupivacaine, prilocaine and lignocaine. *British Journal of Anaesthesia* 1970; **42**: 335–339.

Thorn-Alquist A-M. Intravenous regional anesthesia. *Acta Anaesthesiologica Scandinavica* 1971; 40 (suppl.): 1–35.

Tillement JP, Lhoste F, Giudicelli JF. Diseases and drug protein binding. *Clinical Pharmacokinetics* 1978; **3**: 144–154.

Tucker GT. Pharmacokinetics of local anaesthetics. *British Journal of Anaesthesia* 1986; **58**: 717–731.

Tucker GT, Boyes RN, Bridenbaugh PO, Moore DC. Binding of anilide-type local anesthetics in human plasma. I. Relationships between binding, physicochemical properties, and anesthetic activity. *Anesthesiology* 1970; **33**: 287–303.

Tucker GT, Mather LE. Clinical pharmacokinetics of local anaesthetics. *Clinical Pharmacokinetics* 1979; **4**: 241–278.

Tucker GT, Wiklund L, Berlin-Wahlen A, Mather LE. Hepatic clearance of local anaesthetics in man. *Journal of Pharmacokinetics and Biopharmaceutics* 1977; **5**: 111–122.

Von Anrep B. Ueber die physiologische Wirkung des Cocain. *Archiv für die gesammte Physiologie des Menschen und der Thiere (Pflügers)* 1880; **21**: 38–77.

Wildsmith JAW. Peripheral nerve and local anaesthetic drugs. *British Journal of Anaesthesia* 1986; **58**: 692–700.

Wildsmith JAW, Gissen AJ, Gregus J, Covino BG. Differential nerve blocking activity of amino-ester local anaesthetics. *British Journal of Anaesthesia* 1985; **57**: 612–620.

Wolff AP, Hasselström L, Kerkkamp HE, Gielen MJ. Extradural ropivacaine and bupivacaine in hip surgery. *British Journal of Anaesthesia* 1995; **74**: 458–460.

Wood M, Wood AJ. Changes in plasma drug binding and alpha-1 acid glycoprotein in mother and newborn infant. *Clinical Pharmacology and Therapeutics* 1981; **29**: 522–526.

Chapter 10
Drugs Acting on the Neuromuscular Junction

Structure of the neuromuscular junction

Motor nerve fibres branch extensively within skeletal muscle, and each anterior horn cell normally innervates 10–150 muscle fibres (the motor unit). As the motor nerve terminal approaches skeletal muscle it loses its myelin sheath; the neuromuscular junction (designated the 'final common pathway' by the eminent neurophysiologist Sir Charles Sherrington) commences at the unmyelinated nerve ending that is distal to the last node of Ranvier. Each axonal terminal lies in a junctional fold or gutter on the surface of the muscle fibre (the motor endplate). In most mammalian muscles, each muscle fibre has a single motor endplate, i.e. it is innervated near its midpoint by one axonal terminal (focal innervation). This usually forms an elevation on the surface of the fibre, which is called an *en plaque* neuromuscular junction. These focally innervated fibres are supplied by fast-conducting Aα axons, and have rapid rates of contraction and relaxation. Conversely, some other muscle fibres are densely innervated at numerous sites by slower-conducting Aγ axons. This type of innervation (known as multiple innervation) occurs in extraocular, intrinsic laryngeal and some facial muscles. The termination of motor nerves in multiply innervated fibres in these muscles resembles a bunch of grapes (an *en grappe* neuromuscular junction). In contrast to the fast fibres, the multiply innervated fibres are unable to propagate action potentials and require a series of impulses to produce a muscle response. The resultant contraction and subsequent relaxation is slower than in focally innervated fibres and is sometimes described as a contracture.

The subcellular features of the motor endplate can be demonstrated by electron microscopy (Fig. 10.1). The axonal terminal lies in a cleft in the sarcolemmal membrane, and contains numerous mitochondria and synaptic vesicles. Many of these vesicles are associated with specialized zones in the axonal membrane that correspond to sites of neurotransmitter release. The synaptic vesicles are synthesized in the anterior horn cells of the spinal cord, and are transported to the motor nerve terminal through the intraneuronal microtubular system. The external surface of the axonal membrane is covered by processes of Schwann-cell cytoplasm, which surround the motor nerve terminal. The axolemmal membrane is separated from the postsynaptic membrane by a gap of approximately 50 nm; this includes a basement lamina approximately 20 nm wide, and mainly consists of

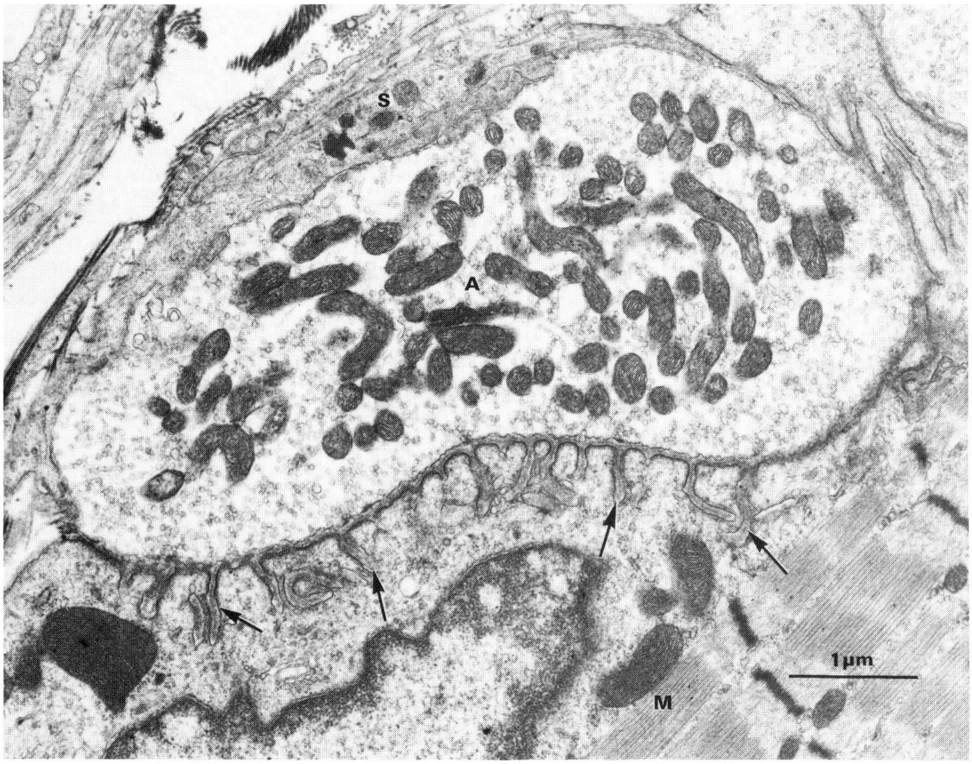

Fig. 10.1 Electron micrograph of part of a normal neuromuscular junction. The axonal terminal (A) lies in a deep indentation of the sarcolemmal membrane and contains abundant mitochondria and synaptic vesicles. The external surface of the axon is covered by processes of Schwann cell cytoplasm (S). There are numerous infoldings (arrowed) of the sarcolemma beneath the axon, and basal lamina material lies between nerve and muscle (M) and fills these subneural folds (× 30 000). (Courtesy of Professor L. W. Duchen.)

mucopolysaccharides. The sarcolemmal postsynaptic membrane is convoluted, forming junctional folds. Acetylcholine receptors are primarily present in discrete groups on the shoulders of the junctional folds; the distal valleys are mainly associated with the hydrolytic enzyme acetylcholinesterase (AChE). Both acetylcholine receptors and AChE are also present at presynaptic sites on the motor nerve terminal.

The synthesis, storage and release of acetylcholine

Neuromuscular transmission depends on the synthesis, storage and release of acetylcholine by the motor nerve terminal. At the motor endplate extracellular choline is partly derived from dietary and plasma choline and partly produced by the hydrolysis of acetylcholine. It is transported from extracellular fluid into the axoplasm by a high-affinity carrier system that is present in all cholinergic nerves (Fig. 10.2). Choline transport is usually the rate-limiting step in the synthesis of acetylcholine in the axoplasm by the enzyme choline acetyltransferase, according to the reaction:

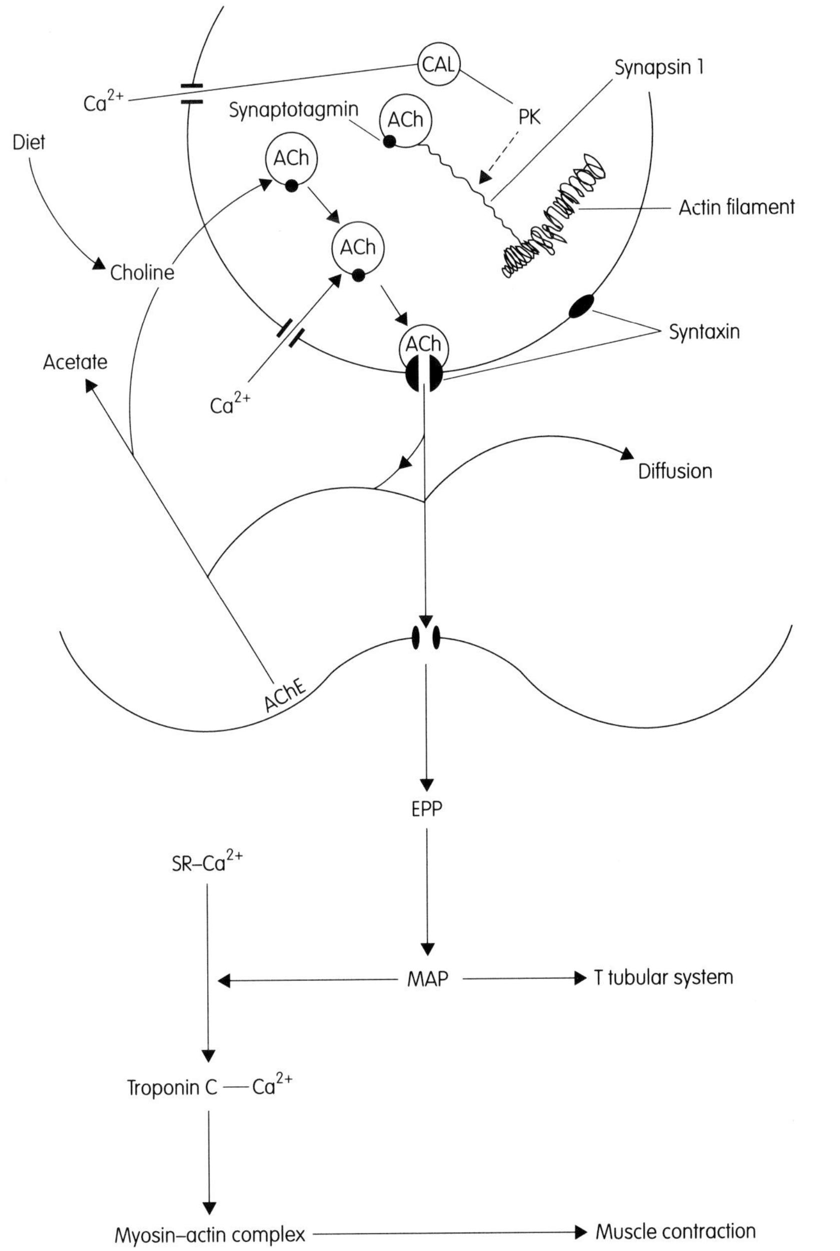

Fig. 10.2 Diagrammatic representation of neuromuscular transmission. ACh, Acetylcholine; AChE, acetylcholinesterase; EPP, endplate potential; MAP, muscle action potential; SR, sarcoplasmic reticulum; PK, protein kinase; CAL, calmodulin.

Choline + acetyl-coenzyme A → acetylcholine + coenzyme A.

In general, the synthesis of acetylcholine is increased by the release of the neurotransmitter; it is not usually possible to deplete the nerve ending of acetylcholine by choline deficiency, or by rapid and unphysiological rates of nerve stimulation.

Approximately 50% of the acetylcholine which is synthesized in the axoplasm of the nerve terminals is then transferred to small synaptic vesicles (about 50 nm in diameter), where it is stored as multimolecular packages or quanta. Some of the remaining acetylcholine leaks across the axonal membrane and may be present in significant amounts in terminal Schwann cells and in the sarcoplasm of muscle fibres, although its function at these sites is unknown. Each synaptic vesicle contains 10 000–12 000 molecules of acetylcholine, as well as Ca^{2+}, adenosine triphosphate (ATP) and a proteoglycan similar to that found in the electroplaque organs of certain fishes. In addition to the vesicles which contain acetylcholine, a small number of large dense-core vesicles have been detected at motor nerve terminals. These vesicles contain the transmitter calcitonin gene-related peptide (CGRP) which is released into the synaptic gap following high-frequency stimulation. The function of CGRP is not entirely clear, but it may be involved in the synthesis of acetylcholine receptors and the regulation of receptor density.

A small number (probably about 1%) of the acetylcholine-containing vesicles are located at release sites on the axolemma of the motor nerve terminal, and constitute the 'easily available' store of the neurotransmitter. The remaining vesicles are distributed throughout the axoplasm, where they may be bound to microtubules and actin filaments, as a large reserve store.

Integral proteins contained in the nerve terminal appear to play an important role in the 'docking' of vesicles at the release site in the motor nerve terminal, and in the formation of an extrusion pore which allows the escape of acetylcholine into the synaptic gap; these proteins may also be involved in the reforming of the vesicles. In addition they can be affected by certain neurotoxins. Synapsin I is a phosphoprotein which encircles the vesicles and anchors them to intracellular structures. Membrane calcium channels which are opened by the arrival of an action potential allow Ca^{2+} to enter the axoplasm and combine with calmodulin. Protein kinase II is subsequently activated and phosphorylates serine residues in the tail region of synapsin I which frees the vesicle. Cyclic adenosine monophosphate (cAMP) may be involved as an intermediate messenger in these events (Fig. 10.2.)

Ca^{2+} also combines with another protein, synaptotagmin, which is bound to the vesicles and allows them to fuse with the docking proteins (syntaxins) in the nerve membrane. This allows the contents of the vesicles to escape into the junctional gap. Other integral proteins (synaptobrevin and synaptophysins) may also have important roles in the storage and subsequent release of acetylcholine.

Acetylcholine receptors

At the neuromuscular junction, acetylcholine receptors are mainly present in discrete groups on the shoulders of the junctional folds of the postsynaptic membrane.

They are also present at presynaptic sites on the motor nerve terminal. During the past 25 years, there has been considerable progress in their isolation and purification; more recently, their precise structure has been determined by molecular biological techniques. Similar acetylcholine receptors are present in abundance in the electroplaque organs of certain fishes (e.g. the South American freshwater eel, the giant electric ray). These receptors are irreversibly bound by the toxins of certain snakes (e.g. α-bungarotoxin derived from the Taiwan banded krait, α-cobra toxin from the cobra). Consequently, nicotinic acetylcholine receptors in electroplaque tissues and mammalian muscle can be irreversibly bound by radiolabelled α-bungarotoxin, and the receptors can then be isolated and purified by affinity chromatography. In addition, acetylcholine receptors have been sequenced and inserted into artificial and amphibian oocyte membranes by molecular biological techniques.

These studies have shown that the acetylcholine receptor at the neuromuscular junction is an integral membrane protein with a molecular weight of approximately 250 kDa (250 000). In adults, it consists of five subunits (2 α subunits, β, ε and δ) which traverse the postsynaptic membrane and surround the ion channel or ionophore. The structure of the receptor is slightly different in fetal life; the ε subunit is replaced by a partly homologous but distinct entity (the γ subunit). In the adult, the ε subunit appears to be responsible for the short channel opening time and higher ionic conductance. Two of the receptor subunits (the α subunits) have a molecular weight of approximately 40 kDa (40 000) and contain acetylcholine-binding sites at the amino acid residues cysteines 192 and 193, tyrosines 93 and 190 and tryptamine 149. There is some evidence that the phospholipid composition of the surrounding membrane may influence the activation of these receptors by acetylcholine. Combination of the neurotransmitter with the binding sites on the α subunits results in conformational changes that open the ion channel; the probability of this occurring is considerably increased when both the sites are occupied by acetylcholine (positive cooperativity). The diameter of the acetylcholine receptor complex is approximately 10 nm, and causes a slight elevation of the postsynaptic membrane. Acetylcholine receptors on the motor nerve terminal (presynaptic receptors) have a slightly different molecular structure, since they are not bound by α-bungarotoxin or cobra toxin, and are differentially affected by neuromuscular blockade.

Neuromuscular transmission

In the absence of nerve impulses, the receptors on the postsynaptic membrane display spontaneous electrical activity. This occurs as discrete, randomly distributed miniature endplate potentials (mepps) with an amplitude of 0.5–1.5 mV. Each mepp is considered to arise from the release of a single quantum (containing 10 000–12 000 molecules) of acetylcholine, and reflects the activity of isolated vesicles which may have been 'lined up' at, or which collided with, extrusion sites on the membrane.

In contrast, when a nerve action potential reaches the axonal terminal, the contents of 100–200 synaptic vesicles are released into the synaptic gap. The quantal release of acetylcholine can be described in statistical terms by the Poisson distribution; the average number of quanta released by each nerve impulse (m) is given by $m = np$, where n is the number of quanta of acetylcholine immediately available for release, and p is the probability of quantal release when the nerve terminal is depolarized. The amount of acetylcholine released is greater than that required to produce endplate depolarization (i.e. there is a considerable safety margin in neuromuscular transmission).

Released acetylcholine diffuses across the synaptic cleft and combines with the α subunits of acetylcholine receptors which surround the ion channel on the postsynaptic membrane. Ion-channel opening is an extremely rapid all-or-none phenomenon that lasts for 5–10 ms, and causes a non-specific increase in permeability to small ions (mainly sodium, potassium and calcium ions). In experimental conditions, it has been estimated that acetylcholine causes the transfer of 10 000 ions per ionophore during each millisecond that the channel is open. These ionic changes result in multiple single-channel currents; each of these has an amplitude of approximately 4 pA (i.e. 4×10^{-12} A). The single-channel currents summate to produce the endplate current, which tends to depolarize the postsynaptic membrane. A small and localized endplate potential is produced; if this reaches a critical amplitude (which normally requires a change of 10–15 mV), voltage-sensitive sodium channels open, the muscle fibre is depolarized and a propagated muscle action potential is conducted along its surface. (The quantal content of the endplate potential (m) can be calculated from the equation: m = amplitude of endplate potential/amplitude of mepps.) The propagated muscle action potential is conducted along the electrically excitable muscle membrane and enters the transverse tubular system (T-tubular system) at the end of the sarcomere (Fig. 10.2). Depolarization of the T-tubular system causes the release of calcium ions from the sarcoplasmic reticulum (possibly by increasing the synthesis of the intermediate messenger inositol trisphosphate). Released calcium ions are bound by troponin C, producing conformational changes in other troponins and tropomyosin. Simultaneously, myosin ATPase is activated and ATP is hydrolysed to adenosine diphosphate (ADP); this provides an abundant supply of intracellular energy. In these conditions, cross-bridges are formed between actin and myosin, resulting in the phenomenon of muscle contraction. The sequence of physiological and biochemical changes between depolarization of the T-tubular system and muscle contraction is known as excitation–contraction (EC) coupling.

The action of acetylcholine at receptors on the postsynaptic membrane is rapidly terminated by the enzyme AChE. Normally, each molecule of acetylcholine only activates a single receptor before its hydrolysis to choline and acetate ions (or its removal by diffusion). The enzyme is primarily present on the junctional clefts of the postsynaptic membrane, although some is also present at presynaptic sites (i.e.

on the motor nerve terminal and in the axoplasm). AChE has two binding sites for acetylcholine — the anionic site and the esteratic site, which are approximately 0.5 nm apart (Fig. 10.3). The anionic site is negatively charged, and probably consists of aspartate or glutamate groups; consequently, it forms an electrostatic (ionic) bond with the quaternary nitrogen atom of acetylcholine, which is supplemented by London–van der Waals dispersion forces. In contrast, the esteratic site consists of the hydroxyl group of serine and the imidazole group of histidine. Hydrogen bonding between these groups enhances the nucleophilic properties of serine, and allows it to react with the ester group in acetylcholine. A covalent bond is formed and choline is released, resulting in the production of the acetylated enzyme; this is rapidly hydrolysed, causing the regeneration of the enzyme and the formation of acetic acid. The reactions involved are extremely rapid, and the half-life of the acetylated enzyme is approximately 40 μs (4×10^{-5} s). The rapid destruction of the neurotransmitter is essential in order to prevent the repetitive firing of the motor endplate.

AChE is present at all cholinergic junctions, and is probably synthesized at these sites. It is also found in red blood cells (where its function is unknown) and in many regions of the central nervous system (CNS). In contrast, butyrylcholinesterase (pseudocholinesterase, plasma cholinesterase; ChE) is synthesized in the liver, and found in plasma, skin, intestine and other tissues. Although ChE can metabolize acetylcholine, it may have a more important function in the regulation of other choline esters (e.g. propionylcholine, butyrylcholine) which are present in the gut wall. In anaesthetic practice ChE has an important function in the hydrolysis of certain muscle relaxants (e.g. suxamethonium, mivacurium) which are unaffected by AChE. ChE also contains two binding sites, and has identical linkage with choline esters at the esteratic site to AChE; however, at the anionic site it forms a dipolar rather than an anionic bond.

When acetylcholine is released from the motor nerve terminal, it mainly produces its effects at nicotinic receptors on the postsynaptic membrane. Nevertheless,

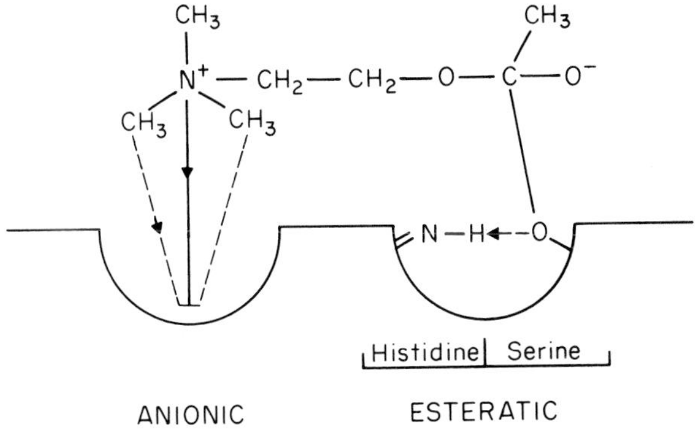

Fig. 10.3 Binding sites of acetylcholinesterase (AChE).

there is some evidence that acetylcholine receptors are also present on the motor nerve terminal, and at the most distal node of Ranvier. Acetylcholine receptors on the motor nerve terminal may play an important part in maintaining transmitter output at high rates of nerve stimulation; their blockade by non-depolarizing neuromuscular-blocking agents may be responsible for the phenomenon of decrement or fade (p. 329). In contrast, acetylcholine receptors at the last node of Ranvier may induce retrograde or antidromic firing of the motor nerve. Thus, the injection of acetylcholine into the popliteal artery of experimental animals not only produces activity of the appropriate muscle groups, but also gives rise to action potentials in the motor nerve which are conducted in a retrograde manner. These antidromic potentials can be recorded from the ventral nerve roots by appropriate electrophysiological techniques. Similar effects can be produced by repetitive nerve stimulation, anticholinesterase drugs or suxamethonium. These results suggest that drugs that act at the neuromuscular junction may also affect the motor nerve terminal. Nevertheless, the functional importance of these effects is a matter of conjecture, and most of the evidence suggests that the main effects of acetylcholine occur at postsynaptic sites.

Drugs that affect neuromuscular function

In general, drugs that modify neuromuscular transmission may affect:

1 Acetylcholine release.
2 Acetylcholine action.
3 Acetylcholine breakdown.
4 EC coupling.

Drugs that affect the release of acetylcholine

The release of acetylcholine from the motor nerve terminal may be affected by:

1 Drugs affecting calcium transport.
2 Local and general anaesthetics.
3 Neurotoxins.
4 Guanidine and aminopyridine.
5 Miscellaneous drugs.

Drugs affecting calcium transport

The release of acetylcholine from the motor nerve terminal is dependent on the entry of calcium ions from extracellular fluid to the axoplasm (p. 320). Consequently, alterations in extracellular calcium might be expected to affect neurotransmitter release from the motor nerve terminal. In practice, although hypocalcaemia and hypercalcaemia have important effects on the excitability of tissues and cardiac contraction, they do not usually modify acetylcholine release (except in experimental conditions).

Nevertheless, drugs that prevent the entry of calcium ions into the motor nerve terminal may decrease acetylcholine release (and thus prolong non-depolarizing neuromuscular blockade). Thus, calcium antagonists (e.g. verapamil, diltiazem, nifedipine) occasionally prevent the entry of calcium ions into the axoplasm; in these conditions they may impair neurotransmitter release and interact with muscle relaxants. Similarly, certainly antibiotics may impair neuromuscular transmission and prolong non-depolarizing blockade by decreasing the entry of calcium ions into the motor nerve terminal. Although this phenomenon has been mainly reported with the aminoglycosides and the polymyxins, it may also occur with other antibiotics (e.g. colistin, tetracyclines, lincomycin).

Although the primary action of these antibiotics is presynaptic, effects on the motor endplate and voluntary muscle may also occur. Classically, neuromuscular function was impaired in tuberculous patients on long-term streptomycin; alternatively, neostigmine-resistant curarization occurred after abdominal surgery in which large doses of intraperitoneal aminoglycoside antibiotics were used. Calcium salts (e.g. calcium gluconate) may cause the reversal of antibiotic-induced neuromuscular blockade; less commonly, anticholinesterase drugs are useful. The problem is not frequently encountered in current anaesthetic practice. A similar phenomenon may occur when antibiotics are given to patients with myasthenia gravis.

Magnesium ions compete with calcium ions for transport into the motor nerve terminal, and thus decrease the release of acetylcholine. Consequently, parenteral magnesium sulphate, or magnesium-containing antacids, may reduce neurotransmitter release and interact with muscle relaxants (particularly in patients with renal failure).

Local and general anaesthetics

Most local anaesthetics can decrease the release of acetylcholine from the motor nerve terminal. After systemic administration or absorption, they may affect conduction in unmyelinated nerve endings; alternatively, conduction blockade of major or minor nerve trunks may prevent the transmission of nerve impulses from anterior horn cells.

General anaesthetics (particularly inhalational agents) may also decrease the release of acetylcholine from the motor nerve terminal. They produce depression of the CNS and thus decrease the generation of nerve impulses by anterior horn cells. In addition, some fluorinated anaesthetics may have direct effects on the muscle cell membrane. Consequently, many volatile anaesthetic agents may profoundly affect the degree of non-depolarizing neuromuscular blockade. Diethylether classically potentiates the effects of muscle relaxants; similar effects are produced by the fluorinated ethers. Halothane is a fluorinated hydrocarbon, and has less potent effects on neuromuscular transmission. Nevertheless, it can still prolong the effects of non-depolarizing drugs. The cardiovascular effects of inhalation anaesthetics may also modify the pharmacokinetics of muscle relaxants.

Neurotoxins

Certain neurotoxins also prevent the release of acetylcholine by the motor nerve terminal. Black widow spider venom contains α-latrotoxin which affects transmitter release in all cholinergic nerves. At the neuromuscular junction, α-latrotoxin initially produces the irreversible fusion of synaptic vesicles with the terminal axonal membrane. Subsequently, the synaptic vesicles become disorganized, and lose their ability to concentrate newly synthesized acetylcholine; the mechanism involved relates to an effect of the toxin on synaptotagmin, which fuses the synaptic vesicles to the docking proteins in the nerve terminal. Botulinus toxin also affects all cholinergic nerves. This toxin is actually an enzyme, a zinc endopeptidase, which cleaves synaptobrevin and prevents the release of acetylcholine from synaptic vesicles, although the neurotransmitter content of the nerve terminal is unaffected.

Guanidine and aminopyridine

Both guanidine and aminopyridine prolong the duration of the neuronal action potential, increase calcium ion entry and thus facilitate the release of acetycholine from the motor nerve terminal (and other cholinergic nerve endings). Their mode of action is slightly different; guanidine delays the inactivation of sodium channels, while aminopyridine tends to inactivate potassium channels (and thus prevent repolarization). Both drugs have been used to increase the release of acetylcholine from the motor nerve terminal in botulism and the Eaton–Lambert syndrome. (This condition is a rare disorder of neuromuscular transmission which is usually associated with a small cell carcinoma of the bronchus.) In Bulgaria, aminopyridine has been used to reverse non-depolarizing neuromuscular blockade. Unfortunately, both guanidine and aminopyridine readily cross the blood–brain barrier, and may cause convulsions; this has severely restricted their clinical use.

Miscellaneous drugs

Many other drugs can affect acetylcholine release in experimental conditions (e.g. dendrotoxin, catechol, phenol, tetraethylammonium, adenosine). Theophylline and other xanthine derivatives can enhance the release of acetylcholine (either by adenosine receptor blockade, or by phosphodiesterase inhibition and accumulation of cAMP). This phenomenon may also explain the improvement which occurs in myasthenia gravis when sympathomimetic drugs (e.g. ephedrine) are administered.

Vesamicol is a novel drug which is used in experimental studies of the neuromuscular junction. It is a tertiary amine which is effective orally and yet blocks neuromuscular transmission. Evidence suggests that vesamicol inhibits the uptake of newly synthesized acetylcholine into synaptic vesicles.

Drugs that affect the action of acetylcholine

Drugs can modify the action of acetylcholine by combining with nicotinic receptors on the postsynaptic membrane. These compounds are traditionally referred to as neuromuscular blocking agents (or muscle relaxants).

They are commonly divided into two groups:

1 Depolarizing agents (e.g. suxamethonium, decamethonium).

2 Non-depolarizing agents (e.g. tubocurarine, atracurium).

As their name implies, depolarizing agents produce depolarization of the motor endplate immediately before the onset of neuromuscular blockade. In contrast, non-depolarizing agents do not produce depolarization (except in experimental conditions in embryonic and cultured muscle cells).

Mode of action

Both depolarizing and non-depolarizing agents have non-specific effects, and may influence neuromuscular transmission at different sites. Consequently, the interpretation of their actions on neuromuscular function in terms of their molecular and electrophysiological effects is imprecise and controversial.

Depolarization blockade is probably due to the rapid inactivation of voltage-sensitive sodium channels in the muscle cell membrane, immediately adjacent to the motor endplate. The intra-arterial injection of small doses of acetylcholine near the motor endplate normally produces a brief contraction of voluntary muscle. In these conditions, the hydrolysis of acetylcholine is extremely rapid, and subsequent stimulation of the motor nerve produces little change in the twitch response. When larger doses of acetylcholine are injected (or its activity is prolonged by anticholinesterase drugs), the initial muscle contraction is followed by neuromuscular blockade, resulting in the depression of the maximal twitch response to nerve stimulation. Similar effects can be produced by other drugs that are structurally related to acetylcholine, but are less rapidly removed from the motor endplate (e.g. suxamethonium, decamethonium).

In normal conditions, depolarization of the motor endplate by acetylcholine activates voltage-sensitive sodium channels in the adjacent muscle fibre, resulting in the generation and propagation of a muscle action potential. If depolarization is maintained, several action potentials may be produced. However, persistent depolarization is rapidly followed by the generation of local current circuits and the inactivation of voltage-sensitive sodium channels in the adjacent muscle fibre, immediately peripheral to the motor endplate. In the inactivated stage, these channels are closed, and cannot be opened by the persistent depolarization of the motor endplate. This phenomenon occurs within several milliseconds, and produces a zone of electrical inexcitability surrounding the motor endplate, which extends for 1–2 mm along the muscle fibre membrane. This zone will not transmit or propagate impulses, although the remainder of the muscle fibre is normally excitable. Consequently neuromuscular blockade is a direct consequence of persistent depolarization of the motor endplate.

In contrast, non-depolarizing neuromuscular blockade is primarily due to competition of drugs with acetylcholine for receptor sites on the postsynaptic membrane. Consequently, these drugs are sometimes referred to as 'competitive' neuromuscular blocking agents (although it is difficult to be certain that all of their effects are due to the competitive antagonism of acetylcholine). The reversible combination of non-depolarizing agents with postsynaptic receptors does not produce any change in membrane conductance or ionic permeability, so that depolarization by acetylcholine is progressively diminished (due to a reduction in the available receptors). Since the number of effective agonist–receptor complexes is reduced, the amplitude of the endplate potential gradually decreases. Eventually, it fails to generate a propagated muscle action potential, resulting in neuromuscular blockade. Normal neuromuscular function is restored when adequate redistribution and/or elimination of the muscle relaxant occurs, or when sufficient acetylcholine accumulates to displace the non-depolarizing agent from postsynaptic receptors.

In normal conditions, the amount of acetylcholine released by nerve stimulation exceeds that required to produce an endplate potential and its subsequent muscle action potential. Consequently, there must be considerable receptor occupation by the antagonist before there is evidence of neuromuscular blockade. Experimental evidence suggests that approximately 80% of receptors must be occupied by non-depolarizing agents before any reduction in neuromuscular transmission occurs; 90–95% receptor occupation is required for complete neuromuscular blockade.

In addition to their effects on acetylcholine receptors on the postsynaptic membrane, non-depolarizing agents affect neuromuscular transmission in at least two additional ways. In the first place, they may combine with receptors on the motor nerve terminal which are normally responsible for the maintenance of transmitter output at high rates of stimulation (and are likely to be activated by the prejunctional effects of acetylcholine itself). Consequently, during partial neuromuscular blockade, the amount of acetylcholine released is diminished during repetitive nerve stimulation, resulting in decrement or fade. Second, non-depolarizing relaxants (and some other drugs) may physically occlude ion channels on the postsynaptic membrane (and possibly at presynaptic sites as well). This type of blockade is most likely to occur when ion-channel opening is most frequent (i.e. when acetylcholine or anticholinesterase drugs are also used). Its contribution to non-depolarizing blockade in current clinical practice is uncertain.

Characteristic features of neuromuscular blockade

Depolarizing and non-depolarizing blockade have characteristic and distinctive features, which may be of clinical significance. These differences are classically seen after the administration of suxamethonium and tubocurarine in humans (Table 10.1).

1 Depolarization blockade is preceded by muscle fasciculations; in non-depolarizing blockade, muscle activity does not occur.

Muscle fasciculations are incoordinated contractions due to the repetitive firing of muscle fibres, and are associated with increased electromyographic activity in voluntary muscle. It is unlikely that muscle fasciculations simply reflect the depolarization of the motor endplate. Acetylcholine receptors are present at presynaptic sites on the motor nerve ending, and their depolarization may initiate a local antidromic axon reflex within the terminals of an entire motor unit. Consequently, fasciculations are probably due to the synchronous release of acetylcholine from a number of motor nerve terminals, and thus reflect the presynaptic actions of depolarizing drugs. Reflex effects mediated by acetylcholine receptors in muscle spindles may play a secondary role.

In contrast, during non-depolarizing blockade muscle fasciculations are absent, since presynaptic receptors are occupied by acetylcholine antagonists. Indeed, non-depolarizing drugs may decrease suxamethonium-induced fasciculations by preventing prejunctional depolarization and the occurrence of local axon reflexes, thus reducing the rate of motor unit firing. Consequently, pretreatment with non-depolarizing relaxants may prevent suxamethonium-induced fasciculations and muscle pain.

2 In depolarization blockade, there is a decrease in potential amplitude during repetitive indirect stimulation, but no evidence of fade (i.e. the progressive decrease in the electrical or the mechanical response to continuous nerve stimulation). In contrast, in non-depolarizing blockade there is a gradual decrease in the amplitude of the muscle action potential or the twitch height during repetitive indirect stimulation (decrement or fade; Fig. 10.4).

Table 10.1 Differences between depolarizing and non-depolarizing neuromuscular blockade.

	Depolarizing blockade	Non-depolarizing blockade
Preceded by muscle fasciculations	Yes	No
Neuromuscular decrement ('fade')	Absent	Present
Posttetanic potentiation	Absent (usually)	Present
Effect of anticholinesterase drugs	Increased	Antagonized
Effect of non-depolarizing drugs	Antagonized	Increased
Tachyphylaxis and dual blockade	May occur	Absent

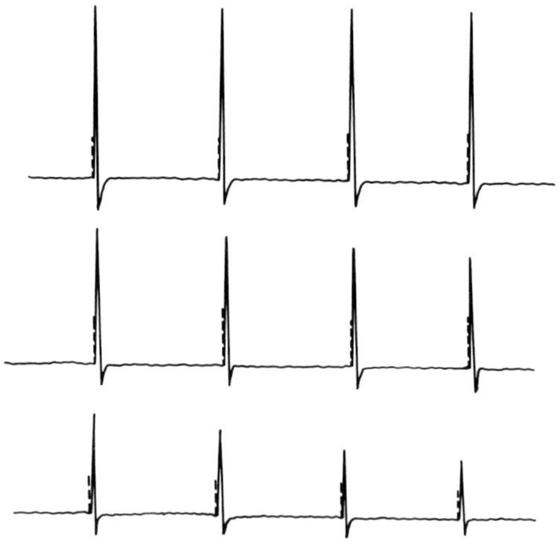

Fig. 10.4 Muscle action potentials evoked by indirect nerve stimulation during the induction of neuromuscular block. A train-of-four was used in each instance.

In depolarization blockade, acetylcholine output is probably maintained during subtetanic or tetanic stimulation, due to the effects of depolarization on presynaptic receptors that preserve transmitter output at high rates of impulse conduction. In any case, variations in acetylcholine release are unlikely to affect the degree of neuromuscular blockade, since this is due to persistent depolarization of the motor endplate. During partial recovery from depolarization blockade, the amplitude of the potential (compared to unaffected muscle) evinced by single or repetitive indirect stimulation is low, but there is no evidence of fade. This presumably reflects a summation of electrical potential in those muscle fibres which have completely recovered from neuromuscular blockade and other fibres which are still refractory to the effects of released acetylcholine.

By contrast, in non-depolarizing blockade there is a progressive decrease in the quantal release of acetylcholine during rapid indirect stimulation, which is probably related to blockade of prejunctional receptors. As postsynaptic receptors are also affected, the 'safety factor' of neuromuscular transmission is compromised, and is reflected by a fall in the amplitude of the muscle action potential or the twitch height during repetitive stimulation. This phenomenon of decrement (fade) is characteristically seen during the onset or recovery from non-depolarizing blockade. It is widely used to monitor the effects of drugs on neuromuscular transmission; the train-of-four method, which compares the amplitude of the first and the last responses to four successive stimuli administered at 2 Hz for 2 s is commonly employed in this context (Fig. 10.4).

3 During the onset or partial recovery from depolarization blockade, significant posttetanic potentiation does not occur. In contrast, in non-depolarizing blockade posttetanic potentiation can usually be demonstrated (in both the electromyogram and the mechanical response to indirect stimulation; Fig. 10.5).

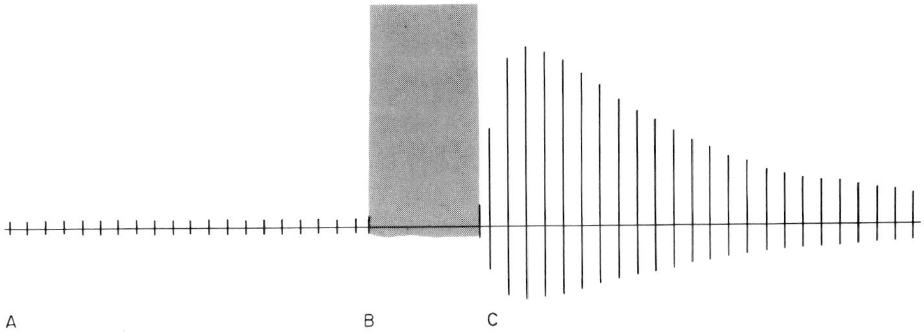

Fig. 10.5 Posttetanic potentiation during partial recovery from non-depolarizing neuromuscular blockade. (A) Compound muscle action potentials evoked by repetitive indirect stimulation. (B) Conditioning tetanus; its amplitude is due to the presence of a stimulus artefact. (C) Posttetanic potentiation after reversion to original rate of stimulation.

Subtetanic or tetanic stimulation of motor nerves results in a progressively diminishing release of acetylcholine per stimulus; this is rapidly followed by enhanced synthesis and transmitter mobilization. Consequently, when the tetanus ends, acetylcholine output per stimulus is increased. In normal circumstances, this does not affect neuromuscular function, due to the presence of the safety margin for synaptic transmission (p. 328); consequently, posttetanic potentiation is not observed on the electromyogram. Nevertheless, some posttetanic potentiation may be present in the twitch response; this probably reflects increased muscle contractility, possibly due to the enhanced entry of calcium ions into muscle cells during tetanic stimulation. The phenomenon is sometimes referred to as augmentation of muscle contraction.

During onset and recovery from depolarization blockade, the enhanced transmitter release per stimulus produced by a conditioning tetanus does not significantly affect the degree of depolarization or the depth of neuromuscular blockade. Consequently, significant posttetanic potentiation does not usually occur (although some augmentation of contraction may be seen in the twitch response, as in normal circumstances).

In contrast, posttetanic potentiation is an established feature of non-depolarizing blockade; the increase in transmitter output produced by the conditioning tetanus increases endplate depolarization above the threshold level in a proportion of partially blocked muscle fibres. In this instance, posttetanic potentiation is due to facilitation of transmission, i.e. a temporary increase in acetylcholine output which displaces non-depolarizing relaxants from their postsynaptic sites. During profound neuromuscular blockade, the 'posttetanic count' can be used to monitor the effects of muscle relaxants on the motor endplate.

4 Anticholinesterase drugs can increase the depth and duration of depolarization blockade. The effects of suxamethonium are prolonged due to inhibition of ChE by anticholinesterase drugs. In the case of decamethonium (which is not metabolized by the enzyme ChE), inhibition of AChE by an anticholinesterase drug will allow accumulation of acetylcholine in the synaptic cleft and augment the depolarization block.

In contrast, during non-depolarizing blockade, accumulation of acetylcholine at the motor endplate allows the neurotransmitter progressively to displace non-depolarizing muscle relaxants from postsynaptic and presynaptic sites, resulting in the antagonism of neuromuscular blockade.

5 Non-depolarizing drugs reverse or antagonize depolarization blockade; in contrast, they invariably potentiate non-depolarizing blockade produced by other drugs.

Non-depolarizing drugs compete for and combine with acetylcholine receptors on the postsynaptic membrane. Consequently, in depolarization blockade they tend to reduce endplate depolarization, and may restore normal neuromuscular transmission. In practice, they are not used clinically for this purpose since their effects are rather unpredictable.

In contrast, non-depolarizing drugs invariably increase the depth and duration of non-depolarizing blockade produced by other drugs. In some instances, synergic or potentiating effects have been reported.

6 Depolarization blockade may be associated with the development of tachyphylaxis and dual block. These complications do not occur in non-depolarizing blockade.

Tachyphylaxis is usually recognized by a decreased response to successive doses of the drug. This phenomenon may precede the gradual development of a second phase of neuromuscular blockade. Changes consistent with non-depolarizing blockade occur, and are usually referred to as dual block or phase II block. In humans, this is most commonly seen when large doses or prolonged infusions of suxamethonium are used, or when drug elimination is compromised by enzyme abnormalities or other drugs.

The explanation for the development of dual block is not entirely clear. It may reflect the continual presence of depolarizing drugs at the motor endplate, resulting in receptor desensitization or ion-channel blockade. Receptor desensitization effectively reduces the number of functional receptors on the postsynaptic membrane. If this reduction is profound, neuromuscular blockade occurs, which is potentiated by non-depolarizing drugs and antagonized by anticholinesterase agents. Similar features might be present if depolarizing drugs progressively blocked open ion channels at the motor endplate. Unfortunately, there is no definite evidence that either receptor desensitization or ion channel blockade can occur in humans.

Depolarizing agents

In general, all depolarizing agents have a similar chemical structure. They are slender, elongated, and flexible molecules (leptocurares) with methyl or ethyl groups attached to their quaternary heads, which are separated by a distance of 1.2–1.4 nm. In the past, decamethonium and suxamethonium have been used to produce neuromuscular blockade; in current practice, only suxamethonium is used for this purpose.

Suxamethonium

[333]
CHAPTER 10
*Drugs Acting on
the Neuromuscular
Junction*

Suxamethonium is a quaternary amine ester (Fig. 10.6); chemically, it consists of two molecules of acetylcholine, joined together at their non-quaternary ends (i.e. through their acetyl groups). The ability of suxamethonium to produce de-polarization blockade in humans was first recognized in 1949–1951 (although its pharmacological properties were first investigated in curarized animals in 1906).

Acetylcholine

$$CH_3-CO-O-CH_2-CH_2-\overset{\overset{\displaystyle CH_3}{|}}{\underset{\underset{\displaystyle CH_3}{|}}{N^\pm}}-CH_3$$

Suxamethonium

$$CH_2-CO-O-CH_2-CH_2-\overset{\overset{\displaystyle CH_3}{|}}{\underset{\underset{\displaystyle CH_3}{|}}{N^\pm}}-CH_3$$

$$CH_2-CO-O-CH_2-CH_2-\overset{\overset{\displaystyle CH_3}{|}}{\underset{\underset{\displaystyle CH_3}{|}}{N^\pm}}-CH_3$$

Decamethonium

$$CH_3-\overset{\overset{\displaystyle CH_3}{|}}{\underset{\underset{\displaystyle CH_3}{|}}{N^+}}-(CH_2)_{10}-\overset{\overset{\displaystyle CH_3}{|}}{\underset{\underset{\displaystyle CH_3}{|}}{N^\pm}}-CH_3$$

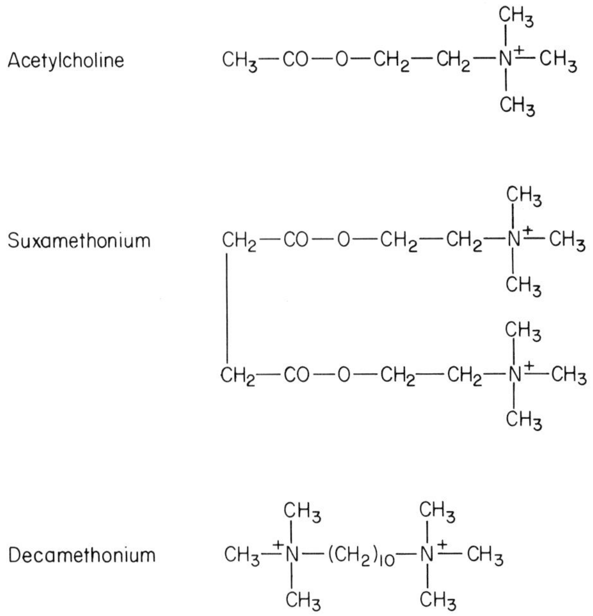

Fig. 10.6 The chemical structure of acetylcholine, suxamethonium and decamethonium.

After the intravenous injection of suxamethonium, profound muscle relaxation preceded by observable muscle fasciculations normally occurs within 1 min. The duration of neuromuscular blockade after normal doses of suxamethonium ($1.0-1.5$ mg kg^{-1}) is usually 4–6 min; during this time there is a rapid fall in the plasma concentration of the drug. Neuromuscular blockade is due to the persistent depolarization of the motor endplate, which rapidly inactivates voltage-sensitive sodium channels in the adjacent muscle fibre (p. 327). Unfortunately, suxamethonium produces a number of additional undesirable effects (Table 10.2).

1 Muscle fasciculations. Muscle fasciculations may be slight (usually involving the small muscles of the hand and the facial muscles), moderate (involving larger muscle groups in the limbs) or severe (involving most muscle groups in the body). Moderate and severe fasciculations can facilitate venous return and cause an increase

Table 10.2 Undesirable effects of suxamethonium.

Muscle fasciculations
Postoperative myalgia
Hyperkalaemia
Tachyphylaxis and dual blockade
Increased intraocular pressure
Malignant hyperthermia
Parasympathomimetic effects
Bradycardia
Increased respiratory secretions
Increased intragastric pressure
Increased uterine tone
Prolonged paralysis due to delayed metabolism

in cardiac output; arterial blood pressure may rise and an increase in intracranial tension can occur. Fasciculations that involve the abdominal muscles may cause an increase in intragastric pressure.

2 Myalgia. Postoperative muscle pains are a frequent complication of the administration of suxamethonium, and occur chiefly in the subcostal region, the trunk and the shoulder girdle. Women are more susceptible than men, and symptoms are more frequently encountered in patients who have been mobilized soon after surgery, and in subjects unaccustomed to muscular exercise. The frequency of postoperative myalgia after suxamethonium varies between 6 and 60%; creatine kinase levels are significantly raised, and myoglobinuria occasionally occurs. These findings suggest that suxamethonium myalgia may be related to muscle damage caused by drug-induced fasciculations. Nevertheless, in many studies the incidence of muscle fasciculations is not directly related to the occurrence of postoperative pain (although pretreatment with a small dose of a non-depolarizing agent can modify the fasciculations and reduce the incidence of pain).

3 Hyperkalaemia. Depolarization of the motor endplate, and the resulting muscle contraction, causes the efflux of intracellular potassium ions into the extracellular fluid. In normal conditions, plasma potassium rises by approximately 0.5 mmol l^{-1}; this increase is rarely of clinical significance (although it may accentuate the cardiac effects of subsequent doses of suxamethonium).

In contrast, in patients with severe burns, peripheral nerve injuries or neurological conditions, much greater increases in serum potassium concentrations may occur. Rises of 4–9 mmol l^{-1} have been reported; in neurological conditions, the major hyperkalaemic response can be demonstrated in the venous blood draining the paralysed or injured limbs. A latent period may be required between the time of injury and the development of an excessive hyperkalaemic response. This suggests that the rise in serum potassium may be related to receptor up-regulation after muscle damage or peripheral denervation (denervation supersensitivity). In peripheral denervation (and during fetal life), acetylcholine receptors on the postsynaptic membrane are not just localized to the motor endplate, but extend along the entire surface of the muscle fibre. In these conditions, the increased loss of potassium from muscle is related to the extensive area of the muscle membrane depolarized by suxamethonium.

There have been numerous reports of cardiac arrest after the use of suxamethonium in patients with severe burns and neurological conditions (particularly between 20 and 60 days after the initial injury). Although clear evidence of muscle damage or denervation may not be present, hyperkalaemia is probably the main causal factor. Hypovolaemia, acidosis and autonomic imbalance may also be involved.

When pre-existing hyperkalaemia is present (e.g. in renal failure or severe acidosis), undesirable cardiac effects should be anticipated if suxamethonium is used.

4 Tachyphylaxis and dual blockade (phase II blockade). Suxamethonium (and decamethonium) may cause tachyphylaxis (a decreased response to successive doses of the drug). This may precede the gradual development of dual blockade (phase II blockade), in which changes consistent with non-depolarizing blockade may occur. This phenomenon is most commonly seen when large doses or prolonged infusions of suxamethonium are used, or when the elimination of the drug is compromised (e.g. by enzyme abnormalities or other drugs). The cause of tachyphylaxis and phase II blockade is uncertain.

5 Increased intraocular pressure. Suxamethonium causes a rise in intraocular tension, which may last for several minutes. Consequently, the drug should be used with caution in patients with penetrating eye injuries, and during open ocular surgery.

In humans, the extrinsic muscles of the eye are multiply innervated by relatively slowly conducting Aγ axons (i.e. each muscle fibre is innervated by more than one axonal terminal). In this respect, their innervation is similar to avian muscle. In many birds, suxamethonium characteristically produces a slow and sustained contraction (contracture) of voluntary muscle. Similar effects are probably produced in human extraocular muscles, causing a transient rise in intraocular pressure.

6 Malignant hyperpyrexia (malignant hyperthermia) is a genetic disorder which affects myoplasmic calcium regulation. In susceptible individuals, malignant hyperpyrexia may be triggered by suxamethonium. The initial dose of suxamethonium may fail to produce muscle relaxation; there may be generalized muscle rigidity, associated with a rapidly rising temperature, which may develop within a few minutes. Suxamethonium probably precipitates the release of calcium ions from the sarcoplasmic reticulum of susceptible individuals, leading to sustained contraction and subsequent muscle damage.

7 Parasympathetic effects. Suxamethonium is chemically related to acetylcholine, and has some activity at muscarinic receptors. Thus, bradycardia or atrioventricular nodal rhythm may occur after a large single dose, or with repeated administration (especially in children). Potentiation of these muscarinic effects on the heart may occur with digoxin or with other drugs that alter autonomic balance in favour of parasympathetic activity (e.g. β-adrenoceptor antagonists). Other muscarinic effects are not uncommon. Increased production of bronchial and salivary secretions are frequently observed, especially with repeated dosage. Gastric tone is increased, and a rise in intragastric pressure occurs (although this is partly related to fasciculations involving the abdominal muscles). Repeated doses of suxamethonium may cause a marked increase in uterine tone during Caesarean section. All these parasympathetic effects can be prevented or attenuated by premedication with atropine or other antimuscarinic drugs.

8 Prolonged apnoea. Occasionally, prolonged paralysis and apnoea are related to the delayed metabolism of suxamethonium. In general, problems may be due to the presence of genetic variants of plasma ChE, or to the concurrent use of other drugs that can inhibit the enzyme.

The transient effects of a single dose of suxamethonium are due to its rapid hydrolysis by ChE. The breakdown of the drug occurs in two stages. Initially, succinylmonocholine is formed, and this has weak neuromuscular blocking activity (approximately 5% of the potency of suxamethonium). Subsequently, succinylmonocholine is broken down to succinic acid and choline. Prolongation of the effects of suxamethonium may be due to genetic polymorphism, decreased availability or inhibition of ChE.

ChE is synthesized by the liver; severe hepatic dysfunction, usually associated with marked hypoalbuminaemia, may cause abnormally low levels of this enzyme, and some prolongation of the action of suxamethonium is likely. More significant problems can arise from genetically determined abnormalities of the enzyme. Genetic polymorphism is present, and at least four allelomorphic genes have been identified at a single locus of chromosome 3. These genes are called E_1^u, E_1^a, E_1^f and E_1^s; they produce the normal (usual) enzyme, the atypical enzyme, the fluoride-resistant enzyme and the absent (silent) enzyme respectively. The commonest genetic variant (the atypical enzyme) can be distinguished from the usual enzyme by its resistance to inhibition by the local anaesthetic cinchocaine (dibucaine). The dibucaine number is defined as the enzyme inhibition (%) produced by dibucaine (10^{-5} mol l^{-1}), using benzoylcholine as the substrate. Normal homozygotes ($E_1^u E_1^u$) have dibucaine numbers of 80; homozygotes for the atypical enzyme ($E_1^a E_1^a$) have dibucaine numbers of 20. Since four allelomorphic genes are present, 10 genotypes have been identified; three of these genotypes will show a greatly prolonged response to suxamethonium (Table 10.3). Their total incidence in the general population is about 1 in 2000. In recent years, at least six additional allelomorphic genes have been identified. In addition, a second distinct locus is associated with two further genetic variants ($E_{Cynthiana}$ and C_5), which may be responsible for increased cholinesterase activity.

Drugs that inhibit ChE may extend the duration of action of suxamethonium. Some agents (i.e. tetrahydroaminacrine and hexafluorenium) have been intentionally used for this purpose, although their action is unreliable and unpredictable. More serious drug interactions (e.g. prolongation of neuromuscular blockade,

Table 10.3 The classical genetic variants of plasma cholinesterase.*

Genotype	Approximate incidence per 1000 population	Dibucaine number	Prolonged response to suxamethonium
$E_1^u E_1^u$	950	80	No
$E_1^u E_1^a$	40	60	Occasionally
$E_1^u E_1^f$	4	75	Occasionally
$E_1^u E_1^s$	6	80	Occasionally
$E_1^a E_1^a$	< 1	20	Yes
$E_1^a E_1^f$	< 1	50	Occasionally
$E_1^a E_1^s$	< 1	20	Yes
$E_1^f E_1^f$	< 1	65	Occasionally
$E_1^f E_1^s$	< 1	65	Occasionally
$E_1^s E_1^s$	< 1		Yes

* During the past decade, this system of classification has been extended by the use of DNA-cloning techniques. At least 10 allelomorphic genes (and a possible 28 phenotypes) have been identified; some genetic variants (e.g. the K-variant, the J-variant and the H-variant) are quantitative variants in which reduced enzyme activity is associated with normal kinetic properties. The amino acid sequence of the normal and the atypical enzyme has also been determined. The atypical (dibucaine-resistant) enzyme is associated with a single mutation at nucleotide 209 (GAT to GGT), which changes amino acid 70 from aspartate to glycine. This substitution at the active site of the acidic (anionic) amino acid aspartate by neutral glycine accounts for the resistance to dibucaine inhibition and the reduced affinity for the quaternary amine suxamethonium.

tachyphylaxis and the increased likelihood of phase II block) may be due to the concurrent use of drugs that are substrates or inhibitors of ChE. These include edrophonium, neostigmine, organophosphorus compounds, alkylating agents, trimetaphan, pitocin and local anaesthetic esters.

Decamethonium

Decamethonium was first used clinically in 1949, after the investigation of several bisquaternary compounds for curare-like activity. It was originally considered to cause less depression of respiration because of a diaphragm-sparing activity; however, it soon became apparent that the production of effective relaxation also produced respiratory paralysis. After the administration of a single dose (usually 4–6 mg), there is a relatively slow onset of action (3–5 min) and a moderate duration of action (10–20 min); its effects are potentiated by passive hyperventilation. The drug is almost entirely excreted in urine unchanged. The effects of decamethonium may be antagonized by other methonium compounds (e.g. pentamethonium, hexamethonium); these drugs may cause considerable hypotension due to ganglion blockade. Decamethonium has been extensively used in experimental studies, but has not been generally available in the UK since 1958. Nevertheless, it may be imported, or a suitable preparation may be made up by a hospital pharmacist from decamethonium powder, and the drug is still occasionally used in clinical anaesthesia. Some of the advantages claimed for decamethonium include a marked degree of cardiovascular stability, little or no histamine release and a lower incidence of muscle fasciculation and postoperative myalgia than occurs with the use of suxamethonium.

Non-depolarizing agents

The classical non-depolarizing muscle relaxant curare is a generic term for various South American arrow poisons; it is used correctly to describe the crude extracts obtained from certain species of the plants *Chondrodendron* and *Strychnos*. The impure extracts, containing several different alkaloids, have been used for many centuries by South American Indians as an arrow or blow-dart poison, in order to kill wild animals for food. Their preparation of curare was shrouded in mystery and ritual, and the samples of the drug which first reached civilization were classified by the containers in which they had been transported; pot curare was carried in earthenware jars, tube curare in bamboo tubes and calabash curare in gourds. Scientific interest in curare dates from the classical observations of Claude Bernard in 1856; he correctly localized the muscle-paralysing effects of curare to the neuromuscular junction, since the drug did not affect nervous conduction or the response of voluntary muscle to direct stimulation. Its clinical use dates from 1932, when purified fractions were used in the treatment of tetanus and spastic disorders. Subsequently, the *d*-isomer of tubocurarine was isolated, and its provisional chemical formula (which was later revised) was established by King in 1932. The drug was later used to control pentylenetetrazole-induced convulsions during the treatment of psychiatric disorders. It was finally introduced into anaesthetic practice in 1942.

Since then, other drugs have been widely used to produce neuromuscular blockade. The first synthetic relaxant, gallamine, was introduced by Bovet in 1947, and alcuronium (a semisynthetic derivative of a curare alkaloid) has been used in the UK since 1962. The bisquaternary aminosteroid pancuronium has been widely employed during the past 25 years, while two agents with significant advantages (i.e. vecuronium and atracurium) were introduced in the early 1980s. Vecuronium is the monoquaternary analogue of pancuronium, while atracurium is a bisquaternary ester with a novel molecular structure, which is spontaneously broken down in the body. Other drugs have recently been introduced, or are currently under development for clinical use (p. 346). All these compounds contain quaternary amine groups, but have a bulky molecular structure and are sometimes described as pachycurares (Fig. 10.7).

Although all these drugs have similar effects on the neuromuscular junction, they differ in certain other respects (Table 10.4). In general, these differences are related to:

1 Effects of extracellular pH on their activity.

2 Histamine release.

Tubocurarine

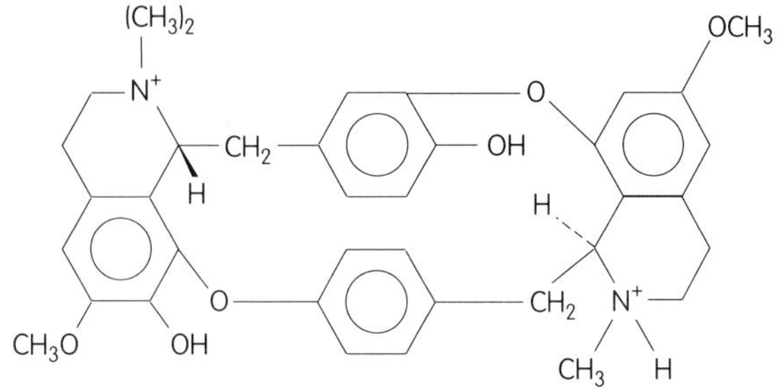

Alcuronium

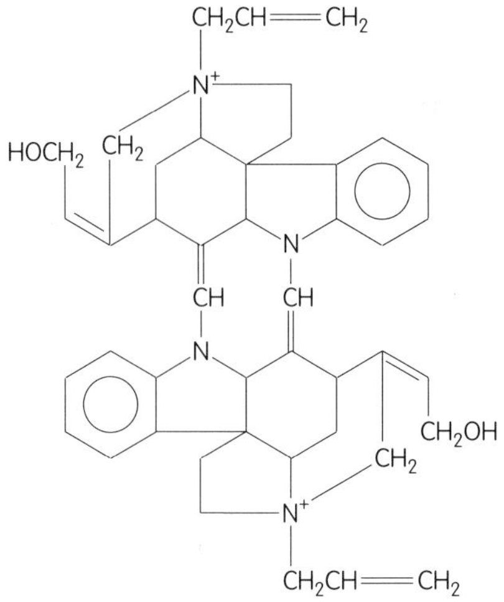

Gallamine

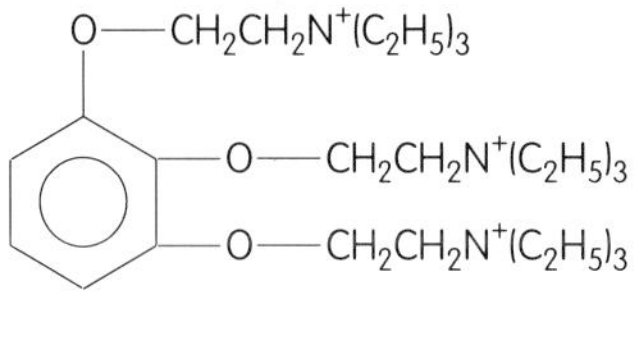

Pancuronium

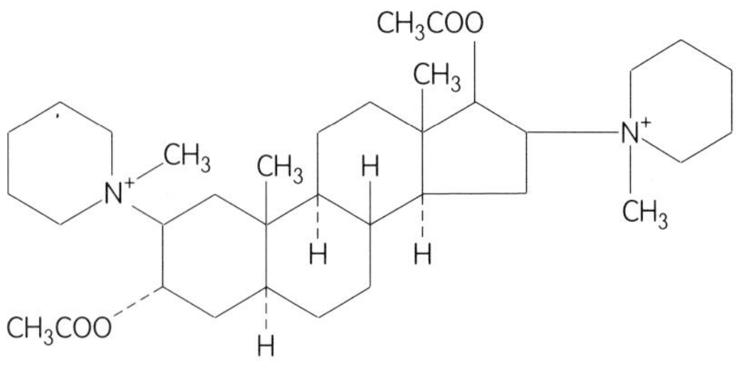

Fig. 10.7 The chemical structure of non-depolarizing muscle relaxants in current clinical use. (The associated anions have been omitted.)

Vecuronium

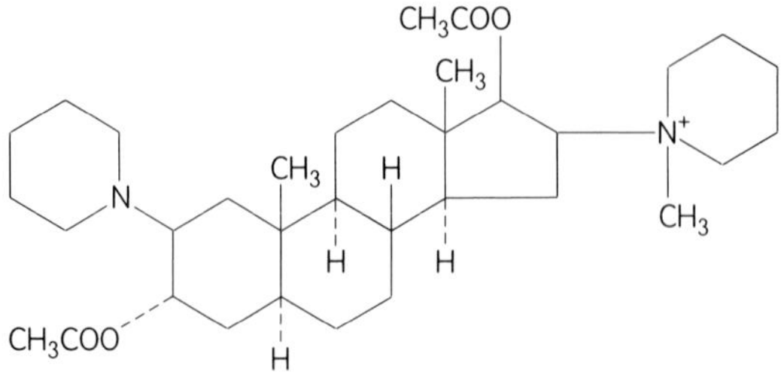

Atracurium

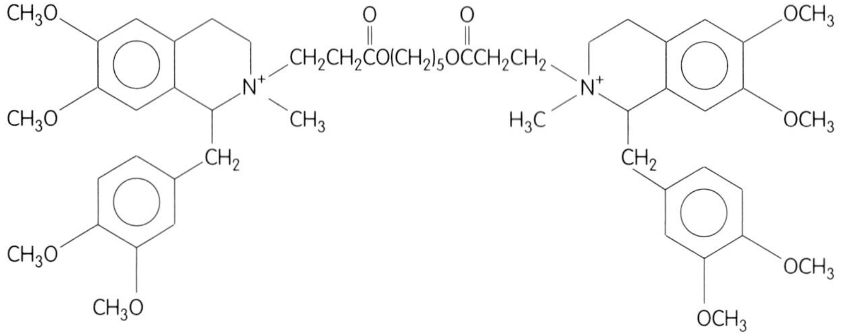

Mivacurium

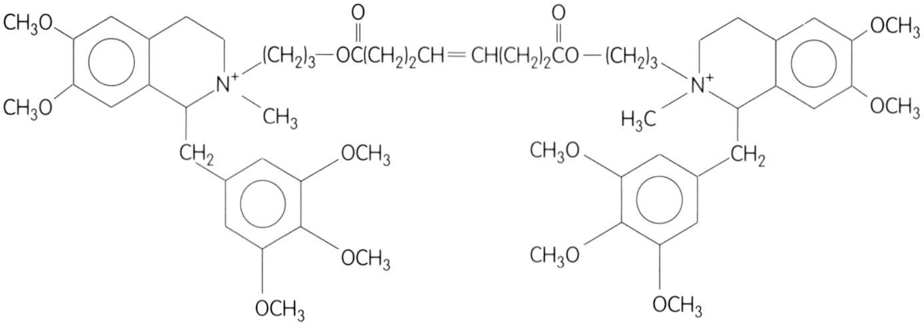

Rocuronium

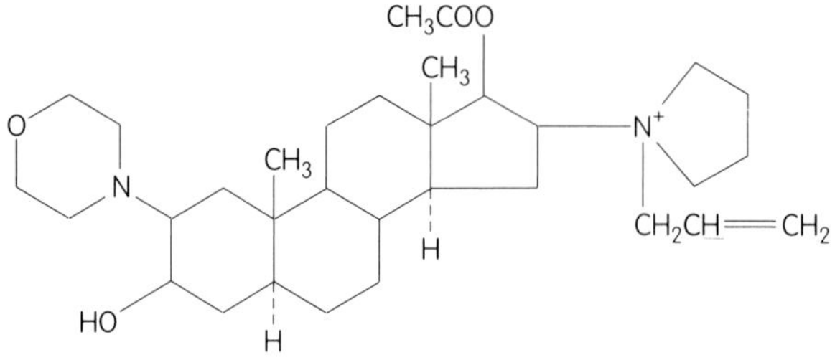

Fig. 10.7 (*continued*)

Table 10.4 Pharmacological differences between non-depolarizing relaxants.

	Onset of action	Histamine release	Cardiovascular effects	Duration of action	Plasma protein binding (%)	Volume of distribution (ml kg^{-1})	Clearance (ml min^{-1} kg^{-1})	$t_{1/2}$ (min)	Elimination
Tubocurarine	Slow	Common	Hypotension	Long	30–50	290	1.5	190	Not metabolized; eliminated in urine (70%) and bile (30%)
Alcuronium	Moderate	? Rare	Hypotension	Long	< 20	300	1.5	200	Not metabolized; eliminated in urine (70%) and bile (30%)
Gallamine	Rapid	Rare	Tachycardia	Medium	< 20	230	1.2	150	Not metabolized; eliminated in urine (100%)
Pancuronium	Moderate	Rare	Tachycardia	Medium	20–60	270	1.5	130	Metabolized (30%) to three deacetylated metabolites; 70% eliminated unchanged (mainly in urine)
Vecuronium	Moderate	Rare	None	Short	< 20	230	4.0	60	Metabolized (20%) to deacetylated metabolites; 80% eliminated unchanged (mainly in bile)
Atracurium	Moderate	Rare	None	Short	< 20	160	5.5	20	Metabolized (95%) to laudanosine, a quaternary acrylate, acid and alcohol; 5% eliminated unchanged
Mivacurium	Moderate	Rare	None	Short	< 20				Metabolized (95%) by plasma cholinesterase to quaternary alcohol and quaternary acid; 5% eliminated unchanged
cis–cis						320	5.5	55	
cis–trans						210	90	2	
trans–trans						210	90	2	
Rocuronium	Rapid	Rare	None	Medium	< 20	210	4.5	85	Eliminated in bile (55%) and urine (35%); deacetylated metabolites may be produced

Values for the volume of distribution, clearance and $t_{1/2}$ (terminal half-life) are median values obtained in patients without hepatic or renal impairment.

3 Effects on the cardiovascular system.
4 Distribution and pharmacokinetics.
5 Metabolism and elimination.

Extracellular pH

The potency and duration of action of individual muscle relaxants may be modified in different ways by changes in plasma and extracellular pH. In particular, the effects of tubocurarine may be enhanced and prolonged by respiratory acidosis, and decreased by respiratory alkalosis. This phenomenon may be related to the effects of pH on the physicochemical properties of tubocurarine, which has one tertiary and one quaternary amine group (Fig. 10.7). In acidic conditions, the ionization of the tertiary amine group ($pK_a = 8$) is increased due to protonation; the ionization of the two hydroxyl groups ($pK_a = 8$ and 9.3) may also be modified. These changes increase the potency of tubocurarine. Similar effects on ionization may occur in metabolic acidosis and metabolic alkalosis. However, in these conditions the shift of K^+ between cells and extracellular fluid may be a complicating factor. Hypokalaemia may prolong non-depolarizing blockade, since it tends to increase the resting membrane potential and prevent depolarization.

The effects of gallamine may be potentiated by alkalosis and antagonized by acidosis; the action of other muscle relaxants is not usually affected by pH changes within the physiological range. Any alterations that do occur are probably related to the effects of pH on electrolyte balance, rather than to an inherent effect on the activity of the drugs.

Histamine release

In common with many other basic drugs (e.g. opioid analgesics, trimetaphan) muscle relaxants have the ability to release histamine and other autocoids from mast cells, either by displacement or by exocytosis. A localized effect (a wheal and flare response, resulting in oedema, erythema and vasodilatation) is commonly observed following the intravenous injection of tubocurarine or atracurium and is considered to be due to displacement of histamine from mast cells in the adjacent vessel wall by localized high concentrations of the drug. Such phenomena are rarely associated with any systemic manifestations.

However, generalized hypersensitivity reactions, sometimes leading to life-threatening bronchospasm and hypotension (with or without generalized erythema), are associated with the use of muscle relaxants in anaesthetic practice. In approximately 65% of these cases a classical anaphylactic (type 1 hypersensitivity) reaction is the causal factor; a history of atopy, previous exposure to the drug, and the subsequent detection of specific immunoglobulin E (IgE) antibodies and positive responses to intradermal testing are common features.

In the remaining cases an anaphylactoid reaction is thought to be the likely cause. In some instances this may be mediated by a direct effect of the drug on circulating basophils (and depend upon the dose and speed of injection of the drug). Another mechanism is the activation of the alternative complement pathway by the protein properidin and the subsequent release of histamine (Chapter 6). Anaphylactoid reactions do not require previous exposure to the drug, but their clinical presentation is usually less severe than a true anaphylactic response.

Tubocurarine, alcuronium (and suxamethonium) have been associated with anaphylactic and anaphylactoid responses. However, atracurium, gallamine and even the aminosteroids (which do not apparently cause histamine release in humans) have also been implicated. The polypharmacy which is associated with current anaesthetic practice undoubtedly inhibits the identification of the drug responsible in many cases. The treatment of hypersensitivity responses which occur in anaesthetic practice is discussed in Chapter 7.

Effects on the cardiovascular system

Most non-depolarizing agents may cause a fall in blood pressure immediately after their administration. This may be related to histamine release, a decrease in venous return caused by loss of muscle tone or other effects.

Tubocurarine commonly causes a fall in blood pressure of 20–30 mmHg or more. Reflex tachycardia is rare; indeed, a slight decrease in pulse rate (less than 10 beats min^{-1}) is usually present. The fall in blood pressure is partly due to histamine release, and partly to blockade of sympathetic ganglia; the absence of reflex tachycardia suggests that ganglion blockade is the most important factor. In general, alcuronium has similar effects to tubocurarine, although significant histamine release is uncommon. A slight fall in blood pressure may occur, probably due to blockade of sympathetic ganglia.

In contrast, both gallamine and pancuronium commonly produce tachycardia. Gallamine usually increases pulse rate by 20–30 beats min^{-1}; blood pressure is usually unaltered or raised. After injection of atropine (whose effects are principally mediated by antagonism of postsynaptic M_3-receptors), a further rise in pulse rate may occur. Gallamine produces selective antagonism of cardiac M_2-receptors by causing conformational changes that reduce their affinity for acetylcholine. In addition, the release of noradrenaline by cardiac sympathetic nerves is increased; this may be due to antagonism of presynaptic M_2-receptors on sympathetic fibres which normally regulate the release of noradrenaline.

Similarly, pancuronium commonly increases pulse rate, blood pressure and venous return, although these effects are usually less marked than with gallamine. Pancuronium has complex effects on cardiac autonomic nerves; it inhibits $Uptake_1$ (i.e. the uptake of noradrenaline by sympathetic nerve endings), and may also have antimuscarinic effects which indirectly increase noradrenaline release. Both these actions tend to increase pulse rate and blood pressure.

Vecuronium and atracurium do not usually affect the cardiovascular system. They may apparently induce bradycardia and hypotension, but this is probably due to the unopposed effects of other drugs on cardiac vagal tone. Occasionally atracurium causes profound bradycardia during halothane anaesthesia.

Distribution and pharmacokinetics

Since all non-depolarizing relaxants are quaternary amines, they are not significantly absorbed from the gut. After intravenous administration, they are mainly distributed in extracellular fluid, and may be partly bound to plasma proteins. *In vitro* techniques (e.g. plasmapheresis, equilibrium dialysis, ultrafiltration) have been widely used to assess the protein binding of individual relaxants. Most of the results suggest that 30–50% of tubocurarine and 20–60% of pancuronium are bound by IgG and by albumin, but that only minor amounts of other relaxants are bound to plasma proteins. Changes in the binding of muscle relaxants to plasma proteins are probably of little practical significance. Patients in whom IgG concentrations are raised (e.g. those with severe burns or liver disease) may be resistant to tubocurarine and pancuronium; it is unclear whether this phenomenon is related to altered plasma protein binding. In the past, attempts have been made to correlate the individual dosage requirements of different relaxants with the concentration of different plasma proteins. In general, there is a positive correlation between tubocurarine dosage and IgG levels and between alcuronium dosage and albumin. The requirements of pancuronium were not related to any fraction of plasma proteins.

Due to their chemical structure, non-depolarizing relaxants do not cross the blood–brain barrier or the placental barrier in appreciable amounts. Nevertheless, small concentrations of muscle relaxants (usually less than 5% of the maternal level) can be detected in the fetal circulation or cord blood after administration to the mother. However, fetal apnoea is only rarely associated with the use of these drugs during anaesthesia for Caesarean section (although paralysis has occurred following repeated dosage during long-term ventilation in pregnancy). Gallamine is more liable to cross the placenta than other relaxants, and its use in anaesthesia for Caesarean section is avoided.

After intravenous administration of non-depolarizing agents, there is a rapid fall in plasma concentration during the first 2–10 min, mainly due to the uptake of the drug by renal and hepatic cells. Small concentrations are localized at the motor endplate and are non-specifically bound at anionic sites in the junctional cleft and at the basement membrane of muscle fibres. Subsequently, there is a further slower phase of exponential decline, which reflects the removal of the muscle relaxant by renal or biliary excretion, or by metabolism. Consequently, the disposition of most muscle relaxants has usually been represented in terms of models containing two compartments. Constants derived from these models can be used to calculate pharmacokinetic parameters; alternatively they may be derived by model-independent methods (Chapter 2). The total apparent volume of distribution of most muscle relaxants is similar to, or slightly greater than, extracellular fluid volume (i.e. 200–400 ml kg^{-1}). Their clearance is more variable, ranging from 1–2 ml min^{-1} kg^{-1} (tubocurarine, alcuronium, gallamine and pancuronium) to 5–6 ml min^{-1} kg^{-1} (vecuronium and atracurium). These differences in clearance are reflected in the terminal half-lives of different relaxants, which in general are ranked in the order tubocurarine = alcuronium > pancuronium > gallamine > vecuronium > atracurium > mivacurium (Table 10.4). This order also corresponds to the relative duration of neuromuscular blockade after the administration of equipotent doses. Indeed, with many relaxants (e.g. tubocurarine) there is a close relation between their steady-state plasma concentration and the degree of neuromuscular blockade. In the past, it has been suggested that the main factor determining the duration of action of muscle relaxants is the rate of dissociation of the drug–receptor complex at the neuromuscular junction. These views are not now generally accepted.

The pharmacokinetics of muscle relaxants may be modified in renal and hepatic disease. In renal failure, the half-life of most non-depolarizing relaxants is increased, due to a reduction in their clearance. However, the half-life and the clearance of atracurium and vecuronium are not significantly affected. In hepatic disease, the pharmacokinetics of muscle relaxants that are mainly eliminated by the liver (e.g. vecuronium) may be modified.

Metabolism and elimination

Most muscle relaxants are partly excreted unchanged in urine, and are not readily metabolized by hepatic enzyme systems. Nevertheless, they all appear to enter liver cells, and some may be significantly secreted in bile (depending on the number of quaternary centres and their molecular weight).

Tubocurarine is not significantly metabolized by the liver or by other tissues. Normally, it is eliminated unchanged in urine (although small amounts are also present in bile, since it is a monoquaternary compound with a molecular weight of more than 400 Da). In renal failure, the amount of tubocurarine eliminated in bile is greatly increased. Similarly, the related drug alcuronium is probably not metabolized, but is mainly eliminated from the body in urine and in bile.

Gallamine is almost entirely eliminated unchanged in urine. Only trace amounts are excreted in bile, since gallamine is a low molecular weight compound with more than one quaternary group. Consequently, in renal failure its clearance is greatly decreased and its half-life prolonged 10–20 times.

Pancuronium is mainly eliminated unchanged in urine, although 15–40% may be metabolized by the liver to three deacetylated compounds (3-hydroxy-pancuronium, 17-hydroxypancuronium and 3,17-dihydroxypancuronium). At least one of these metabolites (3-hydroxypancuronium) has non-depolarizing actions, and is half as potent as pancuronium; it was at one time used as a muscle relaxant (dacuronium). Only trace amounts of pancuronium are eliminated in bile. In contrast, the related aminosteroid vecuronium is mainly eliminated from the body by active secretion in bile, since it is a monoquaternary compound. Vecuronium is also eliminated in urine, and small amounts are deacetylated by the liver.

Atracurium is a unique muscle relaxant, since its chemical structure allows the partial termination of its action by spontaneous degradation *in vivo*. Atracurium is stable in solution in acid conditions (pH 4) at 4°C; in contrast, at pH 7.4 and 37°C, it is rapidly broken down to a tertiary amine (laudanosine) by a spontanous chemical reaction (Hofmann elimination). Since atracurium is a bisquaternary ester, it is also metabolized by lung and plasma esterases to a monoquaternary alcohol and a monoquaternary acid. Although laudanosine has effects of its own (e.g. it is a glycine antagonist), its accumulation in renal or hepatic disease is unlikely. The spontaneous recovery from the effects of atracurium is a marked advantage, and the drug is the relaxant of choice in patients with renal or liver disease.

New neuromuscular blocking agents

The search for the perfect neuromuscular blocking agent continues. It is probably accepted that an ideal muscle relaxant would have a non-depolarizing mode of action and allow optimal intubating conditions within 1 min. Total paralysis should last 5–10 min and complete spontaneous recovery (95% twitch height and a train-of-four value >0.7) should occur within 15–20 min of drug administration (the block should be antagonized by an anticholinesterase drug in the event of slow recovery). The ideal drug would not cause histamine release and be devoid of significant haemodynamic effects. Interactions with other drugs would not occur, and the pharmacological effects of the muscle relaxant would not be influenced by metabolic dysfunction or pH disturbances.

A number of studies have suggested that a rapid onset of non-depolarizing block can only be achieved by large doses of a drug. If a relatively potent drug is administered, this advantage will only be gained at the expense of a prolonged duration of blockade; with less potent drugs, commercial factors and the propensity to produce side-effects may be important.

Mivacurium

Mivacurium is a benzylisoquinoline ester which is structurally related to atracurium, but subject to degradation by plasma cholinesterase activity rather than by Hofmann elimination. Mivacurium demonstrates a relatively slow onset, but a shorter duration of action than atracurium. These effects are essentially dose-related, in that a larger dose will produce a shorter latency period but at the expense of a more prolonged effect. Mivacurium appears to be devoid of cardiovascular side-effects, but shares a weak histamine-releasing property with atracurium.

Mivacurium is a chiral mixture of three stereospecific isomers (*cis–trans* 36%, *trans–trans* 58%, *cis–cis* 6%). The *cis–cis* isomer has only one-tenth of the potency of the other two isomers but is not subject to enzymatic activity; this is reflected in the pharmacokinetic data (Table 10.4).

Clearance of the two principal isomers has been shown to be significantly reduced in hepatic cirrhosis and may reflect decreased availability of ChE; genetic variations of this enzyme have also been associated with a markedly prolonged duration of action. The clearance of the *cis–cis* isomer appears to be reduced in renal failure.

Recovery from neuromuscular blockade may be hastened by the administration of an anticholinesterase drug (in association with an antimuscarinic agent). In these circumstances edrophonium would appear to be advantageous. In contrast to neostigmine, edrophonium rapidly dissociates from ChE (due to hydrogen bonding, rather than covalent bonding, with the esteratic site on the enzyme) and should not prolong the elimination of the two principal isomers. Monitoring of neuromuscular function and some evidence of spontaneous recovery are advisable before reversal is contemplated. Mivacurium was introduced into the UK in 1993 and has achieved a role in day-case surgery and for other short elective procedures requiring endotracheal intubation.

Doxacurium

Doxacurium is a closely related drug, which has been available in the USA since 1992. It is the most potent muscle relaxant available. However, it does not appear to convey any advantages over other established agents, and wide variations in both onset and duration of action have been observed with its use.

Cisatracurium

Cisatracurium is one of the 10 stereoisomers present in the commercially available preparation of atracurium. Its pharmacokinetic profile is similar to that of atracurium, and Hofmann elimination and ester hydrolysis are significant mechanisms for elimination. It is three to five times more potent than atracurium in producing a 95% depression of the electromyogram response (ED_{95}), but the onset of action is predictably slower. Haemodynamic effects and histamine release appear to be minimal, even with relatively high dosage, and the drug has recently been developed commercially.

Rocuronium

Rocuronium is an aminosteroid which has now been introduced into clinical practice. It is structurally related to vecuronium, but has only one-eighth of the potency of the parent drug. The low potency is considered to be responsible for the rapid onset of action (60–90 s), although the duration of action is similar to that of atracurium and vecuronium in equipotent doses. There is some evidence that rocuronium may produce mild vagolytic effects.

The elimination half-life of rocuronium is 70–95 min. The drug is mainly excreted unchanged in bile (approximately 55% of the dose administered) and urine (35%), although some deacetylated metabolites may be produced. The presence of hepatic cirrhosis may influence the onset and duration of action of the relaxant, and its effect may be slightly prolonged in renal failure.

Pipecuronium

Pipecuronium is a long-acting muscle relaxant with a relatively slow onset of action which has been used in Eastern Europe for many years. It has a steroidal structure and a potency similar to that of vecuronium but no vagolytic side-effects.

Drugs that affect the breakdown of acetylcholine

Anticholinesterase drugs prevent the hydrolysis of acetylcholine by combining with the enzyme AChE. Consequently, they cause the accumulation of acetylcholine at all cholinergic synapses to which they gain access. All anticholinesterase drugs produce effects on neuromuscular transmission and the autonomic nervous system; in addition, some of them (i.e. physostigmine, most organophosphorus compounds) produce central effects. Anticholinesterase drugs also inhibit ChE, and may prolong the effects of drugs that are esters, e.g suxamethonium.

Drugs that inhibit AChE can be classified into three main groups:

1 Edrophonium.

2 Carbamate esters, which include neostigmine, pyridostigmine, distigmine and physostigmine (eserine).

3 Organophosphorus compounds.

Edrophonium

Edrophonium is a phenolic quaternary amine with a simple chemical structure (Fig. 10.8), which combines reversibly with AChE. The quaternary group is attracted to the anionic site on AChE (Fig. 10.3); hydrogen bonding also occurs at the esteratic site, producing a drug–enzyme complex which is reversible and rapidly dissociable. Edrophonium thus inhibits enzyme activity by preventing the access of acetylcholine

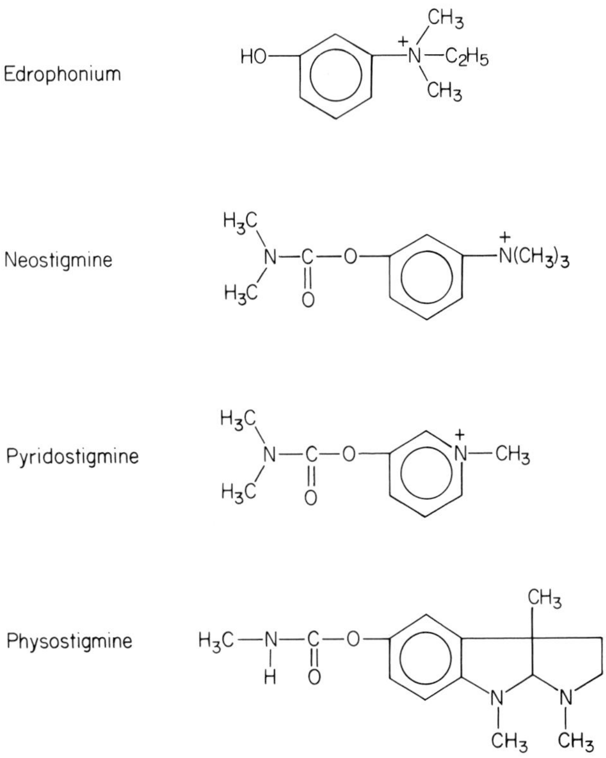

Fig. 10.8 The chemical structure of some anticholinesterase drugs. (The associated anion has been omitted.)

to the active site. At the neuromuscular junction, edrophonium also has direct effects on the motor nerve terminal, resulting in increased acetylcholine release.

After intravenous injection, edrophonium characteristically causes muscle fasciculations which are frequently associated with autonomic effects (e.g. bradycardia, increased secretions and an increase in smooth-muscle tone). Since it is a quaternary amine, it does not cross the blood–brain barrier or the placental barrier. Edrophonium is rapidly distributed in extracellular fluid but may also enter hepatic and renal cells. The plasma concentration of the drug declines in a biexponential manner, with a distribution half-life of less than 2 min, followed by a slower decline (terminal half-life = 25–45 min). As the plasma concentration falls, AChE inhibition is rapidly reversed and the effects of the drug are usually transient. It is mainly eliminated by glucuronide conjugation and by renal excretion of the unchanged drug.

Edrophonium (2–10 mg intravenously) has been widely used as a diagnostic test in suspected cases of myasthenia gravis; it may also be used to distinguish between myasthenic and cholinergic crisis in the established disease. In anaesthetic practice, it has been occasionally used to confirm the development of phase II blockade (dual block) after the administration of suxamethonium or decamethonium.

More recently, the drug has been used in the reversal of non-depolarizing blockade produced by vecuronium or atracurium, since its duration of action is shorter than other anticholinesterase drugs. In these conditions, relatively large doses of edrophonium are required (e.g. 0.5–1.0 mg kg^{-1}) in order to ensure that plasma concentrations and enzyme inhibition persist for long enough to prevent recurarization.

Carbamate esters

All carbamate inhibitors of AChE affect the enzyme in a similar manner. They are attracted to the anionic site by an ionized group, which may be a tertiary amine (physostigmine) or a quaternary amine (neostigmine, pyrodostigmine and distigmine). Subsequently, the methylcarbamyl group (Fig. 10.8) combines with the serine residue at the esteratic site, and the esters are simultaneously hydrolysed to phenolic derivatives which are released from the enzyme. Thus, the combination of carbamate inhibitors with AChE is essentially similar to the physiological substrate acetylcholine (Fig. 10.3). However, the hydrolysis of the methylcarbamylated enzyme (half-time = approximately 30 min) is 10^7–10^8 times slower than the acetylated enzyme (half-time = 42 μs). The formation and hydrolysis of the carbamylated enzyme are mainly responsible for enzyme inhibition. Carbamates are sometimes known as time-dependent, acid transferring or oxydiaphoretic inhibitors of AChE, since they mainly act by transferring a methylcarbamic acid to the enzyme. Carbamates, particularly neostigmine, may also have a direct effect on neuromuscular transmission and autonomic function, probably due to their chemical similarity to acetylcholine. They also inhibit ChE and may prolong the effects of suxamethonium.

In general, neostigmine and pyridostigmine produce similar effects on neuromuscular transmission and the autonomic nervous system. Since both drugs are quaternary amines, they do not significantly cross the blood–brain barrier or the placental barrier. Neostigmine is four to five times more potent than pyridostigmine, since its quaternary group is outside the aromatic ring (Fig. 10.8). The absorption of both drugs from the gut is relatively poor, and their potency after oral administration is only 10–20% of their parenteral potency. Neostigmine is more rapidly absorbed than pyridostigmine, and has a greater first-pass metabolism. It also has the more rapid onset of action after intravenous administration (usually 5–7 min). Its duration of action is less prolonged, since it has a shorter terminal half-life (approximately 30–45 min). Nevertheless, the relatively long duration of action of both neostigmine and pyridostigmine, which far exceeds their removal from plasma and usually prevents recurarization, probably reflects the slow hydrolysis of inhibited AChE in the synaptic gap. Both drugs are partly metabolized by the liver, and partly eliminated unchanged in urine. Pyridostigmine may produce less marked autonomic side-effects than neostigmine; at one time, it was occasionally used to reverse non-depolarizing blockade. Neostigmine, pyridostigmine or the related compound ambenonium are sometimes used orally in the long-term management of myasthenia gravis. Tolerance to their muscarinic side-effects may develop, so that concurrent therapy with anticholinergic drugs is not always necessary. Neostigmine has also been used in the management of supraventricular tachycardias, and to improve smooth-muscle activity in the bladder and the bowel, particularly in the postoperative period.

Distigmine is a combination of two molecules of pyridostigmine, which are joined by a methylene chain at their non-quaternary ends. Distigmine has a relatively long duration of action, and may be used to improve smooth-muscle activity during the postoperative period. It may also be used in the management of the neurogenic bladder.

Physostigmine (eserine) is a naturally occurring anticholinesterase drug derived from the Calabar bean, and was once used by native tribes in West Africa in 'trial by ordeal'. Unlike edrophonium, neostigmine and pyridostigmine, it is a monomethylcarbamate ester and a tertiary amine (Fig. 10.8). Consequently, it is well-absorbed from the gastrointestinal tract, penetrates cellular membranes and crosses the blood–brain barrier and the placental barrier. It has been used in the treatment of poisoning with anticholinergic drugs (e.g. atropine, tricyclic antidepressants). Physostigmine eyedrops are a popular miotic agent, and are sometimes used in the treatment of narrow-angle glaucoma.

Organophosphorus compounds

Organophosphorus compounds inhibit AChE by phosphorylation of the esteratic site of the enzyme (Fig. 10.3), forming an extremely stable complex which is resistant to hydrolysis or reactivation. In some instances, chemical changes take place after phosphorylation which prevent the reactivation of the enzyme (ageing). Consequently, recovery from the effects of inhibition is mainly dependent on the synthesis of new enzyme, and organophosphorus compounds are often considered to be irreversible inhibitors of AChE. Most of these drugs are also potent inhibitors of ChE. The classical organophosphorus compounds are diisopropylfluorophosphonate (DFP; dyflos) and tetraethylpyrophosphate (TEPP). Many of their analogues have been widely used as insecticides, and a number of volatile and lipid-soluble agents were synthesized during World War II as chemical warfare agents. These compounds are readily absorbed by the lungs and through the skin. Exposure leads to numerous toxic manifestations, including nicotinic effects (muscle weakness, paralysis and hypotension) and muscarinic effects (increased smooth-muscle tone and salivary and respiratory secretions). In addition, excitation of the CNS occurs (causing tremors and convulsions), and this may be followed by subsequent depression, with coma and respiratory paralysis. Organophosphorus poisoning is treated with reactivators of AChE (e.g. pralidoxime, obidoxime), which promote the hydrolysis of the phosphorylated enzyme. Repeated administration of atropine (2–4 mg) and anticonvulsant drugs and mechanical ventilation of the lungs may also be necessary. Pretreatment with carbamates has a protective effect against organophosphorus poisoning. Chronic exposure to these agents may lead to the development of a severe polyneuritis.

Ecothiopate is an organophosphorus compound which also has a quaternary amine group. Consequently, it is attracted to the anionic site on AChE, but subsequently phosphorylates the esteratic site, resulting in stable and prolonged inhibition. Proprietary preparations of ecothiopate are no longer available in the UK; an ophthalmic preparation was sometimes used as a miotic in narrow-angle glaucoma, and its chronic administration was associated with prolonged apnoea after suxamethonium.

Drugs that interfere with EC coupling

Normal voluntary muscle contraction depends on the release of calcium ions from the sarcoplasmic reticulum, and their subsequent binding by troponin C. The binding of calcium ions causes conformational changes in the troponin–tropomyosin complex, resulting in activation of myosin ATPase and muscle contraction (EC coupling; p. 322).

Dantrolene prevents the release of calcium ions from the sarcoplasmic reticulum, and thus indirectly prevents the activation of myosin ATPase and muscle contraction. Muscle action potentials are not affected, although the amplitude of the subsequent muscle contraction is reduced. Dantrolene does not usually impair the contractility of cardiac muscle or vascular smooth muscle; in these tissues, muscle contractility is not primarily dependent on the release of calcium ions from the sarcoplasmic reticulum.

Dantrolene sodium is used in the prevention and treatment of malignant hyperpyrexia (p. 358). The drug is also used orally for the treatment of spasticity associated with chronic neurological disorders (e.g. cerebrovascular accidents, multiple sclerosis, spinal cord injury, cerebral palsy). In this context central effects (e.g. dizziness, weakness, fatigue) are not uncommon, and occasional hepatotoxicity can occur. In general, the drug should be administered in gradually increasing doses until the optimum effect is attained.

Practical considerations

Choice of relaxant

Suxamethonium remains the drug of choice to provide optimal conditions for rapid endotracheal intubation, and is also indicated for short procedures in which profound muscle relaxation is required (e.g. electroconvulsive therapy). During longer procedures, suxamethonium has also been administered by intermittent or continuous infusion. This technique is not commonly used, since the development of phase II blockade may occur when the total dose infused is more than 7–8 mg kg^{-1} during nitrous oxide–opioid anaesthesia (or with considerably smaller doses during anaesthesia with volatile anaesthetic agents).

An anticholinergic drug may be given prior to suxamethonium at the discretion of the anaesthetist. However, atropine should always be administered if repeated dosage is contemplated, or in the presence of significant β-adrenoceptor blockade. Small doses of a non-depolarizing relaxant (e.g. atracurium 5 mg, pancuronium 1 mg) are frequently given prior to suxamethonium in order to reduce the muscle fasciculations and subsequent muscle pains, or to modify the sustained activity in the extraocular muscles in cases of penetrating eye injury. In these circumstances, the dose of suxamethonium should be increased by 50%.

Contraindications to the use of suxamethonium include:

1 Major burns and neurological injuries.

2 Hyperkalaemic states (e.g. renal failure).

3 Myasthenic and myotonic diseases.

4 Major qualitative abnormalities of plasma cholinesterase.

5 A family history suggesting susceptibility to malignant hyperpyrexia.

In particular, careful consideration should be given to the use of suxamethonium in children. Reports from the USA and Germany indicate a significant incidence of masseteric muscle spasm, which is sometimes a prelude to malignant hyperthermia, associated with the administration of suxamethonium. Furthermore, there is a possibility of hyperkalaemic cardiac arrest in children with previously undiagnosed myopathies following depolarization blockade.

For a number of years, the choice of a non-depolarizing drug in anaesthetic practice was principally determined by the expected duration of the surgical procedure, with secondary considerations being given to the condition of the patient. However, there is little doubt that the safety factor of atracurium (i.e. spontaneous degradation *in vivo* by Hofmann elimination), coupled with a relative lack of significant side-effects, has led to its widespread use in clinical practice at the present time. It is probably the drug of choice in renal disease, hepatic impairment and in frail and elderly subjects. Atracurium may be administered by single or repeated dosage (or by continuous infusion techniques, depending on the duration of the surgery).

Thus, the use of the older established muscle relaxants has subsequently declined. However, some of these agents may have specific advantages. Tubocurarine has commonly been used to facilitate induced hypotension for certain surgical procedures. It is probably best avoided in patients with a history of asthma, or when its hypotensive effects could be dangerous (e.g. in hypovolaemic states and fixed-output cardiac disease). Alcuronium is an acceptable alternative to tubocurarine, and has a shorter duration of action. It has some histamine-releasing and ganglion-blocking activity, but does not usually decrease blood pressure as much as tubocurarine. It is claimed to be more rapidly and completely reversible than tubocurarine, but this is doubtful. Pancuronium produces muscle relaxation of rapid onset and medium duration. Hypotension and histamine release are uncommon, and the drug may have advantages in asthmatic patients, as well as in cardiac surgery and cardiovascular disease, although tachyarrhythmias can sometimes be a problem. Gallamine has a more rapid onset and a shorter duration of action than pancuronium, and may be useful during short surgical procedures. Unfortunately, its use is limited by the problems of elimination in renal impairment, and the undesirable tachycardia that it commonly induces. Vecuronium has a relatively short duration of action and may have advantages over atracurium if hypersensitivity responses to anaesthesia are predicted or when cardiovascular stability during anaesthesia may be of particular importance. Vecuronium is mainly eliminated in bile, and does not cumulate in patients with renal failure. Both vecuronium and atracurium have been used to provide neuromuscular blockade in patients with myasthenia gravis; in this condition other muscle relaxants may produce prolonged apnoea.

Non-depolarizing blocking drugs may be required to assist long-term ventilatory control (e.g. in the management of tetanus, status epilepticus or chest injuries). It has been considered that the ganglion-blocking activity of tubocurarine may have contributed to the development of paralytic ileus during prolonged intermittent positive-pressure ventilation. Pancuronium has been a logical alternative, although some tachycardia may be expected, particularly in association with the use of inotropic drugs. In recent years, both atracurium and vecuronium have been widely used to assist the control of ventilation; these drugs do not cumulate and offer the advantage of flexibility.

Reversal of neuromuscular blockade

Neostigmine (0.03–0.07 mg kg^{-1}, with a maximum dose of 5 mg) has commonly been used to antagonize non-depolarizing neuromuscular blockade. Atropine (0.01–0.02 mg kg^{-1}, with a maximum dose of 1.2 mg) has normally been administered simultaneously, in order to control the muscarinic effects of neostigmine. However, secretomotor activity appears to be more favourably modified if atropine is given 5 min previously. Full oxygenation and efficient pulmonary ventilation should be maintained during the administration of these drugs, as hypoxia and hypercarbia increase the risk of cardiac arrhythmias. Pyridostigmine was formerly considered to be a useful alternative to neostigmine. It has a longer latency and duration of action than neostigmine, and appears to produce less muscarinic activity; however, pyridostigmine is no longer available as a parenteral preparation.

In order to minimize the possibility of recurarization, anticholinesterase drugs should not be administered less than 20–30 min after full doses of the commonly used non-depolarizing muscle relaxants, and preferably when there is some evidence of return of muscle tone. Clinical evaluation of ventilatory activity and muscle strength have been classically used to measure recovery from neuromuscular blockade. Signs of adequate reversal include an efficient tidal volume with some return of the cough reflex and absence of tracheal tug, a return of jaw tone and ability to protrude the tongue, and a head lift which can be sustained for at least 5 s. These clinical signs are closely correlated with the electrical or mechanical activity in voluntary muscles induced by indirect stimulation. When clinical signs of adequate reversal are present, there is at least 75% recovery from neuromuscular blockade (i.e. the amplitude of the final response to a train-of-four supramaximal stimuli is at least 75% of the amplitude of the first response). It should be recognized that clinical signs of reversal may be difficult to elicit in patients recovering from general anaesthesia without the risk of awareness; undoubtedly, the use of a nerve stimulator is the method of choice in the assessment of residual neuromuscular blockade.

The reversal of neuromuscular blockade, and the doses of the appropriate agents used, is considerably influenced by the pharmacokinetic properties of the non-depolarizing agent used, the amount given and the timing of its administration. The advent of newer muscle relaxants (e.g. atracurium, mivacurium) with novel routes of elimination (e.g. ester hydrolysis, Hofmann degradation) will allow for a further reduction in dosage of neostigmine (or for spontaneous recovery) in many cases, and this could have considerable advantages. There is little doubt that the prolonged muscarinic effects of neostigmine on smooth muscle contribute to postoperative pain; furthermore, the effects of the drug on gastrointestinal activity may increase the incidence of postoperative nausea and vomiting. The development of bradycardia during the postoperative period is also attributed to the muscarinic effects of neostigmine. In this context, an antimuscarinic drug with a longer duration of action (e.g. glycopyrrolate) may be advantageous. In recent years, edrophonium (500–700 $\mu g\ kg^{-1}$) has also been used to antagonize neuromuscular blockade with the newer muscle relaxants. It has a more rapid onset of action than neostigmine, and its duration of action is sufficiently long to prevent residual curarization.

Drug interactions

Clinically significant interactions involving the use of non-depolarizing relaxants in patients on other drugs are uncommon. Many drugs may modify acid–base balance, or influence the plasma concentration of certain cations (e.g. antacids, steroids, chelating agents, diuretics, lithium); in these instances, prolongation of the effects of relaxants, although anticipated, is infrequently present.

Similarly, calcium transport at presynaptic sites may be influenced by many other drugs, e.g. aminoglycoside antibiotics, calcium antagonists and drugs with local anaesthetic properties, including quinidine, propranolol, chlorpromazine and phenytoin; again, the practical implications are usually minimal.

However, interactions with other drugs administered as part of the anaesthetic technique are usually much more important. Many volatile anaesthetic agents may profoundly influence the degree of non-depolarizing neuromuscular blockade. Diethylether has long been known to potentiate this type of blockade, and similar dose-related effects are produced by other volatile agents. The chief mode of action is probably depression of somatic reflexes in the CNS, which consequently reduces transmitter release at the motor nerve terminal. There is some evidence that direct depression at presynaptic sites may also be involved; the effect of inhalational agents on muscle blood flow may also play a part. Diazepam may slightly prolong non-depolarizing blockade by a combination of prejunctional and central effects.

Drugs that block autonomic ganglia, such as trimetaphan, which may be used to produce hypotension during anaesthesia, can complicate neuromuscular blockade. These drugs have some affinity for both acetylcholine receptors and AChE, and in high doses they may prolong non-depolarizing blockade. As mentioned previously, neostigmine-resistant curarization has been observed when large doses of certain antibiotics (particularly streptomycin and neomycin) have been instilled into the peritoneal cavity; calcium salts may partially reverse this type of blockade.

More serious drug interactions are associated with the use of suxamethonium. Prolongation of neuromuscular blockade, and an increased tendency to develop dual blockade, may be due to inhibition of ChE activity (e.g. by anticholinesterase drugs, alkylating agents, trimetaphan, pitocin). Drugs which use ChE for their own metabolism may also prolong the action of suxamethonium (e.g. procaine and possibly other local anaesthetics). Potentiation of the muscarinic effects of suxamethonium (particularly with respect to the cardiac vagus) may also occur with digoxin, or other drugs which alter autonomic balance in favour of parasympathetic activity (e.g. β-adrenoceptor antagonists).

Neurological and muscle diseases

Patients with myasthenia gravis are extremely sensitive to non-depolarizing blockade, but are usually resistant to decamethonium and suxamethonium. Both phenomena have been used as diagnostic tests in myasthenic patients. The differential effects of depolarizing and non-depolarizing drugs in myasthenia are due to the presence of antibodies to acetylcholine receptors at the motor endplate; in these conditions, the endplate potential induced by acetylcholine release is decreased, so that the effects of non-depolarizing agents are enhanced. The thymus gland may play an important role in the pathophysiology of myasthenia gravis. The thymus produces a polypeptide hormone, thymopoietin, which regulates immune function (via T-cell production); in addition, low concentrations of thymopoietin have been shown experimentally to produce a non-depolarizing blockade of acetylcholine receptors at the neuromuscular junction.

In myasthenia gravis, different muscle groups are affected to a variable extent, and the reaction to muscle relaxants is unpredictable. The use of most neuromuscular blocking agents should be avoided in myasthenic patients undergoing major surgery (including thymectomy), since they may induce prolonged postoperative curarization. However, low doses of vecuronium and atracurium have been successfully used to produce neuromuscular blockade in patients with myasthenia gravis undergoing surgical procedures. Suxamethonium has also been used; large doses may be required to produce muscle relaxation, and the elimination of the drug may be retarded by concurrent anticholinesterase therapy.

In the Eaton–Lambert (myasthenic) syndrome, muscle weakness improves with exercise, and an increase in twitch amplitude is observed during tetanic stimulation. The condition may accompany malignant disease, particularly bronchogenic carcinoma. In general, there is a marked sensitivity to non-depolarizing blockade, and resistance to anticholinesterase drugs is present.

In myotonic syndromes (myotonia dystrophica, myotonia congenita and paramyotonia), generalized muscle spasm may occur with depolarizing agents, and is not responsive to tubocurarine. In other genetically determined myopathies (e.g. muscular dystrophy and familial periodic paralysis) the response to muscle relaxants is unpredictable, and their use is best avoided. A similar response may occur in other types of myopathy. In diseases and trauma associated with lower motor neurone lesions, and in patients with severe burns, suxamethonium may cause significant and dangerous hyperkalaemia; increased sensitivity to non-depolarizing drugs can also occur.

In malignant hyperpyrexia, there is an inherited susceptibility to the development of fulminating hyperpyrexia, often associated with muscle rigidity and convulsions. In the established syndrome, there is a mortality rate of 60–70% associated with anaesthesia. The condition has a high familial incidence and is linked to an autosomal dominant gene. Patients at risk may exhibit minor myopathies, and an elevated creatine kinase and qualitative variants of plasma ChE may be present. They may also be identified by muscle biopsy, as they may show an abnormal contractile response to caffeine or halothane in *in vitro* conditions. A similar condition may be induced in susceptible individuals by the administration of suxamethonium, although most inhalational anaesthetics have also been incriminated as triggering agents. Typically, the initial dose of suxamethonium fails to produce adequate relaxation, and generalized muscle rigidity, in association with a rapidly rising temperature, develops within several minutes. The initial event in this hypermetabolic reaction is considered to be a sudden increase in myoplasmic calcium concentration, and a genetic disorder of the calcium-releasing ryanodine receptor in the sarcoplasmic reticulum is postulated. Other views indicate that the triggering agent induces a greatly enhanced influx of extracellular Ca^{2+} by L-type calcium channels, and that calcium antagonists (e.g. diltiazem) may have a protective effect.

Treatment should commence as soon as the diagnosis is suspected. Administration of the suspected triggering agent must be stopped, and surgery discontinued as soon as possible. Active cooling and generalized supportive measures to the cardiovascular and respiratory system should be instituted; blood gases should be estimated and any metabolic acidosis corrected by an infusion of sodium bicarbonate. Previous drug therapy has included the administration of large doses of procaine and steroids, but it is doubtful if they are of any real value. Present evidence suggests that the drug of choice is dantrolene sodium. Dantrolene acts by inhibiting the release of Ca^{2+} from the sarcoplasmic reticulum of striated muscle, thus preventing EC coupling and the abnormal heat production. An intravenous preparation of the drug (sodium dantrolene with mannitol and sodium hydroxide) is available as a powder for reconstitution with water. The initial dose (1 mg kg^{-1}) may be repeated at 5–10-min intervals to a maximum dose of 10 mg kg^{-1}. Dantrolene sodium is also available as an oral preparation for the treatment of various spastic disorders; its prophylactic use has been proposed in patients with a susceptibility to malignant hyperpyrexia who require general anaesthesia.

Monitoring of neuromuscular blockade

Individual responses to muscle relaxants vary widely, and may be modified by age, body temperature, plasma and extracellular pH, electrolyte changes, the presence of other drugs and pathological conditions. Consequently, in individual patients the response to muscle relaxants or their antagonists may be unpredictable, and the effects of some drugs (particularly vecuronium and atracurium) may change rapidly during recovery from neuromuscular blockade. Methods of monitoring the effects of muscle relaxants are therefore desirable; in certain circumstances they may be essential. The most commonly used methods depend on indirect supramaximal stimulation of the ulnar nerve, and the recording of the compound muscle action potential or the mechanical twitch response of adductor pollicis. A square-wave stimulus of short duration (0.1–0.2 ms) is frequently employed in order to prevent repetitive muscle firing. In anaesthetized patients, tetanic rates of stimulation (> 50 Hz) may be used; more frequently, a train-of-four stimulus (2 Hz for 2 s) is employed. Neuromuscular blockade may be monitored by comparing the amplitude of the first response in the train (T1) with the control response before the administration of the relaxant (T0). This ratio (T1 : T0) is probably the most accurate measurement of postsynaptic neuromuscular blockade. More commonly, transmission is monitored by observing the amplitude (or presence, absence or reappearance) of the fourth response (T4) compared to the first response (T1) within train-of-four stimuli (i.e. the ratio T4 : T1). This method avoids the necessity for a control response, although it may reflect the presynaptic effects of muscle relaxants, rather than their postsynaptic actions. In practice, the difference is probably unimportant, since there is usually a close relation between the ratios T1 : T0 and T4 : T1.

Further reading

Ali HH. Monitoring of neuromuscular function. *Seminars in Anesthesia* 1984; **3**: 284–292.

Ali HH, Savarese JJ. Monitoring of neuromuscular function. *Anesthesiology* 1976; **45**: 216–249.

Ali HH, Savarese JJ, Embree PB *et al.* Clinical pharmacology of mivacurium chloride (BW B1090U) infusion: comparison with vecuronium and atracurium. *British Journal of Anaesthesia* 1988; **61**: 541–546.

Azar I. The response of patients with neuromuscular disorders to muscle relaxants: a review. *Anesthesiology* 1984; **61**: 173–187.

Beemer GH, Cass NM. Monitoring the neuromuscular junction. *Anaesthesia and Intensive Care* 1988; **16**: 62–65.

Bell CF, Florence AM, Hunter JM *et al.* Atracurium in the myasthenic patient. *Anaesthesia* 1984; **39**: 961–968.

Bevan DR. Newer neuromuscular blocking agents. *Pharmacology and Toxicology* 1994; **74**: 3–9.

Bevan DR. Succinylcholine. *Canadian Journal of Anaesthesia* 1994; **41**: 465–468.

Bowman WC. *Pharmacology of Neuromuscular Function.* Bristol: John Wright, 1980; 1–186.

Bowman WC. Prejunctional and postjunctional cholinoceptors at the neuromuscular junction. *Anesthesia and Analgesia* 1980; **59**: 935–943.

Bowman WC. New developments at the neuromuscular junction. Proceedings of the JB Stenlake Symposium, University of Strathclyde, Glasgow. September 1993; 15–22.

Buckett WR. Steroidal neuromuscular blocking agents. *Advances in Drug Research* 1975; **10**: 53–92.

Budd A, Scott RFP, Blogg CE, Goat VA. Adverse effects of suxamethonium. *Anaesthesia* 1985; **40**: 642–646.

Caldwell J. New muscle relaxants. *Current Opinion in Anaesthesiology* 1995; **8**: 356–361.

Calvey TN. Assessment of neuromuscular blockade by electromyography: a review. *Journal of the Royal Society of Medicine* 1984; **77**: 56–59.

Calvey TN, Wareing M, Williams NE, Chan K. Pharmacokinetics and pharmacological effects of neostigmine in man. *British Journal of Clinical Pharmacology* 1979; **7**: 149–155.

Calvey TN, Williams NE, Muir KT, Barber HE. Plasma concentration of edrophonium in man. *Clinical Pharmacology and Therapeutics* 1976; **19**: 813–820.

Calvey TN, Wilson H. Muscle relaxant drugs and their antagonists. In: Gray TC, Nunn JF, Utting JE (eds) *General Anaesthesia*, 4th edn. London: Butterworths, 1980; 319–335.

Ceccarelli B, Hurlbut WP. The vesicle hypothesis of the release of quanta of acetylcholine. *Physiological Reviews* 1980; **60**: 351–396.

Changeux J-P, Giraudat J, Dennis M. The nicotinic acetylcholine receptor: molecular architecture of a ligand-regulated ion channel. *Trends in Pharmacological Sciences* 1987; **8**: 459–465.

Collier C. Suxamethonium pains and fasciculations. *Proceedings of the Royal Society of Medicine* 1975; **68**: 105–108.

Cooper R, Mirakhur RK, Clarke RSJ, Boules Z. Comparison of intubating conditions after administration of Org 9426 (rocuronium) and suxamethonium. *British Journal of Anaesthesia* 1992; **69**: 269–273.

Cullen DJ. The effect of pretreatment with nondepolarizing muscle relaxants on the neuromuscular blocking action of succinylcholine. *Anesthesiology* 1971; **35**: 572–578.

Desaki J, Uehara Y. The overall morphology of neuromuscular junctions as revealed by scanning electronmicroscopy. *Journal of Neurocytology* 1981; **10**: 101–110.

Drachman DB, Adams RN, Josifek LF *et al.* Antibody-mediated mechanisms of ACh receptor loss in myasthenia gravis: clinical relevance. *Annals of the New York Academy of Sciences* 1981; **337**: 175–188.

Dundee JW, Gray TC. Resistance to *d*-tubocurarine chloride in the presence of liver damage. *Lancet* 1953; **ii**: 16–17.

Durant NN, Katz RL. Suxamethonium. *British Journal of Anaesthesia* 1982; **54**: 195–208.

Ebashi S. Muscle contraction and pharmacology. *Trends in Pharmacological Sciences* 1979; **1**: 29–31.

Eccles JC. *The Understanding of the Brain*. New York: McGraw-Hill, 1973; 1–238.

Endo M. Calcium release from the sarcoplasmic reticulum. *Physiological Reviews* 1977; **57**: 71–108.

Fambrough DM. Control of acetylcholine receptors in skeletal muscle. *Physiological Reviews* 1979; **59**: 165–216.

Fleming NW, Lewis BK. Cholinesterase inhibitors do not prolong neuromuscular block produced by mivacurium. *British Journal of Anaesthesia* 1994; **73**: 241–243.

Ghonheim MM, Long JP. The interaction between magnesium and other neuromuscular blocking agents. *Anesthesiology* 1970; **32**: 23–27.

Gronert GA, Mott J, Lee J. Aetiology of malignant hyperthermia. *British Journal of Anaesthesia* 1988; **60**: 253–267.

Gwinutt CL, Meakin G. Use of the post-tetanic count to monitor recovery from intense neuromuscular blockade in children. *British Journal of Anaesthesia* 1988; **61**: 547–550.

Harrison GG. Dantrolene — dynamics and kinetics. *British Journal of Anaesthesia* 1988; **60**: 279–286.

Head-Rapson AG, Devlin JC, Parker CJR, Hunter JM. Pharmacokinetics of the three isomers of mivacurium and pharmacodynamics of the chiral mixture in hepatic cirrhosis. *British Journal of Anaesthesia* 1994; **73**: 613–618.

Head-Rapson AG, Devlin JC, Parker CJR, Hunter JM. Infusion pharmacokinetics and pharmacodynamics of the three isomers of mivacurium in health, in end-stage renal failure, and in patients with impaired renal function. *British Journal of Anaesthesia* 1995; **75**: 31–36.

Hilgenberg JC. Comparison of the pharmacology of vecuronium and atracurium with that of other currently available muscle relaxants. *Anesthesia and Analgesia* 1983; **62**: 524–531.

Hohlfeld R, Sterz R, Peper K. Prejunctional effects of anticholinesterase drugs at the endplate mediated by presynaptic acetylcholine receptors or by postsynaptic potassium efflux. *Pflugers Archiv fur die gesamte Physiologie* 1981; **391**: 213–218.

Holmstedt B. Pharmacology of organophosphorus cholinesterase inhibitors. *Pharmacological Reviews* 1959; **11**: 567–688.

Holst-Larsen H. The hydrolysis of suxamethonium in human blood. *British Journal of Anaesthesia* 1976; **48**: 887–892.

Hunter JM. Adverse effects of neuromuscular blocking drugs. *British Journal of Anaesthesia* 1987; **59**: 46–60.

Karlin A, Kao PN, DiPaola M. Molecular pharmacology of the nicotinic acetylcholine receptor. *Trends in Pharmacology Sciences* 1986; **7**: 304–308.

Katz B, Thesleff S. A study of the 'desensitization' produced by acetylcholine at the motor endplate. *Journal of Physiology* 1957; **138**: 63–80.

Kharkevich DA (ed.) *New Neuromuscular Blocking Agents. Handbook of Experimental Pharmacology* vol. 79, Berlin: Springer-Verlag, 1986; 1–717.

La Du BN. Identification of human serum cholinesterase variants using the polymerase chain reaction amplification technique. *Trends in Pharmacological Sciences* 1989; **10**: 309–313.

Lambert JJ, Durant NN, Henderson EG. Drug-induced modification of ionic conductance at the neuromuscular junction. *Annual Review of Pharmacology and Toxicology* 1983; **23**: 505–539.

Lee C, Chen D, Katz REl. Characteristics of non-depolarising neuromuscular block. (1) Postjunctional block by alpha-bungarotoxin. *Canadian Anaesthetists Society Journal* 1977; **24**: 212–219.

Lee C, Katz RL. Neuromuscular pharmacology. *British Journal of Anaesthesia* 1980; **52**: 173–188.

Lenzen C, Roewer N, Wappler F *et al.* Accelerated contractures after administration of ryanodine to skeletal muscle of malignant hyperthermia susceptible patients. *British Journal of Anaesthesia* 1993; **71**: 242–246.

Lu Z, Smith DO. Adenosine 5′triphosphate increases acetylcholine channel opening time in rat skeletal muscle. *Journal of Physiology* 1991; **436**: 45–46.

Meistelman C, Lienhart A, Leveque C *et al.* Pharmacology of vecuronium in patients with end-stage renal failure. *European Journal of Anaesthesiology* 1986; **3**: 153–158.

Meretoja OA, Taivainen T, Wirtavouri K. Pharmacodynamic effects of 51W89, an isomer of atracurium, in children during halothane anaesthesia. *British Journal of Anaesthesia* 1995; **74**: 6–11.

Mortier E, Moulaert P, De Somer A, Rolly G. Comparison of evoked electromyography and mechanical activity during vecuronium-induced neuromuscular blockade. *European Journal of Anaesthesiology* 1988; **5**: 131–142.

Newton DEF. Measurement of neuromuscular function. *Baillière's Clinical Anaesthesiology* 1988; **2**: 133–156.

O'Sullivan EP, Williams NE, Calvey TN. Differential effects of neuromuscular blocking agents on suxamethonium-induced fasciculations and myalgia. *British Journal of Anaesthesia* 1988; **60**: 367–371.

Parker CJR, Jones JE, Hunter JM. Disposition of infusions of atracurium and its metabolite, laudanosine, in patients in renal and respiratory failure in an ITU. *British Journal of Anaesthesia* 1988; **61**: 531–540.

Paton WDM. The effects of muscle relaxants other than muscular relaxation. *Anesthesiology* 1959; **20**: 453–463.

Paton WDM, Waud DR. The margin of safety of neuromuscular transmission. *Journal of Physiology* 1967; **191**: 59–90.

Payne JP, Hughes R. Evaluation of atracurium in anaesthetized man. *British Journal of Anaesthesia* 1981; **53**: 45–54.

Payne JP, Utting JE (eds) Atracurium. *British Journal of Anaesthesia* 1983; **55** (suppl. 1): 1S–139S.

Popper P, Miceyvych PE. Localisation of calcium gene-related peptide and its receptors in striated muscle. *Brain Research* 1989; **496**: 180–186.

Quik M, Collier B, Audhya T, Goldstein G. Thymopoietin inhibits function and ligand binding to nicotinic receptors at the neuromuscular junction. *Journal of Pharmacology and Experimental Therapeutics* 1990; **254**: 1113–1119.

Ridley SA, Hatch DJ. Post-tetanic count and profound neuromuscular blockade with atracurium infusion in paediatric patients. *British Journal of Anaesthesia* 1988; **60**: 31–35.

Robertson EN, Booij LHDJ, Fragen RJ, Crul JF. Clinical comparison of atracurium and vecuronium (Org NC 45). *British Journal of Anaesthesia* 1983; **55**: 125–129.

Rosenberg H, Gronert GA. Intractable cardiac arrest in children given succinylcholine. *Anaesthesiology* 1992; **77**: 1054.

Scott RPF, Norman J. Newer agents. *Current Opinion in Anaesthesiology* 1989; **2**: 493–496.

Shanks CA. Pharmacokinetics of the nondepolarizing neuromuscular relaxants applied to calculation of bolus and infusion dosage regimens. *Anesthesiology* 1986; **64**: 72–86.

Spencer AA, Payne JP. (eds) Proceedings of a symposium on atracurium. *British Journal of Anaesthesia* 1986; **58** (suppl. 1): 1S–113S.

Stanski DR, Sheiner LB. Pharmacokinetics and dynamics of muscle relaxants. *Anesthesiology* 1979; **51**: 103–105.

Sudhof TC, Jahn R. Proteins of synaptic vesicles involved in exocytosis and membrane recycling. *Neurone* 1991; **6**: 665–667.

Tammisto T, Wirtavuori K, Linko K. Assessment of neuromuscular block; comparison of three clinical methods and evoked electromyography. *European Journal of Anaesthesiology* 1988; **5**: 1–8.

Tobey RE, Jacobsen PM, Kahle CT *et al.* The serum potassium response to muscle relaxants in neural injury. *Anaesthesiology* 1972; **37**: 332–337.

Tolmie JD, Joyce TH, Mitchell GD. Succinylcholine danger in the burned patient. *Anaesthesiology* 1967; **28**: 467–470.

Torda TA. The 'new' relaxants. A review of the clinical pharmacology of atracurium and vecuronium. *Anaesthesia and Intensive Care* 1987; **15**: 72–82.

Viby-Mogensen J, Howardy-Hansen P, Chraemmer-Jorgensen B, Ording H, Engback J, Nielsen A. Post-tetanic count (PTC); a new method of evaluating an intense nondepolarising neuromuscular blockade. *Anaesthesiology* 1981; **55**: 458–461.

Weber S, Brandom BW, Powers DM *et al.* Mivacurium chloride (BW B1090U0)-induced neuromuscular blockade during nitrous oxide–isoflurane and nitrous oxide–narcotic anaesthesia in adult surgical patients. *Anesthesia and Analgesia* 1988; **67**: 495–499.

Whittaker VP. The storage and release of acetylcholine. *Trends in Pharmacological Sciences* 1986; **7**: 312–315.

Wierda JMKH, de Wit APM, Kuizenga K, Agoston S. Clinical observations on the neuromuscular blocking action of Org 9426, a new steroidal non-depolarising agent. *British Journal of Anaesthesia* 1990; **64**: 521–523.

Williams NE, Webb SN, Calvey TN. Differential effects of myoneural blocking drugs on neuromuscular transmission. *British Journal of Anaesthesia* 1980; **52**: 1111–1115.

Wilson IB, Harrison MA. Turnover number of acetylcholinesterase. *Journal of Biological Chemistry* 1961; **236**: 2292–2295.

Wilson IB, Hatch MA, Ginsburg S. Carbamylation of acetylcholinesterase. *Journal of Biological Chemistry* 1960; **235**: 2312–2315.

Zaimis E (ed.) *Neuromuscular Junction. Handbook of Experimental Pharmacology*, vol. 42. Berlin; Springer-Verlag, 1976; 1–746.

Chapter 11
Analgesic Drugs

Anatomy and physiology of pain transmission

Pain pathways

Peripheral nociceptive receptors do not have a distinct histological structure, but are interwoven plexiform arrangements of free nerve endings which are widely distributed in interstitial tissues and around blood vessels; they respond specifically to painful stimuli of chemical, mechanical or thermal origin.

Two types of pain have been described. Fast pain allows the injury to be identified in time and space, initiates the rapid reflex withdrawal from the painful stimulus and is of short duration. Slow pain occurs after fast pain and is less localized and more persistent.

Afferent pain fibres can be divided into two groups:

1 Small myelinated Aδ fibres, 2–5 μm in diameter, which conduct first or fast pain and enter the deeper part of the dorsal horn (Rexed laminae IV and V).

2 Unmyelinated C fibres less than 2 μm in diameter, which have a higher threshold and a lower conduction velocity. These fibres conduct second or slow pain and synapse in the superficial area of the dorsal horn (Rexed laminae I and II).

Integration of the impulses in these two types of fibres takes place in lamina II of the dorsal horn (the substantia gelatinosa) and this may influence the quality and intensity of pain that is experienced. The input of nociceptive impulses may be further modified by collateral branches from the larger A fibres which ascend in the posterior columns; these conduct other sensory impulses, and have a lower threshold of activity and a greater conduction velocity than Aδ or C fibres.

Descending tracts from central grey matter (via the reticular formation) may also inhibit activity in the cells of the substantia gelatinosa (Fig. 11.1). Thus, a form of gate control of nociceptive input appears to exist; this may explain why counterirritation by heat or touch, or distraction of the individual, can reduce the intensity of the pain.

Second-order neurones relay in the dorsal horn, decussate in the spinal cord and ascend in the spinothalamic tract and the more diffuse spinoreticular pathways. They eventually terminate in the ventroposterior and medial nuclei of the thalamus, which is probably the main region associated with the appreciation of pain. However, further projections to the postcentral gyri are undoubtedly associated with the

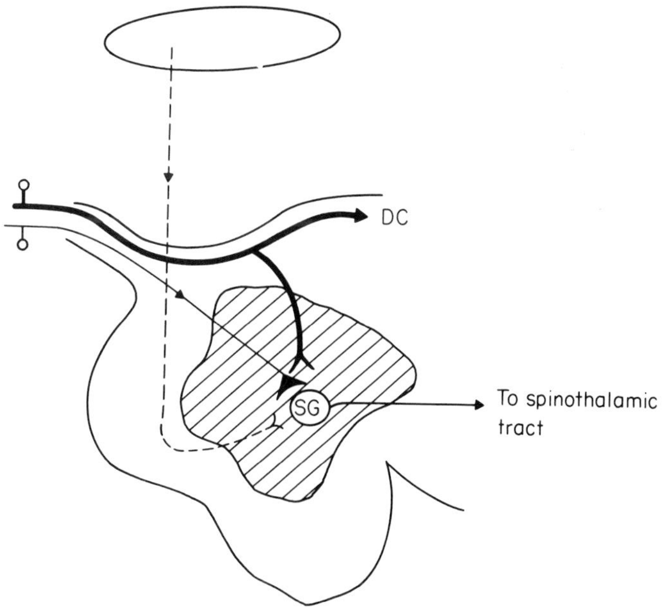

Fig. 11.1 Hemisection of spinal cord showing integration of pain impulses via the substantia gelatinosa. SG, Substantia gelatinosa; DC, dorsal column; ⫱ A δ and C fibres conducting first and second pain impulses. ⫯ Large sensory A fibres sending collateral branch to inhibit (? presynaptically) pain transmission. (Broken line) descending fibres via reticular formation inhibiting (? postsynaptically) pain transmission.

localization of nociceptive impulses, while connections with the prefrontal and temporal lobes and the limbic areas are related to the affective component and the memory of pain. Thus, it is not surprising that pain has been described as an unpleasant emotional state rather than as a simple sensory modality.

Pain production

Pain is produced by mechanical or thermal damage to superficial or deep tissues, ischaemia of somatic or visceral structures, spasm of smooth or striated muscle, and dilatation of blood vessels at the base of the brain. Many endogenous chemical substances are well-known excitants of peripheral nerve endings. These substances include H^+, K^+, acetylcholine, histamine, 5-hydroxytryptamine, cholecystokinin and bradykinin; phosphate ions may also be implicated in the production of bone pain. Other substances which are produced at peripheral sites, in particular certain prostaglandins and leukotrienes, can sensitize the afferent nerve endings to the effects of chemical or mechanical stimuli by lowering the threshold of the nociceptors.

A complex series of events appear to be initiated in the development of pain associated with trauma, inflammation and peripheral nerve damage. Afferent nerves produce sensory neuropeptides such as substance P, neurokinin A and calcitonin gene-related peptide (CGRP). These neuropeptides can migrate both peripherally, leading to an increase in the excitability of sensory fibres and adjacent postganglionic sympathetic fibres, and centrally, to enhance nociceptive transmission in the substantia gelatinosa. Nerve growth factor (NGF) is released by Schwann cells following peripheral damage. NGF will induce changes in cell phenotype and facilitate axoplasmic transport of the sensory neuropeptides. This will further enhance the hyperexcitability of the sensory neurones, so that eventually light touch or pressure may induce a painful sensation (allodynia) mediated by large A fibres.

Central transmission of nociceptive impulses in chronic pain may be further augmented by an increase of glutamate-mediated transmission in the dorsal horn (an up-regulation of *N*-methyl-D-aspartate (NMDA) receptors) resulting in a prolonged and enhanced production of nitric oxide (NO) within the central nervous system (CNS). Although sensory neurones normally synthesize NO and this appears to promote antinociceptive effects by indirect mechanisms, it is postulated that a grossly excessive production of NO may paradoxically promote pain transmission. Cholecystokinin (CCK) may also influence pain pathways. Increased production of CCK in the dorsal horn occurs in neuropathic pain which antagonizes morphine analgesia.

It has been proposed that these central hyperexcitability changes (described as an increased plasticity of the CNS) may be at least partly obtunded by the use of 'pre-emptive' analgesia in relation to surgical procedures. The outcome of a number of studies incorporating local and systemic analgesics has been controversial, but may reflect the inadequacy of nociceptive block provided, either in duration or intensity. Recent advances in histochemistry have demonstrated that increased nociceptive sensitization within the CNS, and the associated behavioural hyperalgesia in animals, are linked to an increase in the expression of the proto-oncogene c-*fos*. By using immunoreactive methods, the number of *fos*-like (*fos*-LI) labelled neurones can be used as an index to quantify the antinociceptive activity of drugs. Experimental evidence suggests that the prior administration of opioid analgesics, NMDA antagonists (e.g. ketamine) and α_2-agonists (see below) can suppress *fos*-LI reactivity. Results also indicate that inhalational anaesthetic agents do not possess any pre-emptive analgesic action.

Compensatory mechanisms also come into play following tissue damage. Opioid receptors are synthesized in the cell body of sensory neurones, and are transported in central and peripheral directions. The centrally directed receptors become the presynaptic receptors on the C-fibre terminals in the substantia gelatinosa, whilst the peripheral receptors become activated only after local tissue damage. Immunocompetent cells, which possess opioid receptors and the ability to synthesize opioid peptides, also arrive at the site of damage. It is considered that all three types of opioid receptor (μ, κ and δ; see p. 367) become available at the periphery, since their respective agonists produce a receptor-selective reduction in the excitability of afferent somatic and sympathetic fibres. Furthermore, when peripheral inflammation occurs and there is no evidence of nerve damage, the central production of CCK is decreased, thus facilitating opioid effects.

Activation of the descending inhibitory noradrenergic pathways may also be important and provide some explanation of the role of tricyclic antidepressants (which inhibit reuptake of catecholamines) in the treatment of chronic pain. The analgesic properties of α_2-agonists (e.g. clonidine, dexmedetomidine) may be synergistic with μ-receptor agonists.

Classification of analgesic drugs

Analgesic drugs may be classified as:

1 Primary, general or non-specific analgesics. These drugs may be subdivided into:

(a) Opioid analgesics, as typified by morphine. The term opiate has previously been used to refer to naturally occurring substances with properties similar to morphine. Opioid is a more specific term which encompasses all naturally occurring or synthetic drugs which can exert stereospecific effects at clearly defined receptors and is used to describe drugs which exert full or partial agonist activity, as well as pure antagonistic effects at these sites.

(b) Simple analgesics, e.g. aspirin and paracetamol. Many of these drugs also have anti-inflammatory and antipyretic effects (e.g. non-steroidal anti-inflammatory drugs or NSAIDs).

2 Secondary or specific analgesics. These drugs may be useful in specific painful conditions (e.g. antacids, vasodilators, carbamazepine).

Opioid analgesics

History

Opioid analgesics are classically known as narcotic analgesics (a name derived from the Greek word *narkoo*, to benumb). Opium (in Greek, *opion* or poppy juice) was first obtained from the capsules of the unripe oriental poppy seed (*Papaver somniferum*) in the 4th century BC. Early writings suggested that it was principally used for its antidiarrhoeal activity, but by the 16th century the analgesic, sedative and antitussive properties of opium had become well-recognized throughout Europe. The principal active ingredient, morphine, was isolated in 1806, and named after Morpheus, the Greek god of dreams.

Opium smoking became popular in the Orient in the 18th century. The invention of the hypodermic syringe and needle in 1853, the ready availability of morphine and its increased usage in the treatment of battle injuries, and the migration of Chinese labourers all contributed to the development of the problem of compulsive drug usage and drug dependence in western civilization. The semisynthetic opioid heroin (diamorphine or diacetylmorphine) was produced at St Mary's Hospital in 1874, with the aim of curing morphine dependence; it was many years before it was appreciated that it provided a cure by replacing morphine with a more powerful drug of addiction. The search for agents with the analgesic effects of morphine, but without its disadvantages of dependence and tolerance, has continued for many years; the introduction of drugs that appeared to be chemically dissimilar to morphine, e.g. pethidine (in 1939) and methadone (in 1942) was of little or no value in this respect.

The mode of action of opioid analgesics remained unclear for many years. It was evident that such drugs could considerably influence the reactive component of pain (i.e. anxiety, fear and suffering) and the ability of patients to tolerate painful conditions. In some experimental studies, the pain threshold (i.e. the intensity at which a stimulus is first appreciated as pain) has been shown to be minimally affected by opioid analgesics.

Various neurochemical changes (e.g. the increased utilization of brain amines, and cholinesterase inhibition) may be induced by opioid analgesics in experimental conditions. However, in the early 1970s it was suggested that specific opioid receptors were present in the CNS. This arose from three observations:

1 Most opioid analgesics are stereospecific; almost invariably, analgesic activity is associated with the levorotatory isomer.

2 The development of highly potent opioid analgesics (e.g. etorphine) indicated that receptor mechanisms may be involved.

3 The pure antagonist naloxone had been synthesized; most of its actions were consistent with the displacement of opioid analgesics from receptor sites.

Subsequently, the rate of uptake of various radiolabelled opioids by animal brain preparations was shown to accord closely with the clinical potency of the drugs concerned. Regional localization of opioid receptors was later demonstrated using autoradiographic techniques. In the spinal cord, the uptake is principally confined to a dense band corresponding to the substantia gelatinosa. In the brainstem, opioid receptors are localized to solitary nuclei which receive afferent vagal fibres, and are present in the area postrema (which is associated with the chemoreceptor trigger zone). Opioid receptors are also present in the periaqueductal grey matter, the amygdaloid nuclei, the cerebral cortex and the thalamus.

The discovery of opioid receptors led naturally to a search for endogenous ligands, and three main families of opioid peptides (enkephalins, endorphins and dynorphins) were subsequently identified in various regions of the CNS, the gastro-intestinal tract and at other peripheral sites.

Further evidence accumulated to indicate that opioid analgesics do not act at a single receptor site. Initial observations were based on nalorphine, a long-established drug with a mixed agonist–antagonist profile. Nalorphine can produce analgesia *per se*, but also arouse withdrawal symptoms in morphine-dependent individuals, reverse the effects of morphine overdose and often lead to dysphoria and other psychotomimetic effects rather than euphoria and sedation. Subsequently, the concept of receptor dualism was advanced, which postulated the existence of two distinct receptors for morphine and nalorphine. By acting as a classical competitive antagonist at the morphine receptor, nalorphine antagonized the analgesic and respiratory depressant effects of morphine; in addition, it acted as an agonist at the nalorphine receptor, producing analgesia.

In subsequent studies, the pharmacology of various opioid analgesics was studied in the chronic spinal dog. Different syndromes were produced and were interpreted in terms of the actions of these drugs at three different receptor sites:

1 μ-Receptors (prototype agonist morphine) mediating euphoria, supraspinal analgesia and morphine-like physical dependence.

2 κ-Receptors (prototype agonist ketocyclazocine) were associated with spinal analgesia, sedation and signs of nalorphine-like dependence.

3 σ-Receptors (prototype agonist *N*-allyl-normetazocine) producing mydriasis, tachypnoea, tachycardia, delirium and mania.

At a later stage, the existence of δ-receptors was proposed, based on the relative potencies of various opioid peptides and drugs to inhibit contractions of the isolated guinea-pig ileum and the rat vas deferens (these peripheral receptors show a high affinity for the endogenous opioid peptide leu-enkephalin). Further studies incorporating animal models suggest that there are highly specific δ-agonists which exhibit analgesic activity (e.g. deltorphin II, which can be isolated from frog skin) and which are not affected by specific μ-antagonists (e.g. β-funaltrexamine). δ-Receptors thus appear to exist within the CNS and were originally implicated in spinal (but not supraspinal) analgesic mechanisms, although functional coupling with μ-receptors was suggested.

σ-Receptors can no longer be classified as opiate receptors:

1 They demonstrate high-affinity binding for phencyclidine and related compounds (e.g. ketamine).

2 σ-Receptor-mediated effects are not reversed by high concentrations of opioid antagonists (e.g. naloxone).

3 σ-Receptors are stereoselective for the dextrorotatory isomers of opioid agonists, whereas μ-, κ- and δ-receptors all evince specificity for the laevorotatory isomers.

σ-Receptors are now subclassified into σ_1- and σ_2-receptors; the dextrorotatory enantiomer of pentazocine binds readily to σ_1-receptors, whilst other drugs (e.g. haloperidol) show a high affinity for both subgroups. Binding sites for phencyclidine are part of the NMDA receptor complex.

Current status of opioid receptors

Present views indicate the presence of three major classes of opiate receptors, namely μ, κ and δ, within the CNS, and that various subgroups exist within each class. All three of the principal receptors have now been cloned, and their amino acid sequence defined. Each of the three arises from a separate gene, although receptor subtypes may result from posttranslational modification of the specific protein.

In general, there is significant correlation between the analgesic potency of opioids and their affinity for μ-receptors. Experimental evidence suggests that only a small degree of receptor occupation is required to produce significant analgesia. Larger doses of opioid analgesics may 'spill over' on to other receptor subtypes and produce additional pharmacological effects. Studies incorporating animal models and highly selective opioid antagonists (β-funaltrexamine, naloxonazine) have indicated that μ-receptors may exist as two distinct subtypes. μ_1-Receptors are responsible for supraspinal analgesia, whilst effects mediated via μ_2-receptors include spinal analgesia, respiratory depression and constipation.

Three subtypes of the κ-receptor have been proposed. κ_1 Subtypes are thought to be involved in spinal analgesia, whilst the pharmacological effects mediated via κ_2 subtypes have not been defined. κ_3-Agonists produce supraspinal analgesia, and it has been suggested that this receptor subtype corresponds to the original nalorphine receptor.

The enkephalins are the endogenous ligands for δ-receptors and a specific antagonist for this receptor (naltrindole) has been developed. Studies with experimental agonists indicate that there may be two subtypes of the δ-receptor: δ_1 activity is mediated at spinal levels, whilst δ_2 effects may also occur supraspinally.

Opioid receptors are principally located at presynaptic sites and their stimulation leads to inhibition of neurotransmitter release. The receptors are linked to G_i proteins which themselves are coupled to transmembrane potassium channels. Increased potassium conductance leads to hyperpolarization; calcium-channel inactivation and inhibition of adenylyl cyclase are mechanisms which are also involved in this inhibitory response. Experimental studies have suggested that very low doses of morphine may produce paradoxical hyperalgesia. In these circumstances stimulation of the opioid receptor will lead to depolarization (either by decreased potassium conductance or by activation of calcium channels and subsequent activation of G_s proteins). In this context morphine itself could be regarded as a partial agonist.

The presence of opioid receptors outside the CNS may account for some other effects of analgesic drugs (e.g. constipation, increased biliary tract pressure). Many physiological functions, as well as analgesia, may be dependent on complex interactions between the different receptors. In addition, opioid receptors are subject to up-regulation and down-regulation by alterations in agonist concentration (Chapter 3). Indeed, receptor down-regulation may be an important cause of tolerance to opioids during their chronic administration.

Endogenous opioid peptides

Endogenous opioid peptides are usually classified as:

1 Enkephalins.

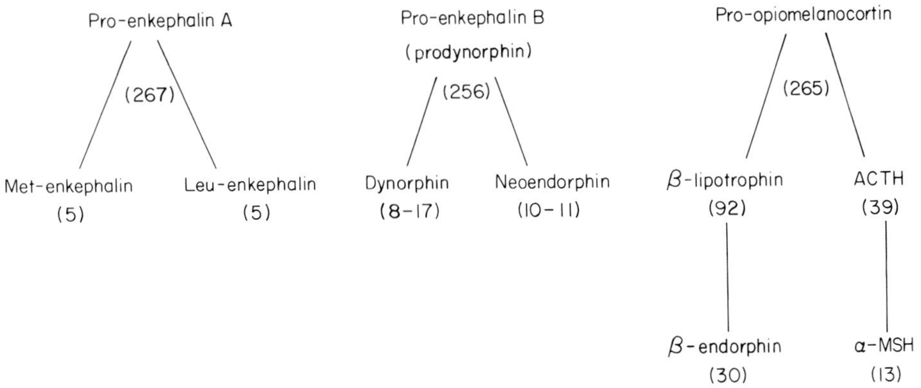

Fig. 11.2 Probable derivation of endogenous opioid peptides and related hormones. The number of amino acid residues in each polypeptide is shown in parentheses.

2 Endorphins (β-endorphins).

3 Dynorphins.

These endogenous peptides have differential potencies and are preferentially bound by different opioid receptors. Enkephalins are most active at δ-receptors; endorphins mainly act at μ-receptors, while dynorphins act on κ-receptors.

Although endogenous opioid peptides have been isolated from many sites in the body and have different molecular weights, they are all derived from three inactive precursors (proenkephalin A, proenkephalin B or prodynorphin, and pro-opiomelanocortin; Fig. 11.2). These peptides derivatives are widely distributed throughout the CNS, and are frequently found in the same region of the brain, but they do not occur in the same groups of neurones.

Enkephalins

In 1975, two similar pentapeptides (methionine (met-) enkephalin and leucine (leu-) enkephalin) were isolated from brain extracts. They were shown to produce analgesia, and to compete with the opioid antagonist naloxone for some brain receptor sites. The initial pentapeptide sequence of all endogenous opioids contains the structure of met-enkephalin or leu-enkephalin (Table 11.1).

Subsequent studies showed that regional variations in enkephalin levels reflected the distribution of opioid receptors. Enkephalins are widely distributed throughout the CNS, particularly in the spinal cord, the hypothalamus, the posterior pituitary, the globus pallidus and the limbic system. They are also present in the gastrointestinal tract, sympathetic ganglia, the adrenal medulla, the eye and the skin. Enkephalins have a selective affinity for δ-receptors, and are present in the cerebrospinal fluid (CSF) after some pain-relieving procedures (e.g. placebo analgesia, acupuncture and electric stimulation of the periaqueductal grey matter). Naloxone antagonizes the analgesia produced by these procedures.

Table 11.1 Amino acid sequences of some endogenous opioid peptides.

Opioid peptide	Amino acid sequence
Leu-enkephalin	H-**Tyr-Gly-Gly-Phe-Leu**-OH
Met-enkephalin	H-**Tyr-Gly-Gly-Phe-Met**-OH
β-Endorphin	H-**Tyr-Gly-Gly-Phe-Met**-Thr-Ser-Glu-Lys-Ser-Gln-Thr-Pro-Leu-Val-Thr-Leu-Phe-Lys-Asn-Ala-Ile-Ile-Lys-Asn-Ala-Tyr-Lys-Gly-Glu-OH
Dynorphin A	H-**Tyr-Gly-Gly-Phe-Leu**-Arg-Arg-Ile-Arg-Pro Lys-Leu-Lys-Trp-Asp-Asn-Gln-OH

All enkephalins are derived from the inactive precursor proenkephalin A, and fulfil the accepted criteria for a classical neurotransmitter. They are rapidly hydrolysed in the body, partly by specific peptidases such as the enzyme enkephalinase. Their action may be prolonged by some enzyme inhibitors (e.g. D-phenylalanine). Due to the susceptibility of the natural peptides to proteolytic attack, many synthetic analogues with amino acid substitutions have been synthesized. Unfortunately, many of these analogues (as well as the endogenous pentapeptides) may produce tolerance and dependence.

Endorphins

The β-endorphins are derived from the inactive precursor pro-opiomelanocortin. Each β-endorphin molecule contains about 30 amino acids and binds preferentially to μ-receptors. Their distribution in the CNS is more restricted than the enkephalins, and is mainly limited to the hypothalamus, the pituitary gland and their connections. In general, the β-endorphins are far more potent and stable compounds than the enkephalins, and can produce profound and long-lasting analgesia (i.e. for several hours) when injected by the intraventricular or intrathecal routes. The endorphins appear to be independent of the enkephalins, since extirpation of the hypothalamopituitary axis in experimental animals does not lead to a decrease in enkephalin synthesis.

The inactive β-endorphin precursor pro-opiomelanocortin, which consists of 265 amino acid residues, is also the precursor of three non-opioids (i.e. adrenocorticotrophic hormone (ACTH), α-melanocyte-stimulating hormone and β-lipotrophin). In response to acute pain and stress, both ACTH and β-endorphin are secreted in increased concentrations. Although β-endorphin contains the same amino acid sequence as met-enkephalin, it does not act as its precursor; all enkephalins are derived from proenkephalin A.

Dynorphins

The dynorphins (and the neoendorphins) are derived from the inactive precursor proenkephalin B, which is mainly present in the posterior pituitary and the hypothalamus. The dynorphins are a group of peptides containing 8–17 amino acids, and are preferentially bound by κ-receptors (although they also interact with μ- and δ-receptors). These peptides differ from other endogenous opioids, since they have no analgesic effects in the brain or the spinal cord. Their function appears to be the modulation of the effects of other opioids, such as analgesia, respiratory depression and cardiovascular function. Some dynorphins may produce flaccid paralysis when injected intrathecally; it is possible that they have a role in the pathophysiology of spinal cord injuries. Thus, experimental studies have shown that dynorphin levels in the CNS are increased after spinal trauma. Administration of dynorphins may prolong survival and improve neurological deficits after cerebrovascular accidents.

Clinical significance of endogenous opioids

Current evidence suggests that endogenous opioids have important physiological roles in humans. Opioid receptors may be involved in other physiological functions as well as nociception; these may include the regulation of body temperature, immunity, gastrointestinal motility, renal and hepatic function, behaviour patterns, extrapyramidal motor activity, cardiac and respiratory function, stress responses, appetite and thirst and some endocrinological effects (e.g. those dependent on hypothalamic and pituitary function). There are high concentrations of μ- and κ-receptors in the vagal nuclei, and this may be related to the bradycardia frequently seen after opioid administration in anaesthetic practice.

Endogenous opioids have an important role in autonomic function, and there are similarities between the signs of opioid overdosage and those of circulatory shock. This has led to the hypothesis that endogenous opioid peptides are directly or indirectly linked to the manifestations of shock. Circulating levels of enkephalins and β-endorphin are elevated in experimental shock; in addition, opioids inhibit catecholamine-induced changes in myocardial contractility and heart rate in the intact heart. These effects may be related to interference with calcium influx across myocardial cell membranes. Although the administration of large doses of opioid antagonists (especially naloxone, 1–3 mg kg^{-1}) may elevate blood pressure in experimental animals and human volunteers, clinical experience in shocked patients is unimpressive; in general, there has been little or no change in survival rates in patients with circulatory shock who have received naloxone. Furthermore, there are many potential disadvantages; reported complications of large doses of naloxone include grand mal seizure, pulmonary oedema and ventricular fibrillation. Some of these complications may be related to activation of the sympathetic nervous system. At present, there is insufficient clinical evidence to support the routine use of naloxone in patients with shock.

Table 11.2 Principal sites of action of endogenous and exogenous opioids and their antagonists at the various classes of opioid receptors.

Receptor	Agonist	Partial agonist	Antagonist
μ	β-Endorphin	Buprenorphine	Naloxone‡
	Morphine*	Butorphenol	Naltrexone
	Pethidine		Naloxonazine
	Methadone		β-Funaltrexamine
	Fentanyl		Nalorphine
	Etorphine		Pentazocine†
κ	Dynorphin	Nalbuphine	Naloxone‡
	Morphine*		Naltrexone
	Pentazocine		
	Nalorphine		
	Nalbuphine		
	Etorphine§		
δ	Leu-enkephalin		Naloxone‡
	Met-enkephalin		Naltrindole
	Deltorphin II		
	Etorphine§		

* Morphine has an affinity 200 times greater at μ-receptors than at κ-receptors.
† Some authorities consider that pentazocine may exert partial agonist effects at μ-receptors.
‡ Naloxone is more effective at the μ-receptor than at other receptors.
§ Etorphine is a highly potent agonist at all three levels of receptors.

The affinity of the various endogenous opioid peptides, opioid analgesics and antagonists for the major classes of opioid receptors is illustrated in Table 11.2.

Classification of opioid analgesics

Opioids are principally classified into those drugs which exhibit pure agonist activity and those demonstrating partial agonist properties. A third group, those described as pure antagonists, and which appear to have no intrinsic opioid activity in humans, will also be considered below. Further subdivisions are related to chemical structure.

Pharmacokinetics of opioid agonists

After oral administration, most opioid analgesics are well-absorbed from the small intestine. Since most opioids are weak bases and have high pK_a values (range = 6.5–9.3), they are mainly present in the stomach as ionized compounds; consequently, their absorption by the gastric mucosa is insignificant. By contrast, in the small intestine the pH is relatively alkaline, and opioid analgesics are mainly present in a non-ionized form; thus, they are rapidly and well-absorbed in the upper small intestine. However, almost all opioid analgesics (with the single exception of methadone) undergo significant first-pass metabolism in the gut wall and the liver so that their oral bioavailability is low (typically 20%; range 15–30%). Consequently, this route of administration is only appropriate in situations where parenteral administration is undesirable or impractical. Opioid analgesics are more usually given by intramuscular administration. Their absorption from muscle is relatively rapid, and maximum plasma concentrations occur 15–60 min after administration. However, absorption will be prolonged by peripheral vasoconstriction (e.g. due to pain, hypovolaemia, hypotension or hypothermia). In this situation, a reservoir of drug may remain in the tissues for some time.

The distribution of opioid analgesics is affected by several factors, including lipid solubility, ionization and binding to plasma proteins and tissue components. Lipid solubility is the most important factor determining the rate of drug entry into, and exit from the CNS (Table 11.3). Highly lipid-soluble drugs such as fentanyl are able to equilibrate rapidly across the blood–brain barrier, and therefore have a rapid onset of action. By contrast, less lipophilic drugs such as morphine enter the CNS more slowly, leading to a delay in peak effect. The degree of ionization of opioid analgesics affects their lipid solubility, binding to plasma proteins, and their partitioning between tissues and plasma. This may be altered by changes in plasma pH. Finally, the uptake of lipid-soluble analgesics by tissues can be appreciable. If they are administered by repeated injections or infusions over a long period of time, they will accumulate and recovery will be prolonged. Changes in the fraction of drug bound to plasma protein usually have very little effect on the amount of drug entering the CNS, as the volumes of distribution of these drugs are very large; any small change in free drug concentration consequent to alterations in protein binding is of little or no significance.

The biotransformation of opioid analgesics mainly occurs in the liver; in general, drug metabolites are inactive, or are much less potent than the parent drug. Most pharmacokinetic studies of opioid analgesics have been based on intravenous drug administration, as this avoids the variability of drug absorption and simplifies the kinetic interpretation of the data. Nevertheless, there is a significant degree of interindividual variability in the main pharmacokinetic constants; typical values for some commonly used analgesics are shown in Table 11.3. It should be recognized that the terminal plasma half-lives of opioid analgesics are not necessarily related

Table 11.3 Typical pharmacokinetic and physicochemical parameters of some opioid analgesics.

	Relative lipid solubility	Terminal half-life (h)	Clearance (ml min^{-1} kg^{-1})	Total volume of distribution (l kg^{-1})	pK_a	% ionized at pH 7.4
Morphine	1	3	15	3.5	7.9	76
Pethidine	28	4	12	4.0	8.7	95
Fentanyl	580	3.5	13	4.0	8.4	91
Alfentanil	90	1.6	6	0.8	6.5	11

to their duration of action; for example, morphine has a shorter terminal half-life than pethidine or fentanyl, but a longer duration of action. The volume of distribution of most opioids is several times greater than total body water, while their clearance is usually similar to liver blood flow (i.e. they are eliminated by flow-dependent hepatic clearance).

Agonists

Pure agonists may be classified as:

1 Morphine.
2 Analogues or derivatives of morphine.
3 Phenylpiperidine derivatives.
4 Methadone and its congeners.
5 Benzomorphan derivatives.

Morphine

Morphine is the principal phenanthrene derivative in opium (which contains 9–17% by weight of morphine base), and is the standard agent with which all other opioids are compared. It has a complex chemical structure (Fig. 11.3); part of this structure (the 'chair' or piperidine ring) is a common feature of many other opioid analgesics.

Route of administration and pharmacokinetics

Morphine is usually administered (as a sulphate or hydrochloride salt) by intramuscular injection; less commonly, it is given subcutaneously. It is well-absorbed from these sites, and produces blood levels which are usually as high as after intravenous injection. The adult dose is normally 10–15 mg, but this should be reduced in frail and elderly subjects, or those with underlying respiratory disorders. A peak effect will be achieved after 30–60 min, and its duration of action is approximately 3–4 h. The onset of action is only slightly more rapid following intravenous administration, as the main factor governing its latency is the permeability of the blood–brain barrier.

Morphine may also be administered orally. However, it undergoes extensive first-pass effects, so that only 10–30% of an orally administered dose reaches the systemic circulation; large doses have to be given to achieve adequate analgesia. Nevertheless, oral therapy with morphine solutions is commonly used in the long-term management of pain associated with malignancy. A slow-release preparation and a suppository form of the drug are also available.

After the intravenous administration of a bolus dose of morphine, plasma concentrations decline in a triexponential manner. Distribution occurs rapidly at

Morphine
$R_1 = H;\ R_2 = H$

Morphine-6-glucuronide
$R_1 = H;\ R_2 = C_6H_9O_6$

Codeine
$R_1 = CH_3;\ R_2 = H$

Diamorphine
$R_1 = CH_3CO;\ R_2 = CH_3CO$

Monoacetyl-morphine (MAM)
$R_1 = H;\ R_2 = CH_3CO$

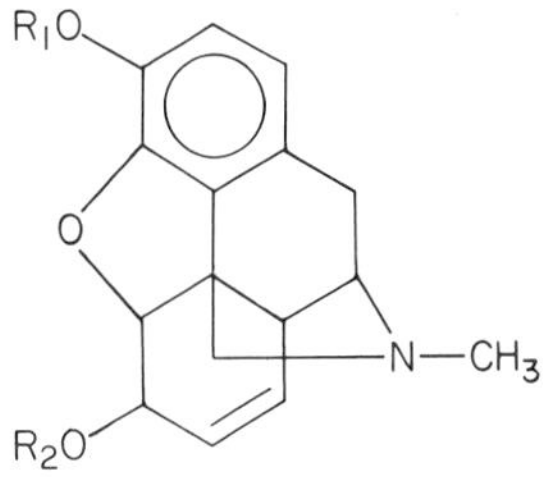

Pethidine

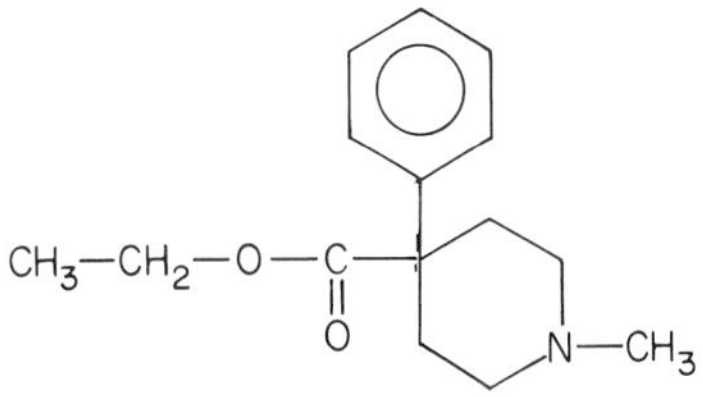

Fentanyl

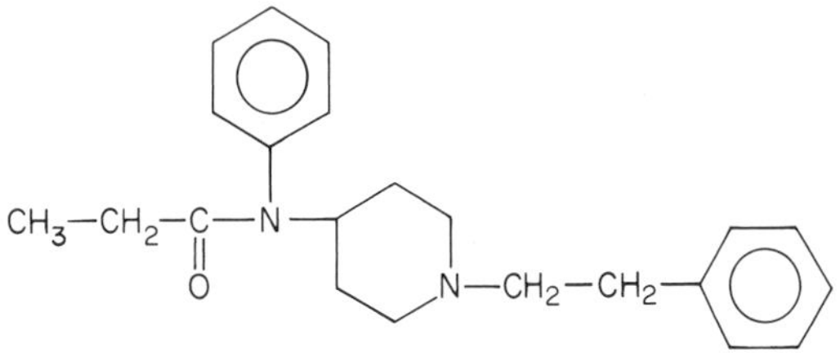

Methadone

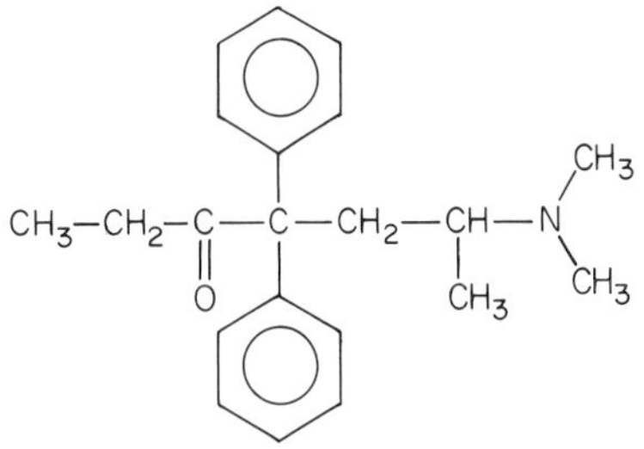

Fig. 11.3 The chemical structure of some opioid analgesics.

first, and then the plasma concentration declines more slowly. During this period, morphine enters the CNS; this occurs gradually, due to its low lipid solubility. These phases are followed by a slower phase of exponential decline, corresponding to the terminal half-life of the drug (approximately 3 h). Although the terminal half-life of morphine in plasma is shorter than that of pethidine or fentanyl, its duration of action is longer, because the decline in morphine concentrations in the brain is slower (due to the lower lipid solubility of the drug). Thus, there is no direct relationship between the plasma concentration of morphine and its clinical effects, such as respiratory depression (in contrast to lipid-soluble drugs such as fentanyl).

Morphine is almost entirely metabolized by the gut wall or the liver to a number of active or inactive compounds; 90% of the dose is excreted within 24 h. The principal metabolite (accounting for 70% of the dose) is morphine-3-glucuronide. This metabolite is partly excreted in bile, but can be broken down by intestinal bacteria; morphine is released, which may then be reabsorbed and metabolized by enterohepatic recirculation. Glucuronidation also takes place at the 6-carbon position, producing morphine-6-glucuronide. This metabolite has pharmacological effects indistinguishable from those of the parent drug, and appears more potent (particularly when administered directly into the CSF in animal studies). Furthermore, high plasma levels of this metabolite are found in patients who receive continuous administration of morphine by the oral route, and morphine-6-glucuronide may be principally responsible for the analgesic activity in these circumstances.

Various factors may affect the pharmacokinetics of morphine. Neonates are more sensitive to the effects of morphine, because the conjugating capacity of the liver is not fully developed. In the elderly, the volume of distribution is about half that of younger subjects, so that peak plasma levels are higher. Morphine clearance is not altered in cirrhosis, since glucuronidation is largely unaffected. Any increased effects of the drug in hepatic cirrhosis are therefore likely to be due to increased sensitivity to morphine (i.e. a pharmacodynamic rather than a pharmacokinetic phenomenon). The accumulation of morphine-6-glucuronide in patients with renal failure may account for their increased sensitivity to morphine. The clearance of morphine administered parenterally appears to be reduced during halothane anaesthesia, due to a reduction in hepatic blood flow. This is unlikely to be of practical significance unless very large doses are administered.

Pharmacological effects

The principal pharmacological effects of morphine (Table 11.4) are almost entirely mediated by μ-receptors.

1 Analgesia. Morphine relieves most forms of pain. However, in clinical practice it is most valuable for the treatment of continuous, dull, poorly localized pain arising from deeper structures, and where there are associated symptoms of fear and anxiety. Patients frequently report that the pain is still present but that they feel more comfortable. Thus, it is most useful for the management of pain arising from acute abdominal catastrophes, postoperative pain, major trauma, myocardial infarction and the management of pain associated with malignant disease. It is less effective in experimentally induced pain, and in acute pain arising from superficial structures.

2 Sedation. Drowsiness usually occurs in humans after the administration of morphine. Sleep is less commonly induced, although there is a shift of the electroencephalogram towards increased voltage and lower frequencies (a δ rhythm), and

Table 11.4 Principal pharmacological effects of morphine and related drugs.

Desirable effects	Undesirable effects
Effective analgesia	Tolerance
Relief of anxiety	Dependence
Sedation*	Dysphoria
Euphoria*	Nausea and vomiting
	Spasm of smooth muscle
	Constipation*
	Respiratory depression*
	Depression of cough reflex*
	Muscle rigidity

* These effects will vary according to circumstances. For example, respiratory depression will be an advantage during intermittent positive-pressure ventilation, whilst sedation and euphoria may be undesirable in the treatment of chronic pain in the ambulant patient.

rapid eye movement sleep is suppressed in animals. Some patients will experience euphoria (an unrealistic sense of well-being); however dysphoria (an unpleasant sensation associated with mild anxiety or fear) may occur, especially when morphine is administered in the absence of pain. In anaesthetic practice, this may also be seen if the drug is administered a few minutes before the induction of anaesthesia.

3 Respiratory depression. Therapeutic doses of morphine will depress the depth — and, more especially, the rate — of respiration by a direct effect on the respiratory centres in the brainstem. Maximal respiratory depression is seen within 7 min of intravenous administration, but may occur up to 30 min after intramuscular administration. In both cases, it may last for 4–5 h. Responsiveness to carbon dioxide is decreased, as shown by a shift to the right and a flattening of the ventilation–response curve (although hypoxic stimulation may still be effective).

However, when the main stimulus to respiration is hypoxia, oxygen therapy may potentiate respiratory depression by suppressing reflex chemoreceptor stimulation. When other CNS depressants, particularly halogenated anaesthetic agents, are used concurrently, marked bradypnoea and periodic breathing may be anticipated. The fetal respiratory centre appears to be highly sensitive to morphine, which precludes the use of the drug as an analgesic during labour.

4 Nausea and vomiting. Nausea and vomiting are common and unpleasant side-effects of morphine. They are primarily due to stimulation of the dopamine and 5-HT_3 receptors associated with the chemoreceptor trigger zone in the area postrema of the medulla; the activity of the vomiting centre may actually be depressed (particularly after repeated doses of morphine). Effects on the vestibular apparatus and on the smooth muscle of the gut may also be involved.

5 Cardiovascular effects. After administration of morphine, a mild bradycardia often ensues. This may be due to the decreased sympathetic drive associated with sedation, or a direct effect on the vagal nuclei. However, a direct action on the sino-atrial node cannot be excluded, and halothane may potentiate this effect. Hypotension may occur, but is not usually significant in the normovolaemic supine patient; it is probably due to some reduction in sympathetic tone leading to peripheral vasodilatation, and the release of histamine from mast cells. Morphine causes no direct myocardial depression, and doses up to 3 mg kg^{-1} are well-tolerated (for example, in patients with aortic valve disease undergoing open heart surgery).

Morphine has a particularly beneficial effect in the treatment of paroxysmal nocturnal dyspnoea, since it produces sedation, reduces preload and depresses abnormal respiratory drive.

6 Histamine release. Morphine releases histamine from mast cells and may produce bronchospasm and hypotension in susceptible patients. Its use should be avoided, if possible, in patients with obstructive airways disease. Nasal pruritus (or even generalized pruritus) may occur; this phenomenon may also be related to histamine release. Atropine may partially antagonize some of these effects.

7 Effects on gastrointestinal function. In general terms, morphine diminishes propulsive contractions and reduces secretory function throughout the gastrointestinal tract. However, the resting tone in smooth muscle is increased (particularly in most gastrointestinal sphincters). This can result in a prolonged gastric emptying time, delayed passage through the intestine and constipation. An important exception is lower oesophageal sphincter tone, which is decreased by morphine in patients with pre-existing reflux.

Spasm of the smooth muscle of the biliary tract and the sphincter of Oddi can also occur. The resulting rise of intraluminal pressure may lead to reflux of bile into the pancreatic duct; elevated levels of serum amylase and lipase are sometimes found following the administration of morphine. Therapeutic doses of the drug increase the tone and amplitude of contraction of the ureters.

8 Miosis. Miosis is due to stimulation of the Edinger–Westphal nucleus, depression of supranuclear pathways or effects on central sympathetic activity. Pinpoint pupils are characteristic features of morphine overdosage.

9 Hormonal effects. The release of ACTH, prolactin and gonadotrophic hormones is inhibited by morphine; by contrast, antidiuretic hormone (ADH) secretion is increased. These effects may be mediated via dopamine receptors in the hypothalamus.

10 Muscle rigidity. Morphine (as well as all other opioids) may occasionally produce rigidity of the thoracic wall (or even generalized muscle rigidity). These effects are thought to be mediated via opioid receptors in the substantia nigra and striatum interacting with dopaminergic and γ-aminobutyric acid (GABA) pathways, and can resemble convulsions. However, true convulsions only rarely occur, and are usually associated with gross overdosage or morphine.

11 Tolerance and dependence. Tolerance is characterized by decreased intensity and shortened duration of the usual effects of morphine, after repeated administration of the same dose of the drug. It may occur in subjects who have become socially habituated to the drug, or in patients who require continuous therapy for chronic pain. The pharmacokinetics of morphine are not altered by its repeated use; however, a negative-feedback system may result in decreased production of endogenous opioids, and there may also be down-regulation of opioid receptors.

The development of morphine dependence can be demonstrated when the drug is suddenly withdrawn after repeated dosage. Various physical and psychological phenomena may develop, the severity of which are related to the total amount administered. Symptoms and signs include restlessness and irritability, frequent yawning, excessive sweating, lacrimation and salivation, painful muscle cramps and intense and uncontrolled vomiting, diarrhoea and urination. Mild symptoms have been reported after only 48 h treatment.

Analogues and derivatives of morphine

Papaveretum (Omnopon)

Papaveretum is a semisynthetic mixture of the hydrochlorides of the opium alkaloids which has been available for many years. More recently one constituent, noscapine, has been shown to exhibit teratogenic effects in animal studies and is no longer incorporated into the formulation. The current preparation contains the three alkaloids morphine, codeine and papaverine (which is a smooth-muscle relaxant). The morphine content is approximately 60–70% of the prescribed or stated amount of papaveretum. Papaveretum may be given by intramuscular, intravenous or subcutaneous administration.

Diamorphine (diacetylmorphine; heroin)

Unchanged diamorphine has little or no affinity for opioid receptors. However, diamorphine is rapidly metabolized to monoacetylmorphine by esterases in plasma and tissues; both diamorphine and monacetylmorphine are more lipid-soluble than morphine, and they consequently penetrate the blood–brain barrier more easily. In the CNS, both diamorphine and monoacetylmorphine are rapidly converted to morphine. Some clinicians consider that diamorphine has a greater euphoriant effect than morphine, and that it may cause less vomiting, although almost all of the drug is eventually hydrolysed to morphine (both *in vivo* and in prepared solutions). In many countries, the manufacture or importation of heroin, even for medical use, is illegal.

When patients with terminal malignant disease require large doses of morphine for pain relief, diamorphine can be administered (usually as the hydrochloride salt), by intramuscular injection (or preferably by continuous subcutaneous infusion with a syringe driver) in a smaller volume of solution than the equivalent dose of morphine. This is an important consideration in patients with muscle wasting and cachexia, and is the only significant advantage of diamorphine.

Codeine

Codeine (methylmorphine) and its derivatives has a higher oral bioavailability than morphine. This is presumably due to the presence of a methyl group in the C3 position, which protects the drug from the activity of conjugating enzymes. Codeine is less effective against severe pain than morphine, although about 10% is metabolized to the parent drug by *O*-demethylation, which depends upon the activity of the CYP 2D6 isoform (Chapter 1). This enzyme exhibits polymorphism and it has been suggested that poor metabolizers may experience less pain relief when codeine is used as an analgesic.

Codeine has a low abuse potential, and large doses tend to produce excitement rather than central depression. Varying doses of the drug (8–30 mg) are commonly incorporated with NSAIDs in analgesic compounds which are used in the treatment of pain of moderate intensity; codeine is also used in antitussive and antidiarrhoeal preparations. Dihydrocodeine, a related compound, is a valuable drug for the management of chronic pain. Oxycodone is even more effective, but has a higher abuse potential. This drug is now only available in suppository form for the management of pain in terminal care.

Levorphanol

Levorphanol is about 10–15 times as potent as morphine when used orally; it may also be given parenterally. Clinical reports suggest that nausea and vomiting are uncommon side-effects. The *d*-isomer (dextrorphan) is devoid of analgesic effects and possesses considerable antitussive activity. Levorphanol is no longer available in the UK.

Etorphine

Etorphine (an analogue of thebaine) is about 400 times more potent than morphine in humans, and is considered to have significant agonist effects at all three classes of opioid receptors. It is frequently used in veterinary practice, and is a particularly valuable drug for immobilizing large animals in zoos and game reserves. It has undergone limited clinical trials in cancer patients, and tolerance and respiratory depression may be less pronounced than with equipotent doses of morphine. However, the development of etorphine has been discouraged by the World Health Organization; it is considered that its high potency conveys an increased risk of accidental overdosage and drug abuse.

Phenylpiperidines

Phenylpiperidine derivatives include pethidine, phenoperidine, fentanyl, alfentanil and diphenoxylate. They are structurally related to morphine and its derivatives (Fig. 11.3).

Pethidine

Although pethidine was originally developed as an anticholinergic agent, it was shown to have analgesic properties and was the first synthetic analgesic used in clinical practice (in 1939). Its apparent chemical dissimilarity to morphine suggested that it might not be associated with undesirable side-effects. However, there is little, if any, difference between the effects of equipotent doses of morphine and pethidine with regard to analgesia, respiratory depression, nausea and vomiting, and tolerance and dependence. Pethidine is more lipid-soluble than morphine, and penetrates the blood–brain barrier more readily. Consequently, there is a clear relationship between the plasma concentration of pethidine and its effects (unlike morphine). There are certain pharmacological differences between morphine and pethidine, some of which may reflect the anticholinergic activity of pethidine, and these are summarized in Table 11.5. More importantly, pethidine may produce serious adverse

Table 11.5 Principal differences between morphine and pethidine.

	Morphine	Pethidine
Equipotent adult dosage	10 mg	100 mg
Cortical effects	Sedation: δ rhythm on EEG	Sedation less marked; no EEG change with single dosage; hallucinations
Pupillary effects	Miosis (see text)	Miosis less marked; ? atropine-like effect on sphincter pupillae
Cardiovascular effects	Bradycardia; slight fall in BP	Significant fall in BP may occur in elderly; tachycardia sometimes
Atropine-like effects	Nil	Dry mouth
Duration of action (i.m. or s.c.)	3–4 h	2–3 h
Use during labour	Generally contraindicated	Opioid of choice if administered > 4 h prior to delivery
Metabolism and excretion	Glucuronide conjugation; excretion in bile (enterohepatic circulation) and mainly via kidneys	Extensive metabolism in liver; two major pathways; one metabolite, norpethidine, may produce hallucinations and convulsions in toxic dosage or in combination with monoamine oxidase inhibitors

EEG, Electroencephalogram; BP, blood pressure; i.m. intramuscular; s.c., subcutaneous.

effects in patients receiving a monoamine oxidase inhibitor (MAOI), including coma, hypotension or hypertension, convulsions and hyperpyrexia. The mechanism of this interaction is unclear; excessive activation of certain cerebral and spinal 5-hydroxytryptamine (5-HT) receptors has been proposed, although the inhibition of pethidine metabolism by MAOIs has also been implicated. Pethidine should not be given if an MAOI has been taken in the preceding 2 weeks; although other opioids are probably safe, it may be preferable to withhold these drugs altogether. If this is not possible, a small test dose (10% of the usual dose) should be given initially and titrated upwards.

Pethidine is almost entirely metabolized by phase I reactions in the liver; its main metabolites are norpethidine, pethidinic acid and pethidine-*N*-oxide. Little or no unchanged pethidine is eliminated. About 70% of the dose is excreted in urine (as metabolites) within 24 h, and this is enhanced by urinary acidification (and reduced by alkalinization). In patients with normal renal function, the elimination half-life of norpethidine is 14–21 h; the clearance of pethidine is reduced in liver disease, in the elderly and in the perioperative period. In renal failure, both pethidine and norpethidine accumulate, and this may be associated with certain neurological sequelae, including grand mal seizures, particularly when the ratio of the metabolite to the parent compound is greater than one.

Pethidine is often used during labour. Since it is relatively lipid-soluble, it readily crosses the placenta and significant amounts reach the fetus over a period of several hours. By contrast, little norpethidine (or other metabolites) crosses the placenta from the maternal circulation. The elimination of both pethidine and norpethidine is considerably prolonged in the neonate; their terminal half-lives are about three times longer than in adults (mainly due to a reduction in their clearance).

Phenoperidine

Phenoperidine is a potent analgesic and respiratory depressant, with a relatively short duration of action and considerable sedative effects. It is approximately five times more potent than morphine. It is invariably administered intravenously, and has been particularly popular in the management of patients requiring prolonged mechanical ventilation in the intensive care unit.

The effects of phenoperidine on respiratory function are maximal in 5–15 min, and the duration of action is usually less than 60 min. After intravenous administration, the plasma concentration shows a secondary peak after 30–40 min, which may be abolished by concurrent antacid therapy. This phenomenon is characteristic of other basic drugs (e.g. pethidine and fentanyl), and is due to their elimination into acidic gastric fluid and subsequent reabsorption from the small intestine. Phenoperidine is mainly metabolized to pethidine and norpethidine; both these metabolites (and traces of the unchanged drug) can be identified in urine.

Fentanyl

Fentanyl is the most potent analgesic used in the UK; it is approximately 100 times more potent than morphine. When given in small intravenous doses (1 μg kg^{-1}), it has a rapid onset and a short duration of action (about 30 min). Although it is structurally related to pethidine, it has little sedative activity at low doses; by contrast, when high doses are administered (50–150 μg kg^{-1}) sedation and unconsciousness are profound, and it may be used as the sole anaesthetic. However, awareness during surgery has been reported and this technique should be used with care. When given in high doses, muscular rigidity, particularly of the chest wall, may be a problem.

In many respects, fentanyl is similar to morphine. It depresses respiration in a dose-dependent manner. Cardiovascular stability is present even when the drug is administered in high dosage, and the role of fentanyl in cardiovascular anaesthesia is well-established. During high-dose fentanyl anaesthesia, bradycardia can occur and may require treatment with atropine. High-dose fentanyl anaesthesia also reduces or eliminates the metabolic stress response to surgery.

Since fentanyl is highly lipid-soluble, it is rapidly and extensively distributed in tissues. Its duration of action is dose-dependent. In small doses (1–2 μg kg^{-1}), its duration of action is short and there is rapid recovery; in these conditions, the plasma (and CNS) concentrations of the drug fall to below an effective level during the rapid distribution phase. However, after multiple or large doses of the drug, the duration of action is significantly prolonged. In these circumstances, the distribution phase is complete while the plasma concentration of fentanyl is still high. Recovery from the effects of the drug then depends on its relatively slow elimination from the body, and profound respiratory depression may be present for several hours during the postoperative period.

Many factors can affect the disposition of fentanyl, and a number of pharmacokinetic studies have shown considerable interindividual variability. After an intravenous bolus dose of fentanyl, plasma levels decline quickly (distribution half-life = approximately 13 min). The terminal half-life is 3–4 h in normal subjects, but may be as long as 7–8 h in some groups of patients. The volume of distribution is relatively large (approximately 4 l kg^{-1}), indicating considerable tissue uptake, and the clearance is slightly less than hepatic blood flow. Fentanyl is predominantly metabolized in the liver; about two-thirds of the administered dose is excreted in the urine as inactive metabolites over 4 days.

Alfentanil

Alfentanil is a synthetic opioid structurally related to fentanyl; it has approximately 10–20% of its potency, and has a shorter duration of action. Its effects on the respiratory and cardiovascular systems are similar to fentanyl, and it is used in similar situations. However, small doses of the drug can cause apnoea in some patients. Although this is usually very short-lasting, it is unpredictable; careful monitoring is essential, particularly in the elderly who are more sensitive to respiratory depression.

There are important pharmacokinetic differences between alfentanil and fentanyl (Table 11.3). Although it has a much lower lipid solubility than fentanyl, more alfentanil in plasma is present in the non-ionized form (89% compared to 9% for fentanyl); consequently, its onset of action is more rapid than fentanyl. Alfentanil has a short distribution half-life (approximately 11 min), and a shorter terminal half-life than fentanyl (approximately 1.6 h); complete recovery is therefore more rapid, and aflentanil provides very little postoperative analgesia. The clearance of alfentanil is about half that of fentanyl, although its lower lipid solubility results in a much smaller volume of distribution, thus reflecting the shorter terminal half-life.

Alfentanil is extensively metabolized in the liver, and less than 2% of the parent drug is excreted unchanged. Its clearance is unaffected by renal disease, but is prolonged in cirrhosis and in patients taking cimetidine.

Alfentanil may be administered in either bolus doses or as a continuous infusion. Bolus doses (10 $\mu g\ kg^{-1}$) are useful to attenuate the cardiovascular responses to intubation and stimulation during surgery. However, the pharmacokinetics of alfentanil are consistent with administration by continuous intravenous infusion; it may be used as the sole anaesthetic agent, or for sedation in the intensive care unit in patients on mechanical ventilation. Typically, a loading dose of 25–50 $\mu g\ kg^{-1}$ is given, followed by an infusion of 0.5–2.0 $\mu g\ kg^{-1}\ min^{-1}$.

Sufentanil

Sufentanil is closely related to fentanyl in chemical structure, but has five to 10 times its potency. It produces excellent cardiovascular stability and has a shorter duration of action than fentanyl. Sufentanil has been widely used in the USA; it is particularly useful in patients undergoing cardiac surgery. More recently, it has been used in low dosage as a premedicant administered by intranasal spray. Carfentanil and lofentanil are other highly potent analogues of fentanyl.

Remifentanil

Remifentanil, which is approximately equipotent to fentanyl, contains an ester linkage which is susceptible to cleavage by non-specific plasma enzymes. Remifentanil has a rapid onset of action (similar to that of alfentanil) and a very short elimination half-life (10–21 min). Evidence suggests that the unique metabolism of remifentanil does not appear to be affected by genetic abnormalities of plasma cholinesterase or the concomitant administration of anticholinesterase drugs.

Furthermore, studies indicate that the offset of activity following continuous infusion of remifentanil is considerably more rapid than with fentanyl or alfentanil. Remifentanil is likely to achieve a role in anaesthetic practice and in intensive care situations. At present, remifentanil is formulated in glycine, and cannot be recommended for spinal or extradural administration.

Tramadol

Tramadol is the phenylpiperidine analogue of codeine and, in common with the latter drug, has a demethylated metabolite which shows a higher affinity for opioid receptors. Tramadol has been available in Germany since 1977 and was recently introduced into the UK. It appears to be a weak agonist at all types of opioid receptor, with some selectivity for μ-receptors. Experimental studies indicate that tramadol also inhibits neuronal reuptake of noradrenaline and 5-HT. This action suggests an additional non-opioid mechanism for analgesia involving descending inhibitory pathways in the CNS; the antinociceptive effects of tramadol are only partially antagonized by naloxone. Tramadol is a racemic mixture and it appears that the two enantiomers have separate effects at opioid and non-opioid sites.

Tramadol has undergone trials for postoperative pain relief, and a similar potency and efficacy to that of pethidine has been demonstrated when both drugs are given by the intravenous route using patient-controlled analgesia. In addition, it has been shown to have a considerable sparing effect on the respiratory centre when compared with equianalgesic doses of morphine. However, it shares many of the common side-effects of other opioids (e.g. nausea, vomiting, drowsiness and ambulatory dizziness). At present tramadol is not subject to controlled drug regulations and it is also available as an oral preparation for the treatment of mild to moderate pain. The concomitant administration of carbamazepine may considerably reduce the plasma concentration and the analgesic efficacy of tramadol.

Diphenoxylate

Diphenoxylate is chemically related to pethidine, and produces constipation in humans. It has an extremely low abuse potential, since its salts are virtually insoluble in aqueous solution. It is commonly incorporated (with atropine salts) in an anti-diarrhoeal preparation (Lomotil).

Loperamide

Loperamide, like diphenoxylate, is a piperidine derivative that is poorly absorbed from the gastrointestinal tract and does not penetrate the blood–brain barrier. Its only use is in the treatment of diarrhoea.

Methadone and its congeners

Methadone

Methadone was synthesized by German chemists during World War II. It is active at μ-receptors, and has similar properties to morphine. Methadone and morphine are approximately equipotent.

Unlike most other opioid analgesics, methadone has a high oral bioavailability, and the oral and parenteral doses (range 5–15 mg) usually equate. Consequently, methadone is a particularly useful drug when oral dosage is preferred. Methadone has a long duration of action (terminal half-life = 15–20 h), and miosis and respiratory depression can be detected for more than 24 h. It is bound to tissue proteins, so that cumulative effects may be observed with repeated dosage, especially in elderly patients (who may experience marked sedation). Methadone is metabolized in the liver by the mixed-function oxidase system (cytochrome P-450). Drugs that induce this enzyme system (e.g. rifampicin) can produce withdrawal symptoms in patients on chronic methadone treatment.

Tolerance develops more slowly to methadone than to morphine; consequently, the drug is used in the treatment of morphine dependence. Thus, methadone may be substituted for morphine without precipating an abstinence syndrome. However, the overall abuse potential of methadone is comparable to that of morphine, and this limits its use for this purpose.

Dextromoramide and dipipanone

Dextromoramide and dipipanone are analogues of methadone, and have similar properties and potency; however, they have a shorter duration of action than the parent drug. Dipipanone is usually used with the antiemetic drug cyclizine in a proprietary preparation (Diconal). Both dextromoramide and dipipanone may provide valuable oral therapy in the management of chronic pain associated with malignancy.

Dextropropoxyphene

Propoxyphene occurs as a racemic mixture (although only the dextrorotatory isomer possesses analgesic activity). It is about 50–65% as potent as oral codeine, and has been used alone or in compound preparations. A popular formulation in the UK has been co-proxamol (Distalgesic); each tablet contains paracetamol (325 mg) and dextropropoxyphene (32.5 mg). Co-proxamol has been prescribed for a wide variety of painful conditions. Unfortunately, its use is associated with several disadvantages; some degree of dependence to dextropropoxyphene can occur, and a number of incidents of drug abuse, particularly in combination with alcohol, have been reported.

In addition, overdosage or drug interaction involving co-proxamol may lead to the rapid development of profound respiratory depression which precedes the manifestations of paracetamol hepatotoxicity. One of the metabolites of dextropropoxyphene (norpropoxyphene) has a longer half-life than the parent drug; it has some analgesic activity, but also has cardiotoxic properties.

Benzomorphan derivatives

Phenazocine

In the UK, phenazocine is the only available benzomorphan derivative that is a pure opioid agonist. It is approximately three times as potent as morphine, and is effective when administered orally or sublingually. There is some evidence that it may be useful in the treatment of biliary colic, since it has little or no spasmogenic effect on the sphincter of Oddi.

Partial agonists

Analgesics in this group can be broadly defined as drugs which do not display full agonist activity at all types of opioid receptors. The term partial agonist can be used to describe two disparate types of drugs in this context (Chapter 3):

1 Drugs which produce antagonistic effects at μ-receptors, but exert their analgesic activity by agonist effects at κ-receptors. The drugs in this group may be subdivided into those in which agonist (i.e. analgesic) activity predominates (e.g. pentazocine, butorphanol, nalbuphine and meptazinol), and those in which antagonist activity predominates (e.g. nalorphine, levallorphan and cyclazocine). Some authorities consider that pentazocine and butorphanol exert partial agonist effects, rather than antagonistic effects, at the μ-receptor.

2 Drugs which do not display antagonistic effects but which have a diminished effect at μ-receptors due to low intrinsic activity (e.g. buprenorphine).

Both categories of partial agonists show important differences to pure agonists with regard to their dose–response relationships. In the case of pure agonists, increasing the dose causes an increase in analgesia and respiratory depression, and the maximum effect is only obtainable with doses well in excess of those used in routine clinical practice. By contrast, the dose–response curve of partial agonists generally shows a plateau or ceiling effect, with the top of the plateau representing the maximum effect possible (Fig. 11.4).

Pentazocine

Pentazocine was the first drug in this group developed for clinical use as an analgesic.

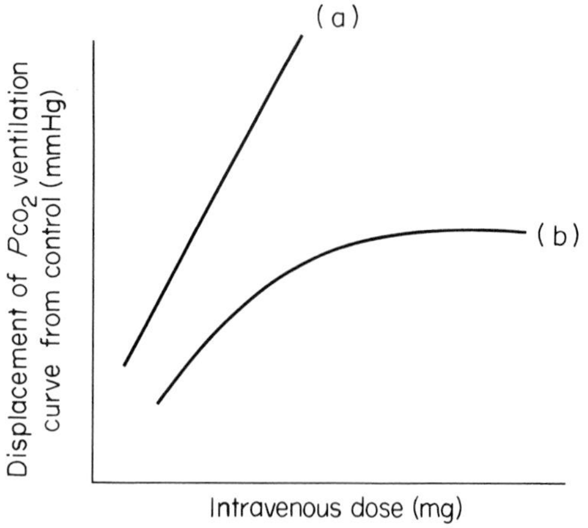

Fig. 11.4 The effects of (a) pure agonists and (b) agonist/antagonists on the Pco_2 — ventilation response. In the case of agonist/antagonists, a plateau (ceiling) effect occurs, so that further increases in dosage do not enhance respiratory depression.

It is a benzomorphan derivative, chemically related to phenazocine, and has approximately 25% of the analgesic potency of morphine. The principal differences between pentazocine and morphine are as follows:

1 Pentazocine has a much lower abuse potential than most pure agonists. Nevertheless, there have been occasional reports of withdrawal symptoms occurring after prolonged use of the drug, particularly by parenteral administration. Consequently, it is now a controlled drug (Schedule 3) in the UK.

2 Pentazocine is not very effective in relieving severe pain. This may be partly due to the absence of the euphoriant effects of morphine.

3 Psychotomimetic effects (e.g. bizarre dreams and hallucinations) occur in about 6% of patients after parenteral administration.

4 Intravenous pentazocine invariably produces an increase in both systemic blood pressure and heart rate, and an increase in circulating catecholamine levels. A rise in pulmonary vascular resistance and mean pulmonary artery pressure is not uncommon; the drug should not be used after myocardial infarction, in pulmonary or systemic hypertension, or in patients with heart failure.

5 The effects of an overdose of pentazocine will not be reversed by nalorphine.

6 Combined therapy with pentazocine and a μ-receptor agonist in chronic pain states may produce unpredictable results. Pentazocine may antagonize the analgesic effects of the μ-agonist, while the full agonist may enhance the psychotomimetic side-effects of pentazocine. Since pentazocine has an antagonist action at the μ-receptor, the technique of sequential analgesia was devised. Pentazocine was used at the end of surgery to antagonize the respiratory depression caused by large doses of introperative fentanyl without affecting the level of analgesia. This technique has not gained widespread acceptance.

Butorphanol

Butorphanol is approximately 20 times more potent than pentazocine, but has a similar profile of activity (particularly on the cardiovascular system). Therapeutic doses (1–2 mg) produce effective analgesia for 3–4 h. Butorphanol produces fewer dysphoric reactions than pentazocine; the drug is no longer available in the UK (although it is still used in the USA).

Nalbuphine

Nalbuphine is structurally related to naloxone. It is a partial agonist at κ-receptors, but is also a potent μ-antagonist which can precipitate withdrawal symptoms in patients who are physically dependent on opioid analgesics. It has also been used effectively in the techniques of sequential analgesia. Nalbuphine undergoes extensive first-pass metabolism in the liver, and its oral bioavailability is low (about 10%). Consequently, it is only available as a parenteral preparation.

Nalbuphine and morphine are equipotent, and both drugs have a similar duration of action. It is similar to other partial agonists, and has a plateau or ceiling effect; increasing the dose has variable effects on the degree of analgesia. Unlike pentazocine, it causes no significant haemodynamic changes, and is a suitable analgesic for patients with heart disease.

Meptazinol

Meptazinol is only one-tenth as potent as morphine; unlike many opioids that are racemates, both of its enantiomers possess analgesic activity. Its mode of action is not clearly understood. It has been stated that meptazinol may have a selective agonist effect at μ_1-receptors; however, in opioid-dependent subjects, it may produce withdrawal symptoms. Cholinergic activity may contribute to the analgesic effect. Meptazinol may produce less respiratory depression than other opioids; although it rarely causes dysphoria, it may produce nausea and vomiting. This may be related to its effects on central cholinergic pathways in the cerebellum, labyrinth and vestibular apparatus. The incidence of emetic complications can be reduced by anticholinergic drugs (although theoretically the analgesic effect could also be diminished).

Buprenorphine

Buprenorphine is chemically related to thebaine, and is approximately 30 times more potent than morphine. Thus, 300 μg buprenorphine and 10 mg morphine produce the same degree of analgesia. It is a highly lipid-soluble drug, and is well-absorbed sublingually.

Buprenorphine is a partial agonist at μ-receptors (and may have some affinity for κ-receptors). Thus, theoretical considerations suggest that if buprenorphine is given with morphine or similar drugs, the level of analgesia will decrease to the ceiling level of buprenorphine. In practice, this interaction will only occur if all the available receptors are already occupied by the μ-agonist, or if extremely large doses of buprenorphine are given. These conditions are only present in subjects who receive large doses of morphine (e.g. cancer patients or drug abusers). In the more usual perioperative situation, the majority of opioid receptors are unoccupied and available for combination with other drugs; in these conditions, no significant interactions should occur.

In general, buprenorphine and morphine produce similar effects and side-effects (e.g. drowsiness, nausea, vomiting, dizziness, sweating). Since buprenorphine has an extremely high affinity for μ-receptors, its effects are not completely reversed by naloxone. Buprenorphine can produce respiratory depression; although a plateau or ceiling for this effect has been described, this can still become clinically significant and should be managed with doxapram. Dysphoria is uncommon, and untoward haemodynamic effects mediated by CNS stimulation are rare. Although it was initially believed to have a low abuse potential, dependence may occur; in the UK, buprenorphine is now a controlled drug (Schedule 3).

Buprenorphine is extremely lipid-soluble, and is absorbed after sublingual administration; it has an extremely low oral bioavailability (due to its high first-pass effect). Buprenorphine is metabolized by the liver, and 70% of a dose is eliminated in the faeces. Although its terminal half-life is similar to pethidine (3–4 h), it has a much longer duration of action (up to 8 h); this may be related to its slow dissociation from the μ-receptor. The clearance of buprenorphine is not affected by renal failure.

Other partial agonists with mixed effects, such as nalorphine and levallorphan, are now only of historical interest. They were formerly used in the treatment of opioid overdosage. At one time levallorphan was incorporated in a preparation containing pethidine (Pethilorfan). This had a popular vogue in the treatment of labour pains, in the mistaken belief that fetal respiratory depression could be diminished without an associated decrease in analgesic efficacy. A related compound, cyclazocine, was also used in the treatment of opioid dependence.

Spinally administered opioid analgesia

The discovery of the existence of opiate receptors in the substantia gelatinosa led to a developing interest in the administration of opioid analgesics by intrathecal and extradural routes. Selective uptake of these drugs by spinal cord receptors at the appropriate dermatomal level suggested that:

1 A localized effect would be produced by a relatively small amount of the drug; the effect would also be enhanced and prolonged by the unavailability of systemic enzyme activity at these sites.

2 Undesirable side-effects should be minimal due to lack of supraspinal activity.

Radiolabelled studies using morphine have indicated a rapid uptake of the drug into laminae of the dorsal horn following intrathecal administration. Subsequently, clinical and experimental evidence in both animals and humans confirmed that a small dose (1 mg in humans) produced prolonged and effective analgesia, whilst other opiates in doses approximately 10% of those used parenterally were shown to produce similar effects. It is probable that spinal analgesic activity is principally mediated via μ-receptors which are found in abundance adjacent to C-fibre terminals in lamina 1 and in the substantia gelatinosa (δ-receptors may also be implicated). However, supraspinal effects also occurred and appeared to be more prominent when less lipid-soluble drugs (e.g. morphine, pethidine) were used.

The intrathecal route has not gained widespread popularity in the UK. The administration of single doses appears to provide little advantage over the use of more conventional routes, whilst continuous infusion techniques can present problems associated with spinal cord infection and catheter breakage; preservative-free preparations must always be used in this context to avoid neurological sequelae (chlorocresol, which is normally present in commercial preparations of morphine, has been used as a neurolytic agent in the management of cancer pain).

In contrast, the use of extradural opiate regimes has become a generally accepted technique. A significant increase in dosage is required compared with the intrathecal route (the bioavailability of morphine, reflecting uptake from the extradural space to the CSF, has been reported as 2–4%). In many instances, opiates are used in combination with local anaesthetic amides, where their differential effects on pain pathways, i.e. neuronal and synaptic transmission, may produce additive or possibly synergistic effects. The reduced dosage requirement of either drug will tend to diminish side-effects such as motor weakness and hypotension with local anaesthetic agents, and opiate-induced respiratory depression and vomiting.

The resultant effects of the specific opiates injected into the extradural space are principally related to their physical and chemical properties. The dura mater is not a lipid membrane, and the rate of diffusion of drugs into the CSF will be inversely related to molecular size. The lipid solubility of the drug is also important, and influences the rate of uptake into peridural fat and to adjacent veins.

The kinetic activity of various opioid analgesics used in this context can be illustrated by comparing the extradural administration of fentanyl and morphine, where the relative lipid solubilities are approximately 500 to 1.

Fentanyl will traverse the dural membrane more rapidly (because of its lower molecular weight) and uptake into the spinal cord will be facilitated because of its greater lipid solubility (peak levels occur within 15 min). At the same time vascular uptake (via the perivertebral fat) will be greater in the case of fentanyl, resulting in more significant plasma levels. The effects of fentanyl administered extradurally would thus more closely equate with those observed following intravenous administration, with the likelihood of supraspinal effects (e.g. respiratory depression, nausea and vomiting) occurring at an earlier stage.

In comparison, the properties of morphine indicate a slower onset of action because of reduced dural diffusion and uptake by the spinal cord, but with less uptake into the systemic circulation (peak CSF levels 1–2 h after administration, with 50% still present after 12 h). The longer latency of morphine in the CNS will enhance rostral spread, allowing uptake of morphine at higher segmental levels, but with a greater likelihood of delayed supraspinal effects. The predicted responses are confirmed by numerous clinical reports. Late-onset respiratory depression is more closely associated with the use of morphine, whereas the effects of fentanyl more parallel those observed following intravenous administration. Furthermore, the analgesic effects of morphine at higher spinal segments (e.g. in producing thoracic analgesia following lumbar extradural injection) are more prominent than in the case of fentanyl.

Diamorphine is frequently administered by the extradural route. Diamorphine has a slightly greater molecular weight than the parent drug, and would presumably traverse the dura at a similar rate. However, diamorphine is approximately 200 times more lipid-soluble than morphine and about one-third as soluble as fentanyl (Table 11.3). Thus, diamorphine could be predicted to have intermediate effects (in relation to morphine and fentanyl) both with regard to systemic and CNS uptake, and to spread within the CSF.

Specific side-effects related to administration of opiates by spinal routes are urinary retention and pruritus. Itching is not confined to the segmental area involved in analgesia, but also occurs in the head and neck. This may be related to enhancement of C-fibre activity and activation of G_s proteins; local release of histamine is also postulated. The mechanisms involved in the production of urinary retention are unclear, although the rapid onset (especially in young men) suggests spinal effects on the parasympathetic sacral outflow. These side-effects are readily reversed by naloxone (although analgesia is similarly affected).

There is no conclusive evidence that opioids injected extradurally or intrathecally provide analgesia which is qualitatively superior to that produced by more conventional routes of administration. An undisputed advantage is their ability to produce more prolonged analgesia, usually with lower doses.

These techniques have been used with considerable success in the management of pain associated with surgery, myocardial infarction, chest injuries and in low-dose combinations with local anaesthetics in the relief of labour pains.

Pure opioid antagonists

Naloxone

Naloxone is the *N*-allyl derivative of oxymorphone. Unlike the *N*-allyl derivatives of other opioids, it has no agonist activity (i.e. it is a pure antagonist). It has a higher affinity for μ-receptors than for other opioid receptors; nevertheless, it can still displace most agonists from other receptor sites. Naloxone was originally designed and developed for the treatment of opioid overdosage, and for the prevention of opioid dependence; at first, it was considered to be devoid of any other inherent actions or effects. Nevertheless, antanalgesic effects may be observed in naive subjects who are given naloxone. Hypertension, pulmonary oedema and cardiac arrhythmias can also occur. Some of these effects may be related to antagonism of specific opioid receptors, or they may reflect generalized central excitation. Both these concepts are possible; thus, naloxone will reverse analgesia produced by classical Chinese acupuncture or placebo analgesia, and can be effective in the treatment of overdosage with CNS depressants (e.g. ethyl alcohol). Naloxone may produce beneficial effects in patients with thalamic pain; its mechanism of action is obscure.

Naloxone is the current drug of choice for the treatment of opioid overdosage. In mild or moderate cases, a single dose (0.4 mg) may be sufficient to antagonize the effects of opioid analgesics. The terminal half-life of naloxone is 2.5 h; the duration of effective antagonism is limited to about 30–45 min. Long-acting agonists will outlast this effect and further bolus doses (or naloxone infusion) will then be required to maintain reversal. Smaller doses (0.5–1.0 μg kg^{-1}) may be titrated to reverse respiratory depression without significantly affecting the level of analgesia. By contrast, very large bolus doses (up to 2 mg) may be required to antagonize severe opioid overdosage. Naloxone has a low oral bioavailability, due to a large first-pass effect. The drug has also been used in the treatment of septic shock (p. 371).

Naltrexone has an identical mode of action, but has two important pharmacokinetic advantages compared to naloxone. It has a longer duration of action, due to its longer half-life; and it has a low first-pass effect (i.e. it is effective after oral administration). It is available in tablet form, and a single dose (50 mg) will remain effective for 24 h. Naltrexone is of value as maintenance therapy for detoxified morphine-dependent subjects; in particular, it will block the euphorogenic effects of high doses of opioids in relapsing cases.

Naloxonazine and β-funaltrexamine are irreversible μ-receptor antagonists, although β-funaltrexamine also has reversible κ-agonist activity. Naltrindole appears to be a highly selective agonist at δ-receptors. These agents are principally used in experimental studies to determine the various opioid receptors and their subtypes.

Doxapram

Doxapram is a non-specific analeptic which may also be of some value in the prevention or treatment of opioid-induced respiratory depression, particularly in the immediate postoperative period. It is also useful in the management of respiratory depression due to buprenorphine, whose effects are only partially antagonized by naloxone. Doxapram mainly acts by affecting reflex mechanisms mediated via chemoreceptors in the carotid body; it also produces some direct medullary stimulation of the respiratory centre. Doxapram has a higher therapeutic ratio than many other analeptics (e.g. nikethamide), since very high doses are required to produce cortical stimulation. However, it should be used cautiously in patients with hypertension, ischaemic heart disease, thyrotoxicosis and epilepsy.

Doxapram may antagonize opioid-induced respiratory depression without abolishing analgesia, and its use in combination with opioid analgesics reduces the incidence of postoperative chest complications. It has a short duration of action (5–12 min) and may need to be given by intravenous infusion. The usual intravenous dose (1.0–1.5 mg kg^{-1}) is administered over 30 s. It is also available as a ready-made solution (2 mg ml^{-1}) which should be infused at a rate of 2–3 mg min^{-1}. The drug may be of some value in the management of respiratory failure in patients with chronic obstructive pulmonary disease.

Choice of analgesic

The use of opioid analgesics is indicated in a wide variety of conditions.

Acute pain states

Acute pain states include abdominal catastrophes, major trauma, the pain of myocardial infarction and pain associated with labour. In most cases, morphine is the drug of choice, although pethidine is preferred in obstetrics. Morphine should be administered by slow intravenous injection in the shocked patient to produce an optimal effect. In the undiagnosed acute abdomen, half the usual dose of morphine or pethidine may be given; some analgesic effect will be attained without masking vital signs.

Although diamorphine has been widely used to relieve the pain of myocardial infarction, its advantages are doubtful; some clinicians consider that it produces more sedation and euphoria and less vomiting than other analgesics. Codeine and its derivatives are commonly used for the management of traumatic pain associated with head injury, since they are less likely to disturb levels of consciousness and have minimal effects on pupillary signs.

In general, partial agonists have significant disadvantages compared with pure agonists. The quality of analgesia is often inferior due to the ceiling effect, and dysphoria is more common. Finally, their actions at the μ-receptor (either antagonistic or high-affinity with low intrinsic activity) may complicate any subsequent change of therapy.

The perioperative period

When pain is present, morphine or pethidine is indicated for premedication.

Pethidine, morphine and fentanyl are most frequently used as analgesic supplements. Alternatively, phenoperidine or fentanyl, often in combination with droperidol, may be used at induction to supplement (or even replace) intravenous anaesthetic agents. The undoubted value of pre-emptive analgesia on the course of postoperative pain suggests that the careful timing of opioid premedication, or the use of highly lipid-soluble analgesics at induction, may confer considerable advantages. Alfentanil is particularly useful during induction, in order to suppress the cardiovascular responses to intubation; it may also be given as an infusion during surgery.

Morphine and pethidine are still the most frequently used opioids for the relief of postoperative pain. Intramuscular injection is not the most effective way of ensuring good postoperative analgesia; during the past decade, numerous techniques have been developed in an attempt to provide more effective pain relief. Current methods now include spinally administered opioids, patient-controlled analgesia, computer-assisted infusions and transdermal and transmucosal drug delivery by sublingual, buccal, gingival and nasal administration. The partial agonist buprenorphine has a longer duration of action than most other opioids, and may have possible advantages (as well as several disadvantages) as a postoperative analgesic.

Prolonged intermittent positive-pressure ventilation (IPPV)

During prolonged IPPV, analgesics are often necessary, both to provide adequate pain relief and to facilitate compliance with mechanical ventilation. In the past, phenoperidine has been extensively used, as it produces marked respiratory depression, analgesia and sedation. In recent years, alfentanil has also been used for this purpose. When administered by infusion, it provides good analgesia and the rate of administration can be increased to cover periods of enhanced stimulation (e.g. physiotherapy). When the infusion is stopped, there is a much more rapid recovery from its effects than from any other opioid in current use.

Chronic pain

Opioid analgesics are widely used for the management of intractable pain associated with malignant disease. In most situations, effective analgesia can be provided by oral or sublingual administration of drugs.

Morphine is the most useful opioid analgesic for the management of terminal pain. It may be given orally as an elixir (e.g. morphine hydrochloride in chloroform water, 4-hourly), or as slow-release tablets. The initial dose should be the minimum that is compatible with adequate pain relief; frequent readjustment may be necessary. It is important to ensure that the drug is given at regular intervals in sufficient dosage to prevent the return of severe pain. Respiratory depression is not usually a problem, although nausea and constipation may require concurrent treatment with other agents (e.g. phenothiazines and laxatives). The oral bioavailability of morphine is poor due to the large first-pass effect; nevertheless, small doses of regular oral morphine may be remarkably effective in the management of terminal pain. It has been suggested that the first-pass effect of morphine gradually decreases with its chronic oral administration, or that accumulation of the active metabolite (morphine-6-glucuronide) occurs. Although compound elixirs containing diamorphine (e.g. cocaine and diamorphine elixir) have been widely used in the past, they have no significant advantages compared with oral morphine.

Other opioid analgesics are sometimes given by oral administration in terminal pain due to malignant disease. Methadone and its analogues (e.g. dipipanone) may be useful, since they have a relatively long half-life and a high oral bioavailability. Drugs that are effective by sublingual administration (e.g. phenazocine and buprenorphine) may be particularly useful due to their rapid onset of action.

In advanced malignant disease, problems with swallowing may occur; in these conditions, morphine suppositories can be used, or opioids can be given parenterally. Thus, morphine (or preferably diamorphine because of its high aqueous solubility) can be given by continuous subcutaneous infusion, using a battery-driven syringe driver.

Simple analgesics

Simple analgesics (also known as antipyretic or non-opioid analgesics) are commonly used in the treatment of mild or moderate pain. Since most of them also possess a variable degree of anti-inflammatory activity, they are frequently referred to as NSAIDs. Nevertheless, it should be recognized that not all of these drugs have anti-inflammatory effects; for example, paracetamol has little or no effect on inflammatory processes, and may not be an effective analgesic when pain is associated with inflammation. Similarly, relatively high doses of aspirin (> 3 g per day) are usually necessary to produce significant anti-inflammatory effects (Table 11.6). NSAIDs mainly act at peripheral sites, and are usually administered orally. They are principally used in the treatment of mild or moderate pain associated with somatic structures; they are of limited value in the treatment of severe visceral pain. Nevertheless, some NSAIDs may be used in the management of renal colic, and are increasingly used in the control of pain during the perioperative period. In minor surgery, they may eliminate the need for additional analgesia, and they can significantly reduce opioid requirements after major procedures.

Mode of action

Many NSAIDs modify nociceptive responses induced by certain polypeptides (e.g. bradykinin). Bradykinin is rapidly synthesized during tissue injury from an α_2-globulin in plasma (bradykininogen; plasma kininogen I), which is converted to a decapeptide (lysyl-bradykinin) by a plasma or tissue enzyme (kallikrein).

Table 11.6 The analgesic, antipyretic and anti-inflammatory activity of simple analgesic drugs.

Drug	Analgesic activity	Antipyretic activity	Anti-inflammatory activity
Aspirin (< 3 g day^{-1})	++	++	–
Aspirin (> 3 g day^{-1})	+++	+++	++
Paracetamol	++	++	–
Phenylbutazone	+	+	+++
Indomethacin	+	+	+++
Naproxen	+	+	++
Ibuprofen	+	+	+
Diclofenac	+	+	+++

–, Absent; +, slight; ++, moderate; +++, marked.

Subsequently, lysyl-bradykinin is converted to the active nonapeptide bradykinin. In the circulation and most tissues, bradykinin has a half-life of 10–20 s; it is rapidly broken down by the enzyme kininase II, also known as angiotensin-converting enzyme (ACE). Consequently, ACE inhibitors (Chapter 14) may prolong the half-life of bradykinin.

The hyperaemia, pain and oedema of the inflammatory response are partly mediated by bradykinin and related polypeptides; high concentrations of bradykinin can be identified in inflammatory exudates and synovial fluid from arthritic joints. Bradykinin stimulates sensory nerve endings, and subcutaneous administration in humans causes intense, evanescent pain. Approximately 25 years ago, it was shown that these effects could be antagonized by aspirin (although the drug has no direct action on the synthesis, degradation or action of bradykinin). It was subsequently shown that aspirin inhibited the synthesis of prostaglandins (PGs), which normally sensitize nerve endings to the action of bradykinin; the synthesis of both mediators is usually increased by tissue injury. In particular, PGE_2 sensitizes nerve endings to bradykinin and similar peptides that stimulate peripheral sensory pathways (as well as histamine and 5-HT). Consequently, subcutaneous infusion of PGE_2 in humans produces oedema and lowers the pain threshold to artificial stimuli, although spontaneous pain does not occur. When bradykinin or histamine is subsequently infused into the site, intense pain is produced.

In the 1930s, human seminal fluid was shown to cause contraction of isolated smooth muscle. Approximately 30 years later, the active agents were isolated as a series of unsaturated fatty acid derivatives, and given the name prostaglandins; they are sometimes known as eicosanoids, since they are related to the 20C acid, eicosanoic acid. Prostaglandins were subsequently identified in almost all tissues in the body. They are synthesized in increased amounts after tissue injury (from the inactive precursor arachidonic acid) by the enzyme prostaglandin synthetase or

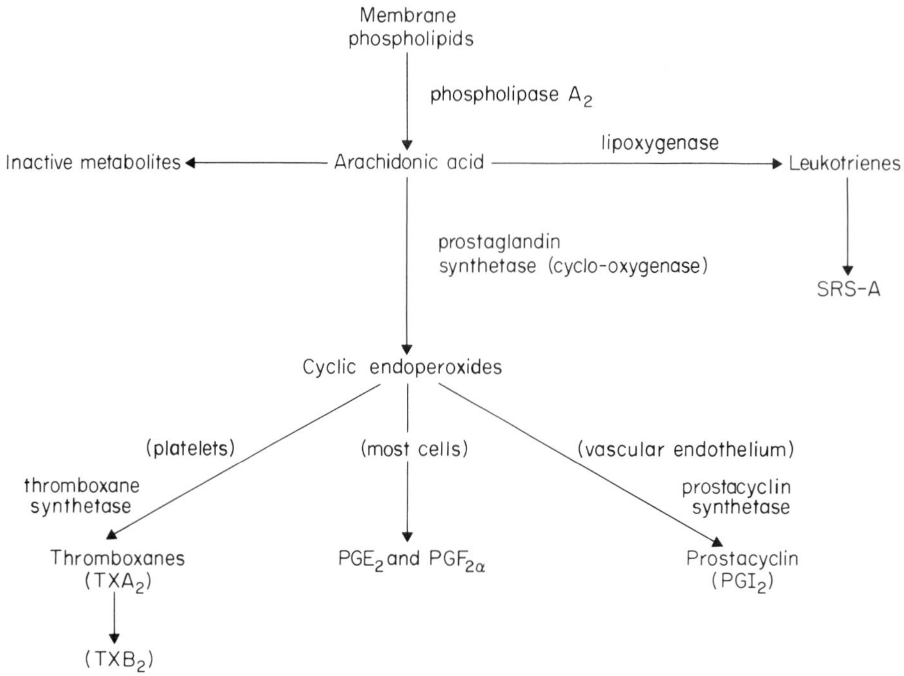

Fig. 11.5 The synthesis of prostaglandins from membrane phospholipids.

cyclooxygenase (Fig. 11.5); the conversion of arachidonic acid to precursor prostaglandins (PGG_2 and PGH_2, also known as cyclic endoperoxides) is inhibited by aspirin and all NSAIDs. The inactive precursor arachidonic acid is present in the phospholipid membrane of almost all cells, from which it is released by the lysosomal enzyme phospholipase A_2; this step is inhibited by lipocortin, a protein whose synthesis is controlled by glucocorticoids (Chapter 17). Thus, glucocorticoids inhibit the formation of arachidonic acid, while NSAIDs inhibit its conversion to prostaglandins (Fig. 11.5).

The subsequent formation of prostaglandins depends on the tissue concerned. In most tissues, cyclic endoperoxides are converted to prostaglandins of the D_2, E_2 and $F_{2\alpha}$ series; these prostaglandins have complex effects on inflammation, smooth-muscle activity, glandular secretions, renal function, peripheral blood vessels and bone resorption. Some of them are formed in bone, and are synthesized in bone metastases.

In platelets, a series of prostaglandin derivatives, the thromboxanes, are formed by the enzyme thromboxane synthetase; thromboxane A_2 (TXA_2) induces platelet aggregation and adhesion, and causes vasoconstriction. By contrast, in vascular endothelial cells, prostacyclin (PGI_2) is formed by the enzyme prostacyclin synthetase; in general it has opposite effects to the thromboxanes (i.e. it inhibits platelet aggregation and causes vasodilatation). It is believed that the balance between the formation of thromboxanes (by the platelets) and PGI_2 (by the vascular endothelium) plays an important role in maintaining the integrity of platelets in circulating blood. When this balance is disturbed, thrombosis may occur. In gastric mucosal cells, PGI_2 and other prostaglandins are synthesized; they may have a protective role in preventing mucosal damage. A series of related compounds, the leukotrienes, are synthesized in white cells (and other tissues) from arachidonic acid by the enzyme lipoxygenase (Fig. 11.5); slow-reacting substance of anaphylaxis (SRS-A) is probably identical with leukotrienes C_4 and D_4. This substance plays an important role in mediating bronchoconstriction in allergic and anaphylactic conditions.

Many prostaglandins are highly unstable, and have extremely short half-lives; for example, TXA_2 and PGI_2 have a half-life of approximately 30 s. Prostaglandins of the series E_2 and $F_{2\alpha}$ are almost entirely metabolized in a single passage through the pulmonary circulation. Other prostaglandins are removed to a lesser extent.

Most of the actions of aspirin and other NSAIDs can be explained in terms of their effects on prostaglandin synthesis. Their anti-inflammatory activity is at least partly due to decreased synthesis of PGE_2 and $PGF_{2\alpha}$. Their effects on platelet aggregation and adhesiveness may reflect the inhibition of thromboxane synthesis, whilst their side-effects in promoting gastric irritation and ulceration may relate to decreased prostaglandin synthesis by gastric mucosal cells.

Two isoenzymes of cyclooxygenase have now been identified. Cyclooxygenase-1 (COX-1), the constitutive form, is considered to be responsible for the production of prostaglandins which regulate renal and haemostatic function (PGE_2, PGI_2, TXA_2) and for the mucosal protective barrier effect. In contrast, cyclooxygenase-2 (COX-2) is an inducible enzyme which is produced in response to tissue trauma (probably via intermediates such as cytokines) and is thus responsible for the inflammatory chain of events.

It has been proposed that the inhibition of COX-1 is principally responsible for the side-effects of NSAIDs, whilst inhibition of the other isoenzyme accounts for their anti-inflammatory properties. The various NSAIDs available would appear to block the two isoenzymes to differing extents; naproxen and diclofenac affect both equally, whilst indomethacin and aspirin have a 50-fold greater effect on COX-1, which would account for the enhanced toxicity of the latter two drugs. The development of selective inhibitors of COX-2 appears to offer significant therapeutic advantages.

Not all the effects of NSAIDs are related to the suppression of the synthesis of prostaglandins at peripheral sites. It is postulated that some of the beneficial effects of such drugs in rheumatoid arthritis and related diseases are due to direct inhibition of neutrophil activity and function. NSAIDs may also have analgesic effects unrelated to cyclooxygenase inhibition which may involve an increase in plasma β-endorphin and inhibition of phosphodiesterase. Prostaglandins are present in the CNS; the antipyretic effects of these agents are largely due to suppression of PGE_2 in the hypothalamic region. Experimental evidence also suggests that NSAIDs may also exert antinociceptive effects at thalamic levels.

Aspirin

Aspirin (acetylsalicylic acid; Fig. 11.6) is a derivative of salicylic acid, which is produced from the glycoside salicin obtained from willow bark. It was introduced into medicine in 1899; since then, it has become one of the cheapest and most widely used drugs in the world.

Aspirin is most commonly used for its analgesic, antipyretic and anti-inflammatory effects. It is most effective in low-intensity somatic pain, rather than severe visceral pain. Aspirin has little or no effect on normal body temperature, although it characteristically reduces temperature rapidly in febrile patients. Toxic doses frequently cause hyperthermia accompanied by an increased metabolic rate and raised oxygen consumption, associated with abnormal cellular respiration. The anti-inflammatory actions of aspirin are closely related to the decreased production of prostaglandins (particularly PGE_2); however, relatively high doses of aspirin are required to produce these effects. In general, daily dosage of 3–6 g per day usually decreases inflammatory responses, but may produce unacceptable side-effects.

Aspirin produces complex effects on acid–base balance. Therapeutic doses of aspirin commonly increase oxygen consumption and carbon dioxide production; this is mainly due to the uncoupling of oxidative phosphorylation (i.e. the conversion of adenosine diphosphate to adenosine triphosphate and the conservation of energy during cellular respiration). There is usually a compensatory increase in alveolar ventilation so that $P\text{aco}_2$ remains constant. When the plasma concentration of salicylate is higher (e.g. with high dosage or overdosage), a CSF acidosis occurs; this may affect the activity of the medullary centres, producing hyperventilation and respiratory alkalosis. In addition, high concentrations of salicylates directly stimulate the respiratory centre, producing increased ventilation and respiratory alkalosis, with a rise in pH and a fall in $P\text{aco}_2$. This may be partially compensated for by the increased renal excretion of bicarbonate. Hyperventilation and respiratory alkalosis

Aspirin (acetylsalicylic acid)

Paracetamol (*p*-acetylaminophenol)

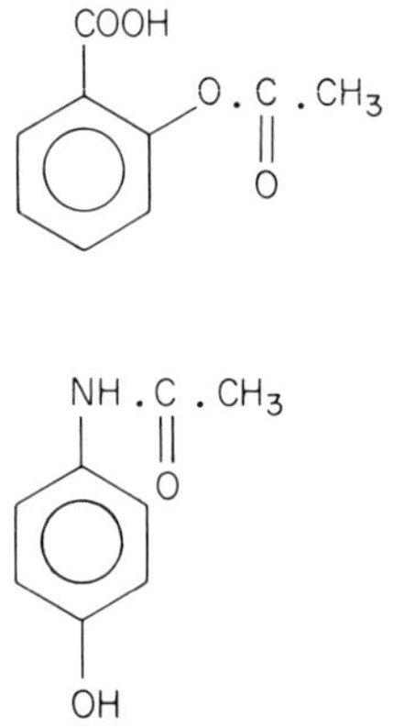

Fig. 11.6 The chemical structure of aspirin and paracetamol.

are common presenting features of aspirin overdosage in adults; terminally, an acidotic state (due to respiratory and metabolic changes) may supervene.

In children, a different clinical picture frequently occurs during aspirin overdosage. Hyperventilation is rare, and the rise in plasma salicylate levels usually depresses the respiratory centre (causing respiratory acidosis). In addition, a true metabolic acidosis develops (due to salicylate dissociation, and the accumulation of lactic and pyruvic acid). These changes are partly due to the uncoupling of oxidative phosphorylation, and partly to vasomotor depression and reduced renal perfusion. Consequently, in childhood, aspirin overdosage usually presents as a combination of respiratory and metabolic acidosis.

Aspirin also reduces platelet adhesion and aggregation; these effects occur with small single doses (as little as 40 mg), and may last for 4–7 days. Aspirin irreversibly acetylates the cyclooxygenase enzyme present in platelets. Consequently, new platelets must be formed from megakaryocytes before normal thromboxane production is restored. For this reason, aspirin has been widely studied for its possible role in preventing vascular thrombosis. In theory, it should only be of value when the production of thromboxanes and PGI_2 is imbalanced, since these two mediators produce opposing effects on platelets and blood vessels. However, this situation may be present when the vascular endothelium is damaged (e.g. by atheroma). Aspirin is sometimes used after cardiopulmonary bypass surgery to prevent graft occlusion, and may help prevent thrombotic episodes associated with mitral stenosis. In recent years, it has also been used in patients with transient ischaemic attacks, in order to prevent the occurrence of major cerebrovascular embolism or thrombosis. In addition to its effects on platelets, aspirin may also decrease prothrombin synthesis (and possibly that of other clotting factors); however relatively high doses (more than 3 g per day) may be required to produce hypoprothrombinaemia.

Aspirin may also affect renal function. In low doses (1–2 g per day), it may cause urate retention (due to inhibition of the tubular secretion of urate anions). In high dosage (> 5 g per day), it is an effective uricosuric agent, since it also inhibits the tubular reabsorption of urates. Unfortunately, these doses usually produce unacceptable side-effects. Aspirin can also produce complex effects on carbohydrate metabolism. In therapeutic doses, it may lower blood glucose (due to increased tissue utilization), and can potentiate the effects of insulin or oral hypoglycaemic agents. Conversely, high doses may cause hyperglycaemia by increasing adrenal cortical and medullary activity.

Unfortunately, the side-effects of aspirin frequently limit its dosage and its therapeutic use. High doses (more than 5–6 g per day) frequently cause the condition of salicylism, with confusion, dizziness, nausea and vomiting, tinnitus, deafness, sweating, tachycardia and hyperventilation. These effects are usually associated with plasma concentrations of 300 $\mu g\ ml^{-1}$ or above. In particular, tinnitus may be produced by high therapeutic doses, and may be used as a guide to the plasma concentration of the drug in patients on high-dose aspirin. In addition, aspirin frequently produces gastrointestinal side-effects which limit its dosage (e.g. dyspepsia, gastric erosions, reactivation of peptic ulceration). Approximately 70% of patients on aspirin lose 5–15 ml of blood daily. Occasionally, aspirin causes haematemesis or severe gastrointestinal haemorrhage, which is probably due to a hypersensitivity reaction. Some of these effects may be related to the inhibition of prostaglandin production (particularly PGI_2) by gastric mucosal cells. However, physicochemical factors suggest that high concentrations of acetylsalicylate or salicylate ions may be present in gastric mucosal cells due to non-ionic diffusion and salicylate trapping (Chapter 1).

Hypersensitivity reactions to aspirin occasionally occur, particularly in atopic individuals with a history of infantile eczema or asthma. These may present as bronchospasm, angioedema, skin rashes or rhinitis; rarely, blood dyscrasias and thrombocytopenia may occur. Drug interactions may occur with oral anticoagulants or with uricosuric drugs (e.g. probenecid and sulphinpyrazone).

In recent years, it has been suggested that the incidence of Reye's syndrome is commoner in children with febrile illnesses who are given aspirin. Reye's syndrome is a rare condition that produces hepatic damage and encephalopathy, and has a high mortality rate. Consequently, aspirin should not be given to children under the age of 12 years.

Aspirin poisoning is not uncommon; after aspirin overdosage, patients are usually conscious and the effects on acid–base balance are often an important clinical feature. Gastric lavage may be worthwhile for up to 12 h after overdosage; in addition, forced alkaline diuresis, using intravenous bicarbonate, may accelerate the renal elimination of salicylates. Haemodialysis and charcoal haemoperfusion may also be of value.

Absorption, distribution and elimination

Aspirin is usually administered orally, and is well-absorbed from the gastrointestinal tract. Absorption from the stomach is favoured by the presence of salicylate in a non-ionized form ($pK_a = 3.5$); however, significant amounts may be trapped as salicylate anions in the relatively alkaline mucosal cells. Absorption from the small intestine is probably more important, due to its larger surface area (Chapter 1).

After absorption, aspirin is rapidly hydrolysed by esterase enzymes in the intestinal mucosa and the liver to salicylate ions; consequently, in the systemic circulation most of the drug is present as salicylate. Both aspirin and salicylate ions are rapidly distributed throughout most tissues, and readily cross most cellular barriers. Binding to plasma proteins occurs; 80–90% is bound to plasma albumin, although the free fraction is increased in patients with hypoalbuminaemia. Salicylates are mainly metabolized in the liver to salicyluric acid, a phenolic glucuronide and an ester glucuronide. Some steps in the metabolism of salicylates are saturable — in particular, the conversion of salicylate to salicylurate (glycine conjugation).

The unchanged drug and its metabolites are eliminated by the kidney and their excretion is enhanced by an alkaline urine. The terminal half-life depends on the dosage, since saturation of glycine conjugation occurs; with normal therapeutic doses, the half-life of salicylate is approximately 4–12 h. In drug overdosage, the half-life may increase due to zero-order metabolism, and it can be up to 30 h.

Clinical uses

Aspirin is commonly used for its analgesic and anti-inflammatory effects. It is particularly useful for the non-specific relief of many types of pain of moderate intensity, and for the symptomatic relief of painful conditions associated with inflammatory processes (e.g. rheumatic diseases and musculoskeletal disorders). Its antipyretic effects may provide increased comfort in febrile conditions, but are unlikely to alter the course of the underlying disease.

Aspirin may also be used for its antiplatelet and antithrombotic effects (e.g. in the secondary prevention of myocardial infarction and the prevention of cerebrovascular accidents).

Aspirin is sometimes used in other conditions. Salicylates and related drugs may be used in the management of diarrhoea associated with irradiation of pelvic tumours, or certain bacterial toxins. In these conditions, there may be increased release of prostaglandins from the damaged gut wall. Similarly, certain malignant tumours may synthesize substantial amounts of prostaglandins and their derivatives. These compounds may influence the uptake of metastatic deposits in bone, and the subsequent bone resorption, destruction and pain. In these conditions, aspirin and related inhibitors of prostaglandin synthesis may be extremely valuable.

Other preparations of aspirin

In the high dosage required to produce anti-inflammatory effects, aspirin may produce unacceptable and intolerable effects on the gastrointestinal tract. Whenever possible, aspirin should be given in the form of dispersible tablets and dissolved before administration. In addition, various formulations and buffered preparations of aspirin are available. Some of these may increase the pH of gastric juice, and increase the ionization of the parent drug, thus decreasing its absorption from the stomach. The ionized drug dissolves readily in gastric secretions, rapidly passes into the small intestine and is distributed over the large absorptive surface. Enteric-coated preparations that dissolve in the higher pH of the small intestine are also available (e.g. Nu-Seals). Benorylate is an ester of aspirin and paracetamol, which is hydrolysed after absorption. These drugs may have an improved gastric tolerance, and a reduced tendency to produce gastrointestinal side-effects.

Phenylbutazone and indomethacin

Phenylbutazone and indomethacin have pronounced anti-inflammatory effects (due to inhibition of cyclooxygenase). Unfortunately, they are both toxic drugs, and are less effective analgesics than aspirin for pain of non-specific origin. In particular, phenylbutazone produces serious adverse effects, such as agranulocytosis and aplastic anaemia; it may also cause sodium retention and precipitate cardiac failure. In the UK, its use is now restricted to hospital practice, and it is only used in the treatment of ankylosing spondylitis. Indomethacin causes headaches and gastrointestinal side-effects; it is less likely to cause blood dyscrasias, and is sometimes used in the treatment of acute gout. Both drugs are extensively bound by plasma proteins, and may be involved in significant drug interactions. Phenylbutazone may also induce or inhibit hepatic enzyme systems. In recent years, the use of both drugs has significantly declined.

Other NSAIDs

In recent years many other NSAIDs have been synthesized and used in the treatment of rheumatic conditions and injuries (Table 11.7). All of these drugs inhibit cyclooxygenase and have anti-inflammatory effects; however, most of them are relatively poor analgesics and antipyretics. Many of them were developed as possible alternatives to aspirin, but without its tendency to produce gastrointestinal side-effects. However, since their anti-inflammatory effects and gastrointestinal side-effects may both be related to the inhibition of both forms of cyclooxygenase, they all, to some extent, have these disadvantages. All drugs that decrease the synthesis of PGI_2 by the gastric mucosa may affect the normal balance between gastric acid secretion and mucus production, and may thus be poorly tolerated.

In general, NSAIDs should not be prescribed for patients with a history of peptic ulceration; however, many patients who develop ulcers when given NSAIDs

Table 11.7 A chemical classification of simple analgesics and non-steroidal anti-inflammatory drugs.

Enolic acids		Carboxylic acids			
Oxicams	Pyrazolones	Acetic acid derivatives	Fenamates	Salicylates	Propionates
Piroxicam Tenoxicam	Phenylbutazone Azapropazone	Diclofenac Etodolac Ketorolac Indomethacin Sulindac Tolmetin	Mefenamic acid Flufenamic acid	Aspirin Diflunisal Benorylate	Fenbufen Fenoprofen Flurbiprofen Ibuprofen Ketoprofen Naproxen Tiaprofenic acid

have no previous history of dyspepsia. Complications are much commoner in the over-60s (particularly in women). The incidence of gastrointestinal side-effects may be considerably reduced by the use of histamine (H_2) antagonists. Alternatively, the prostaglandin analogue misoprostol may provide some protection against the development of gastric ulceration in susceptible patients. In addition, NSAIDs should always be taken with food or milk.

Inhibition of prostaglandin synthesis may also cause impairment of renal function. NSAIDs reduce renal blood flow and glomerular filtration rate in some groups of patients, particularly elderly subjects. Other predisposing factors are chronic heart failure, hepatic cirrhosis, hypovolaemia and concurrent treatment with diuretics and certain antihypertensive agents. NSAIDs may also cause hyperkalaemia and fluid retention. Some of the individual agents are highly protein-bound and can potentiate the action of anticoagulants, hydantoins, lithium and certain sulphonamides; in addition, various adverse effects such as blood dyscrasias and skin rashes have been reported with their use.

The main differences between individual NSAIDs are concerned with the incidence and the occurrence of side-effects (which in general resemble those produced by aspirin). In addition, there is a marked variability in patient response. In the UK, approximately 15 of these drugs are available; naproxen, ibuprofen, sulindac, azapropazone and diclofenac are among the most commonly used NSAIDs.

Naproxen is an effective anti-inflammatory drug, but has a relatively low incidence of gastrointestinal side-effects. Since it has a relatively long half-life, it can be given twice daily. It is commonly used in the treatment of acute gout.

Ibuprofen is a relatively mild anti-inflammatory drug that produces fewer side-effects than naproxen. Although it is widely used in certain conditions (e.g. in dental pain), it has a low affinity for cyclooxygenase, and is not suitable for the management of conditions in which inflammation is a prominent feature (e.g. ankylosing spondylitis).

Sulindac has similar properties to naproxen (although it is closely related chemically to indomethacin). The parent drug is inactive (i.e. it is a prodrug), and only produces slight effects on prostaglandins in the gastrointestinal tract. However, sulindac is metabolized to a sulphide metabolite that is a potent inhibitor of cyclooxygenase. It undergoes extensive enterohepatic recirculation, and thus provides a reservoir of the active drug. It is usually given twice daily.

Azapropazone is chemically related to phenylbutazone; however, it does not appear to cause blood dyscrasias (although it may cause skin rashes). It is commonly used in the treatment of gout. It is not extensively metabolized.

NSAIDs in anaesthetic practice

The use of NSAIDs in the management of postoperative pain has gained considerable popularity in recent years. In this context both diclofenac and ketorolac have been widely used.

Diclofenac is a potent inhibitor of the cyclooxygenase pathway, but in addition the production of leukotrienes is decreased. This implies that diclofenac may reduce the availability of arachidonic acid or exhibit an inhibitory effect on the lipoxygenase pathway, which may enhance its anti-inflammatory properties. Diclofenac is available both as an oral (including a slow-release formulation) and an intramuscular preparation and in four different strengths in suppository form. Diclofenac injections may cause pain and should always be administered at deep intramuscular sites.

Ketorolac, in contrast, appears to demonstrate a minimal anti-inflammatory effect at its analgesic dose. The drug is available in tablet form and as a parenteral preparation which may be administered both intramuscularly and intravenously (it is the only NSAID currently available which may be given by the latter route).

Both drugs have been widely used, both as 'pre-emptive' analgesics and in the treatment of postoperative pain. They appear to be particularly beneficial in relation to ear, nose and throat, plastic and minor gynaecological surgery and in certain orthopaedic procedures (especially when supplementary local anaesthetic techniques are used).

Obvious advantages include a lack of respiratory depression and a low incidence of nausea and vomiting when compared with opioid analgesics. Furthermore, no significant drug interactions are likely with opioids used concomitantly. Nevertheless, the perioperative use of NSAIDs must be viewed with caution. Problems may be encountered when these drugs (particularly ketorolac) are administered to patients with a history of asthma; these drugs must be used sparingly, if at all, where there is impairment of renal function or if attenuation of antihypertensive therapy (e.g. with diuretics or ACE inhibitors) could ensue. The usual haematological disorders and bleeding tendencies are an absolute contraindication to their use and significant haemorrhage during and after surgery has resulted when these NSAIDs have been used concomitantly with low-dose heparin regimes; ketorolac is specifically contraindicated in this respect.

Paracetamol

Although paracetamol was synthesized more than 100 years ago, it has only been widely used as an analgesic since 1949. Paracetamol has analgesic and antipyretic effects that are similar to aspirin; however, it has little if any anti-inflammatory activity. It has been suggested that it only inhibits prostaglandin synthesis in the CNS, although it has little effect on cyclooxygenase in *in vitro* conditions. Nevertheless, it is usually classified with the NSAIDs, since it has similar effects to aspirin on non-specific pain. Paracetamol is widely used in the treatment of pain of moderate intensity such as headache, toothache, dysmenorrhoea and pains of musculoskeletal origin. Similarly, it is incorporated into many compound preparations containing aspirin, pentazocine, dextropropoxyphene or codeine and its derivatives.

Paracetamol is well-absorbed from the gastrointestinal tract and does not cause gastric irritation or bleeding. Although it is an active metabolite of phenacetin and acetanilide, in normal doses it is relatively free from toxic effects. Occasionally, skin rashes, methaemoglobinaemia and haemolytic anaemia may occur; in some cases, haematological side-effects may be related to a deficiency of erythrocyte glucose-6-phosphate dehydrogenase.

After absorption, paracetamol is not significantly bound to plasma proteins. It is almost completely metabolized by the liver; approximately 60% is eliminated as a glucuronide conjugate, and the remainder as sulphate and cysteine conjugates. Only trace amounts are eliminated unchanged in urine.

Paracetamol overdosage can produce potentially fatal hepatic necrosis; in the UK, it is involved in approximately 15% of all hospital admissions for drug overdosage (and 7% of all deaths, mainly due to its delayed presentation). Liver damage due to acute overdosage has been reported after the ingestion of as little as 5 g. More commonly, it is produced by more than 10–15 g (i.e. 20–30 tablets) of the drug. Small amounts of paracetamol are metabolized to an aryl metabolite with a high affinity for sulphydryl groups (*N*-acetyl-*p*-amino-benzoquinoneimine). After normal doses, this toxic metabolite is innocuous, since it is inactivated by conjugation with hepatic glutathione. In paracetamol overdosage, the hepatic reserves of glutathione (and other sulphydryl donors, e.g. methionine) are conjugated and depleted; in these conditions, the toxic metabolite combines covalently with sulphydryl groups in liver macromolecules, producing subacute hepatic necrosis (Fig. 11.7). If patients are on enzyme-inducing drugs, the risk of significant hepatic damage is considerably greater.

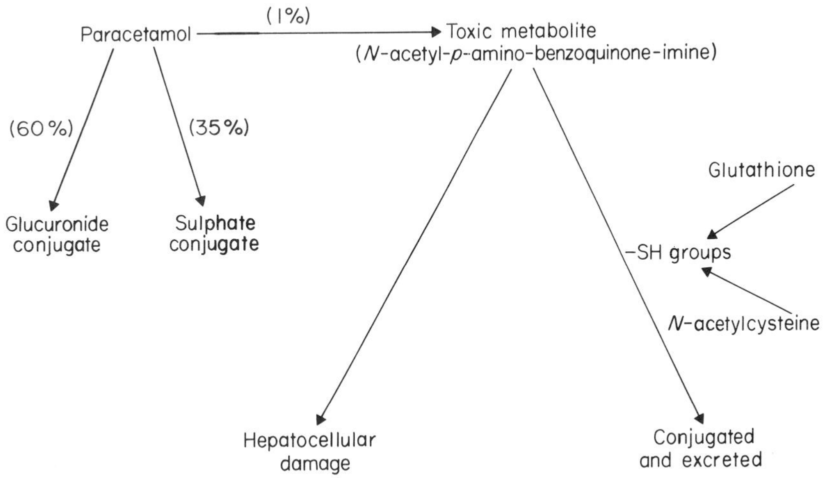

Fig. 11.7 The metabolism of paracetamol. In overdosage, a toxic metabolite produces hepatocellular damage, unless it is conjugated by sulphydryl (—SH) groups.

Unless specific therapy is given, some degree of centrilobular hepatic necrosis will occur in 10–20% of poisoned patients, and 2–3% will die in hepatic failure. Signs of liver damage are usually delayed for 2–5 days after overdosage; the initial symptoms (e.g. nausea, vomiting, abdominal pain) may regress, thus engendering a false sense of security.

Immediate treatment is essential in paracetamol overdosage, since sulphydryl donors (e.g. methionine, cysteamine and *N*-acetylcysteine) can conjugate the toxic metabolite and prevent liver damage if given soon after an acute overdose. Treatment includes gastric lavage (if the patient is seen within 4 h of paracetamol ingestion), intravenous fluids and the cautious use of antiemetics (if there is persistent nausea and vomiting). The sulphydryl donor *N*-acetylcysteine is the treatment of choice; however it must be given by intravenous infusion within 12–15 h of ingestion of the drug, since it is ineffective and may be dangerous if given at a later stage. Plasma paracetamol levels are invaluable in the assessment of the severity of overdosage, and provide a guide to the possible effectiveness of treatment with *N*-acetylcysteine. Vitamin K and other clotting factors may be necessary for the management of coagulation defects.

Analgesic nephropathy

Renal papillary necrosis and chronic interstitial nephritis may occur following the prolonged intake of some NSAIDs, particularly compound proprietary analgesic preparations. In the past, phenacetin was frequently implicated as the causative agent; however, nephropathy will probably occur when any analgesic drug is continually used over a long period of time. Renal complications produced by analgesic drugs may be related to impaired synthesis of prostaglandins, since many prostaglandins are produced by the kidney (e.g. PGE_2, PGI_2). After administration of NSAIDs, the response to renal vasoconstrictors (e.g. noradrenaline and angiotensin II) may be enhanced. In practice, analgesic nephropathy is commoner in compulsive drug users who show mild personality disorders, rather than in patients with rheumatic disorders who are on continuous therapy. The prognosis is good, and renal function may completely recover if all analgesics are withdrawn.

Nefopam

Nefopam is chemically related to diphenhydramine. Its mode of action is unknown, and it is not usually classified as an opioid or a simple analgesic. It is normally free from opioid side-effects such as respiratory depression and drug dependence. Nefopam blocks the uptake of noradrenaline by sympathetic nerve endings, and can also produce numerous atropine-like side-effects. However, it may also induce excessive sweating, and its antimuscarinic effects may be mediated within the CNS, rather than peripherally. Nefopam has been successfully used in musculoskeletal and cancer pain.

Specific analgesics

In specific circumstances, many drugs that are not primarily analgesics may be beneficial in the management of pain. Thus, anticholinergic drugs are of value in the treatment of smooth-muscle spasms. Similarly, pain which arises due to spasm of striated muscle (e.g. upper motor neurone lesions, spasmodic torticollis, muscle tension headaches), may be relieved by centrally acting muscle relaxants. These agents, which increase the effectiveness of the inhibitory transmitter GABA, include the benzodiazepines and the GABA agonist baclofen (Chapter 13). Drugs that affect the calibre of blood vessels are also important. Vasodilators will provide symptomatic relief of pain due to ischaemia of somatic or visceral structures; conversely, the ergot alkaloids, which have partial agonist effects on α-adrenoceptors in extracranial blood vessels, play an important role in the treatment of migraine.

Some of the chemical excitants of a painful impulse may be inactivated or antagonized by specific drugs. Examples include antacid therapy for peptic ulcer, and the use of 5-HT antagonists in the prophylaxis of migraine. The hormone calcitonin produces symptomatic relief in patients with Paget's disease, and occasionally in other forms of bone pain; it has been suggested that these effects are related to a translocation of phosphate ions.

Psychotropic drugs are often used as adjuncts in pain therapy. In addition to their action on the reactive components of pain (e.g. anxiety and misery), they may have more specific effects. Phenothiazines potentiate the effects of opioid analgesics, and may produce analgesia as part of a generalized deafferentation. Tricyclic antidepressants are thought to facilitate transmission in descending fibres that release 5-HT; consequently, they may modify C-fibre input at the substantia gelatinosa.

Treatment of migraine

The aetiology of migraine is complex. It has been suggested that attacks of migraine are caused by the initial release of 5-HT, which triggers the cerebral vasoconstriction and the associated prodromal symptoms. Further release of 5-HT may occur, due to platelet aggregation. The headache corresponds to the phase of dilatation of extracranial vessels, and may be mediated by the increased production of histamine and plasma kinins, while plasma 5-HT levels are decreasing. Current views implicate the triggering of neurogenic inflammation, resulting in plasma extravasation in the dura with resultant nociceptive responses relayed to the most caudal part of the trigeminal nucleus and the dorsal horn of C1 and C2 segments of the spinal cord.

Acute attacks are commonly managed with NSAIDs; the inhibitory effects on platelet aggregation may be an added advantage. These drugs are often combined with ergot alkaloids, which maintain vessel tone by stimulating α-adrenoceptors. For continuous prophylaxis, drugs which antagonize the peripheral effects of 5-HT, histamine and the kinins have been used; these include methysergide, cyproheptadine and pizotifen.

More recently, attention has been diverted to the maintenance of 5-HT receptor activity during the acute phase of migraine. Sumatriptan is an agonist at receptors of the 5-HT_1 subtype (groups B and D) which reduces vasodilatation in the carotid circulation without compromising cerebral blood flow. Sumatriptan is available in tablet and injection form, and a single dose may often ablate an attack. However, if symptomatic relief does not occur, a further dose should not be administered during the same attack, nor should ergotamine be used until 6 h have elapsed. Cardiac pain and transient hypertension are side-effects.

The β-adrenoceptor antagonist propranolol may be used in the management of migrainous neuralgia and atypical facial pain. The mode of action in this context is unclear but it may be related to antagonistic effects on β_2-adrenoceptors in the extracranial vessels, or possibly to inhibitory effects on the synthesis and release of 5-HT from the pineal body. There is some evidence that calcium-channel blockers which principally affect the peripheral vasculature (e.g. nifedipine) may have a role in the prophylaxis of migraine; presumably these effects are related to attenuation of changes in tone of vascular smooth muscle.

Treatment of trigeminal neuralgia

In trigeminal neuralgia, the sudden attacks of severe lancinating pain are inadequately managed by conventional analgesic therapy. The aetiology of the condition is unknown, but the paroxysmal nature of the pain suggests that it is a type of focal sensory epilepsy. It is therefore not surprising that several drugs that were originally introduced into clinical practice for the treatment of epilepsy are effective in the condition; their membrane-stabilizing activity may be of prime importance (particularly on the spinal trigeminal nucleus). The mechanism may involve the reduction of ectopic responses, at concentrations that do not block nerve conduction, involving activated Na^+ channels.

Carbamazepine is the drug of choice. When taken regularly, it is highly effective in controlling the attacks of pain, and 70% of patients gain relief. The development of drug tolerance may be due to an alteration in its pharmacokinetics, since it is known that carbamazepine induces its own metabolism. Side-effects such as drowsiness and ataxia are common, although these may disappear with continued dosage, and gastrointestinal intolerance may occur; blood dyscrasias are an occasional but more serious problem. Other anticonvulsant agents, such as phenytoin and valproate, are logical alternatives to carbamazepine when unacceptable side-effects are present; however, they are not quite as effective. If the symptoms of trigeminal neuralgia are abolished by a surgical procedure or a radiofrequency lesion to the Gasserian ganglion or its appropriate branches, anticonvulsant therapy should be gradually withdrawn, since sudden cessation may induce epileptiform attacks.

Further reading

Akil H, Watson SJ, Young E *et al*. Endogenous opioids; biology and function. *Annual Review of Neuroscience* 1984; **7**: 223–255.

Behar M, Magora F, Olshwang D, Davidson JT. Epidural morphine in the treatment of pain. *Lancet* 1979; **i**: 527–528.

Bovill JG. The opioids in intravenous anaesthesia. In: Dundee JW, Wyant GM (eds) *Intravenous Anaesthesia*. Edinburgh: Churchill Livingstone, 1988; 206–247.

Brunk SF, Delle M. Morphine metabolism in man. *Clinical Pharmacology and Therapeutics* 1974; **16**: 51–57.

Bullingham RES. Synthetic analgesics. In: Atkinson RS, Adams AP (eds) *Recent Advances in Anaesthesia and Analgesia*, no. 15. Edinburgh: Churchill Livingstone, 1985; 43–62.

Carr DB. Opioids. *International Anesthesiology Clinics* 1988; **26**: 273–287.

Carr DB, Murphy MT. Operation, anesthesia, and the endorphin system. *International Anesthesiology Clinics* 1988; **26**: 199–205.

Dray A, Urban L, Dickenson A. Pharmacology of chronic pain. *Trends in Pharmacological Sciences* 1994; **15**: 190–197.

Duggan AW. Nociception and antinociception; physiological studies in the spinal cord. In: Brena SF, Chapman SL (eds) *Chronic Pain: Management Principles. Clinics in Anaesthesiology*, vol. 3. Philadelphia: WB Saunders, 1985; 17–40.

Durant PAC, Yaksh TL. Epidural injections of bupivacaine, morphine, fentanyl, lofentanil, and DADL in chronically implanted rats: a pharmacologic and pathologic study. *Anesthesiology* 1986; **64**: 43–53.

Etches RC, Sandler AN, Daley MD. Respiratory depression and spinal opioids. *Canadian Journal of Anaesthesia* 1989; **36**: 165–185.

Finck AD. Opiate receptors and endogenous opioid peptides. *Current Opinion in Anaesthesiology* 1989; **2**: 428–433.

Fleetwood-Walker S, Mitchell R. Role of substance P in nociception. *Current Opinion in Anaesthesiology* 1989; **2**: 645–648.

Gillman MA. Analgesic (sub-anesthetic) nitrous oxide interacts with the endogenous opioid system; a review of the evidence. *Life Science* 1986; **39**: 1209–1221.

Glass PSA, Hardman D, Kamiyama Y *et al*. Preliminary pharmacokinetics and pharmacodynamics of an ultra-short acting opioid remifentanil (G187084B). *Anesthesia and Analgesia* 1993; **77**: 1031–1040.

Glynn CJ. Intrathecal and epidural administration of opiates. In: Budd K (ed.) *Update in Opioids. Clinical Anaesthesiology*, vol. 1. Edinburgh: Baillière Tindall, 1987; 915–923.

Goodchild CS, Serrao JM. Analgesics and the spinal cord dorsal horn. In: Kaufman L (ed.) *Anaesthesia Review* no. 6. Edinburgh; Churchill Livingstone, 1989; 215–229.

Gregg R. Spinal analgesia. In: Oden RV (ed.) *Management of Postoperative Pain. Anesthesiology Clinics of North America*, vol. 7. Philadelphia: WB Saunders, 1989; 79–100.

Gustafsson LL, Post C, Edvardsen B, Ramsay CH. Distribution of morphine and meperidine after intrathecal administration in rat and mouse. *Anesthesiology* 1985; **63**: 483–489.

Gustafsson LL, Wiesenfeld-Hallin Z. Spinal opioid analgesia. A critical update. *Drugs* 1988; **35**: 597–603.

Hinds CJ, Donaldson MDJ. Endogenous opioids in shock. In: Ledingham IMcA (ed.) *Recent Advances in Critical Care Medicine*. Edinburgh: Churchill Livingstone, 1988; 175–194.

Hug CC Jr. Pharmacokinetics and dynamics of narcotic analgesics. In: Prys-Roberts C, Hug CC Jr (eds) *Pharmacokinetics of Anaesthesia*. Oxford: Blackwell Scientific Publications, 1984; 187–234.

Itzhak Y, Alernand S. Differential regulation of δ and PCP receptors after chronic administration of haloperidol and phencyclidine in mice. *Faseb Journal* 1989; **3**: 1868–1872.

James MK, Feldman PL, Schuster SV. Opioid receptor activity of G187084B a novel ultra-short-acting opioid, in isolated tissues. *Journal of Pharmacology and Experimental Therapeutics* 1991; **259**: 712–718.

Jordan CC. Opioid receptors. In: Kaufman L (ed.) *Anaesthesia Review*, no. 3. Edinburgh: Churchill Livingstone, 1985; 36–48.

Kaufman L. Pain. In: Kaufman L (ed.) *Anaesthesia Review*, no. 4. Edinburgh: Churchill Livingstone, 1987; 194–206.

Kaufman L. Pain. In: Kaufman L (ed.) *Anaesthesia Review*, no. 6. Edinburgh: Churchill Livingstone, 1989; 203–213.

Konieczko KM, Jones JG, Barrowcliffe MP *et al*. Antagonism of morphine-induced respiratory depression with nalmefene. *British Journal of Anaesthesia* 1988; **61**: 318–323.

Mansour A, Khatchaturian H, Lewis ME *et al*. Autoradiograph differentiation of mu, delta, and kappa opioid receptors in the rat forebrain and midbrain. *Journal of Neuroscience* 1987; **7**: 2445–2464.

Martin WR, Eades CG, Thompson JA *et al*. The effects of morphine- and nalorphine-like drugs in the non-dependent chronic spinal dog. *Journal of Pharmacology and Experimental Therapeutics* 1976; **97**: 517–532.

Melzack R. Hyperstimulation analgesia. In: Brena SF, Chapman SL (eds) *Chronic Pain: Management Principles. Clinics in Anaesthesiology*, vol. 3. Philadelphia: WB Saunders, 1985; 81–92.

Melzack R, Wall PD. Pain mechanisms: a new theory. *Science* 1965; **150**: 971–979.

Merrell WJ, Gordon L, Wood AJJ *et al*. The effects of halothane on morphine disposition: relative contributions of the liver and kidney to morphine glucuronidation in the dog. *Anesthesiology* 1990; **72**: 308–314.

Mitchell JA, Akaraseenont P, Thiermann C *et al*. Selectivity of nonsteroidal antiinflammatory drugs as inhibitors of constitutive and inducible cyclooxygenase. *Proceedings of the National Academy of Science USA* 1994; **90**: 11693–11697.

Mitchell RWD, Smith G. The control of acute postoperative pain. *British Journal of Anaesthesia* 1989; **63**: 147–158.

Morgan M. Use of intrathecal and extradural opioids. *British Journal of Anaesthesia* 1989; **63**: 165–188.

Munglani R, Fleming BG, Hunt SP. Remembrance of times past: the significance of c-*fos* in pain. *British Journal of Anaesthesia* 1996; **76**: 1–4.

Nishio Y, Sinatra RS, Kitahata LM, Collins JG. Spinal cord distribution of ^{3}H-morphine after intrathecal administration: relationship to analgesia. *Anesthesia and Analgesia* 1989; **69**: 323–327.

Olson GA, Olson RD, Kastin AJ. Review of endogenous opiates: 1985. *Peptides* 1986; **7**: 907–933.

Olson GA, Olson RD, Kastin AJ. Review of endogenous opiates: 1986. *Peptides* 1987; **8**: 1135–1164.

Pasternak GW. Multiple morphine and enkephalin receptors and the relief of pain. *Journal of the American Medical Association* 1988; **259**: 1362–1367.

Pasternak GW. Pharmacological mechanisms of opioid receptors. *Clinical Neuropharmacology* 1993; **16**: 1–18.

Pert CB, Snyder SH. Opiate receptor; demonstration in nervous tissue. *Science* 1973; **179**: 1011–1014.

Pinnock CA. Endorphins. In: Kaufman L (ed.) *Anaesthesia Review*, no. 3. Edinburgh: Churchill Livingstone, 1985; 49–62.

Pleuvry BJ. Opioid receptors and their relevance to anaesthesia. *British Journal of Anaesthesia* 1993; **71**: 119–126.

Raja SN, Meyer RA, Campbell JN. Peripheral mechanisms of somatic pain. *Anesthesiology* 1988; **68**: 571–590.

Rance MJ. Multiple opiate receptors — their occurrence and significance. In: Brena SF, Chapman SL (eds) *Chronic Pain: Management Principles. Clinics in Anaesthesiology*, vol. 3. Philadelphia: WB Saunders, 1985; 183–199.

Reisine T, Bell GI. Molecular biology of opioid receptors. *Trends in Neurosciences* 1993; **16**: 506–510.

Richmond CE, Bromley LM, Woolf CJ. Preoperative morphine pre-empts postoperative pain. *Lancet* 1993; **342**: 73–75.

Roscow C. Newer opioid analgesics and antagonists. In: Fragen RJ (ed.) *New Anesthetic Drugs. Anesthesiology Clinics of North America* 1988; **6**: 319–333.

Simon EJ, Hiller JM, Edelman I. Stereospecific binding of the potent narcotic analgesic [^{3}H]etorphine to rat-brain homogenate. *Proceedings of the National Academy of Science USA* 1973; **70**: 1947–1949.

Smith AP, Lee NM. Pharmacology of dynorphin. *Annual Review of Pharmacology and Toxicology* 1988; **28**: 123–140.

Smythe DG. Opioid peptides and pain. In: Bullingham RES (ed.) *Opiate Analgesia. Clinics in Anaesthesiology*, vol. 1, Philadelphia: WB Saunders, 1983; 201–218.

Sorkin LS. Pain pathways and spinal modulation. In: Oden RV (ed.) *Management of Postoperative Pain. Anesthesiology Clinics of North America*, vol. 7. Philadelphia: WB Saunders, 1989; 17–32.

Staren ED, Cullen ML. Epidural catheter analgesia for the management of postoperative pain. *Surgery, Gynecology and Obstetrics* 1986; **162**: 389–403.

Sun WZ, Shyu BC, Shieh JY. Nitrous oxide or halothane, or both, fail to express c-*fos* activity in rat spinal cord dorsal horn neurones after subcutaneous formalin. *British Journal of Anaesthesia* 1996; **76**: 99–105.

Tempel A, Zukin RS. Neuroanatomical patterns of the μ, δ, and κ opioid receptors of rat brain as determined by quantative *in-vitro* autoradiography. *Proceedings of the National Academy of Science USA* 1987; **84**: 4308–4312.

Terenius L. Stereoscopic interaction between narcotic analgesics and a synaptic plasma membrane fraction of rat cerebral cortex. *Acta Pharmacologica et Toxicologica* 1973; **32**: 317–320.

Thorpe DH. Opiate structure and activity — a guide to understanding the receptor. *Anesthesia and Analgesia* 1984; **63**: 143–151.

Vane J. Towards a better aspirin. *Nature* 1994; **367**: 215–216.

Vane JR, Botting RM. New insights into the mode of action of anti-inflammatory drugs. *Inflammation Research* 1995; **44**: 1–10.

Vickers MD, O'Flaherty D, Szekely SM *et al.* Tramadol: pain relief by an opioid without depression of respiration. *Anaesthesia* 1992; **47**: 291–296.

Walker JM, Bowen WD, Walker FO *et al.* Sigma receptors: biology and function. *Pharmacological Reviews* 1990; **42**: 355–398.

Wang JK, Nauss LA, Thomas JE. Pain relief by intrathecally applied morphine in man. *Anesthesiology* 1979; **50**: 149–151.

Woolf CJ. Recent advances in the pathophysiology of acute pain. *British Journal of Anaesthesia* 1989; **63**: 139–146.

Yaksh TL, Al-Rodhan NRF, Mjanger E. Sites of action of opiates in production of analgesia. In: Kaufman L (ed.) *Anaesthesia Review*, no. 5. Edinburgh: Churchill Livingstone, 1988; 254–268.

Yaksh TL, Rudy TA. Analgesia mediated by a direct spinal action of narcotics. *Science* 1976; **192**: 1357–1358.

Chapter 12
Drugs and the Autonomic Nervous System

Anatomy and physiology of the autonomic nervous system

Autonomic nerves constitute all the efferent fibres which leave the central nervous system (CNS), apart from those which innervate skeletal muscle, and the system is thus widely distributed throughout the body. In all cases, the autonomic outflow makes synaptic connections with the cell bodies of peripheral neurones; such synapses normally occur in clusters or ganglia. Postganglionic fibres, usually unmyelinated, then innervate the effector organs.

The autonomic nervous system is also known as the visceral or automatic system, and in general its activity cannot be influenced by individual will or volition. Cellular functions which are influenced by autonomic transmission are smooth-muscle activity in blood vessels and all viscera, the mechanisms of the specialized muscle fibres of the heart and uterus, the secretory role of the salivary, mucous and eccrine sweat glands and the activity of the adrenal medulla.

Afferent fibres from visceral structures are carried to the CNS usually by major autonomic nerves such as the vagus and splanchnic nerves or the pelvic plexus. They are concerned with the mediation of visceral sensation and the regulation of vasomotor and respiratory reflexes. Specialized examples of afferent autonomic fibres arise from the baroreceptors and chemoreceptors in the carotid sinus and the aortic arch; these are important in the control of heart rate, blood pressure and respiratory activity. Autonomic afferent fibres from blood vessels, which transmit pain impulses, may be carried in somatic nerves.

Autonomic reflex activity will occur at a spinal level, as can be demonstrated in animal experiments and observed in humans following spinal cord transection, whilst vital functions such as respiration and the control of blood pressure are mediated via nuclei in the medulla oblongata. However, central integration of autonomic function occurs principally in the hypothalamus. The hypothalamus is itself under regulatory control by the neocortex, has important connections with the limbic system and exerts a modulatory effect by virtue of efferent pathways to the pituitary gland.

The autonomic nervous system is conveniently divided on anatomical and physiological grounds into two divisions — parasympathetic and sympathetic.

Parasympathetic division

The preganglionic outflow of the parasympathetic division is from certain cranial nerves and the sacral region of the spinal cord. The cells of origin of the cranial fibres are in the midbrain and medulla and the axons are contained in the 3rd, 7th, 9th and 10th cranial nerves. They affect ocular accommodation and salivary gland secretion, while the vagus nerve carries fibres to the heart, lungs and bronchi, stomach and upper intestine.

Sacral outflow occurs from the 2nd, 3rd and 4th sacral segments of the spinal cord. These form pelvic plexuses which innervate the distal colon and rectum, bladder and reproductive organs. Minute ganglia are situated at points of union and in the walls of individual viscera, and postganglionic parasympathetic fibres are thus very short.

In physiological terms, the parasympathetic nervous system is concerned with the conservation and restoration of energy. Thus the heart rate is slowed, the blood pressure falls, and the digestion and absorption of nutrients (plus the excretion of waste material) are facilitated.

Sympathetic division

The cells of origin of this system are located in the lateral horns of the thoracic and upper lumbar segments of the spinal cord. Their axons travel a short distance in the mixed spinal nerves and then branch off as white rami to enter the sympathetic ganglia. These consist of bilateral chains which lie anterolateral to the vertebral bodies and extend from the cervical to the sacral region. The preganglionic fibres which enter the chain may:

1 Make a synaptic connection with a cell body at the same dermatomal level.

2 Traverse to a ganglion at a higher or lower level before forming a synapse (in both (1) and (2) the postganglionic fibres usually return to the adjacent spinal nerve via grey rami).

3 Emerge through medial branches of the sympathetic chain to synapse with prevertebral ganglia and plexuses in the abdominal cavity.

Some preganglionic fibres which emerge from the lower thoracic segments travel in the greater splanchnic nerve and directly synapse with chromaffin cells in the adrenal medulla.

Experimental studies suggest that an intact sympathetic nervous system, while not essential to life, enables the body to be prepared for ‘fear, fight or flight’. Sympathetic responses include increased heart rate and blood pressure, diversion of blood flow from skin and splanchnic vessels to those supplying skeletal muscle, an increase in the availability of glucose due to liver glycogenolysis, pupillary and bronchiolar dilatation and contraction of sphincters.

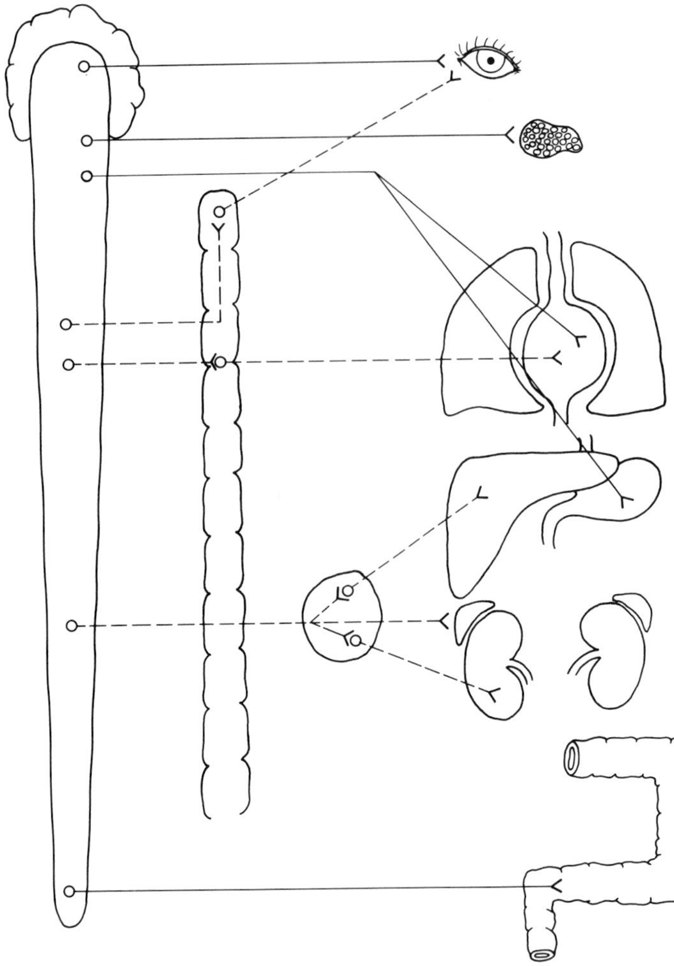

Fig. 12.1 Schematic representation of principal autonomic nerve pathways: parasympathetic (solid line); sympathetic (broken line).

The principal efferent pathways in the autonomic nervous system are illustrated in Fig. 12.1.

Neurotransmitters

Acetylcholine

This neurotransmitter was synthesized by Baeyer in 1868, and in 1914 Dale found that the pharmacological responses to acetylcholine mimicked all the effects of parasympathetic nerve stimulation. The first evidence that neurohumoral transmission occurred was provided by the classical experiments of Otto Loewi in the early 1920s. He stimulated the vagus nerve of a perfused frog's heart and allowed the perfusion fluid to come into contact with a second frog's heart, the rate of which subsequently slowed. He originally called the substance which was released *Vagustoff*, but a few years later it was identified as acetylcholine.

Successive investigations showed that acetylcholine was the neurotransmitter released at the following sites:

1 All postganglionic parasympathetic nerve endings.

2 All autonomic ganglia. All preganglionic fibres (sympathetic or parasympathetic) release acetylcholine at their nerve endings; these include the sympathetic fibres which supply the chromaffin cells of the adrenal medulla.

3 Certain postganglionic sympathetic nerves, such as those supplying the sweat glands.

4 Some vasodilator fibres that supply arterioles in skeletal muscle. However, parasympathetic innervation of vascular smooth muscle appears to be limited, and the mechanism of a vasovagal attack may involve both the direct effects of acetylcholine at non-innervated sites and prejunctional inhibitory effects on sympathetic fibres (see below). It has also been suggested that acetylcholine may act as an intraneuronal precursor in the release of transmitter at all postganglionic sympathetic nerve endings.

In addition, acetylcholine is released at the motor endplate and is an important synaptic transmitter in the CNS.

Nerve fibres that release acetylcholine from their endings are described as cholinergic fibres. The synthesis, storage, release and subsequent fate of acetylcholine is similar at all sites and is more fully described in Chapter 10.

Noradrenaline and adrenaline

In the early years of this century, Langley showed that the actions of an extract of the adrenal gland closely resembled the responses from sympathetic nerve stimulation. He originally suggested that adrenaline was the neurotransmitter involved, although other evidence indicated that the results of stimulation were more accurately mimicked by noradrenaline. Various theories were propounded to explain why injected adrenaline or released 'sympathin' could stimulate some smooth muscle whilst it relaxed others. These included suggestions that the transmitter was modified by receptor substances at the effector site to produce either sympathin I (inhibitory) or sympathin E (excitatory); alternatively it was considered that there were basically two different types of receptors. In the mid 1940s, Von Euler established that noradrenaline was the chemical transmitter released at postganglionic sympathetic nerve endings and that only small quantities of adrenaline (and dopamine) are liberated; these fibres are thus more correctly described as noradrenergic (rather than adrenergic).

Autonomic receptors

Cholinergic receptors

The effects of acetylcholine released from all postganglionic nerve endings (including cholinergic sympathetic fibres) on effector organs can be mimicked by the mushroom alkaloid, muscarine. Such effects have been classically described as muscarinic actions. In clinical practice, the pharmacological effects of parasympathomimetic agents are mediated via muscarinic receptors; similarly, anticholinergic or parasympatholytic agents such as atropine specifically block muscarinic receptors by competitive antagonism.

The cardiovascular responses to muscarinic activity are usually depressant, due to bradycardia and vasodilatation. However, if muscarinic receptors are blocked by adequate doses of atropine, acetylcholine will cause a rise in blood pressure due to stimulation of sympathetic ganglia and the vasoconstrictor and the cardioaccelerator nerves. Release of catecholamines from the adrenal medulla and fasciculation of skeletal muscle will also occur. Similar effects may be produced by administration of the alkaloid nicotine, and postsynaptic receptors in the autonomic ganglia and in the motor endplate have been designated as nicotinic.

Nicotinic receptors

In addition to the classical receptors described at the neuromuscular junction and in autonomic ganglia, experimental evidence suggests that nicotinic receptors may also be present in the CNS and at other neuronal sites, and four subtypes have been proposed. In all instances facilitatory transmission, involving changes in ionic conductance of sodium, calcium and potassium, occurs; the clinical significance of these findings is not evident at the present time.

Muscarinic receptors

Evidence for a diversity of these receptors has accumulated from autoradiographic and radioligand binding studies on cholinergic receptors within the CNS, from observations of the effects of novel muscarinic antagonists (particularly pirenzepine) on lower oesophageal contraction and on gastric acid secretion, and more recently from molecular cloning experiments. Five subtypes of muscarinic receptors (designated M_1 to M_5) have now been identified.

M_1-receptors have a high affinity for the antagonists pirenzepine and telenzepine. It was originally considered that M_1-receptors were mainly located at lower oesophageal and gastric sites. Present opinion suggests that M_1-receptors are present in the CNS and in all autonomic ganglia (in addition to the nicotinic receptors). In general, M_1-receptors have facilitatory effects. Although their physiological role is uncertain, they appear to be responsible for the slow depolarization of autonomic ganglion cells during synaptic transmission.

M_2-receptors are present in the myocardium, the cerebellum and on nerve terminals supplying bronchiolar smooth muscle. They are selectively antagonized by gallamine (and some experimental drugs, e.g. methoctramine). M_2-receptors mainly inhibit the release of noradrenaline from adrenergic nerve terminals (although they may also have a role in the autoregulation of acetylcholine release). Increased acetylcholine release mediated by antagonism at M_2-receptors may be involved in some clinical phenomena (e.g. the initial bradycardia sometimes seen after the administration of atropine and the bronchoconstriction induced by low doses of ipratropium).

M_3-receptors are found at classical postsynaptic sites (e.g. in the smooth muscle of airways and in mucous glands). They are non-selectively antagonized by classical antimuscarinic drugs and selectively antagonized by some experimental drugs (e.g. hexahydrosiladifenidol). When therapeutic doses of atropine or ipratropium are administered, they produce antagonistic effects at M_3-receptors which will overshadow any activity at M_2-receptors. The desired pharmacological result (e.g. antisialogogue activity, bronchodilatation) will thus be achieved.

M_4-receptors have been identified in cerebral, cardiac and pulmonary tissues in experimental animals and are specifically antagonized by tropicamide.

M_5-receptors appear to exist within the CNS.

Intracellular mechanisms resulting from activation of all muscarinic receptor subtypes involve an intermediary linkage to regulatory G proteins. M_1-, M_3- and M_5- receptors are coupled to the G_q family, with activation of phospholipase C and the subsequent production of inositol trisphosphate (IP_3). M_2 and M_4 relate to the G_i family and negatively couple adenylyl cyclase; potassium channels are activated, calcium channels are inhibited and there is a decrease in the intracellular production of cyclic adenosine monophosphate (cAMP).

The clinical significance of the various subtypes of muscarinic receptors in many cases remains a matter of conjecture, but their existence may help to explain certain clinical observations, including the differential effects of atropine and scopolamine at both central and peripheral sites and the superimposed actions of atropine and gallamine on cardiac rate.

Acetylcholine also produces direct inhibitory effects on vascular smooth muscle. These tissues are not innervated by parasympathetic fibres and the receptor has not been clearly identified. Experimental evidence suggests that the intracellular mechanism involved may be unrelated to the production of endothelium-derived relaxing factor (EDRF; now identified as nitric oxide) and the subsequent intracellular accumulation of cyclic guanosine monophosphate (cGMP). An additional factor, termed endothelial-derived hyperpolarizing factor (EDHF), may be important in the initiation of smooth-muscle relaxation, inducing hyperpolarization of the muscle membrane and reducing calcium transport via voltage-dependent channels.

Table 12.1 Distribution of peripheral acetylcholine receptors, effects produced by their stimulation and cellular mechanisms postulated.

Type/site of receptor	Pharmacological effects	Intracellular mechanisms
Nicotinic		
Neuromuscular junction	Voluntary muscle contraction	Mobilization of Ca^{2+} from sarcoplasmic reticulum and binding to troponin C
Autonomic ganglia	Ganglionic transmission (fast channels)	↑ Na^{+} K^{+} Ca^{2+} conductance
Muscarinic		
M_1 (autonomic ganglia)	Ganglionic transmission (slow channels)	↑ Phosphoinositide metabolism
M_2 (prejunctional)	Modulation of release of ACh and ? noradrenaline	K^{+} channel ↑ Ca^{2+} channel ↓ and cAMP ↓
M_3 (postsynaptic)	Smooth-muscle contraction (bronchi); SA slowing; glandular secretion ↑	↑ Phosphoinositide metabolism
M_4 (? inhibitory)	? Relaxation of smooth muscle; ↑ heart rate	K^{+} channel ↑ Ca^{2+} channel ↓ and cAMP ↓
M_5 (? function)	? CNS effects	↑ Phosphoinositide metabolism
Unclassified		
(Vascular smooth muscle)	Vasodilatation	↑ Production of EDHF

ACh, Acetylcholine; cAMP, cyclic adenosine monophosphate; SA, sino-atrial; CNS, central nervous system; EDHF, endothelial-derived hyperpolarizing factor.

The distribution of peripheral acetylcholine receptors is summarized in Table 12.1.

Noradrenergic receptors

In 1948 Ahlquist compared the relative potencies of six different sympathomimetic agents on a variety of peripheral organ systems and on isolated cardiac and smooth muscle. Contraction of smooth muscle was most marked with adrenaline and least with isoprenaline, whilst cardiac stimulation and relaxation of smooth muscle were greatest with isoprenaline and least with noradrenaline. On the basis of these studies Ahlquist suggested that there were two types of receptors (thus supporting Langley's original concept) — the α- and β-adrenoceptors. In general terms, stimulation of α-adrenoceptors produces vasoconstriction, whilst stimulation of β-adrenoceptors results in an increase in the force, rate and conduction velocity of the heart, relaxation of bronchial and intestinal smooth muscle and a vasodilator effect.

There are at least two major subgroups of each type of adrenoceptor. In 1967, Lands and his coworkers subdivided the β-adrenoceptors on the basis of their differing responses to adrenaline and noradrenaline:

1 β_1-adrenoceptors are located in the heart and in the smooth muscle of the intestine, and at these sites adrenaline and noradrenaline have equipotent effects.

2 β_2-adrenoceptors are found in bronchial, vascular and uterine smooth muscle and are far more sensitive to the effects of circulating adrenaline than to noradrenaline (i.e. β_2-adrenoceptors behave as 'hormonal' rather than transmitter receptors).

It has subsequently been shown, using radioligand binding studies, that the myocardium contains both β_1- and β_2-adrenoceptors, which are present in a ratio of 3 : 1 in the normal heart. It is thought that β_2-adrenoceptors in the myocardium are situated extrajunctionally and act as hormonal receptors. The excess sympathetic drive (principally mediated by noradrenaline) which frequently occurs in heart failure may lead to a down-regulation of receptors. In these circumstances β_1-adrenoceptors appear to be principally affected, whilst there is a relative sparing of the β_2 subtype. It has been shown that in severe heart failure the ratio of β_1- and β_2-adrenoceptors may change to 3 : 2. The identification of β_2-adrenoceptors on lymphocytes has also enabled further study of adrenergic receptors to take place. There is considerable evidence that at many sites β_2-adrenoceptors are located presynaptically on the adrenergic neurone; their stimulation appears to promote the release of noradrenaline from the nerve terminal.

A wealth of experimental evidence now indicates the existence of a functional β_3-adrenoceptor in humans. RNA identification and cloning studies have demonstrated β_3-adrenoceptors in omental and subcutaneous tissues, adipocytes in brown fat and in the gallbladder and colon. β_3-Adrenoceptors are stimulated by experimental drugs and by certain β-adrenoceptor antagonists (acting as partial agonists). β_3-Adrenoceptors may become a target for antiobesity and antidiabetic drugs.

Two main groups of the α-adrenoceptor have also been described. α_1-Adrenoceptors are those which subserve the classical vasoconstrictor activity from smooth-muscle stimulation. Physiological evidence suggests that autoregulation of noradrenaline release occurs at sympathetic nerve endings; noradrenaline is considered to inhibit its own neuronal discharge by an effect mediated on α_2-adrenoceptors located at presynaptic sites (Fig. 12.2). A similar (hormonal) effect at α_2-adrenoceptors may be induced by circulating adrenaline.

Studies with radioligands suggest that certain compounds exhibit a selective activity at α_2-adrenoceptors, for example clonidine as an agonist and yohimbine as an antagonist. α_2-Adrenoceptors are also found in platelets (their stimulation results in platelet aggregation) and may exist at other hormonally mediated postsynaptic sites.

It is now generally accepted that the effects of sympathomimetic amines on adrenoceptors are mediated by means of the second messenger system and

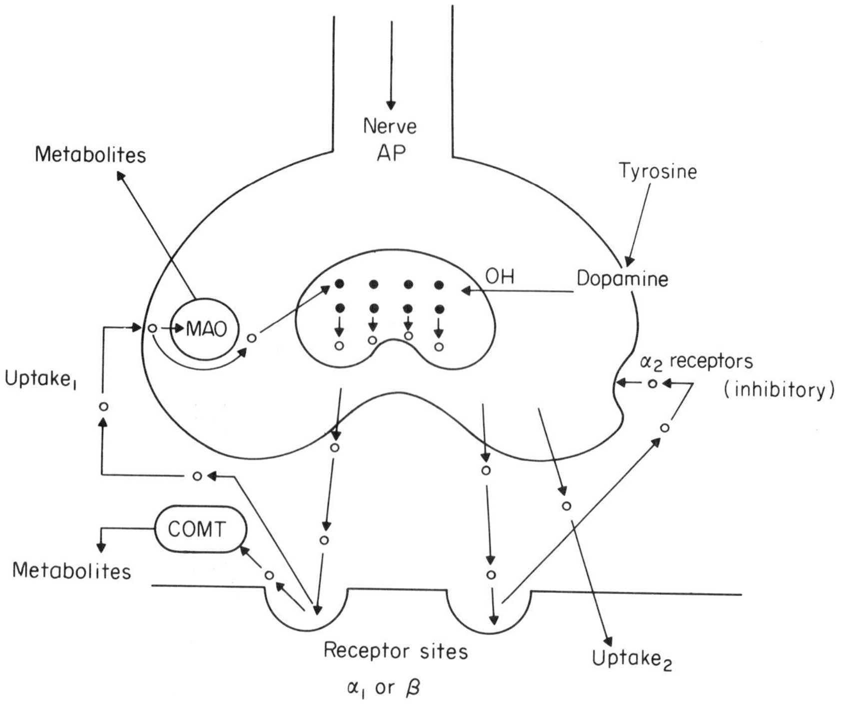

Fig. 12.2 The adrenergic nerve terminal showing the synthesis, release and reuptake of noradrenaline. AP, Action potential; (black circles), bound noradrenaline; (open circles), unbound noradrenaline; MAO, monoamine oxidase; and COMT, catechol-*O*-methyl transferase.

in all cases involve regulatory G proteins. Stimulation of either β_1 or β_2-adrenoceptors (and probably β_3-adrenoceptors) on the surface of the cell membrane (via coupling to the G_s family of proteins) results in the activation of adenylate cyclase, an enzyme present on the cytoplasmic face of the cell membrane. This acts as a catalyst in the conversion of adenosine triphosphate (ATP) into cyclic adenosine-3,5-monophosphate (cAMP). This mediator subsequently activates a specific protein kinase which leads to phosphorylation of a variety of intracellular proteins. The resultant electrophysiological changes (e.g. depolarization or hyperpolarization of the cell membrane) and pharmacological effects (e.g. inotropic activity, smooth-muscle relaxation) can obviously differ. This may be due to a number of factors, including:

1 The type of intracellular protein which undergoes phosphorylation (e.g. troponin C, troponin I, calmodulin, phospholamban).

2 Subsequent effects on calcium transport and release of intracellular calcium.

3 Possible effects on the cell membrane enzyme Na^+/K^+ ATPase.

Current evidence indicates that the effects mediated via α_1-adrenoceptors depend on a different intracellular mechanism. In this case a membrane-bound enzyme (phospholipase C) is activated (via G_q protein coupling) and hydrolyses phosphatidylinositol bisphosphate (PIP_2). Inositol trisphosphate (IP_3) is subsequently produced and this leads to increased calcium mobilization (and possibly enhanced calcium uptake) in the effector cell.

The effects of stimulation of α_2-adrenoceptors are mediated via a reduction in the activity of cAMP (with activation of potassium channels and inhibitory effects on calcium channels) via coupling to an inhibitory regulatory protein (G_i) family.

Currently three subtypes of both α_1- and α_2-adrenoceptors are described. In each group receptor activation appears to result in identical intracellular mechanisms, and their role in human autonomic pharmacology is not yet relevant, although they may herald the arrival of highly specific agonists and antagonists at α_1 and α_2 sites.

Dopaminergic receptors

Dopamine is the immediate precursor of noradrenaline and may also stimulate its release from noradrenergic nerve terminals. Dopamine is also an important transmitter within the CNS, and receptors have been located in the basal ganglia, the nigrostriatal pathway and in areas of the anterior and intermediate lobes of the pituitary gland. Two types of dopaminergic receptors, designated D_1 and D_2, have been identified in the CNS; both groups are thought to be located at presynaptic and postsynaptic sites. Activation of D_1-receptors stimulates various hormonal and neurosecretory functions, leading to a modulation of extrapyramidal activity. These effects are induced by an increase in intracellular cAMP via G_s protein coupling and activation of adenylate cyclase. Stimulation of D_2-receptors results in inhibition of pituitary hormone output, and modulation of the release of acetylcholine and endorphins within the CNS. The mechanism involves G_i protein coupling and inhibition of cAMP.

Functional interaction between the two groups of receptors occurs. Alteration of the receptor population may account for the 'on–off' therapeutic response or for the development of tardive dyskinesia which can occur following the administration of non-selective dopamine agonists in the treatment of parkinsonism.

Two related receptors are found at peripheral sites and are probably identical to their CNS counterparts. D_1-receptors are found in vascular and mesenteric smooth muscle; agonist effects lead to an increase in intracellular cAMP content and subsequent vasodilatation. D_2-receptors appear to be inhibitory autoreceptors and also inhibit the release of noradrenaline from certain postganglionic sympathetic sites.

More recently, five different dopamine receptor subtypes have been cloned and identified using molecular biological techniques. These have also been considered as three subtypes of D_1-receptors and two subtypes of D_2-receptors which exhibit regional variation within the CNS.

The various types of peripheral adrenergic receptors are summarized in Table 12.2, whilst their involvement in different sympathetic responses is shown in Table 12.3.

Table 12.2 Subtypes of peripheral adrenoceptors, principal pharmacological effects and probable intracellular mechanisms involved.

Type of receptor	Principal effects	Intracellular mechanisms
β_1	Positive inotropic and chronotropic	↑ cAMP availability → phosphorylation of phospholamban and ↑ Ca^{2+} mobilization
β_2	Relaxation of smooth muscle	↑ cAMP availability → Increase in cell membrane Na^+/K^+ ATPase activity (? phosphorylation of troponin I in myocardium)
α_1	Contraction of smooth muscle	Activation of phospholipase C → Production of IP_3 and subsequent ↑ Ca^{2+} turnover and binding to calmodulin
α_2	Presynaptic inhibition of adrenergic neurone	K^+ channel ↑ Ca^{2+} channel ↓ ↓ cAMP availability
D_1	Relaxation of renal vascular and mesenteric smooth muscle	↑ cAMP availability and ? membrane stabilization from effects on Na^+/K^+ ATPase
D_2	Presynaptic inhibition of dopamine and noradrenaline release	? ↓ cAMP availability

cAMP, cyclic adenosine monophosphate; IP_3, inositol trisphosphate.

Table 12.3 Types of receptors involved in differing sympathetic responses.

Tissue/organ	Response	Receptor type
Vascular smooth muscle		
Skin	Constriction	α_1
Muscle	Dilatation or	β_2
	constriction	α_1
Splanchnic	Dilatation or	β_2 D_1
	constriction	α_1
Renal	Dilatation or	β_2 D_1
	constriction	α_1
Other smooth muscle		
Bronchial	Relaxation	β_2
Intestinal	Relaxation	α_1 β_2
Sphincters	Contraction	α
Uterine	Relaxation	β_2
Other effects		
Heart	Increased rate and contractility	Mainly β_1 (also β_2 ? α and D_1)
Renin secretion by kidney	Increased	β_1
Liver glycogenolysis	Stimulation	β_2 α
Lipolysis	Stimulation	β_3
Insulin secretion	Stimulation	β (? β_2)
	Inhibition	α

Where α only is cited, the subtype has not been definitely identified.

Many other endogenous compounds can mimic or enhance autonomic activity. These include histamine, 5-hydroxytryptamine, adenosine, endothelins, vasointestinal peptide and substance P. These agents are broadly grouped as autacoids or local hormones and the phenomena described as non-adrenergic non-cholinergic (NANC) transmission. The effects produced following the local release of such substances may be mediated via other known or putative receptors, or may involve the modulation of the synthesis, release or receptor activation of classical neurotransmitters.

Autonomic drugs

Drugs may affect autonomic function in a number of ways:

1 By mimicking or modifying the action of the neurotransmitter on the effector organ.

2 By effects on ganglionic transmission or on release of the appropriate transmitter.

3 By modifying central integration of autonomic activity.

4 Occasionally, by an effect on afferent autonomic input. For example, the veratrum alkaloids, which were used in the early years of the 20th century in the management of eclampsia and were among the original group of drugs used in the treatment of essential hypertension, appeared to induce their cardiovascular depressive responses through stimulation of chemoreceptor sensory mechanisms.

Parasympathomimetic agents

Acetylcholine

The widespread effects and evanescent action of acetylcholine preclude its systemic administration, although it has been used historically to induce convulsions in the treatment of schizophrenia. It may be employed as a topical agent in ophthalmology when a rapid miosis is required.

Synthetic choline esters

These are more stable compounds than the parent drug, and may exhibit a more selective action at certain muscarinic sites. Methacholine is only hydrolysed slowly by cholinesterases; it has been used to decrease the heart rate in cases of supraventricular tachycardia and occasionally as a vasodilator in peripheral vascular disorders. Carbachol and the related compound bethanechol are resistant to enzymatic destruction and have been used in the treatment of postoperative atony of the bladder and the gut, and as locally acting miotics in the treatment of glaucoma.

Naturally occurring cholinomimetic alkaloids

These include muscarine (which is found in various wild mushrooms), arecoline (a constituent of the betel nut) and pilocarpine (an extract of certain South American shrubs) which is employed as a miotic.

Anticholinesterase drugs

These agents may be subdivided into:

1 Simple quaternary amines, e.g. edrophonium

2 Carbamate esters (reversible or acid-transferring inhibitors).

3 Organophosphorus compounds with potentially irreversible effects.

By inhibiting enzymatic degradation of acetylcholine, anticholinesterases will allow accumulation of the neurotransmitter at all its peripheral sites of liberation. In addition the non-polar compounds (e.g. physostigmine, most organophosphorous substances) may induce significant CNS activity.

Anticholinesterase drugs may be employed therapeutically for both nicotinic and muscarinic effects. The nicotinic effects of this group of compounds are essentially dose-related. Thus the carbamates are used therapeutically to reverse the effects of non-depolarizing muscle relaxants and to improve neuromuscular function in myasthenia gravis and related conditions. Conversely, overdosage of the reversible agents, or inadvertent systemic uptake of organophosphorus compounds, can lead to muscular weakness or even paralysis.

Carbamate esters are also employed for their muscarinic effects. They may be used for the treatment of paralytic ileus or for atony of the urinary bladder; distigmine, which is a combination of two molecules of pyridostigmine and has a relatively long duration of action, may be particularly useful in this context. These agents may also be administered by topical instillation in the management of glaucoma. The anticholinesterase agents are further discussed in Chapter 10.

Antagonists of parasympathomimetic activity

Several naturally occurring and synthetic compounds competitively antagonize the muscarinic effects of acetylcholine and other parasympathomimetic drugs. Their principal site of action is at effector organs innervated by postganglionic parasympathetic fibres (M_3-receptors), although some members of the group may inhibit ganglionic transmission or have significant CNS activity. Pharmacological effects at the neuromuscular junction are not significant, although in experimental studies high doses of atropine have been shown to inhibit depolarization of the motor endplate.

Naturally occurring antagonists

These compounds are organic esters which are derived from solanaceous plants and are chemically related to cocaine; an aromatic acid (tropic acid) is combined with a complex base, tropine or scopine, to form atropine or hyoscine respectively.

Atropine

This drug has been used in anaesthetic practice for many years both for premedication and to antagonize the muscarinic effects from the administration of anticholinesterase drugs; these aspects are considered more fully in the appropriate chapters (10 and 13). Atropine is sometimes employed topically as a mydriatic in the treatment of iritis and choroiditis; the effects may last up to 2 weeks and profound cycloplegia (paralysis of accommodation) occurs. Atropine has frequently been administered with opioid analgesics in the treatment of biliary and renal colic in the hope that smooth-muscle relaxation will contribute to pain relief. Likewise, it has been used in the management of acute pancreatitis to reduce the volume and tryptic activity of pancreatic secretion, and thus produce an analgesic effect. There is little evidence that such measures are of value. The use of atropine is indicated in myocardial infarction where there is bradycardia associated with hypotension or where the prolonged atrioventricular conduction results in ventricular 'escape' and multiple extrasystoles ensue. Atropine can also be of value in the management of intra-operative bradycardia during general anaesthesia, or in the treatment of an overdose of local anaesthetic agents. A transient accentuation of the bradycardia is sometimes observed following the administration of atropine under these circumstances. This was historically attributed to a CNS effect, but is now considered to be due to initial responses at M_2-receptors.

Atropine is a specific antidote in the treatment of poisoning caused by the alkaloid muscarine, which is found in the mushroom *Amanita muscaria* and certain other fungi; it is also a valuable agent in the management of organophosphorus poisons.

Therapeutic doses of atropine can produce a slight stimulatory effect on the CNS, and larger doses give rise to excitement, hallucinations and hyperpyrexia, although in the untreated case respiratory depression and coma will supervene. Children are most frequently affected by atropine poisoning as they may accidentally consume deadly nightshade berries. Treatment may include gastric lavage, methods to reduce body temperature, the administration of physostigmine and the use of controlled ventilation.

Hyoscine

In contrast to atropine, hyoscine produces a depressant effect on the CNS when administered in therapeutic doses (suggesting a differing affinity of the two drugs for subtypes of muscarinic or nicotinic receptors within the CNS). The amnesic property may be advantageous when hyoscine is used in combination with morphine to induce 'twilight sleep' or when it is given by intravenous injection after clamping of the cord to minimize awareness during obstetric anaesthesia. When used in anaesthetic practice, hyoscine appears to induce less tachycardia than an equipotent dose of atropine; it also has greater antisialogogue activity and more pronounced ocular effects. However, the administration of hyoscine may lead to undue excitation with confusion and ataxia, or to excessive drowsiness in elderly patients. The term central anticholinergic syndrome has sometimes been used to describe this symptom complex.

Hyoscine is of proven value when used prophylactically in the management of motion sickness and other vestibular disorders. The mechanism of action probably involves inhibition of cholinergic pathways from the labyrinthine apparatus to the medullary centres.

Atropine and hyoscine were the first drugs available for the treatment of Parkinson's disease. The imbalance of cholinergic/dopaminergic activity within the CNS was corrected and tremor and rigidity were particularly benefited. In more recent years, drugs which effectively improve dopaminergic transmission, such as levodopa and bromocriptine, have been developed and found to be more beneficial in alleviating the akinesia (immobility) associated with parkinsonism. However, in patients who are intolerant of the side-effects of dopaminergic agents, and particularly in drug-induced parkinsonism, anticholinergic drugs may still be valuable.

Synthetic antagonists

Benzhexol (Artane), which appears to produce less peripheral antimuscarinic side-effects than atropine, is commonly used as an antiparkinsonian agent. Procyclidine, which is available as a parenteral preparation, is the drug of choice for the reversal of acute dystonia induced by phenothiazines and related drugs.

Homatropine has a shorter duration of action than atropine when applied locally and has been employed as a mydriatic for diagnostic procedures. A related synthetic compound, tropicamide, has an even more evanescent action and is used to facilitate examination of the fundus of the eye.

Many synthetic and semisynthetic drugs have been developed as antispasmodics for the management of various gastrointestinal and genitourinary disorders. They differ from the naturally occurring agents in that they are quaternary ammonium compounds; they are thus poorly absorbed from the gut and do not effectively cross the blood–brain barrier. They also show more affinity for ganglionic (M_1) receptors and may abolish the effects of sympathetic nerve activity on muscle tone, particularly in the sphincters. Drugs in this group include propantheline, dicyclomine and ipratropium; ipratropium is a common constituent of inhalant mixtures used in the treatment of bronchospasm. A similar drug, glycopyrrolate, may confer a number of advantages when used in premedication prior to anaesthesia and during the reversal of neuromuscular blockade. It appears to be devoid of any CNS effects and placental transfer is not significant. It is an effective antisialogogue with a long duration of action; changes in heart rate and pupillary size appear to be minimal.

Pirenzepine, which demonstrates a high affinity for M_1-receptors, has been developed for the treatment of peptic ulceration; pirenzepine appears to reduce gastric acid secretion and prevent reflux without other significant antimuscarinic effects. Both pharmacokinetic (relating to drug distribution) and pharmacodynamic (the variable affinities of anticholinergic drugs for the subtypes of both muscarinic and nicotinic receptors at central and peripheral sites) factors undoubtedly influence the different clinical responses observed with this group of drugs.

Sympathomimetic agents

Endogenous substances

Adrenaline, noradrenaline and dopamine are the sympathomimetic amines which exist in the body as neurotransmitters. The synthesis of adrenaline from the amino acid phenylalanine *in vivo* has been demonstrated using radiolabelled techniques, and the pathway involved in this process also leads to the formation of dopamine and noradrenaline (Fig. 12.3). As 3 : 4 dihydroxybenzene is also known as catechol, these three substances are commonly referred to as catecholamines.

Adrenaline

Adrenaline is considered to have only a minor role in the conduction of peripheral autonomic impulses. However, adrenaline is the major constituent (80–90%) of the adrenal medulla in adults and may produce 'hormonally' mediated effects on both α_2 and β_2-adrenoceptors. Furthermore, adrenaline is an important neurotransmitter within the CNS.

The physiological responses to an infusion of adrenaline are mediated via both α- and β-adrenoceptors. The heart rate, force of contraction and conduction velocity are invariably increased, and arrhythmias are likely. The systolic blood pressure is elevated, but depending on the dose and rate of administration, there may be a fall in diastolic pressure due to effects mediated via β_2-adrenoceptors on splanchnic and muscle blood vessels. At higher dose levels, effects at α_1-adrenoceptors at these sites will predominate and peripheral resistance will be increased. In all instances, skin blood flow will be reduced. Coronary arterioles will be dilated as a consequence of the metabolic changes brought about by the increased work of the heart. This effect will overshadow the responses mediated through α-adrenoceptors in the coronary vascular smooth muscle.

The systemic uses of adrenaline are limited. However, it should be employed as the first-line approach in the treatment of anaphylactic shock; 0.5–1 ml of 1 in 1000 adrenaline (500 μg–1 mg) by intramuscular injection is recommended; the dose may be repeated at 10-min intervals if necessary. Following cardiac arrest, 5–10 ml of a 1 in 10 000 solution (500 μg–1 mg) of adrenaline may be given

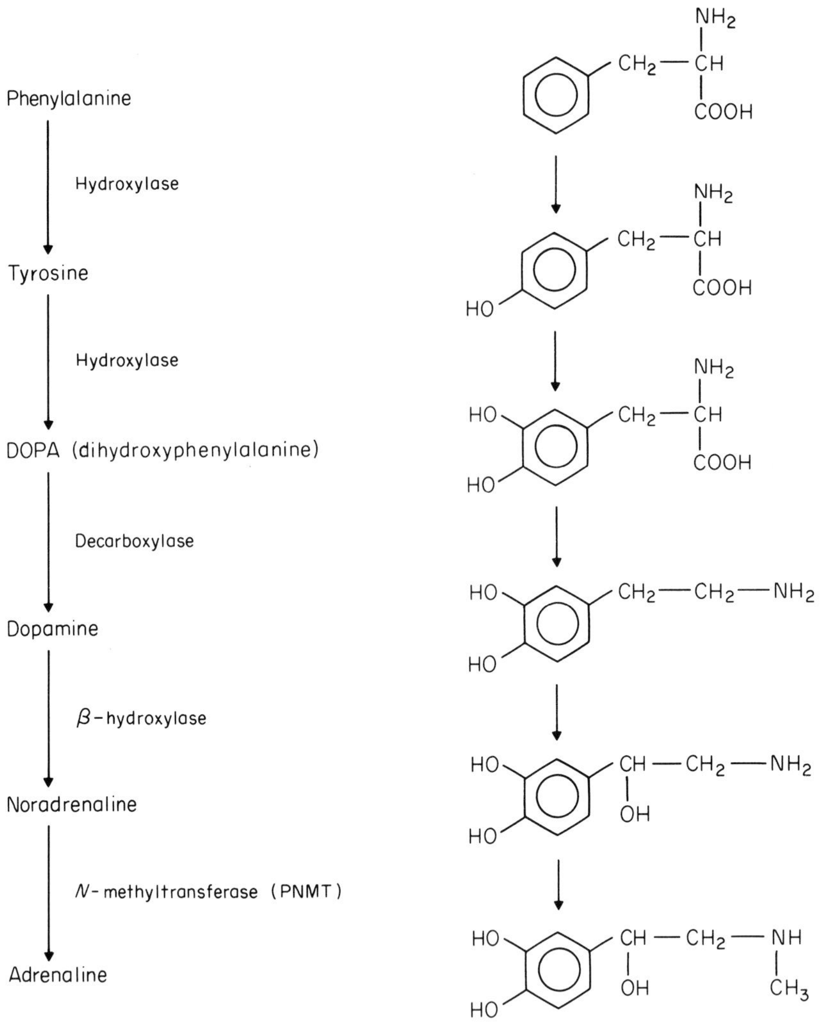

Fig. 12.3 Steps in the enzymatic synthesis of noradrenaline and adrenaline.

intravenously or by the intratracheal route when there is ECG evidence of asystole, or when fine fibrillation (high-frequency, low-amplitude waves) needs to be coarsened prior to direct current cardioversion. The intravenous administration of 1 in 10 000 adrenaline is now recommended as first-line treatment of severe hypersensitivity responses which may occur during anaesthesia (Chapter 7).

Adrenaline is commonly incorporated into local anaesthetic solutions in concentrations varying from 1 in 80 000 (12.5 μg ml^{-1}) to 1 in 200 000 (5 μg ml^{-1}). The vasoconstrictor effect will diminish local blood flow and decrease the rate of absorption of the local anaesthetic agent, thus prolonging its pharmacological action and reducing systemic toxicity.

Adrenaline may be used as a local decongestant or as a topical haemostat, and is also found in various proprietary mixtures used for bronchodilator therapy.

Adrenaline eyedrops may be of value in the treatment of wide-angle glaucoma, where the vasoconstrictor effect will reduce the secretion of aqueous humour.

Noradrenaline

The effects of noradrenaline are exerted almost exclusively via α-adrenoceptors. Peripheral resistance and both systolic and diastolic blood pressure are raised due to generalized vasoconstriction. Although noradrenaline has direct effects on the heart, these are usually obscured by baroreceptor responses (mediated via the vagus nerve) to the increase in blood pressure. In consequence the heart is little affected, although slight bradycardia may occur.

Noradrenaline infusions were formerly used in the treatment of hypotensive shock states. Blood pressure levels were maintained at the expense of reduced tissue perfusion, and the state of shock actually worsened; furthermore, extravasation of the infusion into the tissues often produced severe necrosis. However, noradrenaline has now regained a role, when used in a low-dose combination with other inotropes, in the treatment of cardiogenic shock (p. 436).

Noradrenaline was also employed as a vasoconstrictor in local anaesthetic solutions; this is no longer recommended as severe and occasionally fatal pressor responses have been associated with its use.

Dopamine

Dopamine has developed a role as an inotropic agent in the treatment of low-output states associated with renal insufficiency; clinical indications include endotoxic or cardiogenic shock, refractory congestive cardiac failure, and to improve circulation following cardiac surgery. Dopamine is administered by continuous infusion; when a low-dose regime (1–2 $\mu g\ kg^{-1}\ min^{-1}$) is employed, renal blood flow is enhanced and urinary output increased due to a direct effect (probably mediated via D_1-receptors) on renal vasculature. With higher dose levels (2–10 $\mu g\ kg^{-1}\ min^{-1}$) cardiac output is improved due to an effect mediated via β-adrenoceptors. In these circumstances, dopamine is considered to have a more specific effect on the force of contraction (inotropic) than the heart rate (chronotropic), although tachycardia can sometimes be a problem, particularly in underhydrated patients. If the rate of infusion is further increased, α-adrenoceptor effects may supervene and lead to profound vasoconstriction and decreased renal blood flow; arrhythmias are also likely.

Replenishment of dopamine stores in the CNS is a logical approach to the treatment of parkinsonism. Dopamine does not effectively cross the blood–brain barrier; its precursor, levodopa, is usually prescribed, and may be used in combination with a dopa-decarboxylase inhibitor (carbidopa or benserazide) to minimize side-effects such as nausea, vomiting and cardiac arrhythmias which may occur due to the formation of extracerebral dopamine. Other drugs which may be used to increase dopaminergic activity within the CNS include bromocriptine, which has analogous effects; amantidine, which stimulates the release of dopamine presynaptically; and selegiline, which selectively inhibits the principal enzyme (monoamine oxidase B) concerned in the destruction of dopamine at central sites.

Exogenous substances acting principally via β-adrenoceptors

Isoprenaline

Isoprenaline is a synthetic catecholamine which has a powerful action on β-adrenoceptors. Following infusion of isoprenaline, both heart rate and cardiac output are increased; there does not appear to be a selective inotropic effect and arrhythmias are likely. There is a fall in peripheral resistance, but renal blood flow is not specifically increased as with dopamine; furthermore, coronary perfusion may be embarrassed because of the tachycardia and a reduced diastolic blood pressure.

Isoprenaline infusions (0.5–10 μg min^{-1}) are sometimes used in the management of shock, although dopamine is usually preferred. Isoprenaline is of more value in the short-term management of bradyarrhythmias, in particular those associated with atrioventricular block (e.g. Stokes–Adams attacks).

Isoprenaline exhibits a powerful bronchodilator effect and has been administered by sublingual routes and as an inhalant in the treatment of bronchospasm. However, the excessive use of isoprenaline inhalers has been associated with an increased incidence of sudden death in asthmatic patients. This has been assumed as due to the cardiotoxicity of isoprenaline (although the effects of the propellant have sometimes been implicated); safer drugs are now available.

Selective β_2-adrenoceptor agonists

These agents were developed primarily for their use in bronchial asthma. They are relatively specific for β_2-adrenoceptors and normally have little effect on the heart. Tachycardia and palpitations may occur occasionally, and were previously thought to be compensatory mechanisms following β_2 vasodilatation. Present evidence would indicate that a direct action on the myocardium may be involved. Such effects may be enhanced in heart failure when there is a relative preponderance of β_2-adrenoceptors.

Salbutamol is available as an oral preparation, in tablet and injection form, and as a nebulized solution. Salbutamol may be given intravenously as a bolus dose (250 μg repeated 4-hourly if necessary) or by continuous infusion (3–20 μg min^{-1}) in the treatment of severe bronchospasm. Alternatively, salbutamol may be administered as a respirator solution either intermittently (5 mg ml^{-1}) or continuously

(50–100 μg ml^{-1}) through a suitably driven nebulizer in severe asthmatic states. Closely related drugs include terbutaline and ritodrine. Salmeterol is a longer-acting agent which is usually administered twice daily, in association with inhaled corticosteroids, in the long-term management of obstructive airway disease.

β_2-Adrenoceptor agonists will relax uterine smooth muscle, and may be administered by continuous infusion to delay delivery in premature labour. Drugs of this type will cross the blood–brain barrier and central side-effects, including tremor and nervous tension, are associated with their use.

β_2-Adrenoceptor agonists may cause hypokalaemia. The mechanism involved is the stimulation of membrane-bound Na^+/K^+ ATPase which is linked to the receptor.

Exogenous substances acting via α-adrenoceptors

Phenylephrine

This has a close structural relationship to the endogenous catecholamines and exhibits pharmacological effects which resemble those of noradrenaline. Phenylephrine may be employed as a mydriatic or as a topical decongestant; it may also be incorporated into local anaesthetic solutions as a vasoconstrictor.

Methoxamine

Methoxamine has similar effects mediated via α-adrenoceptors. It is of proven value when administered intravenously (2–10 mg) in the management of untoward hypotension occurring during anaesthesia, particularly following subarachnoid or extradural blockade or when ganglion-blocking drugs have been employed. Metaraminol is an alternative drug of choice in this context.

α_2-Adrenoceptor agonists

Drugs with significant α_2-agonist activity, such as clonidine and methyldopa (via its active metabolite, methylnoradrenaline), have been used in the treatment of hypertension. Their principal therapeutic effects appear to be mediated via α_2-adrenoceptors which inhibit vasomotor responses in the medulla oblongata. More selective α_2-agonists include azepexole and dexmedetomidine. Such agents are achieving an important role in anaesthetic practice (Chapter 13). They appear to have significant hypnotic properties (and may produce synergistic effects with benzodiazepines); they also reduce the minimum alveolar concentration (MAC) requirements of certain inhalational agents. Such effects are presumably due to inhibition of central adrenergic pathways. Furthermore, their peripheral actions at presynaptic receptors could prove valuable in the attenuation of reflex sympathetic responses which may occur during anaesthesia.

α_2-Adrenoceptor activation within the CNS also produces potent analgesic responses mediated at both supraspinal and spinal sites. Both clonidine and dexmedetomidine have been administered by various routes to produce postoperative analgesia, or to enhance other therapy (e.g. opiates, spinal and extradural blockade). Lofexidine, an analogue of clonidine, has recently been introduced for the management of symptoms associated with opioid withdrawal in dependent subjects.

Exogenous synthetic agents with a mixed effect on adrenoceptors

Ephedrine

Ephedrine occurs naturally in various plants but can also be synthesized. The drug exhibits both α and β (β_1 and β_2) effects and its pharmacological actions are partly dependent on the displacement of noradrenaline from sympathetic nerve endings, and partly due to direct stimulation of adrenoceptors. Ephedrine may also inhibit the action of monoamine oxidase on the metabolism of noradrenaline. Tachyphylaxis will occur with the continuous use of ephedrine due to depletion of noradrenergic stores.

Ephedrine readily crosses the blood–brain barrier, and is employed for its effects on the CNS in the management of narcolepsy and nocturnal enuresis. It is still occasionally used in the treatment of bronchospasm and in the management of arrhythmias associated with atrioventricular conduction defects. Ephedrine is usually preferred to methoxamine for the management of hypotensive complications which may occur during obstetric anaesthesia and analgesia, as the combined α and β_2 effects are less likely to compromise placental perfusion and subsequent fetal oxygenation. However, ephedrine is more likely to cross the placental barrier.

Amphetamine and related compounds, such as methylphenidate and phentermine, which may be used as analeptics or anorectics, have a peripheral action which resembles that of ephedrine. Fenfluramine is often used as an appetite suppressant. Drug interactions have been reported in patients who are also receiving monoamine oxidase inhibitors or various antihypertensive agents, and dangerous arrhythmias have been described when halothane has been administered to patients who are also taking fenfluramine.

Miscellaneous agents

Aminophylline

Aminophylline, a mixture of theophylline and ethylenediamine (which is 20 times more soluble than theophylline itself), is a methylxanthine derivative. Although it is not strictly speaking a sympathomimetic amine it is a potent but non-specific inhibitor of the various isoenzymes of phosphodiesterase, and many of its pharmacological effects appear to be due to the accumulation of intracellular cAMP. Other modes of action which may have some import include a reduction in the translocation of calcium ions, blockade of adenosine receptors, effects on the release and subsequent availability of catecholamines and potentiation of prostaglandin synthetase activity.

Aminophylline is a highly effective bronchodilator, and was the drug of choice for the treatment of bronchospasm before the advent of the β_2-selective agonists. Aminophylline has both inotropic and chronotropic effects on the heart and was formerly used in the treatment of asthma when the distinction between a respiratory or cardiac (paroxysmal nocturnal dyspnoea due to acute left ventricular failure) cause was not clear-cut.

Aminophylline may be given by slow intravenous injection (250–500 mg over 20 min) or as an infusion (500 $\mu g\ kg^{-1}\ h^{-1}$). Tachyarrhythmias may occur, and nausea, vomiting and other gastrointestinal disturbances are sometimes encountered. At high dose levels convulsions may be induced and plasma levels should be monitored during such therapy. At one time aminophylline was often administered prior to anaesthesia as a slow-release oral preparation or in suppository form, as a prophylactic measure in patients with a history of bronchospasm.

Ergot alkaloids

Ergotamine appears to have more than 300 times the affinity of noradrenaline for α-adrenoceptors and initially acts as a partial agonist to induce direct stimulation of smooth muscle. Prolonged administration of ergot alkaloids can produce symptoms of vascular insufficiency and may lead to gangrene of the extremities; marked CNS effects, including headache, loss of consciousness and convulsions, may also occur. Endemic episodes of ergotism ('St Anthony's fire') have resulted following the ingestion of rye bread manufactured from grain infected with the ergot fungus.

The agonist effect is followed by α-adrenoceptor antagonism, but this is of little therapeutic value. The principal use of ergotamine is in the treatment of an acute attack of migraine. Some of the beneficial effects may also be due to an interaction with 5-hydroxytryptamine receptors. Ergometrine, which has powerful oxytocic activity, and is used in obstetrics to control postpartum bleeding, has considerably less effect on vascular smooth muscle (either as a partial agonist or as an antagonist) than ergotamine; however, the drug should be administered with special care to hypertensive patients or those with pre-existing cardiac disease.

Drugs used as inotropic agents

The use of dopamine and isoprenaline in this context has been discussed previously. Digitalis and related glycosides also produce a positive inotropic effect. The mechanism involves inhibition of membrane-bound Na^+/K^+ ATPase (with subsequent effects on calcium mobilization) combined with enhancement of vagal activity on the myocardium. Digitalis is discussed more fully in Chapter 15.

Dobutamine

This is a synthetic catecholamine which resembles dopamine. It is also used in the treatment of shock states which result in a low cardiac output; dobutamine appears to have a more selective inotropic action than dopamine, and thus leads to less increase in myocardial oxygen requirements. Unlike dopamine, it does not appear to have any effect on the renal vasculature and does not directly increase urinary output.

Dobutamine has a very short plasma half-life due to rapid metabolism in the liver to inactive conjugates. The drug must therefore be administered by continuous intravenous infusion; the normal dose range which is required is 2.5–10 $\mu g\ kg^{-1}\ min^{-1}$.

Dobutamine is frequently infused in combination with renal doses of dopamine in low-cardiac-output states. More recently, there has been a reappraisal of the use of supplementary noradrenaline infusions in hypotensive patients who are unresponsive to plasma expansion and dopamine alone. The effects of noradrenaline on β_1-adrenoceptors in the myocardium may complement the positive inotropic effect, and when relatively low doses (0.5–1.5 $\mu g\ kg^{-1}\ min^{-1}$) are used, excessive vasoconstriction is not a problem and there are no deleterious effects on renal function.

Dopexamine

Dopexamine hydrochloride, an analogue of dopamine, is a potent β_2-adrenoceptor agonist and also acts on peripheral dopaminergic (D_1) receptors. In contrast to dopamine, it lacks α- and β_1-agonist activity. Dopexamine exerts a positive inotropic effect, presumably due to effects on cardiac β_2-adrenoceptors. Clinical trials of dopexamine in patients with cardiac failure have proved inconclusive.

Enoximone

Enoximone belongs to the imidazole group of cardioactive compounds and is a selective inhibitor of type III phosphodiesterase isoenzyme. This isoenzyme is principally located in the myocardium, smooth muscle and platelets (and may be further inhibited by the intracellular accumulation of cGMP).

Enoximone exerts positive inotropic effects by enhancing cAMP activity in heart muscle, leading to an increase in intracellular calcium levels.

Enoximone has been used in the treatment of congestive cardiac failure which has proved refractory to other therapies (e.g. angiotensin-converting enzyme inhibitors). Enoximone produces an increase in cardiac index and a reduction in ventricular filling pressures with a decrease in systemic vascular resistance (the inhibition of platelet aggregation may also be beneficial in this context); myocardial oxygen requirements are not significantly increased. The associated relaxation of vascular smooth muscle can lead to a fall in blood pressure and the drug is relatively contraindicated in hypotensive patients.

Enoximone is administered by slow intravenous injection or by infusion; the solution provided in the ampoules must be diluted beforehand and mixed in plastic syringes or infusion containers, as crystal formation has been observed when glass apparatus is used. The drug is principally eliminated by the kidney as a sulphoxide metabolite; the elimination half-lives of both the parent drug and the metabolite are approximately 20 times greater in patients with congestive cardiac failure than in healthy volunteers.

Sustained haemodynamic and clinical benefits have been observed in patients treated for up to 48 h, but as yet there is no conclusive evidence of a reduction in mortality. Furthermore, the use of enoximone has been associated with a significant number of side-effects which include tachyarrhythmias, hypotension, thrombocytopenia, nausea and vomiting, fever, oliguria and limb pain. Milrinone is a dipyridone derivative with similar properties to those of enoximone.

Xamoterol

Xamoterol is a selective partial agonist at β_1-adrenoceptors which is available only in tablet form. Clinical responses to this agent are dependent on the resting sympathetic tone. Thus xamoterol appears to exert a moderate inotropic effect at rest, but during exercise can partly attenuate the β-adrenergic response. Xamoterol has been used in patients with mild chronic heart failure due to ischaemic disease, and where there is no evidence of sympathetic overactivity xamoterol augments myocardial contractility, and reduces left ventricular filling pressure. Myocardial relaxation during diastole is enhanced and there is no increase in resting oxygen consumption. However, the use of this drug is absolutely contraindicated in more severe forms of cardiac failure when sympathetic 'drive' is presumed to be high, and the depressant effects of the drug will supervene.

Xamoterol does not exhibit any significant β_2-adrenoceptor agonist activity and tachyphylaxis is not associated with the continued use of the drug.

Glucagon

Glucagon is a polypeptide which is secreted by the α-cells of the pancreatic islets. The positive inotropic effects were first described in 1960. The effects on adenylyl cyclase with subsequent cAMP production and intracellular calcium mobilization are similar to those of catecholamines, although a different receptor may be involved. Glucagon is still used occasionally when an inotropic action is required following cardiac surgery, or in heart failure complicating acute myocardial infarction. Glucagon appears to be relatively ineffective in congestive cardiac failure. Hyperglycaemia and hyperkalaemia are likely problems during its use.

Antagonists of sympathetic activity

Centrally acting agents

There is little doubt that the activity of central catecholamine-containing neurons will determine peripheral sympathetic responses. For example, the tricyclic antidepressant drugs which effectively increase the availability of noradrenaline within the CNS by inhibiting neuronal uptake may produce manifestations of overactivity at peripheral sites, including excessive sweating (which is mediated via cholinergic sympathetic fibres). Conversely, there is evidence that the cardio-accelerator and vasomotor areas in the medulla oblongata are under modulatory control by α_2-adrenoceptors. The antihypertensive properties of both methyldopa and clonidine are considered to be due to agonistic effects on centrally situated receptors.

Ganglion-blocking agents

Drugs in this group act as competitive antagonists to the effects of acetylcholine on postsynaptic (nicotinic) receptors in autonomic ganglia. Originally used in the treatment of essential hypertension, initial members of the group included tetraethylammonium chloride and salts of the bisquaternary ammonium compound hexamethonium (C6); at a later stage secondary (mecamylamine) and tertiary (pempidine) amines were introduced.

Marked disadvantages associated with the use of these compounds included irregular absorption following oral administration, postural hypotension and numerous side-effects (e.g. cycloplegia, intestinal ileus, disturbances of sexual function) due to the indiscriminate blockade of both sympathetic and parasympathetic ganglia.

They are no longer used as antihypertensive agents in the UK. However, the related compound, trimetaphan, is used to produce controlled hypotension in surgery, in the treatment of hypertensive crises and in the management of autonomic hyperreflexia associated with spinal cord injuries.

Drugs that affect postganglionic sympathetic nerve endings

In sympathetic nerve terminals, dopamine and recirculating noradrenaline are taken up from the cytoplasm into storage vesicles by active transport mechanisms. In the vesicles, these catecholamines mainly exist in a bound form and are linked to various proteins described as chromogranins. One type of chromogranin contains the enzyme β-hydroxylase which catalyses the conversion of dopamine to noradrenaline. The arrival of an action potential at the nerve terminal allows the release of noradrenaline into the synaptic gap where it acts on the receptor of the appropriate effector organ (Fig. 12.2). As mentioned previously, the released noradrenaline may inhibit further output from the nerve terminal by an effect on α_2-adrenoceptors located at presynaptic sites. The subsequent fate of the noradrenaline which has been discharged into the synaptic gap involves two alternative mechanisms:

1 Reuptake into the neurone (Uptake$_1$) where some of the noradrenaline is inactivated by the enzyme monoamine oxidase, while the remainder is transported back into the storage vesicles.

2 Uptake into extraneuronal tissue (Uptake$_2$); noradrenaline is then metabolized chiefly by the enzyme catechol-*O*-methyltransferase (COMT).

Both enzymes involved are widely distributed throughout the body and the metabolism of noradrenaline will eventually involve two pathways, as shown in Fig. 12.4.

Urinary metabolites include *O*-methylnoradrenaline and *O*-methyladrenaline (resulting from the conversion of adrenaline by COMT), small amounts of which

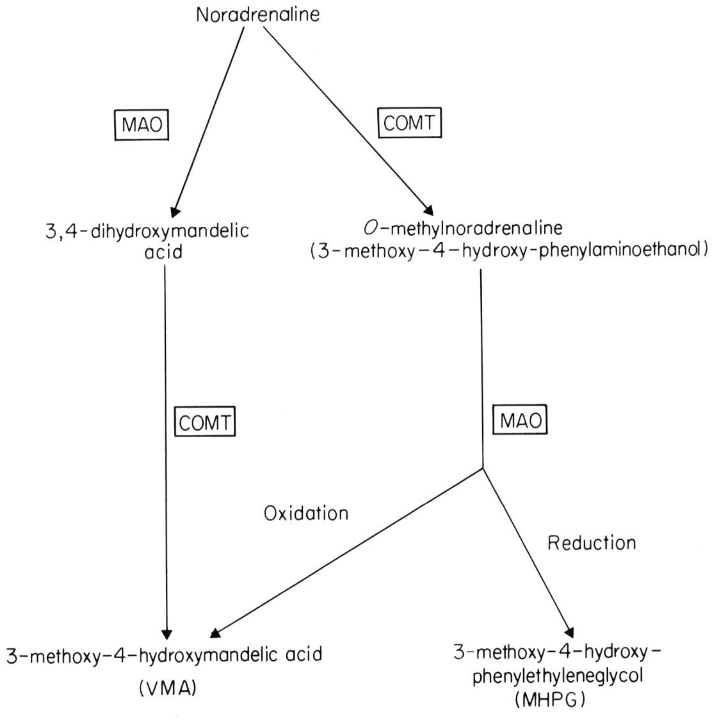

Fig. 12.4 Metabolism of noradrenaline.

are conjugated as sulphates and glucuronides. 3-Methoxy-4-hydroxymandelic acid (VMA) and 3-methoxy-4-hydroxyphenylethylene glycol (MHPG) can also be recovered from urine and changes in urinary MHPG levels may reflect differing activity within the CNS, where it is the major metabolite of noradrenaline. Drugs which are classified as adrenergic neurone-blocking agents are thought to act by interfering with the storage of intraneuronal catecholamines. Reserpine appears to inhibit the transport of noradrenaline (and its precursor dopamine) from the cytoplasm into the storage granules. The action of guanethidine and its analogues (bethanidine, debrisoquine) is probably more complex. They may act partially as 'false transmitters' and also prevent storage of noradrenaline by competing for granular binding sites. Guanethidine requires active transport for neuronal uptake; the pathway involved appears to be identical to that required for the reuptake of noradrenaline. This provides further evidence for the pharmacological action of guanethidine, and explains why its own effects are antagonized in the presence of drugs which block Uptake$_1$ mechanisms (e.g. phenothiazines, tricyclic antidepressants).

Drugs of this type are occasionally employed as antihypertensive agents and this role is discussed more fully in Chapter 14.

Adrenoceptor antagonists

α-Adrenoceptor antagonists

This group of drugs will bind selectively to α-adrenoceptors and inhibit the sympathetic responses involved at these sites. However, they show considerable variation with regard to their affinity for the two subgroups involved. Those agents which indiscriminately block both α_1- and α_2-adrenoceptors (e.g. phentolamine, tolazoline) will facilitate the further release of noradrenaline. As only α-adrenoceptors are blocked, there will be an enhanced response to the circulating catecholamines mediated via β-adrenoceptors and tachycardias are likely; postural hypotension may also be a problem. Such drugs are thus of little use in lowering the blood pressure of patients with essential hypertension, but are of some value in the control of secondary hypertension due to a high level of circulating catecholamines. In particular, phentolamine is a useful drug for the management of hypertensive episodes associated with surgical removal of a phaeochromocytoma, and is occasionally employed to ablate the sympathetic responses to anaesthesia and surgery which may occur in uncontrolled hypertensive patients.

Phenoxybenzamine exhibits more selective α_1-adrenoceptor antagonism. A covalent linkage is formed with the receptor and the effects of a single dose of this agent can last for several days. Phenoxybenzamine is used in the preoperative preparation of patients with phaeochromocytoma and in the long-term management when surgery is precluded. At one time it was employed (usually in combination with an inotropic agent such as dopamine) to improve peripheral perfusion in 'shock' states. Neuroleptic agents (e.g. phenothiazines, butyrophenones) have significant adrenoceptor antagonist activity and have sometimes been used in a similar context.

Prazosin appears to be relatively devoid of α_2-antagonist activity and has been developed as an antihypertensive agent; prazosin has also been used in the management of urinary outflow obstruction. Yohimbine is a selective α_2-adrenoceptor antagonist and has been shown experimentally to block the hypotensive responses to clonidine.

β-Adrenoceptor antagonists

In recent years, many agents with β-adrenoceptor antagonist properties have been introduced into clinical practice for the treatment of cardiovascular disorders. The prototype, dichloroisoprenaline, was not used clinically as it produced considerable partial agonist effects prior to blockade of the receptors. The closely related compound, pronethalol, was developed commercially as an antiarrhythmic and antianginal agent, but was later withdrawn when teratogenic effects had been observed following prolonged administration to mice. Propranolol, which differs chemically from the two aforementioned agents in that it has an oxymethylene (—O—CH_2—) bridge between the benzene ring and the ethanolamine side-chain, was then undergoing clinical trials. Propranolol and other analogues have subsequently been developed commercially and are identified in Table 12.4.

Table 12.4 Properties of β-adrenoceptor antagonists.

Drug	Cardioselectivity	Partial agonist activity	Membrane-stabilizing effect	Lipid solubility
Acebutolol	±	+	+	Moderate
Atenolol	+	–	–	Low
Betaxolol	+	–	+	Moderate
Bisoprolol	+	–	–	Low
Carvedilol*	–	–	?	Moderate
Celiprolol†	+	+	?	Low
Esmolol	+	–	–	High
Labetalol*	–	±	+	High
Metoprolol	+	–	±	High
Nadolol	–	–	–	Low
Oxprenolol	–	+	+	High
Pindolol	–	++	±	Moderate
Propranolol	–	–	++	High
Sotalol	–	–	–	Low
Timolol	–	+	+	High

–, Absent; ± minimal; +, present; ++, marked.
* Combined α- and β-adrenoceptor antagonists.
† Also possesses partial β_2-agonist activity.

Pharmacological properties

The varying members of this group of drugs may differ with respect to three distinct pharmacological actions:

1 Cardioselectivity. The majority of these agents, including propranolol, oxprenolol and alprenolol, are non-selective antagonists of both β_1- and β_2-adrenoceptors. β_2-Adrenoceptor blockade will account for the principal undesirable effects associated with the use of these drugs, notably bronchospasm in susceptible individuals and symptoms of peripheral vascular insufficiency; in addition, β_2-adrenoceptor activity mediates the secretion of insulin following a glucose load and potentiation of the effects of hypoglycaemic agents may occur when these drugs are used concurrently. Relatively specific β_1-adrenoceptor antagonists, such as atenolol and acebutolol, are usually preferred when therapy is required in patients with bronchial asthma, insulin-dependent diabetes and peripheral vascular disorders, although cardio-selectivity should be regarded as a relative and a dose-dependent phenomenon.

2 Intrinsic sympathomimetic activity. Some of these drugs (e.g. acebutolol, pindolol) display a partial agonist effect as well as antagonistic activity at β_1-adrenoceptors. In theory, they should be less likely to induce severe bradyarrhythmias or to induce cardiac failure. However, the significance of this property in clinical practice is less clear, although drugs with a much greater partial agonist effect (e.g. xamoterol) have been introduced and used in the treatment of mild to moderate cardiac failure.

3 Local anaesthetic effect. Some of the drugs in this group can decrease the rate of depolarization and increase the refractory period of cardiac muscle; this is a membrane-stabilizing or local anaesthetic effect. Experimental studies suggest that this effect is only produced by extremely high doses of these agents.

Pharmacokinetic properties

The degree of lipid or water solubility is the most important determinant of the subsequent pharmacokinetic behaviour of the β-adrenoceptor antagonists. In general terms, lipid-soluble agents in this group (e.g. propranolol, metoprolol) are well-absorbed following oral administration but are subject to a considerable first-pass effect due to hepatic metabolism. Thus, the bioavailability of such drugs is susceptible to a number of factors, including pharmacogenetic influences, liver disease and concomitant therapy with other drugs. Subsequently, drugs in this category usually have a short elimination half-life and are subject to wide variations in their plasma levels. Transfer across the blood–brain barrier is also more easily attained and such agents are more likely to induce side-effects such as sedation and bizarre dreams.

In contrast, water-soluble and relatively lipophobic agents (e.g. atenolol, nadolol) are less well-absorbed from the gut, but are unlikely to be subject to first-pass effects in the liver. They are usually eliminated unchanged by the kidney, and thus

Table 12.5 The pharmacokinetics and elimination of some common β-adrenoceptor antagonists.

	Absorption (%)	Bioavailability (%)	Protein binding (%)	Terminal half-life (h)	Significant active metabolites	Eliminated by metabolism (M) or renal excretion (RE)
Alprenolol	90	20	80	3	No	M
Labetalol	70	30	50	4	No	M
Metoprolol	90	50	20	4	No	M
Oxprenolol	80	50	80	2	No	M
Pindolol	90	90	50	4	No	M
Propranolol	90	30	80	5	Yes	M
Timolol	90	50	10	4	No	M and RE
Acebutolol	90	50	20	8	Yes	M and RE
Atenolol	50	50	0	8	No	RE
Nadolol	20	20	30	20	No	M and RE
Sotalol	80	60	0	15	No	RE

The data for absorption, bioavailability, protein binding and terminal half-lives represent median values.

have considerably longer plasma half-lives, so that less frequent dosage regimes are required. They are relatively impermeable to the blood–brain barrier and, in consequence, CNS effects are unlikely. The pharmacokinetic parameters of commonly used β-adrenoceptor antagonists are shown in Table 12.5.

Clinical uses

β-Adrenoceptor antagonists have developed a widespread role in the treatment of hypertension and in the management of angina pectoris and of certain cardiac arrhythmias. In almost all cases the therapeutic benefits achieved are due to blockade of β_1-adrenoceptors.

Hypertension

β-Adrenoceptor antagonists are now regarded as first-line therapy in the treatment of essential hypertension. However, the mechanism of this antihypertensive action is not entirely clear and may involve:

1 A reduction in cardiac output.

2 A resetting of baroreceptor activity at a lower blood pressure level.

3 Inhibition of the renin–angiotensin–aldosterone system.

4 An effect on plasma volume.

5 Presynaptic inhibition of noradrenaline release.

6 A CNS effect by those compounds which can effectively traverse the blood–brain barrier.

Present opinion suggests that the therapeutic benefits achieved in hypertension relate principally to the reduction in cardiac output and to the inhibition of renin release. This topic is also discussed in Chapter 14.

Angina pectoris

The use of β-adrenoceptor antagonists in the prophylaxis of attacks of exertional angina is logical. The negative inotropic effect reduces the work of the heart, whilst the concomitant slowing of the cardiac rate effectively improves coronary perfusion; furthermore, the effect of lowering the blood pressure will reduce the cardiac afterload. Similar pharmacological mechanisms also determine the numerous trials of various β-adrenoceptor antagonists for the prevention of reinfarction and the reduction of mortality following myocardial infarction.

However, not all the effects of β-adrenoceptor antagonists in this context can be considered to be beneficial. The lowering of the heart rate and the decrease in contractility will lead to a prolongation of the systolic ejection time, with a resultant increase in the left ventricular end-diastolic volume; oxygen consumption may therefore be greater. In those cases in which the attacks of angina are primarily due to spasm of the coronary vasculature (Prinzmetal angina), the administration of β-adrenoceptor antagonists can actually worsen the symptoms, as the unopposed effects mediated via the α-adrenoceptors will further reduce coronary perfusion. Finally, there is a danger that these agents may precipitate heart failure in patients with a poor cardiac reserve.

Arrhythmias

β-Adrenoceptor antagonists are essentially defined as class II antiarrhythmic agents. These agents prevent the increase in the rate of diastolic (phase 4) depolarization which is induced by catecholamines and decrease the rate of spontaneous firing of the sinoatrial node in the presence of excess sympathetic activity; of considerable therapeutic import is the increase in the effective refractory period of the atrioventricular node which results from blockade of β-adrenoceptor activity. Sotalol also has class III properties (possibly by specific inhibitory effects on potassium channels during repolarization).

β-Adrenoceptor antagonists are thus particularly useful in the management of tachyarrhythmias related to abnormal catecholamine activity such as those induced by exercise, emotion or thyrotoxicosis. They may also be used in the treatment of dysrhythmias induced by cardiac glycosides; conversely, propranolol is sometimes used in association with digoxin to control the ventricular rate in the presence of atrial fibrillation or flutter.

Other less common uses of β-adrenoceptor antagonists include the control of the peripheral responses to stress, the management of pathological anxiety states, the prophylaxis of migraine and the treatment of schizophrenia. Some drugs in this group (e.g. timolol, betaxolol) are also used as topical preparations in the treatment of chronic simple glaucoma. Intraocular pressure is reduced by a mechanism which is not entirely clear but probably involves a reduction in the rate of production of aqueous humour.

β-Adrenoceptor antagonists in anaesthetic practice

Drugs of this type have been employed in the preoperative preparation and intraoperative management of patients undergoing cardiac or vascular procedures, surgery for the removal of a phaeochromocytoma, thyroidectomy, and in the prevention of dysrhythmias which may occur during dental extractions under general anaesthesia. They may also be used to minimize reflex tachycardia during induced hypotension with ganglion-blocking agents (e.g. trimetaphan). Trimetaphan may release histamine, and its use in combination with a non-cardioselective agent can accentuate the risk of bronchospasm. A β-adrenoceptor antagonist may also be used to suppress the dysrhythmias observed during induced hypothermia.

Those patients who are on established therapy with β-adrenoceptor antagonists should continue to receive their medication until a few hours before surgery and should recommence treatment as soon as is practical in the postoperative period. Acute withdrawal of such therapy may cause ventricular dysrhythmias, severe angina, myocardial infarction and even sudden death. Furthermore, pretreatment with β-adrenoceptor antagonists before surgery and anaesthesia has been advised for patients with uncontrolled or inadequately treated hypertension. Such an approach may considerably modify the pressor responses which can occur, particularly during induction of anaesthesia and endotracheal intubation. Conversely, excessive suppression of β-adrenoceptors during anaesthesia can produce its own complications of bradyarrhythmias and hypotension; the administration of atropine and occasionally the use of a β-adrenoceptor agonist such as isoprenaline may be necessary.

Drugs have been developed which exhibit selective antagonism at β_2-adrenoceptors (e.g. butoxamine, α-methylpropranolol); they are unlikely to achieve a clinical role.

Further reading

Adgey AAJ, Geddes JS, Mulholland HC *et al.* Incidence significance and management of early bradyarrhythmia complicating acute myocardial infarction. *Lancet* 1968; **ii**: 1097–1101.

Ahlquist RP. A study of adrenotropic receptors. *American Journal of Physiology* 1948; **153**: 586–600.

Ask JL, Stene-Larsen G, Helle KB, Resch F. Functional β_1 and β_2 receptors in the human myocardium. *Acta Physiologica Scandinavica* 1985; **123**: 81–88.

Barger G, Dale HH. Chemical structure and sympathomimetic action of amines. *Journal of Physiology (London)* 1910; **41**: 19–59.

Barnett DB. Myocardial β-adrenoceptor function and regulation in heart failure: implications for therapy. *British Journal of Clinical Pharmacology* 1989; **27**: 527–538.

Breckenridge A. Which beta-blocker? *British Medical Journal* 1987; **286**: 1085–1088.

Burn JH, Rand MJ. Sympathetic postganglionic mechanisms. *Nature (London)* 1959; **184**: 163–165.

Chamberlain DA, Williams JH. Immediate care of cardiac emergencies. *Anaesthesia* 1976; **31**: 758–763.

Cohen LH, Thale T, Tissenbaum MJ. Acetylcholine treatment of schizophrenia. *Archives of Neurology and Psychiatry* 1944; **51**: 171–175.

Dale HH. The action of certain esters and ethers of choline, and their relation to muscarine. *Journal of Pharmacology and Experimental Therapeutics* 1914; **6**: 147–190.

DeJong W, Zandberg P, Bohus PH. Central inhibitory noradrenergic cardiovascular control. *Progress in Brain Research* 1975; **42**: 285–298.

Desjars P, Pinaud M, Bugnon D, Tasseau F. Norepinephrine has no deleterious renal effects in human septic shock. *Critical Care Medicine* 1989; **17**: 426–429.

Farah AE, Tuttle R. Studies on the pharmacology of glucagon. *Journal of Pharmacology and Experimental Therapeutics* 1960; **129**: 49–55.

Foex P. Beta-blockade in anaesthesia. *Journal of Clinical and Hospital Pharmacy* 1983; **8**: 183–190.

Furchgott RF. The role of endothelium in the responses of vascular smooth muscle to drugs. *Annual Review of Pharmacology and Toxicology* 1984; **24**: 175–197.

Garland CJ, Plane F, Kemp BK, Cocks TM. Endothelium-dependent hyperpolarisation: a role in the control of vascular tone. *Trends in Pharmacological Sciences* 1995; **16**: 23–30.

Goldberg LI. Dopamine — clinical uses of an endogenous catecholamine. *New England Medical Journal* 1974; **291**: 707–710.

Grant WM. Action of drugs on movements of ocular fluids. *Annual Review of Pharmacology* 1969; **9**: 85–94.

Greenberg MJ, Pines A. Pressurised aerosols in asthma. *British Medical Journal* 1967; **1**: 563.

Gurin S, Delluva A. The biological synthesis of radioactive adrenalin from phenylephrine. *Journal of Biology and Chemistry* 1947; **170**: 545–550.

Hall IP. Isoenzyme selective phosphodiesterase inhibitors: potential clinical uses. *British Journal of Clinical Pharmacology* 1993; **35**: 1–7.

Hammer R, Giachetti A. Muscarinic receptor subtypes; biochemical and functional characterisation. *Life Sciences* 1982; **31**: 2992–2998.

Hirschowitz BI, Hammer R, Giachetti A, Keirns JJ, Levine RR (eds) Subtypes of muscarinic receptors. *Trends in Pharmacological Sciences* (supplement 1): 1984; 1–103.

Hulme EC, Birdsall NJM, Buckley NJ. Muscarinic receptor subtypes. *Annual Review of Pharmacology and Toxicology* 1990; **30**: 633–673.

Jewitt J, Birkhead J, Mitchell A, Dollery C. Clinical cardiovascular pharmacology of dobutamine. *Lancet* 1974; **ii**: 363–367.

Kebabian JW, Agui T, van Oene JC *et al*. The D_1 dopamine receptor: new perspectives. *Trends in Pharmacological Sciences* 1986; **7**: 96–99.

Lands AM, Arnold A, Mcauliff JP *et al*. Differentiation of receptor systems activated by sympathomimetic amines. *Nature* 1967; **214**: 597–598.

Lands AM, Luduena FP, Buzzo HJ. Differentiation of receptors responsive to isoproterenol. *Life Sciences* 1967; **6**: 2241–2249.

Langer SZ. Presynaptic receptors and their role in the regulation of transmitter release. *British Journal of Pharmacology* 1977; **60**: 481–497.

Langer SZ, Hicks PE. Physiology of the sympathetic nerve ending. *British Journal of Anaesthesia* 1984; **56**: 689–700.

Langley JN. On the reaction of cells and of nerve-endings to certain poisons, chiefly as regards the reaction of striated muscles to nicotine and to curare. *Journal of Physiology (London)* 1905; **33**: 374–413.

Leff SE, Creese I. Dopamine receptors re-explained. *Trends in Pharmacological Sciences* 1983; **4**: 483–487.

Lewis RV, McDevitt DG. Adverse reactions and interactions with beta-adrenoceptor blocking drugs. *Medical Toxicology* 1986; **1**: 343–361.

Loewi O, Navratil P. Uber humorale Ubertragbarkeit der Herznervenwirkung. X. Mitterling. Uber das Schickshal des Vagusstoffs. *Pflugers Archives Furdic Gesante Physiologie* 1926; **214**: 678–688.

Maclagan J, Barnes PJ. Muscarinic pharmacology of the airways. *Trends in Pharmacological Sciences* 1989; **10** (suppl. IV): 88S–92S.

Mitchell JR, Oates JA. Guanethidine and related agents I. Mechanisms of the selective blockade of adrenergic neurones and its antagonism by drugs. *Journal of Pharmacology and Experimental Therapeutics* 1970; **172**: 100–107.

Moncada S, Radomski MW. Endothelium derived relaxing factor. Identification as nitric oxide and role in the control of vascular tone and platelet function. *Biochemical Pharmacology* 1988; **37**: 2495–2502.

Okospki JV. Recent advances in pharmaceutical chemistry — review III. A new wave of beta-blockers. *Journal of Clinical Pharmacy and Therapeutics* 1987; **12**: 369–388.

Parker JO, West RO, Digiori S. Haemodynamic effects of propranolol in coronary heart disease. *American Journal of Cardiology* 1968; **21**: 11–19.

Powell CE, Slater IH. Blocking of inhibitory adrenergic receptors by a dichloro analogue of isoprotorenol. *Journal of Pharmacology and Experimental Therapeutics* 1958; **122**: 480–488.

Prys-Roberts C. Developments in adrenergic receptor pharmacology and their relevance to anaesthesia. *Current Opinion in Anaesthesiology* 1990; **3**: 89–97.

Putney JW Jr. Calcium mobilising receptors. *Trends in Pharmacological Sciences* 1987; **8**: 481–485.

Rhoden KJ, Meldrum LA, Barnes PJ. Inhibition of cholinergic neurotransmission in human airways by $beta_2$-adrenoceptors. *Journal of Applied Physiology* 1988; **65**: 700–705.

Rosenblum R. Physiological basis for the therapeutic use of catecholamines. *American Heart Journal* 1974; **87**: 527–530.

Sargent P. The diversity of neuronal nicotinic acetylcholine receptors. *Annual Review of Neurosciences* 1993; **16**: 403–443.

Sen G, Bose KC. *Rauwolfia serpentina*, a new Indian drug for insanity and high blood pressure. *Indian Medical World* 1931; **2**: 194–201.

Sibley DR, Morisma FJ. Molecular biology of dopamine receptors. *Trends in Pharmacological Sciences* 1992; **13**: 61–69.

Smith LDR, Oldershaw PJ. Inotropic and vasopressor agents. *British Journal of Anaesthesia* 1984; **56**: 767–780.

Snow HM. The pharmacology of xamoterol: a basis for modulation of the autonomic control of the heart. *British Journal of Clinical Pharmacology* 1989; **28**: 3S–13S.

Speizer FE, Doll R, Strang LG. Investigation into use of drugs preceding death from asthma. *British Medical Journal* 1968; **1**: 339–343.

Starke K. Regulation of noradrenaline release of presynaptic receptor systems. *Review of Physiology, Biochemistry and Pharmacology* 1977; **77**: 1–124.

Stoof JF, Kebabian JW. Dopaminergic receptors. *Life Sciences* 1984; **35**: 2281–2296.

Sutherland EW, Rall TW. The relation of adenosine-3′5′ phosphate and phosphorylase to the actions of catecholamines and other hormones. *Pharmacological Reviews* 1959; **12**: 265–269.

Von Euler US. A specific sympathomimetic ergone in adrenergic nerve fibres (sympathin) and its relations to adrenaline and nor-adrenaline. *Acta Physiologica Scandinavica* 1946; **12**: 73–97.

Weiner N. Multiple factors regulating the release of epinephrine consequent to nerve stimulation. *Federal Proceedings* 1979; **39**: 2193–2202.

Whyte KF, Addis GJ, Whitesmith R, Reid JF. The mechanism of salbutamol-induced hypokalaemia. *British Journal of Clinical Pharmacology* 1987; **23**: 65–71.

Wilmshurst P. Phosphodiesterase inhibitors. *Current Opinion in Anaesthesiology* 1989; **2**: 83–87.

Yaksh TL. Pharmacology of spinal adrenergic systems which modulate spinal nociceptive processing. *Pharmacology, Biochemistry and Behaviour* 1985; **22**: 845–848.

Yeo J, Southwell P, Hindmarsh E. Preliminary report on the effect of distigmine on the neurogenic bladder. *Medical Journal of Australia* 1973; **1**: 116–120.

Chapter 13
Drugs used in Premedication and Antiemetic Agents

An ever-increasing variety of drugs may be prescribed or used by the anaesthetist prior to the administration of general or regional anaesthesia. The aims of such premedication may be directed at:

1 The allayment of fear and anxiety.

2 A reduction in anaesthetic requirement.

3 The suppression of unwanted parasympathetic or sympathetic activity, including haemodynamic responses to intubation.

4 The prevention or diminution of pain, nausea and vomiting in the postoperative period.

5 The minimization of risks associated with the aspiration of gastric contents, particularly in obstetric anaesthesia.

Development of premedication

For many years opioid analgesics were routinely used as premedicant drugs. Their sedative and analgesic effects had considerable advantages in facilitating the induction and maintenance of anaesthesia in the era prior to the introduction of intravenous barbiturates, neuromuscular blocking agents and potent inhalational anaesthetics. Nevertheless, there are several disadvantages associated with opioid premedication:

1 Dysphoria may occur in the absence of preoperative pain.

2 Gastric emptying time is prolonged, and nausea and vomiting may occur.

3 Interaction with other central nervous system (CNS) depressants may be undesirable.

4 There may be difficulty in timing drug administration to produce an optimal effect during routine operating lists.

5 Parenteral administration is usually essential.

Opioid analgesics are less widely used for premedication in present-day anaesthetic practice, but are still a valuable choice in small children; in these conditions, parenteral administration is frequently necessary, and some 'hangover' analgesia into the postoperative period is particularly desirable. Morphine (0.25 mg kg^{-1}) or pethidine (1 mg kg^{-1}) is commonly used and may be administered with atropine (0.02 mg kg^{-1} up to a maximum dose of 0.6 mg) by intramuscular injection 30–45 min prior to surgery. Some anaesthetists consider that the 'twilight sleep' induced by combination of papaveretum (Omnopon; 20 mg) and hyoscine (scopolamine; 0.4 mg; adult doses) confers marked advantages when used as premedication prior to cardiac surgery.

At one time preanaesthetic sedation or basal narcosis was induced by the rectal administration of powerful CNS depressants during the preoperative period. The agents used included tribromethyl alcohol (bromethol; Avertin), paraldehyde, or thiopentone sodium suspension in large doses (approximately 45 mg kg^{-1}). This method was considered to be particularly useful in uncooperative children, or in patients with uncontrolled thyrotoxicosis ('stealing the thyroid'). However, there is the likelihood of profound depression of vital reflexes and delayed recovery from anaesthesia, and the technique is now considered obsolete. Similarly, the use of orally administered barbiturates as hypnotics or preoperative sedatives has declined. Barbiturates potentiate the CNS effects of anaesthetic agents, and increased restlessness in the presence of pain may be anticipated.

In recent years, benzodiazepine tranquillizers have been widely used for premedication (particularly in adult patients). They may be used as night hypnotics (i.e. to promote drowsiness and sleep), or administered during the day to produce sedation (a state conducive to sleep) or anxiolysis (the reduction of fear, anxiety and apprehension). Benzodiazepines have a low toxicity and do not affect the pain threshold; drug interactions, or potentiation of other agents administered during anaesthesia, are usually of little practical significance.

General hazards of hypnotic and premedicant drugs

Some potential hazards and side-effects are common to all hypnotic and sedative drugs, including those that are commonly used as agents for premedication. All hypnotic drugs characteristically impair judgement and increase reaction time; ambulant patients should always be warned of their hazards in relation to car driving, working at heights and operating dangerous machinery. Even short-acting hypnotics may impair psychomotor performance or produce hangover effects on the day after their administration. In normal dosage, currently used hypnotic drugs do not usually affect respiration (except, perhaps, in elderly patients with impaired lung function). Nevertheless, hypnotic overdosage (particularly with barbiturates and their derivatives) is classically associated with severe respiratory depression. All hypnotic drugs may interact with other central depressants, including ethyl alcohol. Some hypnotic drugs (e.g. barbiturates, dichloralphenazone) are enzyme-inducing agents, and may potentially interact with other drugs (e.g. oral anticoagulants, antidepressants, anticonvulsants, contraceptives). The elimination of all hypnotics may be compromised in hepatic and/or renal impairment, and in patients over 60 years old. In general, hypnotics are poorly tolerated by elderly patients, and drowsiness, disorientation and unsteadiness may result in slurred speech, falls and fractures, poor memory and acute confusional states. The increased susceptibility of elderly patients is partly due to pharmacokinetic factors (i.e. decreased hepatic oxidative drug metabolism) and partly to enhanced sensitivity at neuronal sites in the CNS.

All hypnotics may also induce tolerance and dependence, and they may alter the pattern of physiological sleep. The onset and establishment of sleep can be monitored by continuous measurement of cortical activity using the electroencephalogram (EEG). Four stages of the development of sleep, associated with a gradually decreasing rate of activity accompanied by an increase in electrical amplitude, are recognized. Once sleep is established two distinct patterns may be observed:

1 A fast cortical rhythm of low amplitude (accompanied by slow-wave activity in the hindbrain) which is associated with rapid eye movement (REM) between the closed lids, fluctuations in cardiac and respiratory rates and dreaming. This phenomenon, which occupies approximately 25% of total sleep time, is known as paradoxical or REM sleep.

2 Longer-lasting periods of cortical slow-wave sleep (in which the hindbrain rhythm is faster) when eyeballs are still, cardiac and respiratory rates are regular and dreaming does not occur. This is known as non-REM (NREM) sleep. During the administration of hypnotic drugs, the intensity and duration of stage 3, stage 4 and REM sleep is reduced. When the hypnotic is stopped, a rebound phenomenon occurs, and there is subsequent compensation for the earlier loss of REM sleep. This is sometimes associated with unpleasant dreams and nightmares due to more intense REM mentation. Since the function of non-REM sleep is unknown, the significance of these changes is a matter of conjecture.

Benzodiazepines

Benzodiazepines are the most commonly prescribed drugs in the western world; in the UK alone, there may be 3 million chronic users of these agents. They have significant advantages compared with the barbiturates, which they have largely replaced as hypnotics, sedatives, anxiolytics and premedicant agents. They are less dangerous in overdosage; they are less likely to interact with other drugs (apart from other hypnotic drugs); and their side-effects are less frequent. Nevertheless, performance of psychomotor skills, such as driving a car, may be impaired; and the potentiation of the effects of other CNS depressants, such as ethyl alcohol, may be a problem. At present 15 benzodiazepines are currently available in the UK as hypnotics, sedatives or anxiolytics (Table 13.1), and some of them are widely used as premedicants. Although their pharmacological actions are similar, there are significant differences in their pharmacokinetic properties.

Mode of action

Benzodiazepines are generally considered to produce sedation and hypnosis by

Table 13.1 Relative potencies, terminal half-lives and active metabolites of benzodiazepines.

	Approximate normal hypnotic or sedative dose (mg)	Approximate potency	Terminal half-life of parent drug (h)	Active metabolites	Half-lives of significant active metabolites (h)
Hypnotics					
Flunitrazepam	1	30	12–20	Yes	25–30
Flurazepam	30	1	2–3	Yes	50–100
Lormetazepam	2	15	8–12	No	
Loprazolam	2	15	6–8	Yes	6–8
Nitrazepam	10	3	18–34	Doubtful	
Temazepam	20	1.5	4–10	No‡	
Triazolam	0.25	120	1–3	Yes	3–5
Midazolam	10	3	1–3	No	
Sedatives					
Alprazolam	0.5	60	10–12	Yes	†
Bromazepam	6	5	8–19	Yes	†
Chlordiazepoxide	20	1.5	5–30	Yes	6–25 50–120
Clobazam	20	1.5	10–30	Yes	35–45
Clorazepate	15	2	*	Yes	50–120
Diazepam	10	3	24–48	Yes	4–10 6–25 50–120
Ketazolam	15	2	*	Yes	50–120
Lorazepam	1	30	10–20	No	
Medazepam	10	3	1–2	Yes	50–120
Oxazepam	30	1	6–25	No	50–120
Prazepam	20	1.5	*	Yes	

* Clorazepate, ketazolam and prazepam are rapidly metabolized in the gut or the liver to desmethyldiazepam.
† Alprazolam and bromazepam have active metabolites, but they are probably not clinically significant.
‡ Minor amounts of temazepam (about 2–5%) may be metabolized to oxazepam.

depressing the excitability of the limbic system. This loosely defined area of the brain consists of the hippocampus, the septal region, the amygdaloid nuclei, and part of the cerebral cortex and the hypothalamus, and is believed to be concerned with the integration of emotional responses. In consequence, benzodiazepines generally produce:

1 Modification of emotional responsiveness and behaviour, due to suppression of neuronal activity between the limbic system and the hypothalamus.

2 A decrease in alertness and arousal reactions, since interaction between the limbic system and the reticular activating system is depressed.

3 Anticonvulsant properties, probably due to effects on the amygdaloid nuclei.

4 Suppression of polysynaptic reflexes in the spinal cord. In this context, benzodiazepines may be regarded as centrally acting muscle relaxants.

Although initial electrophysiological studies demonstrated that benzodiazepines depressed the reticular activating system, recent neurochemical evidence suggests that they produce more widespread effects by facilitating effects mediated by γ-aminobutyric acid (GABA), which is the principal inhibitory transmitter within the CNS. Neurones which release GABA are essentially small interneurones which induce hyperpolarization at pre- and postsynaptic sites (probably involving 20–40% of all synapses within the CNS) by an increase in chloride conductance. Two types of GABA-receptors, designated $GABA_A$ and $GABA_B$, have been described. $GABA_A$-receptors are widely distributed at supraspinal levels as well as in the spinal cord, and are closely related to specific high-affinity binding sites for benzodiazepines. There is no evidence to suggest that benzodiazepines affect the synthesis, release or breakdown of GABA. It is considered that benzodiazepines have a modulatory effect on the $GABA_A$–chloride complex, and probably increase the frequency of opening of the ionic gate. A specific antagonist (flumazenil) has been developed for clinical use, whilst β-carbolines, which are found in brain tissue, have been shown to produce inverse agonist effects (e.g. anxiety and convulsions) in experimental animals.

$GABA_B$-receptors have been demonstrated at presynaptic sites on peripheral autonomic nerve terminals and throughout the CNS, with a high concentration found in the dorsal horn of the spinal cord. The principal effects mediated via $GABA_B$-receptors would appear to be a diminished release of amines, neuropeptides and excitatory neurotransmitters (autoreceptors may also inhibit the release of GABA itself). $GABA_B$ effects do not appear to interrelate with those of the benzodiazepines; however, a specific agonist, baclofen, is used to reduce spasticity and prevent flexor spasms in a variety of neurological disorders, presumably by inhibiting spinal reflexes.

Two subgroups of the benzodiazepine receptor (BZ_1 and BZ_2) have also been identified. BZ_1-receptors are found throughout the spinal cord, with large concentrations in the cerebellum; anxiolytic activity has been ascribed to actions at these sites. BZ_2-receptors are located in the cerebral cortex, spinal cord and hippocampus, and may be more closely related to the sedative (and presumably anticonvulsant) effects.

The $GABA_A$-receptor subtype may be a heterogeneous group of different receptors rather than a single entity. Five different $GABA_A$-receptor subunits (α, β, γ, δ and ρ) have been described, with multiple isoforms within each class. Experimental evidence suggests that the distribution of the six isoforms of the α subunit may be the most important determinant of affinity for BZ_1- and BZ_2-agonists.

Benzodiazepines also decrease dopamine and 5-hydroxytryptamine turnover in specific brain regions, and the increase in noradrenaline turnover induced by stress is prevented. It is now believed that these changes represent indirect and secondary effects on brain metabolism.

Benzodiazepines differ greatly in potency (Table 13.1); for instance, alprazolam (normal hypnotic dose = 0.5 mg) is approximately 40 times as potent as temazepam (normal hypnotic dose = 20 mg). These differences in potency appear to be related to the variable affinity of benzodiazepines for receptors in the CNS, and may relate to structural differences between various members of this group.

Pharmacokinetics

In general, benzodiazepines that are used to produce hypnosis and premedication show a wide variation in their half-lives (Table 13.1). In addition, some drugs have metabolites with considerable pharmacological activity which may cumulate during chronic administration. Differences between the terminal half-lives of the benzodiazepines and their metabolites have been used to divide them into hypnotics and sedatives/anxiolytics. Although this distinction is rather artificial and arbitrary, it may be valuable in practice. Benzodiazepines with short terminal half-lives (and whose active metabolites have short half-lives) have considerable advantages as hypnotic or premedicant drugs. They are less likely to produce impaired psychomotor performance and hangover effects (e.g. ataxia, motor incoordination, muscle weakness, poor memory and concentration, mental confusion) on the day after their administration.

Most benzodiazepines have a large apparent volume of distribution due to their high lipid solubility. The majority are extensively bound to plasma proteins; diazepam, for example, is 96–97% bound, mainly by albumin. Only the unbound (free) fraction can cross the blood–brain barrier and affect the CNS. Although protein-displacement reactions can be demonstrated in *in vitro* conditions, little is known of their significance in anaesthetic practice. In general, benzodiazepines are non-polar, lipid-soluble drugs, and are not extensively excreted unchanged in urine. Consequently, they do not usually cumulate in renal failure. Benzodiazepines are almost entirely eliminated from the body by hepatic metabolism. This usually involves oxidative reactions that are primarily carried out by microsomal enzymes associated with the hepatic endoplasmic reticulum. Nevertheless, some benzodiazepines (e.g. oxazepam) are almost entirely eliminated by glucuronide conjugation. Most benzodiazepines have a low intrinsic hepatic clearance which is not restricted by hepatic blood flow (with the possible exception of midazolam). Many of the metabolic pathways of the benzodiazepines are closely interrelated; to some extent, this may account for the similarity in their actions. Thus diazepam and clorazepate are converted to the active compound desmethyldiazepam (nordiazepam), which has a half-life of several days (Fig. 13.1). Elderly patients are more sensitive and vulnerable to benzodiazepines; this is partly due to decreased oxidative metabolism by the liver.

Although most benzodiazepines are extensively bound to plasma proteins, the unbound (free) drug can diffuse across the placental barrier and may affect the fetus. There is little or no definite evidence that benzodiazepines cause fetal abnormalities; nevertheless, some of these drugs can cause complications when used during pregnancy or labour. For instance, when diazepam is used in late pregnancy (e.g. in the treatment of pre-eclampsia and eclampsia), it readily crosses the placenta,

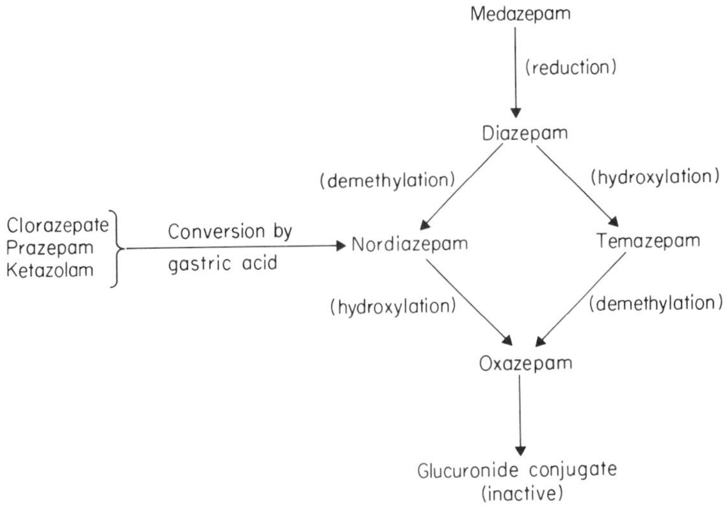

Fig. 13.1 Metabolic relationships between some commonly used benzodiazepines.

and may be metabolized by the fetus. Some of its active metabolites (including desmethyldiazepam, temazepam and oxazepam) may accumulate in fetal tissues, and can cause neonatal depression, hypotonia and hypothermia. In addition, chronic exposure of the fetus to benzodiazepines can result in withdrawal symptoms after birth.

Use in anaesthetic practice

Benzodiazepines are often used as premedicant agents in adult patients prior to elective surgery. Regimes were designed to provide sedation and hypnosis during the preoperative period; they were started on admission to hospital and continued until the morning of operation. Nitrazepam (10 mg at night) and diazepam (5 mg three times daily) were commonly used for this purpose. This combination was shown to be satisfactory as assessed by subjective and objective measurements of the level of anxiety (although either drug, used alone, would probably be equally effective). However, the sedative and amnesic effects of nitrazepam (or diazepam) may persist until the following day, and confusion and ataxia may occur in elderly patients. Temazepam (10–20 mg at night) is now replacing nitrazepam as a hypnotic in this context and may also be prescribed on the morning of operation.

For day-case surgery, including endoscopic procedures and outpatient dental treatment, benzodiazepines with a shorter duration of action are usually preferred. Temazepam (10–20 mg), diazepam (5–10 mg) or lorazepam (1–2.5 mg) may be given orally 1.5–2 h before the procedure. There is little advantage in using the intramuscular route, which is painful and is associated with a reduced bioavailability.

Although benzodiazepines have been used as intravenous induction agents, they have a relatively slow onset of action, and produce variable and unpredictable effects on the level of consciousness. They are generally less satisfactory than intravenous barbiturates, but are occasionally of value in patients known to be hypersensitive to other agents. Nevertheless, benzodiazepines are frequently administered by this route to provide sedation and anterograde amnesia for surgical procedures under local or regional anaesthesia. Intravenous preparations of lorazepam, diazepam and midazolam are mainly used for this purpose.

Intravenous lorazepam has a relatively slow onset of action (usually within 10–20 min) and a prolonged duration of action (up to 6 h) due to its slow distribution to, and redistribution from, the CNS. It usually produces intense and prolonged anterograde amnesia within 30 min which lasts for up to 4 h. It is less likely to cause pain, thrombophlebitis and venous thrombosis than aqueous diazepam. Despite the disadvantage of its slow onset of action, it may be of value in prolonged procedures under local anaesthesia, in intensive care or to diminish the psychotomimetic effects of other drugs.

Diazepam usually acts within 2–3 min, producing sedation (for up to 60 min) and amnesia (for 10–30 min). Nevertheless, active metabolites of the drug can usually be detected for at least 24–48 h, and ambulant patients must be warned of the possible hazards during this period. The drug has often been used before regional anaesthesia, therapeutic nerve blocks, uncomfortable diagnostic procedures, conservative dentistry and sometimes as a prelude to general anaesthetic techniques. There is wide individual variation in the response to this agent, and the injection should be given very slowly (2.5 mg every 30 s) until drooping of the eyelids is observed. Diazepam was sometimes used in this way in combination with opioid agents (e.g. pentazocine) to produce sedation and analgesia during dental treatment. In these conditions, respiratory depression is a real possibility and facilities for artificial ventilation should always be available with this technique.

Like most benzodiazepines, diazepam is poorly soluble in water; in the UK, aqueous preparations are acidic and viscous, and contain various organic solubilizers (e.g. propylene glycol, ethanol and benzoic acid). Local complications can be produced by these preparations; pain on injection, thrombophlebitis and venous thrombosis are not uncommon, particularly when the drug is injected into small-diameter veins on the hand. Occasionally, hypersensitivity reactions may occur. The incidence of local complications can be reduced by appropriate techniques (e.g. the injection of the drug into a fast-running infusion, the use of veins in the antecubital fossa, or by *barbotage*) or by the use of other preparations of diazepam. Diazemuls is a white opaque soybean oil-in-water emulsion of diazepam similar to Intralipid. It rarely causes pain and thrombophlebitis after injection, but in other respects is similar to aqueous diazepam.

Midazolam has several advantages compared with diazepam; in recent years, it has largely replaced diazepam as an intravenous sedative and amnesic agent.

At an acid pH (i.e. pH 4 or less) midazolam is ionized in aqueous solution and is relatively water-soluble. After intravenous injection, the chemical structure of the drug is modified, increasing its lipid solubility and facilitating its diffusion into the CNS. Consequently, pain on injection and thrombophlebitis are infrequent complications. Midazolam has a rapid onset of action, and usually causes more profound amnesia than diazepam. The relatively short terminal half-life of the drug (approximately 2 h) is associated with rapid recovery and the absence of hangover effects. However, there have been occasional reports of respiratory depression (sometimes associated with severe hypotension) following the intravenous administration of midazolam; furthermore, drug interactions in association with macrolide antibiotics and certain antiarrhythmic agents have been described. Midazolam is almost entirely metabolized by the liver. Its metabolism (unlike that of other benzodiazepines) may be partly dependent on liver blood flow; one of its metabolites may have slight hypnotic activity. In the USA, midazolam has been administered by oral, rectal and intranasal routes for premedication in children.

Other uses

Benzodiazepines are the hypnotics and sedatives of choice for short-term oral administration. They are particularly useful in the treatment of insomnia associated with anxiety. In most subjects, they are relatively safe in overdosage, and patients have recovered from as much as 80 times the normal hypnotic dose. Nevertheless, they can produce dangerous respiratory depression in the elderly, or in patients with impaired pulmonary function (for example, in chronic bronchitis). They do not induce hepatic microsomal enzymes, and do not usually interact with other drugs (apart from other hypnotics and sedatives, including ethyl alcohol). Similarly, side-effects (apart from drowsiness and related central phenomena) are rare; occasionally they cause nightmares, nausea, skin rashes or an increase in body weight. Although most benzodiazepines are suitable hypnotics, a drug with a short half-life (e.g. temazepam) may be preferred when hangover effects impair performance. Unfortunately, there is increasing evidence that drug tolerance and dependence are not uncommon, and their use as hypnotics and sedatives should be restricted to less than 1 month, if possible. It is usually stated that tolerance to their hypnotic effects may occur after 3–14 days' continual administration; during their chronic use, physical dependence is said to occur in 15% of patients.

A benzodiazepine withdrawal syndrome is now described and may occur within a few hours or up to 3 weeks after stopping the drug (symptoms will occur more rapidly when a short-acting drug has been administered). Characteristics include insomnia, anxiety, loss of appetite, tremor, perspiration and tinnitus and may persist for several months. Problems with specific drugs have also occurred. The most potent member of the group, triazolam, was withdrawn because of its association with a high frequency of reversible psychiatric side-effects, particularly loss of memory and depression. Temazepam has gained some notoriety as a drug of social abuse; gangrene following the injection of the contents of the gel-filled capsules has been reported.

Benzodiazepines are widely used for other purposes. It is generally accepted that intravenous diazepam is the drug of choice in status epilepticus, whether idiopathic or drug-induced (thiopentone may be a suitable alternative when facilities for artificial ventilation are immediately available). An initial dose of 10–30 mg can be given intravenously, but repeated administration or continuous infusion may be necessary; a total dose of 200 mg in 24 h should not be exceeded, unless controlled ventilation has been instituted. Although benzodiazepines are effective in the prophylaxis of many forms of epilepsy (particularly those associated with a generalized EEG discharge), the doses required often cause an unacceptable degree of sedation and drowsiness. Clonazepam and clobazam have been most widely used for the prophylaxis of seizures. They may be useful for short-term prophylaxis, or as an addition to other anticonvulsant regimes. Clonazepam may be particularly effective in the long-term control of myoclonic disorders, although problems with oversedation can occur. Like certain other anticonvulsant drugs, it may be of value in the management of trigeminal neuralgia and other painful conditions. Clobazam (a 1,5-benzodiazepine) may cause less psychomotor disturbance than clonazepam and other 1,4-benzodiazepines. It should be remembered that most benzodiazepines can provoke seizures, and may cause irritability and hyperactivity in children. Benzodiazepines are also useful in the management of muscle hypertonicity or spasticity, due to their central muscle relaxant effects. Thus, they may be of value in painful spasms associated with spinal cord injury or demyelinating disorders, muscle contraction headaches, and in the management of tetanus. In addition, they are used in the treatment of alcohol withdrawal, and the control of night terrors and sleep walking.

Benzodiazepine antagonists

Flumazenil is an imidazobenzodiazepine which behaves as a competitive, reversible benzodiazepine antagonist; it may also stimulate benzodiazepine receptors, and some of its actions appear to be unrelated to benzodiazepine antagonism. It is mainly metabolized in the liver, and has a rapid onset but relatively brief duration of action, due to its short half-life (approximately 1 h). Consequently, it may require to be given by repeated injection or continuous intravenous infusion in order to antagonize sedation and respiratory depression produced by longer-acting benzodiazepines. It may be used to reverse the effects of benzodiazepines after anaesthesia, or after short diagnostic procedures, although careful supervision will be required until recovery is complete.

The side-effects of flumazenil include nausea, vomiting, flushing, anxiety and agitation, and convulsions can be precipitated in epileptic patients. Some of these effects may be due to inverse agonist activity. The duration of anterograde amnesia produced by benzodiazepines is usually reduced by flumazenil. The initial dose is 0.2 mg, with further 0.1 mg increments at 1-min intervals until recovery is complete.

Other hypnotic drugs

Chlormethiazole

Chlormethiazole is a hypnotic drug that is chemically related to vitamin B_1 (thiamine) and the proprietary name (Heminevrin) reflects this structural similarity. Although its mode of action has not been precisely defined, it is believed to have direct or indirect effects on GABA-dependent pathways in the CNS. Approximately 50% of the drug is normally bound by plasma proteins, and its terminal half-life is usually 3–5 h. After oral administration, it induces sleep within 30–40 min, and is particularly useful for the management of agitation, confusion, restlessness and insomnia in elderly patients. Chlormethiazole has also been used for the control of delirium tremens and acute withdrawal symptoms in alcoholic patients, and as an anticonvulsant for the management of status epilepticus and pre-eclamptic toxaemia. It is available as an oral preparation and as an intravenous infusion (0.8%). The hypnotic dose is 250–500 mg.

Although chlormethiazole is a relatively safe hypnotic drug with a low systemic toxicity, it may potentiate the effects of other CNS depressants, and may cause respiratory embarrassment, especially in acute or chronic pulmonary disease. Nevertheless, hangover effects are infrequent, and acute overdosage is uncommon. Chlormethiazole can cause nasal congestion, increased secretions and conjunctivitis. These effects usually occur within 10–30 min of oral administration, and are commoner in younger patients with an allergic diathesis. They appear to be mainly due to local histamine release from mast cells in the nasal mucosa.

Chloral hydrate and its derivatives

Chloral hydrate is one of the oldest and safest hypnotic drugs. It is a halogenated hydrocarbon, and is closely related to chloroform and trichlorethylene. Indeed, its introduction as a hypnotic drug by Liebreich in 1869 was based on the assumption that chloral would slowly release chloroform in the body. Although this is incorrect, it is believed that chloral hydrate and its derivatives act like general anaesthetics, i.e. they produce hypnosis by acting at non-polar sites on lipid or protein components of neuronal membranes. In this manner, they may interfere with ion transport and prevent depolarization. In electrophysiological studies, both chloral hydrate and its main metabolite reduce synaptic activity in the reticular activating system, causing a deactivating response in the EEG.

When taken orally, chloral hydrate acts within 30–40 min and produces hypnosis for 6–8 h. It has little effect on respiration or on reflex activity in the spinal cord. Although tolerance and dependence may develop, they are uncommon; side-effects are also infrequent. Chloral hydrate is metabolized by the liver to trichlorethanol, which is subsequently eliminated as a glucuronide conjugate (urochloralic acid). Trichlorethanol itself has a considerable hypnotic activity, and is probably mainly responsible for the effects of chloral hydrate.

When used as an oral hypnotic drug, chloral has several important disadvantages. After oral administration it has an unpleasant taste and an irritant effect on the gastric mucosa, and may cause nausea and vomiting. In addition, it is hygroscopic and deliquescent, and cannot be prepared or preserved as tablets. Nevertheless, mixtures, elixirs and capsules of chloral hydrate are sometimes used in children and in elderly patients. Alternatively, stabilized preparations of chloral may be used. These preparations do not have the disadvantages of chloral hydrate, since the drug is present as a complex which is not dissociated until absorption is complete. Dichloralphenazone is a stabilized preparation of chloral and the analgesic phenazone, and generally causes fewer gastrointestinal side-effects than chloral hydrate. Unfortunately, phenazone (antipyrine) may induce drug-metabolizing enzymes in the liver, and can cause interactions with other drugs (e.g. oral anticoagulants). The occasional development of hypersensitivity reactions and blood dyscrasias is probably due to phenazone. An alternative preparation is trichlorethanol phosphate, which is a stabilized form of the main metabolite of chloral hydrate.

Phenothiazines

Some hypnotic and sedative drugs that are chemically classified as phenothiazines (e.g. promethazine and trimeprazine) are used as premedicant drugs, particularly in children. Both these drugs have considerable antimuscarinic (anticholinergic) effects and indirect evidence suggests that their hypnotic activity is related to the antagonism of acetylcholine at central synapses. There are numerous cholinergic neurones in the brain and the spinal cord, and acetylcholine is an important excitatory transmitter at many sites in the CNS (including the reticular activating system and the cerebral cortex). Many drugs that produce sedation have antimuscarinic activity (e.g. antidepressants, antipsychotics, H_1-histamine antagonists, scopolamine). In general, phenothiazines produce varying degrees of sedation that are closely related to their antimuscarinic effects.

Most phenothiazines may antagonize or affect a wide range of central neurotransmitters (as well as acetylcholine). Consequently, they have multiple actions on the CNS, and are generally unsuitable as sedative or hypnotic drugs. Nevertheless, promethazine and trimeprazine have reasonably selective effects and are widely used as hypnotic and premedicant agents in children.

Promethazine (a structural analogue of promazine) is an H_1-histamine antagonist with a prolonged duration of action (up to 24 h). After oral administration it is well-absorbed and widely distributed, and usually acts within 30–60 min. It is relatively safe in overdosage, and therapeutic doses have little effect on the cardiovascular or respiratory system. Promethazine may produce dizziness and disorientation (particularly in the elderly). In addition to its sedative and hypnotic effects, it has antiemetic and antisecretory properties, which contribute to its usefulness as a premedicant drug in children. Promethazine is sometimes indicated as a hypnotic–premedicant drug in asthmatic patients; the drug has bronchodilator effects, and may also prevent responses due to histamine release by certain anaesthetic agents. It may be useful in the symptomatic relief of various hypersensitivity reactions, although hypnotic and antimuscarinic side-effects are common. Promethazine may be valuable in the prophylaxis of motion sickness, and can be used as an antiemetic drug in early pregnancy. Like other antihistamines and certain phenothiazines with marked antimuscarinic activity, promethazine may be used in parkinsonism.

Trimeprazine is an H_1-histamine antagonist with more powerful sedative and hypnotic effects than promethazine. It is widely used as a premedicant agent in children. The palatable apricot-flavoured elixir may be administered in a dosage of 1.5–2.0 mg kg^{-1} (depending on the degree of sedation required) 1.5–2 h prior to surgery. Some delay in the recovery from anaesthesia may be anticipated. Trimeprazine can antagonize the effects of 5-hydroxytryptamine, dopamine and noradrenaline, and high doses may produce extrapyramidal effects, hypothermia and hypotension. Other central side-effects (e.g. disturbing dreams and possibly hallucinations) have also been reported.

Barbiturates

Barbiturates were widely used as hypnotics and premedicant agents for many years, although their use for this purpose is currently considered to be undesirable.

Pentobarbitone is an example of a barbiturate with a medium duration of action which was once a popular choice in this context; its hypnotic effect lasts for up to 6 h. Pentobarbitone is the oxygen analogue of thiopentone, but has a much lower lipid solubility. It is well-absorbed after oral administration, is 50% bound to plasma proteins and undergoes extensive distribution and metabolism. This drug is no longer available in the UK, but has had considerable popularity in the USA as a premedicant drug prior to general or regional anaesthesia.

Newer hypnotic agents

Zolpidem (an imidazopyridine) and zopiclone (a cyclopyrrolone compound) have been introduced into the UK in recent years for the short-term treatment of insomnia. Both these drugs are structurally unrelated to the benzodiazepines.

However, evidence suggests that both drugs have modulatory effects at the $GABA_A$–chloride complex (acting at different subsites to benzodiazepines or producing other conformational changes). The effects of therapeutic or toxic doses of either drug are apparently reversed by flumazenil.

Antimuscarinic drugs

Premedication with antimuscarinic drugs (in particular, atropine and hyoscine) has been an established clinical practice for many years. The main advantages are a reduction in the amount of bronchial and salivary secretions, a diminution in the cardiac responses to inhalational anaesthetics with significant vagomimetic activity, and a decrease in reflex stimulation during endotracheal intubation and visceral traction.

In present-day circumstances, the routine use of these agents may no longer be considered necessary. Anaesthetic agents which induced pronounced salivation and respiratory secretions (diethyl ether) or vagomimetic activity (cyclopropane) are rarely administered, and neuromuscular blocking agents are used to provide optimal conditions for laryngoscopy and intubation. In addition, the subjective discomforts of a dry mouth, palpitations and blurring of vision are obviously undesirable.

Current indications for the use of antimuscarinic drugs as premedicants are not well-defined. In many instances they are omitted, or are given intravenously at the time of induction of anaesthesia. However, they may have some advantages in the following situations:

1 In small children, when the presence of copious secretions in the airway may be a particular embarrassment.

2 When effects mediated through the cardiac vagus may be enhanced:

(a) In patients receiving treatment with β-adrenoceptor antagonists or cardiac glycosides.

(b) During ophthalmic surgery, in order to prevent oculocardiac reflexes.

(c) In other surgical procedures when reflex parasympathetic activity may be pronounced, e.g. haemorrhoidectomy, cholecystectomy.

(d) When techniques involving intermittent suxamethonium are used.

3 In patients with obstructive airways disease, in order to prevent reflex or drug-induced bronchospasm.

The action of antimuscarinic drugs in preventing the regurgitation of stomach contents is less clearly understood. Antagonizing the effects of acetylcholine should theoretically increase the tone of the cardiac sphincter and impede the entry of gastric contents into the oesophagus. However, current concepts suggest that a cardiac 'valve' is produced by the apposition of folds of gastric mucosa at the acutely angled cardio-oesophageal junction. Thus, antimuscarinic drugs which produce relaxation of smooth muscle can facilitate regurgitation by lowering this barrier pressure. In spite of other beneficial effects (e.g. a reduction in the volume of gastric secretion which will enhance the efficacy of antacid therapy), atropine and related drugs should not be used prior to induction of anaesthesia for obstetric procedures.

The antimuscarinic drugs most commonly used as premedicant agents are the naturally occurring alkaloids atropine and hyoscine (Chapter 12). These tertiary amines readily cross the blood–brain barrier; however, they produce different central effects, and also have differential effects on acetylcholine receptors in some effector organs.

Atropine

Systemic administration of the usual premedication dose of atropine (0.6 mg in adults) may produce a transient decrease in heart rate prior to the development of tachycardia. This may be due to central effects on the vagal nucleus, or to a partial agonist effect at peripheral muscarinic receptors (M_2-receptors may be involved in this phenomenon). Moderate antisialogogue effects occur, and some mydriasis may be observed, although significant elevation of intraocular pressure does not occur in normal conditions. Bronchodilatation results in an increase in the physiological dead space. This effect, which is associated with slight stimulation of the cerebral cortex and the medullary centres, can lead to an increase in the rate and depth of respiration.

Atropine has a relatively short duration of action (1–1.5 h); it is extensively metabolized by liver esterases, and only small amounts of the unchanged drug are normally identified in urine. After oral administration, atropine is extensively (60–70%) absorbed from the small intestine; it is frequently administered orally, with a sedative such as trimeprazine, as premedication for elective surgical procedures in children. The recommended dose is 0.05 mg kg^{-1}, up to a maximum dose of 1.2 mg.

Hyoscine

Hyoscine (scopolamine) may also be used as a premedicant drug. In the doses normally used in adults (0.4 mg), it has a shorter duration of action than atropine, and produces less tachycardia; cardiac arrhythmias are unlikely to occur after its use. It is a more powerful antisialogogue than atropine, and has more pronounced effects on the eye.

In contrast, it has less bronchodilator activity. In therapeutic doses, it causes depression of the CNS; drowsiness, amnesia and confusion (particularly in elderly patients) may occur. The central actions of hyoscine may be useful in the management of motion sickness and other vestibular disorders, and it has been used with opioid analgesics to produce 'twilight sleep'. It also has a short duration of action

(1–1.5 h), and is extensively metabolized by liver esterases; only trace amounts of hyoscine (approximately 1% of the dose) are eliminated unchanged in urine. Although hyoscine may be given orally, it is less extensively absorbed from the small intestine than atropine.

Glycopyrrolate

Glycopyrrolate is an antimuscarinic drug which has been widely used in premedication in recent years. Unlike atropine and hyoscine, glycopyrrolate is an ionized quaternary amine, and does not readily cross cell membranes. Thus, it does not readily cross the blood–brain barrier, and does not produce central effects; similarly, placental transfer of the drug is insignificant.

Glycopyrrolate is an effective antisialogogue with a prolonged duration of action (approximately 6 h); sweat-gland activity is also affected for a similar period of time. However, moderate doses do not tend to cause other antimuscarinic effects. Heart rate may not increase; indeed, a slight but insignificant bradycardia may occur, and arrhythmias are rare. Similarly, changes in pupillary size are minimal. Nevertheless, larger doses will cause typical antimuscarinic effects.

Glycopyrrolate may be given by intramuscular or intravenous injection, in doses ranging from 0.1 to 0.4 mg in the adult. It is usually considered that 0.2 mg intramuscularly produces optimal premedicant effects. Larger doses (2–8 mg) may be given orally, but there is a predictable delay in the onset of action.

Neuroleptic drugs

Promethazine (a phenothiazine derivative with antihistamine, sedative and hypnotic properties) was introduced into anaesthetic practice in France in 1952; it was primarily used as a premedicant drug, and to supplement the action of other anaesthetic agents. At that time, the related phenothiazine, chlorpromazine, had recently been synthesized, and its ability to potentiate other anaesthetic agents had been investigated. It was also recognized that chlorpromazine produced profound sedation without loss of consciousness, and the absence of any interest in the immediate environment. Consequently, promethazine and chlorpromazine (in combination with pethidine) were used as a 'lytic cocktail' to induce a state of artificial hibernation or neurovegetative block. This method, with little or no supplementation, was used as an alternative to conventional anaesthetic techniques. The main advantages were said to be the reduction in bleeding, the absence of shock and a decreased requirement of postoperative analgesic drugs. However, a profound degree of hypotension and a prolonged depression of autonomic reflexes tended to restrict the use of this technique.

Chlorpromazine was subsequently shown to have marked antipsychotic properties, and was the first effective drug to be used in the treatment of schizophrenia. The term neuroleptic (supporting the nervous system) was introduced to describe chlorpromazine and its analogues in 1957. At this time, various phenylpiperidine derivatives related to pethidine were shown to have properties similar to chlorpromazine; subsequent chemical modification led to the development of the butyrophenones (i.e. haloperidol and droperidol). Other phenylpiperidine derivatives were shown to be extremely potent analgesics, and had an extremely short duration of action. Some of these drugs (e.g. fentanyl and phenoperidine) were subsequently introduced into clinical practice.

The concept of neuroleptanalgesia was introduced in 1959, and the use of a butyrophenone (e.g. droperidol) and a potent opioid analgesic (e.g. phenoperidine) became popular as an alternative to general anaesthesia. There were frequent problems of respiratory depression associated with the use of these drugs, and the applications and use of neuroleptanalgesia have diminished in recent years. However, a remarkable degree of cardiovascular stability is commonly produced by this technique. Thus, these drugs may be used to supplement light anaesthesia in the elderly or poor-risk patient, during induction and maintenance of anaesthesia for cardiac and vascular surgery and in neurosurgery (although droperidol may cause some reduction in cerebral blood flow). Neuroleptanalgesia may also be valuable as an adjunct to regional anaesthesia, and for procedures in which patient cooperation is an advantage (e.g. percutaneous cordotomy).

In recent years, chlorpromazine and related phenothiazines have assumed a more specific role in anaesthetic practice; in particular, they are widely used for their antiemetic properties (p. 470).

Non-steroidal anti-inflammatory drugs (NSAIDs)

The recent increase in the popularity of NSAIDs as anaesthetic adjuvants has led to their frequent use as premedicant drugs, particularly for minor surgery. In this context diclofenac and ketorolac are commonly used (Chapter 11). Both these drugs are available as tablets and in solution for intramuscular injection; diclofenac is also available in suppository form, whilst ketorolac can be given intravenously. Another NSAID, mefenamic acid, has been incorporated, along with trimeprazine and atropine, into an oral preparation (TAM mixture) which is used for premedication in children.

α_2-Adrenoceptor agonists

Clonidine was first used as a nasal decongestant, but was subsequently developed in clinical practice as an antihypertensive agent. Clonidine inhibits catecholamine release by peripheral and central α_2-agonist effects, although transient hypertension may ensue with intravenous administration due to an effect on postsynaptic vascular receptors. Dry mouth, sedation, depression, bradycardia and rebound hypertension following withdrawal were commonly associated side-effects and clonidine is now rarely used in the treatment of hypertension. Dexmedetomidine, a more highly selective and potent α_2-agonist, has been used for many years in veterinary practice for its sedative, hypnotic and analgesic properties.

It is thus unsurprising that α_2-agonists have more recently established a role as anaesthetic adjuncts. When used in premedication, useful anxiolytic and sedative effects (comparable to those produced by benzodiazepines) have been shown. A reduction of anaesthetic requirements has also been demonstrated; this has allowed a reduction in dosage of intravenous induction agents and more evidently in the minimum alveolar concentration (MAC) requirements of inhalational anaesthetics (e.g. dexmedetomidine can reduce the MAC of halothane by approximately 90%).

Other important advantages include attenuation of sympathoadrenal responses associated with anaesthesia and surgery. In particular, α_2-agonists appear to minimize hypertension and tachycardia associated with endotracheal intubation and to contribute to haemodynamic stability during cardiac surgery (these latter effects may involve additive or synergic mechanisms with other drugs commonly used, such as fentanyl and droperidol). In this context clonidine has been administered orally prior to surgery in doses of 100–300 μg.

α_2-Agonists also produce potent analgesic responses and can enhance the effects of both opioid analgesics and local anaesthetic agents. Clonidine has also been given by extradural and intrathecal routes for postoperative analgesia and in the management of chronic pain.

The sites of action of α_2-agonists within the CNS include the tractus solitarius (leading to hypotension and bradycardia), the locus coeruleus (sedation) and certain vagal nuclei. The analgesic effect appears to involve non-opioid mechanisms at both spinal and supraspinal sites and may encompass thalamic transfer of impulses to the cerebral cortex as well as descending inhibitory pathways to the dorsal horn. In addition to their peripheral inhibitory effects on cardiac rate and vascular smooth muscle tone (including an enhancement of coronary blood flow), α_2-agonists can induce diuresis and platelet aggregation. Oversedation or excessive falls in blood pressure may be associated with the use of these drugs, whilst respiratory depression may occur with high dosage.

Premedication and obstetric anaesthesia

The principal aim of drug therapy before the administration of general anaesthesia for Caesarean section or other operative procedures during late pregnancy and labour is to minimize the risks associated with the aspiration of gastric contents. The avoidance of depressant effects on the fetus is also extremely important.

Opioids should never be used in these circumstances; in addition to their undesirable effects on the fetus, opioids will reduce lower oesophageal sphincter pressure, delay gastric emptying and increase the likelihood of regurgitation. Benzodiazepines are also contraindicated, as cumulative effects leading to oversedation, hypotonia and hypothermia in the baby may occur.

Apomorphine, which is obtained by exposure of morphine to strong mineral acids, has potent effects on dopaminergic receptors and produces a combination of excitatory and depressant effects on the CNS. Apomorphine has been used to produce vomiting (by stimulation of the chemoreceptor trigger zone) before anaesthesia. The procedure is unpleasant for the patient, and cannot be relied upon to empty the stomach efficiently. Apomorphine is rarely used now in this context, but is of some value in the management of refractory problems associated with the drug treatment of Parkinson's disease.

More specific aims have been directed at a reduction in the acidity of the stomach contents; it is suggested that maintaining a pH above 2.5–3 will considerably reduce the severity of pulmonary complications should aspiration occur. Preoperative regimes incorporating the regular administration of an oral suspension of magnesium trisilicate were in vogue for many years. A slow onset of action (silicon dioxide is formed in the stomach and acts as a gelatinous mucosal protectant) and the risks of particulate matter being deposited in the lungs following aspiration now preclude its use.

H_2-Histamine antagonists, which reduce the volume of gastric juice secreted and its hydrogen ion concentration (the output of pepsin also decreases), are now commonly used in preoperative preparation. Ranitidine is the drug of choice and is usually administered (150 mg orally) at 6-h intervals throughout labour; a further 50 mg is given intravenously following a decision to operate. Hypersensitivity responses have rarely been reported and bradyarrhythmias occasionally occur. H_2-Antagonists will not neutralize acid already present in the stomach, so a soluble antacid (30 ml of 0.3 mol l^{-1} sodium citrate) is given prior to induction. Metoclopramide, which increases the tone of the oesophageal sphincter and promotes gastric emptying, may also be given intravenously before induction; atropine, which has the opposite effects, is contraindicated.

Antiemetic drugs

Nausea and vomiting can be induced by many physiological and pathological factors. These include pregnancy, acute pain, raised intracranial pressure, ionizing radiation, psychogenic factors, labyrinthine or vestibular disturbance, metabolic disorders and inflammation or irritation of the gastrointestinal tract. In addition, many drugs or ingested toxins can induce nausea and vomiting. Some of these agents (e.g. ipecacuanha, squill, chloral hydrate, ammonium chloride and other simple salts) act immediately after oral administration. Indeed, ipecacuanha emetic mixtures are sometimes used in the management of acute drug overdosage in children. These drugs have a local irritant effect on the stomach, or they activate abdominal visceral afferent nerves in the intestinal mucosa or the portal vein. Afferent stimuli are mainly conducted to the brain via the vagus nerves. Other emetic drugs (e.g. opioid analgesics, digitalis glycosides, levodopa, bromocriptine, some inhalational anaesthetics) predominantly affect central pathways concerned with the control of nausea and vomiting. Cytotoxic drugs with pronounced emetic properties (i.e. mustine, cisplatin, dacarbazine and streptozotocin) act by both peripheral and central mechanisms.

For many years, it has been generally accepted that nausea and vomiting are primarily controlled and coordinated by the vomiting centre, which is situated in the dorsolateral reticular formation of the medulla. More recent evidence suggests that the existence of a discrete vomiting centre is doubtful; physiologically, it can be considered as the area in the brainstem that integrates emetic responses. Its functions are probably dependent on complex interactions between the reticular formation, the nucleus tractus solitarius and certain autonomic nuclei (particularly the dorsal vagal nucleus). Similarly, its neurochemistry is extremely complex, since almost 40 different neurotransmitters have been identified in this area of the brain. Efferent impulses from these medullary centres influence related brainstem nuclei (e.g. the vasomotor, respiratory and salivary nuclei) and pass to the gastrointestinal tract to initiate the vomiting reflex.

The activity of the vomiting centre is affected by afferent stimuli from chemoreceptors and pressure receptors in the gut and the CNS, as well as peripheral pain receptors (Fig. 13.2). In addition, it has an afferent input from other sites in the CNS (i.e. the cerebral cortex, vestibular and cerebellar nuclei and the chemoreceptor trigger zone). Stimuli from the labyrinths, mediated by vestibular and cerebellar nuclei, increase the excitability of the vomiting centre and may cause nausea and vomiting. At least one of the synaptic connections in this afferent pathway is cholinergic, and is susceptible to antagonism by centrally acting antimuscarinic drugs. There is also some evidence that noradrenaline may be an inhibitory neurotransmitter in the brainstem reticular system and the vestibular nuclei. However, the activity of the vomiting centre is primarily dependent on other neurotransmitters; in particular, it is affected by the activity of the chemoreceptor trigger zone (Fig. 13.2).

The chemoreceptor trigger zone (CTZ) is a group of cells close to the area postrema on the floor of the fourth ventricle; it normally has a tonic effect on the activity of the vomiting centre. The area postrema is a highly vascular area of the brainstem; physiologically, it is outside the blood–brain and cerebrospinal fluid–brain barriers and is extremely sensitive to systemic emetic stimuli. It may also be concerned with the control of blood pressure, sleep and the regulation of food intake. Many emetic drugs increase the excitability of the CTZ and only indirectly affect the vomiting centre. At least two neurotransmitters (dopamine and 5-hydroxytryptamine; 5-HT) play an important functional role in the activity of the CTZ.

Dopamine is probably released physiologically from the peripheral processes of astrocytes that synapse with the CTZ, and can directly influence neurones in the area postrema by the activation of specific receptors. Current concepts suggest that

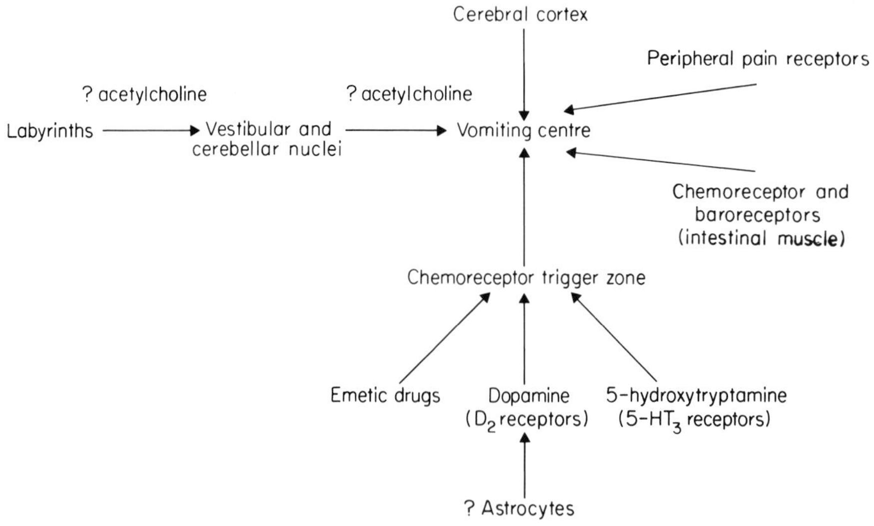

Fig. 13.2 Central and peripheral pathways affecting the activity of the vomiting centre.

the dopamine receptors in the area postrema and the CTZ (principally D_2-receptors) are sensitive to apomorphine and dopaminergic ergots, and are antagonized by metoclopramide and sulpiride. Most centrally acting emetic drugs are D_2-receptor agonists in the CTZ. There is also considerable evidence that dopamine may act as an inhibitory transmitter in the gastrointestinal tract, and may affect peripheral mechanisms concerned with nausea and vomiting.

More recent evidence suggests that 5-HT may also play a crucial role in drug-induced emesis. One subtype of 5-HT receptors (5-HT_3-receptors) appears to play an important part in the mediation of nausea and vomiting induced by high doses of cytotoxic agents. These receptors are present in the small intestine, the CTZ and the area postrema, and can be stimulated by emetic drugs. Preliminary experimental and clinical evidence suggests that 5-HT_3-receptor antagonists are highly effective antiemetic drugs; indeed, the effectiveness of high-dose metoclopramide in cisplatin-induced emesis appears to be due to antagonism of 5-HT at 5-HT_3-receptors.

Thus, experimental evidence suggests that the neurotransmitters acetylcholine (via central cholinergic pathways and vestibular nuclei), dopamine (via D_2-receptors in the CTZ) and 5-HT (via 5-HT_3-receptors in the area postrema and the CTZ) may play an important part in the central control of nausea and vomiting. Consequently, most antiemetic drugs act as antagonists of one or more than one of these neurotransmitters. In addition they may affect peripheral pathways concerned with nausea and vomiting. Unfortunately, most antiemetic drugs do not selectively or specifically antagonize these neurotransmitters (either at vestibular pathways or at the CTZ). Drugs with central antimuscarinic activity invariably produce peripheral parasympathetic blockade, causing pupillary dilatation and cycloplegia, decreased salivary and respiratory secretions, tachycardia and relaxation or decreased motility of smooth muscle in the respiratory tract, the gut and the bladder. Central side-effects, such as drowsiness and sedation, may be due to competitive blockade of cholinergic pathways in the reticular activating system and the cerebral cortex. In contrast, dopamine antagonists may act on the pituitary gland, the hypothalamus, the mesolimbic system and the corpus striatum, causing hyperprolactinaemia, decreased body temperature and extrapyramidal effects (e.g. tremors, dystonias, oculogyric crises). Dopamine antagonists may affect 5-HT_3-receptors in high dosage (e.g. metoclopramide); however, some 5-HT_3-receptor antagonists appear to have relatively specific effects.

Individual antiemetic drugs can be classified pharmacologically as:

1 Antimuscarinic (anticholinergic) drugs.
2 Dopamine antagonists.
3 5-HT_3-receptor antagonists.
4 Miscellaneous agents.

Antimuscarinic drugs

In general, all drugs that antagonize the muscarinic effects of acetylcholine and that can cross the blood–brain barrier may have antiemetic properties (particularly in motion sickness, labyrinthine disease or vestibular disorders). In practice, atropine, hyoscine and some antihistamine drugs (i.e. H_1-antagonists) have been mainly used for this purpose.

The antiemetic effects of atropine and hyoscine are mainly due to their central antimuscarinic effects; however, both drugs decrease muscle tone and secretions in the gut, which may contribute to their effects. In general, atropine is a less potent and less effective antiemetic agent than hyoscine (although its activity on intestinal motility and secretions is greater). Both drugs decrease the opening pressure of the lower oesophageal sphincter (barrier pressure) and thus predispose to gastro-oesophageal regurgitation. They also produce characteristic autonomic side-effects, and hyoscine may cause profound sedation. Both atropine and hyoscine may suppress the emetic effects of therapeutic doses of opioid analgesics, and are used for premedication.

Some antihistamine drugs (i.e. competitive antagonists of histamine at H_1-receptors) have antiemetic properties; in the UK, cinnarizine, cyclizine, diphenhydramine, dimenhydrinate and promethazine have been most widely used in the management of nausea and vomiting. Cyclizine and cinnarizine usually produce less sedation than diphenhydramine and promethazine. Nevertheless, promethazine (a phenothiazine) has a longer duration of action than other antihistamines, and is commonly used for its antiemetic effects. These drugs are frequently of value in the prophylaxis and treatment of motion sickness, and in the management of labyrinthine disorders (e.g. Ménière's disease). When nausea and vomiting are due to other causes, their effectiveness is limited. Nevertheless, antihistamines may suppress the emetic effects of opioid analgesics, and some of them (e.g. cyclizine and promethazine) have been used in anaesthetic practice. In particular, promethazine has been used for premedication in children and cyclizine is commonly used as an antiemetic drug in the preoperative period. The drug is available as a compound preparation with morphine (Cyclimorph), and is also present with the methadone analogue dipipanone in Diconal for use in chronic pain therapy.

Although these drugs are primarily competitive antagonists at H_1-receptors, there is little or no evidence that histamine plays any part in peripheral and central mechanisms concerned with nausea and vomiting. Many antihistamines also have significant antimuscarinic activity, which accounts for many of their side-effects (e.g. dryness of the mouth, urinary retention, drowsiness). Their antiemetic effects (particularly in nausea and vomiting of labyrinthine origin) are almost certainly due to the central antagonism of acetylcholine. Antihistamines that do not cross the blood–brain barrier (e.g. terfenadine, astemizole) are of no value as antiemetic drugs.

Dopamine antagonists

Since dopamine plays an important physiological role in the CTZ and the area postrema, almost all drugs that antagonize its effects at D_2-receptors have anti-emetic properties. The dopamine antagonists that are used clinically for their antiemetic effects are usually phenothiazines, butyrophenones, metoclopramide or domperidone.

Phenothiazines

In general, phenothiazines have many pharmacological effects and can modify responses to a wide range of central and peripheral neurotransmitters. Most phenothiazines antagonize the effects of dopamine at central synapses, and have a variable degree of antimuscarinic activity. Consequently, they are often useful in the control of nausea and vomiting, whether induced by drugs or other causes (e.g. uraemia, neoplastic disease, radiotherapy). Phenothiazines are usually divided into three groups, depending on their chemical structure:

1 Type 1 phenothiazines (e.g. chlorpromazine) cause sedation and have some tendency to produce extrapyramidal side-effects, particularly at high dose levels.

2 Type 2 phenothiazines (e.g. thioridazine) are usually less potent; they have only moderate sedative effects and little tendency to produce extrapyramidal side-effects.

3 Type 3 phenothiazines (e.g. fluphenazine) are more potent drugs with little sedative effect, but have a marked tendency to produce extrapyramidal effects.

The classical type 1 phenothiazine, chlorpromazine, has a wide range of actions (as suggested by its proprietary name, Largactil). These are mainly related to its widespread effects on different central and peripheral receptors. Thus, chlorpromazine can cause antagonism of dopamine (at D_1- and D_2-receptors), acetylcholine (at muscarinic receptors), noradrenaline (at α_1- and α_2-adrenoceptors), histamine (at H_1-receptors), and 5-HT (at some 5-HT receptors). In addition, chlorpromazine has membrane-stabilizing (local anaesthetic) activity and prevents the uptake of noradrenaline at sympathetic neurones ($Uptake_1$). Some of the central effects of chlorpromazine are due to its relatively selective action on the brainstem-alerting system. This consists of ascending neurones in the pontine and medullary reticular formation, which project to thalamic and hypothalamic nuclei and transmit arousal impulses to the sensory cortex. Chlorpromazine does not directly inhibit the reticular activating system, but isolates it from numerous collateral afferents (including auditory and visual impulses) which are constantly impinging on it. The resultant effects are classically described as neurolepsy — sedation, indifference to external stimuli and a reduction in motor activity. The EEG shows a characteristic sleep pattern (although patients can be roused by moderate stimulation). Paradoxically, chlorpromazine may induce epileptic attacks in susceptible individuals, and convulsions may be a prominent feature of phenothiazine overdosage. Reduction in muscle tone may also occur, due to suppression of reticular afferents from proprioceptive fibres in muscle spindles.

Other central effects of chlorpromazine are mainly due to dopamine antagonism. Extrapyramidal effects (e.g. acute dystonia, akathisia, tardive dyskinesia) are usually seen with high and continuous dosage; classical symptoms of Parkinson's disease (i.e. rigidity, tremor and akinesia) are less common. The hypothalamic regulation of pituitary function is modified; the secretion of growth hormone and pituitary gonadotrophins is decreased, and hyperprolactinaemia occurs (dopamine is the prolactin release-inhibitory factor and central dopamine antagonism invariably increases plasma prolactin). Hypothalamic activity is also affected in other ways. Temperature regulation is impaired, and a fall in body temperature may occur. Similarly, interference with autonomic regulation by the hypothalamus (as well as α-adrenoceptor blockade) may cause profound hypotension. In addition, chlorpromazine produces antiemetic effects by competitive antagonism of dopamine D_2-receptors in the area postrema and the CTZ.

Chlorpromazine may potentiate the actions of other central depressants, including analgesics. Indeed, one phenothiazine (methotrimeprazine; levomepromazine) has analgesic effects that are similar to morphine, and schizophrenic patients who are receiving long-term treatment with phenothiazines may have a stoical indifference to pain.

Hypersensitivity reactions to chlorpromazine are not uncommon. Cholestatic jaundice may develop during chronic treatment; it is less common with other phenothiazines. Agranulocytosis can also occur, and skin reactions in patients and nursing staff may be due to handling tablets containing the drug. Photosensitivity and pigmentation of the skin and the cornea occasionally develop. Like other phenothiazines, chlorpromazine may cause the malignant neuroleptic syndrome.

Chlorpromazine is well-absorbed after oral administration. It is extensively metabolized by the liver to a large number of breakdown products; it has been suggested that some of these can be detected in urine for as long as 18 months. Only small amounts of the active drug are eliminated unchanged in bile or urine. After oral administration, the drug has a large and variable first-pass effect, and its metabolism is affected by enzyme-inducing agents. Consequently, it is commonly given by intramuscular injection. Chlorpromazine has a relatively long terminal half-life, and a large volume of distribution.

Chlorpromazine is the classical phenothiazine used in the treatment of psychotic disorders. In schizophrenic patients, it controls violence and hyperactivity, and also has a beneficial effect on other symptoms, such as thought disorders, delusions and hallucinations. It is useful in the treatment of intractable hiccup and in the management of tetanus.

In anaesthetic practice, chlorpromazine may be used with opioid analgesics during the preoperative period, or in the management of pain due to malignant disease. It may also be used as an adjunct to induce hypotension or hypothermia. It is sometimes indicated in the treatment of shock; the α_1-adrenoceptor antagonism results in increased tissue perfusion, and the anti-shivering and deafferentation properties may also be useful.

More commonly, chlorpromazine is used in the symptomatic treatment of nausea and vomiting; it has a protective effect against emesis induced by opioid analgesic drugs. It is less effective in motion sickness or the vomiting which occurs after radiotherapy. In the doses required to control nausea and vomiting, antimuscarinic and extrapyramidal side-effects are usually moderate; unfortunately, sedation and drowsiness may be severe and disabling. Consequently, phenothiazines without marked sedative properties are more commonly used as antiemetic drugs (e.g. perphenazine, prochlorperazine, trifluoperazine). These drugs are all group 3 phenothiazines, and do not usually have significant antimuscarinic effects. Unfortunately, extrapyramidal effects due to dopamine antagonism are relatively common, particularly when high doses are used over a prolonged period. Prochlorperazine is less potent than perphenazine and trifluoperazine, and is widely used for its antiemetic effects during the postoperative period. The usual dose is 12.5 mg, by intramuscular injection; after oral administration, the drug has a large and variable first-pass effect (like most other phenothiazines).

Butyrophenones

Some butyrophenones are relatively selective dopamine receptor antagonists, and have similar effects to group 3 phenothiazines. This may be related to their uptake and localization in the CNS. The chemical structure of the butyrophenones is related to the inhibitory transmitter GABA, and it has been suggested that they may compete with GABA at postsynaptic receptor sites (although it is not clear how this is related to dopamine antagonism).

Butyrophenones have powerful tranquillizing and antiemetic effects. Although they are commonly administered with opioid analgesics, they do not appear to potentiate their analgesic and respiratory depressant effects. In low doses, they do not produce significant sedation or pronounced peripheral antimuscarinic effects; unfortunately, extrapyramidal signs and hypothalamic dysfunction are relatively common. They have less peripheral activity than phenothiazines, and adverse haemodynamic effects are infrequent.

Two butyrophenones (haloperidol and droperidol) have been extensively used in medical practice. Haloperidol is potent, effective and long-acting, and is sometimes used as an antiemetic agent; the effects of a single dose may last for 24–48 h. It is also used in the treatment of various psychoses, behavioural disorders and motor tics. Droperidol has a shorter duration of action (6–12 h) and is often used with opioid drugs to produce neuroleptanalgesia. It should not be used alone, as the occurrence of apparent tranquillization may conceal a state of inner anxiety with psychotic features (e.g. hallucinations and bizarre symptoms of body transference). Droperidol may cause a slight fall in blood pressure, due to α-adrenoceptor blockade. Premedication with droperidol may be of value in preventing the emergence of delirium after the administration of ketamine.

Metoclopramide

Metoclopramide is structurally related to procainamide, and was developed in France in the early 1960s. The antiemetic properties of metoclopramide are mainly due to dopamine antagonism; however, in high doses it also antagonizes the effects of 5-HT at 5-HT_3-receptors in the area postrema and the CTZ. Unfortunately, metoclopramide does not have a selective action at these sites; consequently, it may cause extrapyramidal effects (particularly oculogyric crises). These can be prevented or treated by drugs with antimuscarinic properties (e.g. procyclidine, benztropine). Other toxic reactions, apart from drowsiness, are relatively rare. Metoclopramide also has significant peripheral effects on the gastrointestinal tract. It increases the rate of gastric emptying by enhancing fundal and antral contractility, relaxes the pyloric sphincter, stimulates peristalsis and increases lower oesophageal sphincter pressure (barrier pressure). These effects may be due to the peripheral antagonism of dopamine in the gastrointestinal tract.

Metoclopramide has been used in the prophylaxis of Mendelson's syndrome, and to prevent nausea and vomiting during cancer chemotherapy.

Domperidone

Domperidone is also an antiemetic drug with central and peripheral effects, which are mainly due to dopamine antagonism. Like metoclopramide, it increases the rate of gastric emptying and increases the lower oesophageal sphincter pressure.

Domperidone also prevents the effects of dopamine and dopamine agonists on the CTZ, and may cause increased prolactin secretion. It is less likely to produce acute dystonic reactions than metoclopramide, since it does not cross the blood–brain barrier readily and affect the corpus striatum. In large doses, domperidone may cause cardiac arrhythmias which are sometimes fatal. It is mainly used as an antiemetic drug during chemotherapy with cytotoxic drugs; in these conditions, it may have some advantages over metoclopramide. It is available as an oral preparation and a suppository.

5-HT$_3$-receptor antagonists

Ondansetron

Ondansetron is a potent and selective antagonist at 5-HT$_3$-receptors. Central effects are mediated at medullary sites, including the area postrema and the tractus solitarius, as well as the chemoreceptor trigger zone. Peripheral 5-HT$_3$-receptors have been identified on parasympathetic nerve afferents in the myenteric nerve plexus of the intestinal wall (the cytotoxic agent cisplatin may induce nausea and vomiting by the release of 5-HT from damaged intestinal mucosa). Ondansetron has been used to considerable advantage in the prevention and treatment of emesis associated with chemotherapy and radiotherapy, and has more recently gained popularity in the management of postoperative nausea and vomiting. A number of clinical studies suggest that ondansetron may be superior to conventional antiemetics in this context, particularly in the treatment of established vomiting.

Ondansetron is available in tablet and injection form. A prophylactic dose of 8 mg may be administered by mouth 1 h before anaesthesia, followed by two further doses of 8 mg at 8-hourly intervals if deemed necessary. For the treatment of established nausea and vomiting, ondansetron 4 mg by intramuscular or slow intravenous injection is recommended; this may be repeated at intervals according to the severity of the symptoms. Ondansetron may also be administered by continuous infusion.

Bioavailability following oral administration is approximately 60%. Ondansetron is moderately bound to plasma proteins (60–75%) and has a relatively large volume of distribution (160 l). The terminal half-life is 3 h; only 5% of the drug is excreted unchanged in the urine, with the majority being subjected to hydroxylation and conjugation to inactive metabolites by the liver. The dose of ondansetron should be reduced in patients with significant liver damage. Ondansetron is known to increase bowel transit time and constipation is a common side-effect. Other undesirable effects, which include headache, sensations of warmth or flushing, transient visual disturbances and occasionally chest pain and cardiac arrhythmias, suggest that ondansetron may exert some activity at other subtypes of the 5-HT receptor. Hypersensitivity reactions have also been reported.

Granisetron and tropisetron are closely related drugs with a similar spectrum of activity. They are used in the prophylaxis and treatment of nausea and vomiting associated with cancer chemotherapy; at present neither drug has a product licence for perioperative use.

Other antiemetic drugs

Nabilone is a synthetic cannabinoid with antiemetic properties, and is chemically related to tetrahydrocannabinol. Experimental evidence suggests that it acts on opioid receptors in the area postrema, since its antiemetic effects can be competitively antagonized by naloxone. It has been suggested that the activation of opioid receptors may lead to persistent inhibition of the vomiting centre. Nabilone has been used to prevent nausea and vomiting during cancer chemotherapy, although it is probably less effective than other drugs during cisplatin therapy. Unwanted effects (particularly drowsiness, dizziness and dry mouth) and psychotic reactions (e.g. dysphoria, depression, nightmares, hallucinations) are relatively common. Nabilone should only be used as an antiemetic drug during cancer chemotherapy, due to the possibility of drug dependence and misuse. Recent studies involving molecular cloning have demonstrated specific cannabinoid receptors at both central and peripheral sites, while an endogenous agonist, anandamide, has also been identified.

Lorazepam is a potent benzodiazepine with profound sedative and amnesic properties. It has also been used as an antiemetic drug during cancer chemotherapy. Its mode of action is obscure; presumably it modifies central pathways concerned with the control of nausea and vomiting. In addition, the powerful amnesic action of lorazepam prevents anticipatory vomiting, which occurs in approximately 20% of patients during repeated courses of therapy with cytotoxic drugs.

Some corticosteroids (e.g. dexamethasone) have been used as antiemetic drugs during cancer chemotherapy. In these conditions, dexamethasone is well-tolerated and is as effective as prochlorperazine or metoclopramide. The mode of action of corticosteroids is uncertain. It has been suggested that their action depends on the decreased release of arachidonic acid, reduced turnover of 5-HT or decreased permeability of the blood–brain barrier.

Postoperative nausea and vomiting in anaesthetic practice

Many patients who undergo anaesthesia and surgery experience nausea and vomiting in the early postoperative period. The incidence is variable, but causal factors which may be involved include:

1 Patient susceptibility (e.g. previous experiences of nausea and vomiting in association with anaesthesia, a history of motion sickness).

2 Specific surgical procedures (e.g. abdominal, gynaecological and ear, nose and throat surgery).

3 Anaesthetic agents and procedures. A high incidence of postoperative nausea and vomiting (approximately 80%) was associated with the use of diethylether and cyclopropane. Opioids are now commonly used as anaesthetic adjuvants and are potent emetics. There is some evidence that the use of anticholinesterase drugs to reverse neuromuscular blockade is associated with an increased incidence of postoperative nausea and vomiting. 'Stormy' induction of anaesthesia, hypoxic episodes, insufflation of anaesthetic gases into the oesophagus and inadequate suppression of reflex autonomic activity are other contributory factors.

Antiemetic drugs may be given for the prophylaxis and treatment of postoperative nausea and vomiting. Anticholinergic drugs may confer some protective effect, but antimuscarinic side-effects can be a disadvantage. Dopamine antagonists are most commonly used. Metoclopramide and prochlorperazine are frequently administered; they both inhibit the emetic effects of opioids, but their duration of action is relatively short. Droperidol, which has a longer duration of action, is also a popular choice, and is frequently administered with opioid analgesics during continuous infusion in the postoperative period. These drugs should all be used with care. There is a significant incidence of extrapyramidal reactions even after single dosage; these are particularly prone to develop in young females. Furthermore, the use of droperidol in the absence of an opioid may lead to the development of unpleasant psychotomimetic side-effects.

Ondansetron appears to be as effective as droperidol in the prophylaxis of postoperative nausea and vomiting, and may be more beneficial in the treatment of established vomiting. It does not produce extrapyramidal problems, but the present high cost of the drug tends to limit its use in anaesthetic practice. The intravenous administration of dexamethasone during induction of anaesthesia may reduce the incidence of postoperative nausea and vomiting.

Further reading

Andrews PLR, Rapeport WG, Sanger GJ. Neuropharmacology of emesis induced by anti-cancer therapy. *Trends in Pharmacological Sciences* 1988; **9**: 334–341.

Alon E, Himmelseher S. Ondansetron in the treatment of postoperative vomiting: a randomised double-blind comparison with droperidol and metoclopramide. *Anesthesia and Analgesia* 1992; **75**: 761–765.

Ashton H. Benzodiazepine withdrawal: an unfinished story. *British Medical Journal* 1984; **288**: 1135–1140.

Betts TA, Birtle J. Effect of two hypnotic drugs on actual driving performance next morning. *British Medical Journal* 1982; **285**: 852.

Bowcock SJ, Stockdale AD, Bolton JAR *et al.* Antiemetic prophylaxis with high dose metoclopramide or lorazepam in vomiting induced by chemotherapy. *British Medical Journal* 1984; **288**: 1879.

Braestrup C, Schmiechen R, Nielsen M, Petersen EN. Benzodiazepine receptor ligands, receptor occupancy, pharmacological effect and GABA receptor coupling. In: Usdin E, Skolnick P, Tallman JF, Greenblatt D, Paul SM (eds) *Pharmacology of Benzodiazepines*. London: Macmillan Press, 1982; 71–85.

Brand ED, Harris TD, Borison HL, Goodman LS. The anti-emetic effect of 10-(α-dimethyl-aminopropyl)-2-

chlorophenothiazine (chlorpromazine) in dog and cat. *Journal of Pharmacology and Experimental Therapeutics* 1954; **110**: 86–92.

Brandt AL, Oakes FD. Preanaesthesia medication: double-blind study of a new drug, diazepam. *Anesthesia and Analgesia* 1965; **44**: 125–129.

Breimer DD. Clinical pharmacokinetics of hypnotics. *Clinical Pharmacokinetics* 1977; **2**: 93–109.

Brogden RN, Carmine AA, Heel RC *et al.* Domperidone: a review of its pharmacological activity, pharmacokinetics and therapeutic efficacy in the symptomatic treatment of chronic dyspepsia and as an antiemetic. *Drugs* 1982; **24**: 360–400.

Butler TC. Theories of general anaesthesia. *Pharmacological Reviews* 1950; **2**: 121–160.

Calvey TN. Hypnotics, sedatives and antiemetics. In: Nimmo WS, Smith G (eds) *Anaesthesia*. Oxford: Blackwell Scientific Publications, 1989; 22–33.

Castleden CM, George CF, Marcer D, Hallett C. Increased sensitivity to nitrazepam in old age. *British Medical Journal* 1977; **1**: 10–12.

Clift AD. Factors leading to dependence on hypnotic drugs. *British Medical Journal* 1972; **3**: 614–617.

Conney AH. Pharmacological implications of microsomal enzyme induction. *Pharmacological Reviews* 1967; **19**: 317–366.

Cook P. How drug activity is altered in the elderly. *Geriatric Medicine* 1979; **9**: 45–46.

Correa-Sales C, Rabin BC, Maze M. Hynotic response to dexmedetomidine, an α_2 agonist, is mediated in the locus coraelus in rats. *Anesthesiology* 1992; **76**: 948–952.

Cree JE, Meyer J, Hailey DM. Diazepam in labour: its metabolism and effect on the clinical condition and thermogenesis of the newborn. *British Medical Journal* 1973; **4**: 251–255.

Dahl JB, Kehlet H. The value of pre-emptive analgesia in the treatment of postoperative pain. *British Journal of Anaesthesia* 1993; **70**: 434–439.

Davis CJ, Lake-Bakaar GV, Grahame-Smith DG. *Nausea and Vomiting: Mechanisms and Treatment*. Berlin: Springer-Verlag, 1986.

Dent SJ, Ramachandra V, Stephen CR. Postoperative vomiting: incidence, analysis and therapeutic measures in 3000 patients. *Anesthesiology* 1955; **16**: 564–572.

Devane W. A new dawn of cannabinoid pharmacology. *Trends in Pharmacological Sciences* 1994; **15**: 40–41.

Doughty A. The evaluation of premedication in children. *Proceedings of the Royal Society of Medicine* 1959; **52**: 823–833.

Fenton GW. Clinical disorders of sleep. *British Journal of Hospital Medicine* 1975; **14**: 120–145.

Gee KW, Yamamura HI. Benzodiazepine receptor heterogencity: a consequence of multiple conformational states of a single receptor or multiple population of structurally distinct macromolecules? In: Usdin E, Skolnick P, Tallman JF, Greenblatt D, Paul SM (eds) *Pharmacology of Benzodiazepines*. London: Macmillan Press, 1982; 93–108.

Goodchild CS. GABA receptors and benzodiazepines. *British Journal of Anaesthesia* 1993; **71**: 127–133.

Haefely WE. Central actions of benzodiazepines: general introduction. *British Journal of Psychiatry* 1978; **133**: 231–238.

Hayashi Y, Maze M. Alpha$_2$ adrenoceptor agonists and anaesthesia. *British Journal of Anaesthesia* 1993; **71**: 108–118.

Iversen LL, Bloom FE. Studies on the uptake of ^{3}H-GABA and ^{3}H-glycine in slices and homogenates of rat brain and spinal cord by electron microscopic autoradiography. *Brain Research* 1972; **41**: 131–143.

Joss RA, Goldhirsch A, Brunner KW, Galeazzi RL. Sudden death in cancer patient on high-dose domperidone. *Lancet* 1982; **i**: 1019.

Kanto JH. Use of benzodiazepines during pregnancy, labour and lactation, with particular reference to pharmacokinetic considerations. *Drugs* 1982; **23**: 354–380.

Kawer P, Dundee JW. Frequency of pain on injection and venous sequelae following the i.v. administration of certain anaesthetics and sedatives. *British Journal of Anaesthesia* 1982; **54**: 935–939.

Kebabian JW, Calne DB. Multiple receptors for dopamine. *Nature* 1979; **277**: 93–96.

Kesson CM, Gray JMB, Lawson DH. Benzodiazepine drugs in general medical patients. *British Medical Journal* 1976; **1**: 680–682.

Klotz U, Antonin K-H, Bieck PR. Pharmacokinetics and plasma binding of diazepam in man, dog, rabbit, guinea pig and rat. *Journal of Pharmacology and Experimental Therapeutics* 1976; **199**: 67–73.

Kris MG, Tyson LB, Gralla FRJ *et al.* Extrapyramidal reactions with high dose metoclopramide. *New England Journal of Medicine* 1983; **309**: 433–434.

Kumar A, Bose S, Bhattacharya A *et al*. Oral clonidine premedication for elderly patients undergoing intraocular surgery. *Acta Anaesthesiologica Scandinavica* 1992; **36**: 159–164.

Lader MH. How tranquillisers work. *British Journal of Hospital Medicine* 1976; **16**: 622–628.

Lader MH, Petursson H. Benzodiazepine derivatives — side effects and dangers. *Biological Psychiatry* 1981; **16**: 1195–1201.

Laduron PM. Leysen JE. Domperidone, a specific *in vitro* dopamine antagonist, devoid of *in vivo* central dopaminergic activity. *Biochemical Pharmacology* 1979; **28**: 2161–2165.

Lidbrink P, Corrodi H, Fuxe K, Olson L. The effects of benzodiazepines, meprobamate, and barbiturates on central monoamine neurones. In: Garrattini S, Mussini E, Randall LO (eds) *The Benzodiazepines*. New York: Raven Press, 1973; 203–223.

Lind JF, Crispin JS, McIver DK. The effect of atropine on the gastro-oesophageal sphincter. *Canadian Journal of Physiology and Pharmacology* 1968; **46**: 233–238.

McKay AC, Dundee JW. Effect of oral benzodiazepines on memory. *British Journal of Anaesthesia* 1980; **52**: 1247–1257.

Malegalada J-R. Gastric emptying disorders: clinical significance and treatment. *Drugs* 1982; **24**: 353–359.

Markham A, Sorkin EM. Ondansetron. An update of its therapeutic use in chemotherapy-induced and postoperative nausea and vomiting. *Drugs* 1993; **45**: 931–952.

Marin IL. The benzodiazepine receptor; functional complexity. In: Lamble JW, Abbott AC (eds) *Receptors Again*. Amsterdam: Elsevier Science Publications, 1984; 214–220.

Mazzi E. Possible neonatal diazepam withdrawal: a case report. *American Journal of Obstetrics and Gynecology* 1977; **129**: 586–587.

Mirakhur RK. Anticholinergic drugs. *British Journal of Anaesthesia* 1979; **51**: 671–679.

Mohler H, Okada T. Benzodiazepine receptor: demonstration in the nervous system. *Science* 1977; **198**: 849–851.

Murphy SM, Owen RT, Tyrer PJ. Withdrawal symptoms after six weeks treatment with diazepam. *Lancet* 1984; **ii**: 1389.

Nuotto EJ, Korttila K, Lichtor JL *et al*. Sedation and recovery of psychomotor function after intravenous administration of various doses of midazolam and diazepam. *Anesthesia and Analgesia* 1992; **74**: 265–271.

Olesen AS, Huttel MS. Local reactions to i.v. diazepam in three different formulations. *British Journal of Anaesthesia* 1980; **52**: 609–611.

Olsen RW. Drug interactions at the GABA receptor-ionophore complex. *Annual Review of Pharmacology* 1982; **22**: 245–277.

Owen RT, Tyrer P. Benzodiazepine dependence: a review of the evidence. *Drugs* 1983; **25**: 385–398.

Padfield NL, Twohig M McD, Fraser ACL. Temazepam and trimeprazine compared with placebo as premedication in children. *British Journal of Anaesthesia* 1986; **58**: 487–493.

Patsolas PN, Lascelles PT. Changes in regional brain levels of amino acid putative transmitters after prolonged treatment with the anticonvulsant drugs diphenylhydantoin, phenobarbitone, sodium valproate, ethosuximide and sulthiame in the rat. *Journal of Neurochemistry* 1981; **36**: 688–695.

Patton CM, Moon MR, Dannemiller FJ. The prophylactic antiemetic effect of droperidol. *Anesthesia and Analgesia* 1974; **53**: 361–364.

Przybyla AC, Wang SC. Locus of central depressant action of diazepam. *Journal of Pharmacology and Experimental Therapeutics* 1968; **163**: 439–447.

Reynolds JM, Blogg CE. Prevention and treatment of postoperative nausea and vomiting. *Prescribers Journal* 1995; **35**: 111–116.

Ricou B, Forster A, Bruckner A, Chastonay P, Gemperle M. Clinical evaluation of a specific benzodiazepine antagonist (Ro 15–1788). *British Journal of Anaesthesia* 1986; **58**: 1005–1011.

Rowbotham DJ. Current management of postoperative nausea and vomiting. *British Journal of Anaesthesia* 1992; **69**: 46–59S.

Sage DJ, Close A, Boas RA. Reversal of midazolam sedation with anexate. *British Journal of Anaesthesia* 1987; **59**: 459–464.

Schacht U, Backer G. *In vitro* studies on GABA release. *British Journal of Clinical Pharmacology* 1979; **7**: 25–315.

Skegg DCG, Richards SM, Doll R. Minor tranquillisers and road accidents. *British Medical Journal* 1979; **1**: 917–919.

Smith DE, Wesson DR. Benzodiazepine dependency syndromes. *Journal of Psychoactive Drugs* 1983; **15**: 85–96.

Smith MT, Eadie MJ, Brophy TO'R. The pharmacokinetics of midazolam in man. *European Journal of Clinical Pharmacology* 1981; **19**: 271–278.

Squires RF, Braestrup C. Benzodiazepine receptors in rat brain. *Nature* 1977; **266**: 732–734.

Study RE, Barker JL. Diazepam and (–)pentobarbital: Fluctuation analysis reveals different mechanisms for potentiation of γ-aminobutyric acid responses in cultured central neurones. *Proceedings of the National Academy of Sciences USA* 1981; **78**: 7180–7184.

Study RE, Barker JL. Cellular mechanisms of benzodiazepine action. *Journal of the American Medical Association* 1982; **247**: 2147–2151.

Thomas DL, Vaughan RS, Vickers MD, Mapleson WW. Comparison of temazepam elixir and trimeprazine syrup as oral premedication in children undergoing tonsillectomy and associated procedures. *British Journal of Anaesthesia* 1987; **59**: 424–430.

Watcha MF, White PF. Postoperative nausea and vomiting. *Anaesthesiology* 1992; **77**: 162–184.

Wilkinson GR. Factors influencing the disposition of benzodiazepines. In: Usdin E, Skilnick P, Tallman JF *et al.* (eds) *Pharmacology of Benzodiazepines*. London: Macmillan Press, 1982; 285–297.

Wilson J, Ellis FR. Oral premedication with lorazepam (Ativan); a comparison with heptabarbitone (Medomin) and diazepam (Valium). *British Journal of Anaesthesia* 1973; **45**: 738–744.

Wood CD. Antimotion sickness and antiemetic drugs. *Drugs* 1979; **17**: 471–479.

Wood CD, Graybiel A. A theory of motion sickness based on pharmacological reactions. *Clinical Pharmacology and Therapeutics* 1970; **11**: 621–629.

Young WS, Kurhar MJ. Autoradiographic localisation of benzodiazepine receptors in the brains of humans and animals. *Nature* 1979; **280**: 393–395.

Chapter 14
Antihypertensive Agents: Drugs Used to Induce Hypotension

Hypertension has been recognized as a disease for over a century, but it is only in the last three or four decades that effective pharmacological therapy has become generally available. Prior to this time, treatment was directed principally to those patients with only the most severe forms of the disease; remedies included prolonged bedrest, the use of sedative drugs and surgical attempts to extirpate the sympathetic nervous system.

The World Health Organization has defined hypertension as a condition which exists when the blood pressure persistently exceeds 160/90 mmHg. There appears to be little doubt that specific therapy aimed at reducing diastolic levels will decrease morbidity and mortality resulting from the disease. In particular, large-scale studies have demonstrated that the incidence of renal complications, haemorrhagic stroke and cardiac failure is diminished; recent surveys have also indicated that myocardial infarction is less likely to ensue. Before specific therapy is initiated, the following factors should be taken into consideration:

1 The age of the patient, as the undesirable effects of antihypertensive agents may outweigh the possible benefits in the elderly.

2 The existence of related diseases (e.g. diabetes, hypercholesterolaemia) which if more effectively treated may provide improved control of the hypertensive disorder.

3 The use of non-specific measures (e.g. cessation of smoking and excessive alcohol consumption, reduction of weight and salt intake, regular exercise) where appropriate.

The British Hypertension Society recommends early initiation of drug therapy where blood pressure levels greater than 200 mmHg systolic or 110 mmHg diastolic are confirmed. In relation to lesser degrees of hypertension, the decision when to commence therapy is principally determined by the presence of cardiovascular complications or of end-organ damage (e.g. renal impairment, retinal changes), although drug treatment will always be indicated if the average systolic pressures are >160 mmHg or diastolic pressures are >100 mmHg over a period of 3–6 months. It is now evident that treatment of isolated systolic hypertension (persistent levels greater than 160 mmHg) in patients between 60 and 80 years of age results in a significant reduction in the incidence of cardiac and cerebrovascular complications.

In all cases regular blood pressure measurement is indicated and the use of self-monitoring devices may be a useful adjunct to clinical readings in milder forms of hypertension. 'White-coat' hypertension is thought to occur in approximately 20% of patients, and may be an important factor in preoperative assessment.

In more than 80% of patients with hypertension no aetiology is apparent, although there is some evidence to suggest that morphological changes in the arteriolar wall (due to genetic or environmental influences) may be an important precipitating factor. Alterations in sodium, potassium or calcium balance have also been implicated in having a causal relationship with essential hypertension. The theory that sodium intake will lead to plasma volume expansion and resultant hypertension was originally propounded (although normal sodium balance should be retained in the presence of an intact renin–angiotensin system) and regimes involving drastic reductions in salt intake, which produced little therapeutic benefit, were introduced. However, some individuals may achieve a modest fall of blood pressure with a substantial reduction in salt intake; furthermore, patients who modify their diet whilst taking hypertensive therapy will achieve more sustained periods of normotension. There is also some evidence that increased potassium intake and calcium supplementation may produce beneficial effects in hypertensive patients; the dietary intake of magnesium, which is itself a vasodilator, may prove to have an important role. The endogenous transmitter endothelin 1 (ET-1) appears to have an important regulatory role in ionic transport of calcium (and possibly potassium) and experimental studies with endothelin-receptor antagonists demonstrate an effective hypotensive response in animal models of hypertension.

However, in 10–20% of cases an identifiable and sometimes curable cause of their hypertension may be found. Disease processes resulting in secondary hypertension include coarctation of the aorta, renal artery stenosis, phaeochromocytoma and hyperaldosteronism.

The level of arterial blood pressure is determined by the cardiac output and the impedance of the resistance vessels (arterioles) and is principally maintained by the efficiency of both the sympathetic nervous system and the renin–angiotensin–aldosterone system. Pharmacological methods of reducing blood pressure frequently involve the modification of these pathways at various sites. In addition, drugs which act directly to relax vascular smooth muscle or alter vessel wall compliance by effects on extracellular fluid volumes (thus decreasing peripheral resistance) are effective antihypertensive agents. In some instances drugs of this class may also reduce cardiac output secondary to their effects on capacitance vessels (thus diminishing venous return) or by negative inotropic or chronotropic effects on the heart. The sites of action of the various drugs which may be employed in the treatment of hypertension are shown in Table 14.1. It must be stressed that this physiological classification in no way correlates with their importance in practice. The clinical implications are discussed at a later stage of the chapter.

Table 14.1 Sites of action of the various antihypertensive agents.

Inhibitors of sympathetic nervous system activity
Centrally acting drugs (e.g. methyldopa, clonidine)
Ganglion-blocking compounds (trimetaphan)
Adrenergic neuron-blocking agents (e.g. guanethidine, bretylium)
α-Adrenoceptor antagonists (e.g. prazosin, phenoxybenzamine)
β-Adrenoceptor antagonists (e.g. propranolol, atenolol)
Combined α- and β-antagonists (labetalol)
Inhibitors of the renin–angiotensin–aldosterone system
Reduction of renin secretion (by β-adrenoceptor antagonism)
Angiotensin converting enzyme inhibitors (e.g. captopril, enalapril)
Angiotensin receptor antagonists (losartan)
Aldosterone antagonists (spironolactone, potassium canrenoate)
Drugs with non-autonomic effects on peripheral resistance
Vasodilators (e.g. calcium-channel blockers, hydralazine)
Diuretics (thiazides and loop diuretics)

Centrally acting drugs

Methyldopa

Methyldopa was originally shown to be a dopa decarboxylase inhibitor, and it was considered that the antihypertensive effect was due to failure of conversion of dopa → dopamine → noradrenaline. It was subsequently demonstrated that methyldopa itself acted as a substrate for the enzyme and was converted into methylnoradrenaline which was thought to act as a false transmitter at noradrenergic nerve terminals. Further evidence indicated that this substance displayed significant intrinsic sympathomimetic activity. Methyldopa readily traverses the blood–brain barrier and is converted into α-methylnoradrenaline which subsequently inhibits cardioregulatory centres in the tractus solitarius in the medulla oblongata, through effects mediated via α_2-adrenoceptors situated at these sites.

In recent years the use of methyldopa in the treatment of hypertension has declined. Side-effects include drowsiness and depression, oedema, drug rashes and hepatotoxicity. With prolonged therapy 10–20% of patients show a positive direct Coombs test and in a small proportion of these, haemolytic anaemia will occur. In contrast, postural hypotension rarely occurs with methyldopa therapy.

Clonidine

Clonidine was originally designed as a topical vasoconstrictor and its potent antihypertensive activity was discovered accidentally. The intravenous administration of clonidine produces a transient increase in blood pressure and peripheral vasoconstriction — an effect which appears to be mediated via α_1-adrenoceptors.

The secondary responses of bradycardia and hypotension are principally due to a central nervous system (CNS) effect; clonidine has an agonistic effect on α_2-adrenoceptors in the medulla oblongata and inhibits central vasomotor activity. Clonidine may also act as an agonist on peripheral presynaptic (α_2) adrenoceptors to inhibit the release of noradrenaline.

Clonidine produces some degree of sedation, and a dry mouth (which appears to be due to central inhibition of salivation) is a common side-effect. Postural hypotension is not usually a problem. However, the use of this drug in the therapy of hypertension has been considerably restricted by the severe rebound phenomena which have occurred following the sudden withdrawal of the drug. A life-threatening hypertensive crisis associated with hyperexcitability can ensue and may require treatment with a combination of α- and β-adrenoceptor antagonists.

Clonidine has been used in low dosage in the prophylaxis of migraine; presumably the peripheral vasoconstrictor effect is considered to predominate in these circumstances. The administration of clonidine has also been shown to reduce the minimum alveolar concentration (MAC) value of anaesthetic agents. Furthermore, clonidine appears to exhibit an antinociceptive effect (see Chapter 12) and has been administered by intrathecal routes for the relief of intractable pain. The drug has also been used in the management of the Gilles de la Tourette syndrome.

Ganglion-blocking compounds

These were the first drugs used specifically for the treatment of essential hypertension. Marked disadvantages to the use of these drugs include:

1 Irregular absorption after oral administration.

2 Non-selective blockade of nicotinic receptors in all autonomic ganglia leading to a variety of side-effects, including dry mouth, blurred vision, paralytic ileus and disturbances of sexual function.

3 The problem of postural hypotension; the receptors on the chromaffin cells of the adrenal medulla are also blocked, and adequate compensation for postural changes is not possible.

Mecamylamine is still available in the USA, and pentolinium and hexamethonium are used to a limited extent for the treatment of hypertension in some countries. These drugs are no longer used in the UK, where the role of ganglion-blocking agents is now limited to the more rapid reduction of blood pressure in hypertensive emergencies, or to provide a relatively bloodless field during surgical procedures. Trimetaphan is commonly used in this context and is discussed later in the chapter.

Adrenergic neurone-blocking agents

In sympathetic nerve terminals, noradrenaline, which has reappeared due to Uptake_1 mechanisms, together with dopamine, which is available for its further synthesis, undergo active transport from cytoplasm into storage vesicles. Drugs which lower the blood pressure by acting at postganglionic sympathetic nerve endings appear to have complex mechanisms affecting the transport, storage and subsequent release of noradrenaline.

Guanethidine

Guanethidine is an antihypertensive agent which acts principally on the storage vesicles in sympathetic nerve terminals by displacing noradrenaline from binding sites and preventing its further uptake from the axoplasm. Intravenous administration of guanethidine appears to produce a triphasic effect. Initially there is a fall in blood pressure which is due to a direct effect on resistance vessels (in this respect guanethidine may be regarded as a false transmitter). A slight rise of blood pressure then occurs because noradrenaline is displaced into the synaptic gap. A progressive fall in both systolic and diastolic blood pressure subsequently ensues because of failure of release of further neurotransmitter. Following oral administration of guanethidine, a rise in blood pressure is unlikely to occur; the fall is slow in onset and usually develops over several days. The drug has a long duration of action; the effects of a single dose persist for up to 4 days and cumulation is likely. Side-effects include postural hypotension, diarrhoea and failure of ejaculation; CNS effects are uncommon as guanethidine does not readily penetrate the blood–brain barrier. Transport of the drug into the neurone and the subsequent antihypertensive effect are prevented by drugs which block Uptake_1 mechanisms (e.g. tricyclic antidepressants, cocaine, amphetamines). Conversely, those patients receiving long-term therapy with guanethidine exhibit a marked 'supersensitivity' to pressor amines.

Guanethidine is also used to produce intravenous regional sympathetic blockade in the treatment of intractable pain involving a limb in which there is evidence of autonomic dysfunction; the drug also has significant local anaesthetic activity.

Bethanidine and debrisoquine are closely related drugs with a shorter duration of action. Bretylium, another analogue, has now found a role in the management of ventricular dysrhythmias resistant to other treatment, and is described as a class 3 antiarrhythmic agent.

Reserpine

Reserpine is an alkaloid which has been extensively used in the treatment of hypertension. It acts by preventing the uptake of noradrenaline from the axoplasm into the storage granules. The uptake of dopamine into the vesicles is similarly inhibited and storage of 5-hydroxytryptamine also appears to be impaired. The amines are thus more vulnerable to mitochondrial monoamine oxidase, and eventually depletion of the neurotransmitter occurs. Reserpine readily crosses the blood–brain barrier, and undoubtedly produces similar effects on adrenergic neurones within the CNS. Deficiency of dopamine and noradrenaline at central sites would account for the main side-effects of reserpine which include depression, extrapyramidal disturbances and the manifestations of hyperprolactinaemia, and these effects appear to be dose-dependent. Reserpine is no longer used in the UK.

Metirosine

Metirosine (α-methyl-*p*-tyrosine) is a competitive inhibitor of the enzyme tyrosine hydroxylase. Metirosine thus prevents the conversion of tyrosine $\rightarrow$ dopa with a consequent reduction in the formation of dopamine and noradrenaline at central and peripheral sites, including the adrenal medulla.

Metirosine may be used in the preoperative preparation of patients scheduled for the removal of a phaeochromocytoma, or in the long-term management of those unsuitable for surgery. Side-effects associated with the use of the drug include moderate or severe sedation and the appearance of extrapyramidal disorders; diarrhoea is also a common complaint. Metirosine is not recommended for the treatment of essential hypertension.

Other drugs which can produce a hypotensive effect, which is probably due to the production of a false transmitter at the noradrenergic nerve terminal, include the monoamine oxidase inhibitor pargyline and the experimental agent 6-hydroxydopamine.

α-Adrenoceptor antagonists

In general, drugs of this group have been of more value in treating secondary hypertension due to a high level of circulating catecholamines than for the management of essential hypertension. They have also been used to improve organ blood flow in the treatment of shock, and occasionally as peripheral vasodilators.

Many of these agents indiscriminately antagonize both α_1 and α_2-receptors so that further release of noradrenaline is facilitated. As only the α-adrenoceptors are antagonized, there will be an enhanced response to the circulating catecholamines mediated via β-adrenoceptors and tachycardias are likely; postural hypotension can also be a problem.

Phenoxybenzamine

Phenoxybenzamine forms a covalent linkage with the α-adrenoceptor and a potentially irreversible blockade results. The effects of a single dose of this agent may last for several days. Phenoxybenzamine is used in the preoperative management of patients with phaeochromocytoma or in their long-term treatment when surgery is precluded. The drug has also been employed in the control of hypertensive episodes associated with monoamine oxidase inhibitor (MAOI)–food interactions, or those following the sudden withdrawal of antihypertensive therapy with, for example, clonidine. Phenoxybenzamine has also been used to improve splanchnic and renal perfusion in shock states; in such circumstances monitoring of the central venous pressure is essential.

Phentolamine

Phentolamine was formerly employed as a diagnostic agent for phaeochromocytoma. However, false-positive responses may occur, and a dangerous degree of hypotension may ensue; this effect may be due to a direct action of the drug on vascular smooth muscle. Estimations of the levels of urinary metabolites of catecholamines and radiological techniques, in particular the use of computed tomography (CT scans) to localize the tumour, are more rational approaches to diagnosis. Nevertheless, phentolamine infusions (0.1–2 mg min^{-1}) are still useful in the management of hypertensive crises which may occur with surgical removal of a phaeochromocytoma, especially during manipulation of the tumour.

Indoramin

Indoramin is an α-adrenoceptor antagonist which has local anaesthetic properties (including a quinidine-like effect on the myocardium) and antihistamine activity. It is used in the treatment of hypertension, usually in combination with a thiazide diuretic or a β-adrenoceptor antagonist, and has also been shown to reduce the frequency of migraine attacks in some patients. Indoramin interacts with alcohol; plasma levels of both drugs are enhanced with an increased likelihood of drowsiness. Indoramin may also cause extrapyramidal effects.

Prazosin

Prazosin has a highly selective action on α_1-adrenoceptors. It is therefore about 10 times more potent than phentolamine in controlling the vasoconstrictor responses to noradrenaline, and rarely produces tachycardia. Prazosin is available as an oral preparation for the treatment of essential hypertension. A number of incidents of fainting with loss of consciousness have occurred when a course of treatment with this agent is initiated (first-dose phenomenon). It is unclear whether this effect is due to severe postural hypotension from peripheral adrenoceptor blockade or whether central mechanisms are involved. This untoward response can be minimized by commencing treatment with a low dose which is taken on retiring to bed. Terazosin and doxazosin have similar properties to those of prazosin. Selective α-adrenoceptor antagonists are also used to relax smooth muscle and improve obstructive symptoms in benign prostatic hyperplasia. Other agents which exhibit α-adrenoceptor antagonist activity include the neuroleptic phenothiazines and the ergot alkaloids (see Chapter 11).

β-Adrenoceptor antagonists

The value of β-adrenoceptor antagonists in the treatment of hypertension is well-established and most of the drugs in this group have been used for this purpose. The mechanism of the antihypertensive effect is not entirely clear and it may be that more than one pharmacological action is involved. These may include the following:

1 A reduction in cardiac output which occurs fairly rapidly following the administration of a drug of this type. However, the peripheral resistance will rise initially due to compensatory mechanisms and the hypotensive response will occur more slowly.

2 A resetting of baroreceptor activity at a lower blood pressure level.

3 Inhibition of the renin–angiotensin system particularly in those patients showing high plasma renin activity (PRA).

4 Presynaptic inhibition (via β_2-adrenoceptors) of noradrenaline release from sympathetic nerve terminals.

5 A CNS effect. A hypotensive response can be shown experimentally following the intraventricular injection of a β-adrenoceptor antagonist. However, some drugs in this group (e.g. atenolol, nadolol) have a low lipid solubility and do not cross the blood–brain barrier significantly. Nevertheless, they are effective antihypertensive agents.

Present opinion suggests that the most important effects are those influencing cardiac output and the renin–angiotensin system. The release of renin from the juxtaglomerular apparatus is stimulated via β_1-adrenoceptors and is thus inhibited by propranolol and related compounds. There is evidence to show that hypertensive patients who exhibit elevated high PRA can be more effectively controlled with low doses of β-adrenoceptor antagonists.

Propranolol

Propranolol was the first drug of this type to be widely used for the treatment of hypertension. It is non-selective with regard to β_1 and β_2 effects and is devoid of intrinsic sympathomimetic activity (ISA). Propranolol is a highly lipid-soluble compound which undergoes significant first-pass metabolism. It readily crosses the blood–brain barrier and has a large volume of distribution, a high clearance rate and a relatively short elimination half-life (approximately 4 h). Related compounds which are poorly lipid-soluble (e.g. atenolol, nadolol) can be advantageous when central side-effects (sedation, depression, unpleasant dreams) are a problem; their pharmacokinetic properties also allow blood pressure to be controlled on a once-daily dose regime. One exception is the hydrophilic agent esmolol, which has a plasma half-life of less than 10 min. The relatively evanescent effects of esmolol are due to its rapid destruction by plasma enzymes (p. 497).

Cardioselective agents (e.g. acebutolol, metoprolol) should be chosen for those patients in whom the effects of β_2-antagonism such as bronchospasm, intermittent claudication and hypoglycaemia are likely to occur. However, even selective β_1-antagonists demonstrate significant degrees of β_2-adrenoceptor antagonism at high doses. Drugs with ISA (e.g. oxprenolol, alprenolol) are theoretically superior when there is a risk of heart failure developing.

β-Adrenoceptor antagonists are also discussed in Chapters 12 and 15.

Labetalol

Labetalol produces competitive antagonism at α_1- (postsynaptic), β_1- and β_2-adrenoceptors. When given intravenously it is approximately seven times more potent at β-adrenoceptors than at α-adrenoceptors; following oral administration the relative potencies are 3 to 1. Labetalol is used in the management of hypertensive disorders; it may be administered by mouth in a twice-daily regime. Like propranolol, it is subject to first-pass metabolism and sometimes produces CNS side-effects and occasional skin rashes. Intravenous administration of labetalol may also be of value in hypertensive emergencies, and is occasionally used to produce controlled hypotension during anaesthesia and surgery. It may be given by injection or infusion up to a maximum dose of 200 mg. A fall in peripheral resistance, principally due to a reduction in arteriolar tone, occurs. Reflex tachycardia does not ensue as cardiac β-adrenoceptors are antagonized. The hypotensive effects can be readily reversed by atropine and tachyphylaxis has not been observed. Carvedilol is a closely related drug which has recently been introduced as an oral preparation for the treatment of hypertension. Another relatively new agent, celiprolol, also exhibits β_2-agonist activity and has mild vasodilating properties.

The renin–angiotensin–aldosterone system

Angiotensin II is the most potent pressor substance known. In addition to having a direct vasoconstrictor effect, particularly on arterioles, it promotes the release of catecholamines from the adrenal medulla and facilitates sympathetic nervous system activity by central and peripheral mechanisms. Furthermore, it blocks the reuptake of noradrenaline into the adrenergic nerve terminal and has a stimulatory effect on autonomic ganglia cells. Angiotensin II also stimulates the production of aldosterone by the adrenal cortex. This mineralocorticoid enhances sodium reabsorption and potassium excretion in the distal tubule.

The production of angiotensin II itself depends upon the release of renin, a proteolytic enzyme which is produced in the cells of the juxtaglomerular apparatus of the renal cortex. The substrate for renin is a plasma protein, angiotensinogen, which is present in the α_2-globulin fraction.

Angiotensin I, a decapeptide which has limited intrinsic pharmacological activity, is then formed but is almost immediately converted to angiotensin II; this reaction is catalysed by an angiotensin-converting enzyme (ACE) which is present in the vascular endothelium and lung tissue. Angiotensin II is metabolized under the influence of various peptidases to produce a number of breakdown products, one of which (angiotensin III) retains some pressor activity.

There is now evidence for the existence of at least two types of angiotensin (AT) receptors. AT_1-receptors, which show a greater affinity for angiotensin II, and mediate their effects via G-protein coupling and phosphoinositide metabolism, are thought to subserve the classical pressor role. AT_2-receptors, at which angiotensin II and angiotensin III demonstrate equal potency, are apparently linked to protein tyrosine phosphate activity. They may have an important role in physiological processes such as cell growth and differentiation.

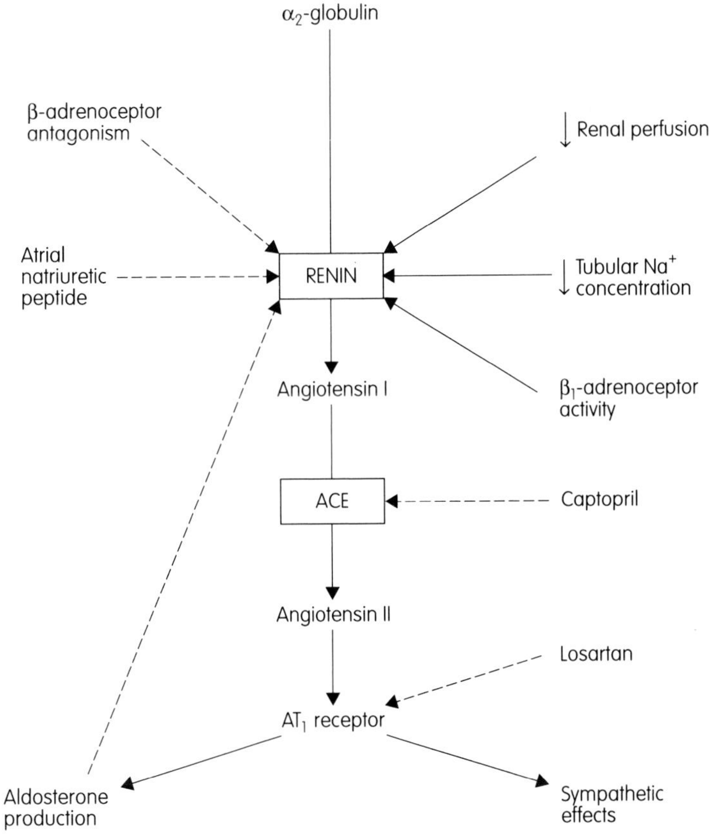

Fig. 14.1 The renin–angiotensin–aldosterone system and its modification by intrinsic and extrinsic factors. Boxes denote enzymes. Solid arrows denote stimulatory effects: broken arrows, antagonistic activity.

There are three principal mechanisms which appear to control the release of renin from the juxtaglomerular apparatus:

1 Mechanical. A fall in renal perfusion pressure will reduce the tension within the wall of the afferent arteriole and signal the release of renin.

2 Ionic. A lowering of the sodium concentration in the distal tubule situated in the adjacent macula densa is considered to stimulate the secretion of renin. This implies that the increased production of aldosterone, which promotes the retention of sodium ions at this site, will result in a negative-feedback effect.

3 Neurogenic. Stimulation of the nerves of the renal plexus will result in the release of renin; this secretomotor effect is mediated via β_1-adrenoceptors.

The renin–angiotensin–aldosterone system can be inhibited at a number of sites and by a variety of mechanisms; these are summarized in Fig. 14.1. The production of both renin and aldosterone appears to be antagonized by *atrial natriuretic peptide* (ANP), a hormone which is stored (in an inactivated form) by atrial myocyte granulocytes and whose rate of secretion into the plasma appears to be dependent on atrial wall tension. Thus, elevated levels have been observed following expansion of the blood volume and in congestive cardiac and renal failure. Specific high-affinity receptors for ANP have been identified in vascular, renal and adrenal tissue. ANP appears to produce an increase in both glomerular filtration rate and fractional excretion of sodium, and experimental evidence suggests that it is an arterioselective vasodilator. Furthermore, there appears to be little doubt now that the antihypertensive effects of the β-adrenoceptor antagonists are at least partially due to inhibition of renin secretion.

Captopril

Captopril is an ACE inhibitor which prevents the conversion of angiotensin I to angiotensin II. Captopril produces a fall in blood pressure initially by reducing peripheral resistance; arteriolar tone is more predominantly affected than venous tone. Heart rate is usually unchanged or slightly increased and postural hypotension is infrequent. Renal blood flow is usually increased; aldosterone secretion is thus further inhibited and sodium excretion is promoted. However, captopril and related drugs may occasionally cause significant renal impairment, particularly in patients with pre-existing kidney disease or renal artery stenosis, and in elderly patients or those receiving non-steroidal anti-inflammatory drugs (NSAIDs). Hyperkalaemia may develop and renal function and electrolytes should be checked prior to treatment and subsequently monitored. Initial dosage may produce a profound fall in blood pressure, particularly when there is a pre-existing deficit of sodium. Side-effects which may be induced by captopril include a persistent dry cough, loss of taste sensation, gastrointestinal disturbances, proteinuria and occasionally bone marrow depression. The use of ACE inhibitors has been associated with increased insulin sensitivity in diabetic patients. A symptom complex including fever, myalgia, eosinophilia, photosensitivity and other skin reactions has also been reported. A number of these undesirable effects may be related to the accumulation of the peptide bradykinin, the metabolic degradation of which is also suppressed by ACE inhibitors.

Captopril is used in the treatment of mild to moderate hypertension, usually as an adjunct to diuretic therapy, and in severe hypertension resistant to other treatment.

ACE inhibitors will undoubtedly produce vasodilatation in patients with normal or low levels of plasma renin. The mechanism of this action is not completely clear but may involve a potentiation of the inhibitory effects of bradykinin and possibly other 'relaxing' factors on smooth muscle. Captopril has thus developed a useful role in the management of chronic congestive cardiac failure by reducing both preload and afterload. Originally used when fluid retention proved refractory to other forms of treatment (e.g. digitalis, diuretics), it is now sometimes introduced as first-line therapy.

Enalapril (a prodrug ester which is hydrolysed to the pharmacologically active parent dicarboxylic acid, enalaprilat), perindopril and lisinopril are related compounds with a more prolonged duration of action.

Losartan potassium, a substituted imidazole compound, has recently been introduced in the UK for the treatment of hypertension and appears to be a specific angiotensin II antagonist (with high affinity and selectivity for the AT_1-receptor). The drug is effective orally, but has a low bioavailability and undergoes significant first-pass metabolism to produce an active metabolite. Losartan is recommended for the treatment of mild to moderate hypertension when other agents have proved to be ineffective or give rise to problems; the drug may be a useful alternative to ACE inhibitors in those patients who develop a troublesome cough. Saralasin is a competitive antagonist of angiotensin II which has been used in the USA as an aid in the differential diagnosis of hypertension, although partial agonist effects would appear to preclude its more general use as a therapeutic agent. Antagonists of renin activity are also being investigated.

Spironolactone is a diuretic which selectively binds to aldosterone receptors in the distal tubule and thus inhibits the mineralocorticoid effect. At one time, it was extensively used in the management of essential hypertension. There is now some evidence that spironolactone is carcinogenic to animals when it is administered over a prolonged period; side-effects such as gastrointestinal disturbances, gynaecomastia and those related to potassium retention can also be a problem. The role of this drug is now normally restricted to the management of primary hyperaldosteronism (Conn syndrome) and in the treatment of refractory oedema associated with cirrhosis of the liver, congestive cardiac failure or the nephrotic syndrome. Potassium canrenoate has similar properties (it is hydrolysed to canrenone, which is the major metabolite of spironolactone) and is available as a preparation for parenteral use.

Vasodilators

Calcium-channel blockers

This class of drugs will antagonize the cardiovascular effects mediated via the high voltage activated and voltage-dependent (L-type) calcium channels, which produce long-lasting calcium currents. They have become widely used in the management of angina pectoris and have developed an established role as antiarrhythmic agents (see Chapter 15). Class 2 calcium-channel blockers (dihydropyridine derivatives), which include nifedipine and nicardipine, do not appear to affect the rate of recovery of the 'slow' calcium channel in the myocardium, in contrast to class 1 phenylalkylamine derivatives (e.g. verapamil), which are also considered to inhibit baroreceptor reflex activity. Thus they will produce arteriolar vasodilatation at concentrations which appear to have little effect on cardiac conduction. Coronary blood flow and subendocardial perfusion are also improved and there is a reduction in the work of the left ventricle.

Nifedipine has been used in the treatment of essential hypertension, usually in combination with a β-adrenoceptor antagonist. Side-effects related to peripheral vasodilatation, such as headache, flushing and postural hypotension, are sometimes a problem and ankle oedema may occur. Amlodipine and felodipine are closely related drugs which have a longer duration of action. Experimental evidence indicates that this group of drugs may antagonize the effects of ET-1 and inhibit the progress of atherosclerosis.

Hydralazine

Initial studies of this agent suggested that its antihypertensive activity was mediated within the CNS. However, present evidence indicates that its major effect is to produce a direct relaxation of smooth muscle. The mechanism is thought to be similar to that of the organic nitrates, as it produces intracellular accumulation of cyclic guanosine monophosphate (cGMP). However, arteriolar tone is more selectively inhibited and postural hypotension does not usually occur during treatment with this agent. Reflex tachycardia and fluid retention are common accompaniments, thus in the treatment of hypertension it is normally administered in combination with a β-adrenoceptor antagonist and a diuretic. Hydralazine is a valuable drug, when administered intravenously, in the treatment of hypertensive emergencies and is a popular agent for the management of severe hypertension associated with pregnancy. Chronic therapy with a high daily dosage may produce a lupus-like syndrome. Hydralazine is subject to pharmacogenetic influences and 'slow acetylators' of the drug are more prone to develop this condition.

Minoxidil has a similar spectrum of activity to that of hydralazine and its mechanism of action is probably identical. One interesting side-effect of this agent is hypertrichosis and it has been used by topical application for the treatment of baldness.

Diuretics

Many drugs which are used as diuretics can induce a moderate fall in blood pressure when the plasma volume decreases consequent to enhanced renal elimination of water and electrolytes. Thiazide diuretics are most commonly employed in the long-term management of oedema associated with congestive cardiac failure, hepatic cirrhosis and the nephrotic syndrome. They are acidic compounds which are structurally related to the sulphonamides and are actively secreted in the proximal tubule. Their principal site of action is in the distal tubule, where they inhibit the active transport (reabsorption) of sodium and chloride ions. Thiazide diuretics may also stimulate the secretion of potassium at a more distal site, and potassium supplementation is sometimes necessary during continuous therapy. Drugs in this group include hydrochlorothiazide, bendrofluazide, hydroflumethiazide and chlorothiazide.

However, thiazide diuretics and closely related analogues (e.g. chlorthalidone, metolazone, indapamide) are commonly used in the long-term therapy of mild to moderate hypertension. They exert this therapeutic effect at doses far lower than those required to induce significant loss of free water, sodium or potassium ions. In this context, thiazide diuretics appear to act as peripheral vasodilators, although the mechanism probably involves a reduction in interstitial fluid volume, resulting in an increase in vascular compliance. The use of low-dose regimes appears to be safe and effective; in particular the many side-effects associated with this group of agents when diuretic doses are required (e.g. hypokalaemia, urate retention, hyperglycaemia, elevated plasma lipid levels) are considerably reduced. Furthermore, thiazide diuretics appear to potentiate the antihypertensive effects of other drugs with different mechanisms of action.

In contrast, both the diuretic and antihypertensive effects of the thiazides may be antagonized in patients who are concomitantly treated with NSAIDs. Inhibition of the synthesis of prostaglandins, which have significant effects on renal blood flow, glomerular filtration and tubular ion transport, is undoubtedly a causal factor.

The carboxylic acid derivatives (frusemide, ethacrynic acid and bumetanide) are highly potent diuretics with a relatively short duration of action. In contrast to the thiazides which produce a diuretic effect by inhibiting reabsorption in the distal tubule, the site of action of frusemide and related compounds is in the ascending loop of Henle and they are commonly referred to as loop diuretics. In addition, an increase in renal blood flow frequently occurs following intravenous administration of these agents. They are most effective for producing a rapid diuresis in severe cardiac failure, pulmonary or cerebral oedema. They are also valuable when administered with blood transfusions for severe anaemia where cardiac failure due to fluid overloading may be anticipated. Loop diuretics are not used for their antihypertensive effects.

Other diuretics of clinical importance include the carbohydrate derivative mannitol. Mannitol is a polyhydric alcohol which is produced by reduction of the monosaccharide mannose and has a molecular weight of approximately 200 Da. Mannitol is widely distributed throughout the vascular bed and interstitial tissues. Its volume of distribution ($0.2\ l\ kg^{-1}$) thus reflects the volume of the extracellular fluid. Mannitol is pharmacologically inert; it is freely filtrable at the glomerulus and is not significantly reabsorbed. When administered intravenously as a hypertonic infusion (usually 250 ml of a 10 or 20% solution given over 20 min) it produces a rapid diuresis due to an osmotic effect which reduces water and electrolyte absorption in the renal tubule. Mannitol is of value in the prophylaxis of renal failure (e.g. during surgery for aortic aneurysm or for operations in the presence of severe jaundice), in the treatment of cerebral oedema and glaucoma, and to promote forced diuresis in cases of drug overdose.

Carbonic anhydrase inhibitors, such as acetazolamide, are now rarely used as diuretics. However, they reduce bicarbonate production and consequently the secretion of aqueous humour, and may be useful in the management of glaucoma.

Potassium-sparing diuretics (e.g. triamterene, amiloride) may be used as an alternative to potassium supplements to prevent the hypokalaemia associated with thiazide or loop diuretic therapy.

Treatment of hypertension

In many patients with moderate or severe essential hypertension, blood pressure can be slowly and gradually controlled by oral therapy. Thiazide diuretics or β-adrenoceptor antagonists are recommended as first-line therapy. The choice of such drugs may be determined by the presence of coexisting disorders (e.g. angina pectoris, obstructive airways disease, peripheral vascular insufficiency, diabetes, gout) but they may be used in combination when they are ineffective alone. A peripheral vasodilator such as hydralazine may be added to this regime in resistant cases and supplementation by centrally acting drugs (e.g. methyldopa) or adrenergic neurone-blocking agents (e.g. bethanidine) is occasionally of some value.

More recently introduced drugs which are proving effective in the treatment of hypertension include ACE inhibitors (e.g. captopril, enalapril), calcium-channel blockers (e.g. nifedipine, nicarpidine) and α-adrenoceptor antagonists (e.g. prazosin, indoramin). Minor side-effects are perhaps more common with these latter agents and their use in long-term management is less well-established. Drugs in this category may be of specific value in the presence of associated disease; examples include the use of ACE inhibitors where there is evidence of incipient heart failure, calcium-channel blockers in patients with peripheral vascular insufficiency, and the use of α_1-adrenoceptor antagonists where there is a history of prostatism.

Thiazide diuretics and β-adrenoceptor antagonists both produce adverse effects on the plasma lipid profile. In contrast, selective α_1-adrenoceptor antagonists slightly reduce the levels of risk factors associated with coronary heart disease, namely, total cholesterol, its low-density subfraction and triglycerides, whilst elevating the high-density cholesterol levels.

In certain hypertensive emergencies, the blood pressure must be lowered immediately. Such situations include hypertensive encephalopathy, intracranial haemorrhage, dissecting aortic aneurysm, acute congestive cardiac failure and severe hypertension associated with toxaemia of pregnancy. Parenteral therapy may be indicated in such cases, although precipitous falls in blood pressure should be avoided to minimize further complications from the reduction in cerebral, myocardial or renal blood flow. Drugs which may be used for this purpose include hydralazine, labetalol, diazoxide, sodium nitroprusside and trimetaphan (the two last mentioned drugs are discussed more fully in a subsequent section of this chapter).

Diazoxide has a close structural resemblance to the thiazide diuretics, although paradoxically the drug itself has sodium-retaining effects. Diazoxide produces its hypotensive effects by relaxation of arteriolar smooth muscle; there appears to be little effect on capacitance vessels. The baroreceptor response evoked by the fall in blood pressure may lead to an increase in heart rate and stroke volume; the release of renin is also enhanced. When used in the treatment of a hypertensive crisis, diazoxide is administered by rapid intravenous injection in a dose of 1–3 mg kg^{-1} to a maximal single dose of 150 mg. The optimal depressor response occurs after a few minutes and if further treatment is not instituted, the blood pressure will return to its original level within 4–24 h. The concomitant use of a rapidly acting diuretic, such as frusemide, may be necessary if the hypertensive emergency is associated with pulmonary oedema or renal failure. As with the thiazide diuretics, diazoxide has diabetogenic properties and may antagonize the effects of insulin and other hypoglycaemic agents. Conversely, it is sometimes used as an oral preparation in the management of chronic hypoglycaemia associated with hyperplasia or tumours of the islet cells of the pancreas.

Hypertension in pregnancy

The presence of hypertension during pregnancy is one of the leading causes of maternal death and of fetal mortality and morbidity. There is a considerable amount of evidence to show that an increase in the incidence of stillbirths and intrauterine growth retardation may be associated with only a moderate increase in the diastolic or mean arterial blood pressure during the middle trimester. Maternal risks appear to correlate with rises in blood pressure which occur during the third trimester.

It is thus important to control an elevated blood pressure which occurs during pregnancy, whether this is due to pre-existing essential or secondary hypertension or to pre-eclampsia. Non-pharmacological methods (e.g. strict bedrest) are sometimes of value, but drug treatment will often be required. However, the choice of an appropriate antihypertensive agent will need careful consideration. Thiazide diuretics are probably not indicated in pregnancy. They do not prevent the development of toxaemia and may lead to hypovolaemia and to a decrease in placental perfusion. In the neonate thrombocytopenia, jaundice, hyponatraemia and an increased risk of hypertension developing at maturity have been reported.

Propranolol readily crosses the placental barrier; a number of fetal complications have been reported in association with its use, including intra-uterine growth retardation, severe neonatal hypoglycaemia, bradycardia and respiratory depression. Reserpine has also been associated with a number of fetal abnormalities, including lethargy, disturbances of temperature control and engorgement of the mucous membranes, whilst clonidine has been shown to be teratogenic in animal studies. ACE inhibitors such as captopril may adversely affect fetal and neonatal blood pressure control and renal function, whilst the use of calcium-channel blockers such as nifedipine may inhibit the progress of labour.

Methyldopa and β-adrenoceptor antagonists with low lipophilic properties (e.g. atenolol) are safe to administer during pregnancy and oral hydralazine is useful as second-line therapy; the intravenous administration of this drug may be necessary to control hypertensive crises associated with eclampsia.

Antihypertensive drugs and anaesthesia

It is evident that many of the agents used in anaesthetic practice can exert significant activity on the autonomic nervous system and can theoretically potentiate the effects of established antihypertensive therapy. At one time it was considered desirable that whenever possible antihypertensive drugs should be withdrawn for up to 14 days prior to anaesthesia and surgery. Various tests were used to assess the magnitude of residual sympathetic activity; these included the measurement of blood pressure responses to the Valsalva manoeuvre or to postural changes, or to the administration of indirectly acting sympathomimetic amines such as ephedrine or tyrosine.

This view is no longer tenable. The attendant dangers of a rising blood pressure are an obvious disadvantage, and the enhanced pressor responses which are observed during laryngoscopy and intubation in uncontrolled hypertensive patients is particularly hazardous. Furthermore, the sudden withdrawal of clonidine, β-adrenoceptor antagonists and possibly other agents may lead to dangerous rebound phenomena.

It is now standard practice to continue antihypertensive therapy until a few hours prior to surgery. However, special vigilance is still necessary to prevent excessive hypertension and tachycardia which may result from airway manipulation or surgical stimulation. In this context, the depth of anaesthesia is of considerable import; however, the concentrations of volatile agents required to suppress such haemodynamic responses are considerably greater than their MAC values, and may lead to depression of an already compromised myocardium.

In such a situation, the use of rapidly acting opioid analgesics (e.g. fentanyl, alfentanil) during induction may be especially valuable. Topical lignocaine applied to the larynx before intubation and, on occasions, the prior administration of glyceryl trinitrate would also appear to be beneficial.

In this context, the ultrashort-acting β-adrenoceptor antagonist esmolol may also prove to be of value. Esmolol is a cardioselective agent with no ISA or membrane-stabilizing activity. Esmolol has a rapid onset of action following intravenous administration; no significant activity can be detected 20 min after termination of treatment. The short half-life (approximately 9 min) is due to rapid biotransformation of the drug, by esterases present in the red blood cells, to an inactive acid metabolite and methyl alcohol (less than 2% is excreted unchanged in the urine). Such properties would suggest that the drug would be particularly suitable for the management of hypertensive responses which may occur during the induction or recovery phases of anaesthesia. Adenosine, which has negative inotropic and chronotropic effects on the heart and a transient duration of action (half-life = 8–10 s) may also be used in this situation.

Esmolol has also been used in the treatment of supraventricular tachycardias, and may be effective in the management of acute myocardial ischaemia and unstable angina. A non-cardioselective analogue flestolol, which may have an even briefer action, is also being developed. α_2-Adrenoceptor agonists (e.g. clonidine, azepexole) which can reduce anaesthetic requirements, and also decrease adrenergic activity by both central and peripheral mechanisms, may also develop a role in the modification of cardiovascular reflex responses which may occur during anaesthesia (Chapter 13).

In both treated and untreated hypertensive patients, untoward changes in cardiovascular parameters are more prone to occur during anaesthesia than in normotensive subjects. Special attention must thus be paid to the maintenance of blood volume, ventilatory parameters and positioning the patient on the operating table.

Induced hypotension

Deliberate hypotension has been employed for many years to reduce bleeding during surgical procedures. Techniques which were originally used included controlled arteriotomy, the application of negative pressures to the lower limbs and the production of high spinal or extradural blockade with local anaesthetic agents. The inhalational agents now in common use (halothane, fluorinated ethers) produce dose-related effects on blood pressure and may be employed to produce moderate and predictable hypotension during anaesthesia. Controlled ventilation is necessary for this technique and the combined use of tubocurarine as the muscle relaxant may be particularly beneficial. Other drugs which have been specifically employed to produce controlled hypotension during surgery include trimetaphan, sodium nitroprusside and glyceryl trinitrate.

Trimetaphan

Trimetaphan is a sulphonium compound containing two tertiary amine groups. When used to produce a bloodless field during surgery, it is usually administered in physiological saline at a rate of 1–4 mg min^{-1}. Trimetaphan is incompatible in solution with some other drugs commonly used in anaesthesia (e.g. intravenous barbiturates, gallamine). The hypotensive effects are due to several different actions of the drug. Trimetaphan causes blockade of both sympathetic and parasympathetic ganglia and releases histamine from mast cells. Furthermore, it decreases peripheral resistance by a direct action on blood vessels; experimental evidence suggests that this may be an important factor in the hypotensive response. Arteriolar and venular tone are decreased, so that both afterload and preload are reduced and venous pooling may occur. These changes are frequently associated with a compensatory tachycardia, the pulse rate may increase by 20% and the cardiac output is variably affected. Although the tachycardia may be controlled by β-adrenoceptor antagonists (e.g. with propranolol), this may result in a fall in cardiac output and the occurrence of bronchospasm in susceptible patients. The administration of trimetaphan is unlikely to lead to a fall in cerebral blood flow unless the mean arterial blood pressure falls below 60 mmHg; however, renal and splanchnic perfusion are usually decreased. Trimetaphan does not cross the blood–brain barrier.

The use of trimetaphan may be associated with several problems:

1 The effects of the drug are often unpredictable. It may cause a dramatic fall in blood pressure in susceptible patients. Conversely, continued infusion of trimetaphan may lead to the occurrence of tachyphylaxis or acute tolerance with a diminution in response to the drug. This may be partially related to the compensatory tachycardia or to increased neurotransmitter release.

2 Trimetaphan can cause the release of histamine from mast cells and produce local oedema, bronchospasm and an accentuated fall in blood pressure. Histamine release may also account for a delay in the return of the blood pressure to normal values which sometimes occurs after the infusion is stopped.

3 Trimetaphan causes pupillary dilatation which may persist and thus complicate observations during recovery from anaesthesia.

4 Postoperative complications such as paralytic ileus and urinary retention may result from the autonomic blockade.

5 Trimetaphan may potentiate and thus prolong the effects of non-depolarizing neuromuscular blocking agents and produce variable responses to reversal by anticholinesterases. Although trimetaphan is not an ester, it may be broken down by plasma cholinesterase and can enhance the effects of suxamethonium. The use of trimetaphan is contraindicated in patients with genetic variants in plasma cholinesterase or in the presence of liver disease and other drugs which may inhibit the enzyme.

Sodium nitroprusside

Sodium nitroprusside (SNP) was first shown to reduce blood pressure in 1929. Over 30 years elapsed before it was used in anaesthetic practice to provide controlled hypotension. SNP causes arteriolar and venular dilatation by a direct action on the blood vessels. This results in a fall in peripheral resistance and an increase in venous capacitance with a reduction in blood pressure which is not posture-dependent. SNP has little or no direct effect on cardiac function, although reflex tachycardia may occur following its administration. Renal blood flow is usually unaltered, but the effects of SNP on the cerebral circulation are complex and controversial. There has been some concern that the drug may increase cerebral blood flow and intracranial pressure and that autoregulation of the cerebral circulation may be impaired. A fall in arterial oxygen tension may also occur.

However, studies incorporating a cerebral function monitor have indicated that cerebral activity is depressed at a higher mean arterial pressure with trimetaphan than with sodium nitroprusside and that brain surface oxygen tension is greater with SNP than with trimetaphan. Recent animal investigations, involving radiolabelled techniques during profound hypotension, suggest that cerebral blood flow is significantly less compromised by nitroprusside than by trimetaphan or by hypotension induced by haemorrhage.

The mechanism of the hypotensive action is probably similar to that of the organic nitrates and is mediated by the nitroso group (—N=O) contained in the drug. Nitroso-thiol derivatives which are formed stimulate guanylyl cyclase, increasing cGMP levels and producing relaxation of vascular smooth muscle.

SNP must be given parenterally. It has a rapid onset and a short duration of action and is an extremely potent and toxic drug. SNP is normally administered as a 0.01% solution in 5% dextrose or normal saline. It is available as crystals (50 mg per ampoule); the solution, which should be freshly prepared, has a faint orange-brownish tint. When exposed to light, SNP is broken down to cyanide ions and other derivatives; solutions become dark brown or blue and must then be discarded. The infusion solution should be protected by wrapping the container in aluminium foil or other opaque material. SNP is normally infused until a mean arterial pressure of 50–60 mmHg (6.7–8.0 kPa) is reached. It is suggested that the dose used to provide controlled hypotension during anaesthesia should not normally exceed 1.5 $\mu g\ kg^{-1}\ min^{-1}$.

The brief duration of action of SNP is due to its rapid breakdown. Initially cyanide ions are produced, but under the influence of the enzyme rhodanase and in the presence of thiosulphate (which provides sulphydryl groups) cyanide is converted into thiocyanate which is excreted by the kidney (an enzyme present in erythrocytes, thiocyanate oxidase, is present in erythrocytes and may reconvert thiocyanate to cyanide). An alternative pathway for removal of cyanide ions is by combination with hydroxocobalamin to form cyanocobalamin.

Cyanide may accumulate when high rates of infusion are employed or when elimination is impaired. Cyanide toxicity inhibits cellular oxidative processes; the resultant metabolic acidosis may be manifested by sweating, hyperventilation, cardiac arrhythmias and an accentuated fall in blood pressure. The appearance of toxic effects is sometimes delayed until 1–3 h after the administration of SNP.

If the diagnosis of cyanide intoxication is clearly established, the infusion should be stopped immediately and an antidote (either sodium thiosulphate to promote conversion to thiocyanate or dicobalt edetate which chelates cyanide ions) given by intravenous injection. The administration of nitrites (e.g. intravenous sodium nitrite or amyl nitrite by inhalation) is also valuable; they induce the formation of methaemoglobin which has a greater affinity for cyanide than the cellular cytochrome oxidases. Calcium salts may help to restore the blood pressure. Hydroxocobalamin is sometimes given prophylactically to provide another route for the removal of cyanide. Conversely the use of SNP should be avoided in patients with disorders of vitamin B_{12} metabolism. Thiocyanate inhibits the uptake of iodide by the thyroid gland; thus SNP is contraindicated in hypothyroid states or in renal failure, when this potentially toxic metabolite can accumulate. Sodium nitroprusside and trimetaphan have been used in combination to provide the best features of both agents and a 1 : 5 mixture appears to provide hypotension with little change in heart rate.

Glyceryl trinitrate

Glyceryl trinitrate (nitroglycerine) can be used to enhance or induce controlled hypotension. This agent causes peripheral vasodilatation by a direct action on vascular smooth muscle. In contrast to SNP, there appears to be a more selective effect on capacitance vessels. Thus venular tone and preload are decreased to a greater extent than arterial tone and afterload; in consequence, the hypotensive action of glyceryl trinitrate is highly susceptible to alterations in posture. Furthermore, glyceryl trinitrate is less likely to induce direct effects on cerebral blood flow than SNP.

Glyceryl trinitrate is normally diluted prior to use, with either normal saline or isotonic dextrose, to produce a 0.01% solution. Loss of activity may occur if glyceryl trinitrate is prepared in packs or bags composed of polyvinyl chloride. The resulting solution is normally infused using a dose range between 10 and 200 μg min^{-1} until the desired level of blood pressure is achieved. The onset of action is usually within 2–3 min, because of rapid formation of the active free radical nitric oxide, and tolerance to the effects of the drug (Chapter 6) is not usually a problem with short-term use.

By virtue of the effects of glyceryl trinitrate (principally on preload), left ventricular end-diastolic pressure and myocardial wall tension are reduced and there is a resultant decrease in myocardial oxygen demand. Glyceryl trinitrate can be administered by a number of routes (sublingual, buccal, percutaneous) in the management of anginal attacks and may also be given by intravenous infusion in the treatment of unstable angina, the management of congestive cardiac failure following myocardial infarction or to control myocardial ischaemia during and after cardiovascular surgery.

Labetalol has occasionally been used to facilitate controlled hypotension during surgery. This drug is discussed more fully with the β-adrenoceptor antagonists.

The use of methods employing deliberate hypotension has undoubtedly declined during the past few years. Improvements in both anaesthetic and surgical techniques and the judicious use of local vasoconstrictor solutions have clearly contributed to this change in practice. Furthermore, the loss of autoregulation and cerebral blood flow associated with profound hypotension and the problems associated with intraoperative haemorrhage or rebound hypertension in the postoperative period have tended to preclude its use. At one time the use of ganglion-blocking agents in association with spontaneous ventilation was commonly employed. In this instance hypercarbia due to respiratory depression from general anaesthetic agents may be accentuated by changes in the ventilation/perfusion ratio due to peripheral pooling, and this technique is now rarely employed.

Induced hypotension is a useful adjunct to middle-ear surgery. Lowering the level to a mean arterial pressure of 50–55 mmHg in otherwise healthy patients appears to be safe and produces no effects on psychomotor function. Induced hypotension appears to be of particular value in reducing the morbidity associated with the removal of cerebral vascular tumours and intracranial arteriovenous malformations; however, in the case of cerebral aneurysms where cerebral vasospasm is a common complication, hypotension may further compromise the cerebral oxygen supply by reducing collateral circulation.

SNP impairs cerebral blood flow to a lesser extent than trimetaphan and would appear to be the drug of choice when brief periods of profound hypotension are required. In this context halothane, which may have detrimental effects on cerebral metabolic rate, should also be avoided; halogenated ethers either have no effect on, or reduce, metabolic requirements.

Induced hypotension is probably best avoided in hypovolaemic states, cardiovascular, hepatic and renal diseases and during pregnancy. In the presence of raised intracranial pressure, cerebral perfusion may be further compromised and deliberate hypotension should not be employed unless the dura is open or intracranial pressure monitoring facilities are available. Hypocarbia, by its effects on cerebral blood flow, may further increase the risk of complications. When such techniques are used, meticulous attention to detail, with accurate drug administration (when possible by means of an infusion pump) and the continuous intra-arterial monitoring of blood pressure are essential.

Further reading

Aitken D. Cyanide toxicity following nitroprusside induced hypotension. *Canadian Anaesthetists Society Journal* 1977; **24**: 651–660.

Alderman MH. Non-pharmacological treatment of hypertension. *Lancet* 1994; **344**: 307–311.

Alper MH, Flacke W, Krayer O. Pharmacology of reserpine and its implications for anaesthesia. *Anaesthesiology* 1963; **24**: 524–542.

Ames RP. The effects of antihypertensive drugs on serum lipids and lipoproteins. II Non-diuretic drugs. *Drugs* 1986; **32**: 335–357.

Andrews G, MacMahon SW, Austin A, Byrne DG. Hypertension: comparison of drug and non drug-treatments. *British Medical Journal (Clinical Research)* 1982; **284**: 1523–1526.

Antonaccio MJ. Angiotensin-converting-enzyme (ACE) inhibitors. *Annual Review of Pharmacology and Toxicology* 1982; **27**: 57–87.

Bagnall WE, Salway JG, Jackson EW. Phaeochromocytoma with myocarditis managed with α-methyl-*p*-tyrosine. *Postgraduate Medical Journal* 1976; **52**: 653–656.

Barlow RB, Ing HR. Curare-like action of polymethylene bis-quaternary ammonium salts. *British Journal of Pharmacology and Chemotherapy* 1948; **3**: 298–304.

Bloor BC, Flacke WE. Reduction in halothane anaesthetic requirement by clonidine, an alpha-adrenergic agonist. *Anesthesia and Analgesia* 1982; **61**: 741–745.

Braunwald E. Mechanism of action of calcium-channel blocking agents. *New England Journal of Medicine* 1982; **307**: 1618–1627.

Chestnut JS, Albin NS, Gonzalez-Aboda E *et al.* Clinical evaluation of intravenous nitroglycerine for neurosurgery. *Journal of Neurosurgery* 1978; **48**: 704–711.

Clive DM, Stoff JS. Renal symptoms associated with non-steroidal anti-inflammatory drugs. *New England Journal of Medicine* 1984; **310**: 563–572.

Conolly ME, Briant RH, George CF, Dollery CT. A crossover comparison of clonidine and methyldopa in hypertension. *European Journal of Clinical Pharmacology* 1972; **4**: 222–227.

Crandell D Le R. The anesthetic hazards in patients on antihypertensive therapy. *Journal of the American Medical Association* 1962; **179**: 495–500.

Deacock AR de C, Hargrove RL. The influence of certain ganglionic blocking agents on neuromuscular transmission. *British Journal of Anaesthesia* 1962; **34**: 357–362.

Enderby GEH. A report on the mortality and morbidity following 9107 hypotensive anaesthetics. *British Journal of Anaesthesia* 1961; **33**: 109–113.

Feneck R. Cardiovascular function and the safety of anaesthesia. In: Taylor TH, Major E (eds) *Hazards and Complications of Anaesthesia*. Edinburgh: Churchill Livingstone, 1987; 11–32.

Folkow B. The haemodynamic consequence of adaptive structural changes of the resistance vessels in hypertension. *Clinical Science* 1971; **41**: 1–7.

Fries ED, Rose JC, Riggins TF *et al.* The haemodynamic effects of hypotensive drugs in man IV. I-Hydrazinophthalazine. *Circulation* 1953; **8**: 188–204.

Fujibyashi T, Sugiura Y, Yanagimoto M *et al.* Brain energy metabolism and blood flow during sevoflurane and halothane anaesthesia: effects of hypocapnoea and blood pressure fluctuations. *Acta Anaesthesiologica Scandinavica* 1994; **38**: 413–418.

Garcia JY Jr, Vidt DG. Current management of hypertensive emergencies. *Drugs* 1987; **34**: 263–278.

Goldberg LI. Current therapy of hypertension — a pharmacological approach. *American Journal of Medicine* 1974; **58**: 489–494.

Goldman L, Caldera DL. Risks of general anaesthesia and elective operation in the hypertensive patient. *Anaesthesiology* 1979; **50**: 285–292.

Gorczynski RJ. Basic pharmacology of esmolol. *American Journal of Cardiology* 1985; **56**: 3F–13F.

Graham RM, Thornell IR, Gain JM *et al.* Prazosin: the first-dose phenomenon. *British Medical Journal* 1976; **2**: 1293–1294.

Hannington-Kiff JG. Intravenous regional sympathetic block with guanethidine. *Lancet* 1974; **i**: 1019–1020.

Heise A, Kroneberg G. Central nervous alpha-adrenergic receptors and the mode of action of α-methyldopa. *Archives of Pharmacology* 1973; **279**: 285–300.

Hellewell J, Potts MW. Propranolol during controlled hypotension. *British Journal of Anaesthesia* 1966; **38**: 794–801.

Janssen PAJ. 5-HT_2 receptor blockade to study serotonin-induced pathology. *Trends in Pharmacological Sciences* 1983; **5**: 198–206.

Johnston CI. Angiotensin receptor antagonists: focus on losartan. *Lancet* 1995; **346**: 1403–1407.

Johnston CI, Arnolde L, Hiwatari M. Angiotensin-converting inhibitors in the treatment of hypertension. *Drugs* 1984; **27**: 271–277.

Lang RE, Unger T, Ganten D. Atrial natriuretic factor: a new factor in blood pressure control. *Journal of Hypertension* 1987; **5**: 255–271.

Larson AG. Deliberate hypotension. *Anaesthesiology* 1964; **25**: 682–706.

Leigh JM. The history of controlled hypotension. *British Journal of Anaesthesia* 1975; **47**: 745–749.

Low J, Harvey J, Prys-Roberts C, Dagnino J. Studies of anaesthesia in relation to hypertension. *British Journal of Anaesthesia* 1986; **58**: 471–477.

McDowall DG. Induced hypotension and brain ischaemia. *British Journal of Anaesthesia* 1985; **57**: 110–119.

Mehta J, Cohn JN. Haemodynamic effects of labetalol, an alpha and beta adrenergic blocking agent, in hypertensive subjects. *Circulation* 1977; **55**: 370–375.

Moss E. Cerebral blood flow during induced hypotension. *British Journal of Anaesthesia* 1994; **74**: 635–637.

Murphy MB, Scriven AJI, Dollery CT. Role of nifedipine in the treatment of hypertension. *British Medical Journal (Clinical Research)* 1983; **287**: 257–259.

Murthy VS, Patel KD, Elangovar RG *et al.* Cardiovascular and neuromuscular effects of esmolol during general anaesthesia. *Journal of Clinical Pharmacology* 1986; **26**: 351–357.

Nakawaza K, Taneyama C, Benson KT *et al.* Mixtures of sodium nitroprusside and trimetaphan for induction of hypotension. *Anesthesia and Analgesia* 1991; **73**: 59–63.

O'Shea PJ. Induced hypotension. In: Taylor TH, Major E (eds) *Hazards and Complications of Anaesthesia* 2nd edn. Edinburgh: Churchill Livingstone, 1993; 527–534.

Paton WDM, Zaimis E. The methonium compounds. *Pharmacological Reviews* 1952; **4**: 219–253.

Peach MJ. Renin–angiotensin system; biochemistry and mechanisms of action. *Physiological Reviews* 1977; **57**: 313–370.

Pickering TG. Blood pressure measurement and detection of hypertension. *Lancet* 1994; **344**: 31–35.

Prichard BNC. Beta-adrenergic receptor blockade in hypertension; past present and future. *British Journal of Clinical Pharmacology* 1978; **5**: 379–399.

Prys-Roberts C, Green LT, Meloche R, Foex P. Studies of anaesthesia in relation to hypertension; II Haemodynamic consequences of induction and endotracheal intubation. *British Journal of Anaesthesia* 1971; **43**: 531–547.

Regoli D, Park WK, Rioux F. Pharmacology of angiotensin. *Pharmacological Reviews* 1974; **26**: 69–123.

Robertson D, Nies AS. Antihypertensive drugs. In: Turner P, Shand DG (eds) *Recent Advances in Clinical Pharmacology* no. 1. Edinburgh: Churchill Livingstone, 1978; 55–92.

Rogers MC, Troystman RJ. Cerebral haemodynamic effects of nitroglycerine and nitroprusside. *Anaesthesiology* 1979; **51**: 199S.

Salem MR. Therapeutic uses of ganglion blocking drugs. *International Anaesthesiology Clinics* 1978; **16**: 171–200.

Sever P, Beevers G, Bulpitt C *et al.* Management guidelines in essential hypertension: report of the Second Working Party of the British Hypertension Society. *British Medical Journal* 1993; **306**: 983–987.

Stamler J, Stamler R. Intervention for the prevention and control of hypertension and arteriosclerotic disease: United States and international experience. *American Journal of Medicine* 1984; **77** (suppl. 12): 13–36.

Stanaszek WF, Kellerman D, Brogden RN, Romankiewitz JA. Prazosin update; a review of its pharmacological properties and therapeutic use in hypertension. *Drugs* 1983; **25**: 339–384.

Tamsen A, Gordh TE. Epidural clonidine produces analgesia. *Lancet* 1984; **ii**: 231–232.

Tinker JH, Michenfelder JD. SNP: pharmacology, toxicology and therapeutics. *Anaesthesiology* 1976; **45**: 340–354.

Tobian L. Why do thiazide diuretics lower blood pressure in essential hypertension? *Annual Review of Pharmacology* 1967; **7**: 399–408.

Turlapaty P, Laddu A, Murthy VS *et al.* Esmolol: a titratable short-acting intravenous beta blocker for acute critical care settings. *American Heart Journal* 1987; **114**: 866–885.

Vanhoutte PM, Auch-Schwelk W, Biondi ML *et al.* Why are converting enzyme inhibitors vasodilators? *British Journal of Clinical Pharmacology* 1989; **28**: 95S–104S.

Vesey CJ, Cole PV, Linnell JC, Wilson J. Some metabolic effects of sodium nitroprusside in man. *British Medical Journal* 1974; **2**: 140–142.

Webb DJ, Benjamin N, Allen MJ *et al.* Vascular responses to local atrial natriuretic peptide infusion in man. *British Journal of Clinical Pharmacology* 1988; **26**: 245–252.

Wilson AL, Matzke GR. The treatment of hypertension in pregnancy. *Drug Intelligence and Clinical Pharmacy* 1981; **15**: 21–26.

Wolf RL, Mendslowitz M, Fruchter A. Diagnosis and treatment of phaeochromocytoma. *Mount Sinai Journal of Medicine NY* 1970; **37**: 549–567.

Chapter 15
Antiarrhythmic and Antianginal Drugs

Antiarrhythmic drugs

Cardiac arrhythmias may be defined as irregular or abnormal heart rhythms. By convention, they also include bradycardias or tachycardias outside the physiological range (i.e. 55–90 beats min^{-1} in adults). Arrhythmias may be present before surgery, and are commonly seen in patients admitted to intensive care units. During anaesthesia, they may be precipitated by surgical stimuli, or by physiological and pharmacological factors. In all these circumstances, the use of antiarrhythmic drugs may be necessary to control cardiac irregularities or maintain cardiac output.

Electrophysiology of normal cardiac muscle

The understanding of the mode of action of antiarrhythmic drugs is dependent on an appreciation of cardiac electrophysiology, and the manner in which this is modified by disease. During recent years, microelectrode studies on single muscle fibres in the heart have clarified these concepts. The heart contains:

1 Conducting pathways (i.e. the sinoatrial (SA) node, the internodal tracts, the atrioventricular (AV) node, the bundle of His and the Purkinje network) which initiate or preferentially conduct cardiac impulses.

2 Contractile cells (atrial and ventricular muscle fibres) which respond to these impulses by depolarization, resulting in muscle contraction.

There are important structural differences between conducting tissues and contractile muscle fibres; these are paralleled by electrophysiological differences that are responsible for the sequential conduction of the cardiac impulse. Conducting pathways consist of elongated, delicate fusiform cells which are usually embedded in dense connective tissue; they contain relatively few myofibrils and are only faintly striated. In contrast, typical cardiac muscle cells contain numerous myofibrils, which are responsible for the prominent striations seen on light microscopy. The myofibrils consist of filaments of myosin and actin, which interact when the intracellular calcium concentration increases above the resting level (excitation–contraction coupling). Each muscle cell is partly divided at numerous sites by the transverse (T) tubular system. The sarcolemmal membrane contains numerous ion channels which regulate the concentration of potassium, sodium and calcium ions in the cytoplasm, and thus control the gradient across the cell membrane. Cardiac muscle fibres form a syncytium; the cells branch frequently and are separated from each other by intercalated discs.

During inactivity, the inside of all conducting tissues and cardiac muscle fibres is electrically negative compared to the outside, i.e. there is a potential difference across the cell membrane (the resting membrane potential). As in all other excitable tissues, the potential difference reflects the balance between two opposing forces; these are first, the tendency of potassium ions to diffuse from cells along selectively permeable potassium channels, and second, the attraction of potassium ions for negatively charged phosphate groups on intracellular proteins. The resting membrane potential represents the balance between these forces, i.e. it is a potassium diffusion potential. In conducting tissues and cardiac muscle fibres, the resting membrane potential is approximately –60 to –80 mV.

In the SA node (and to a lesser extent in the AV node and Purkinje tissue) the changes in electrical potential during the cardiac cycle are different from those in atrial and ventricular muscle. The resting membrane potential is unstable, and decreases from approximately –60 to –40 mV during atrial diastole (Fig. 15.1). This change in potential (sometimes known as the prepotential or the pacemaker potential) is probably due to changes in sodium and/or calcium permeability of the cells in the SA node. When the resting potential reaches –40 mV, depolarization occurs; the action potential in the SA node is usually bell-shaped and lasts for 150–200 ms. The action potential in the SA node during each cardiac cycle is mainly due to the slow entry of calcium ions along specific slow calcium channels (L channels) in the cytoplasmic membrane. The slow calcium channels are voltage-dependent and tend to open at a membrane potential of approximately –40 mV. Repolarization is due to closure of slow calcium channels and the unopposed diffusion of potassium ions, which re-establishes the normal resting potential.

In contrast, in atrial and ventricular muscle the resting potential is stable at approximately –80 mV. The changes in electrical potential during the cardiac cycle are usually divided into five phases (Fig. 15.1). During phase 0, the myocardial cell depolarizes from –80 mV to approximately +30 mV, due to the rapid influx of sodium ions (and to a lesser extent, of calcium ions). This phase usually lasts for less than 1 ms. In phase 1, the amplitude of the action potential transiently decreases as the fast sodium channels are inactivated, and chloride ions are passively extruded. During phase 2 (the plateau phase), the action potential is maintained between 0 and –20 mV, mainly due to the slow influx of calcium ions along voltage-dependent L channels. This phase usually lasts for 100–150 ms. In phase 3 (repolarization), the action potential rapidly returns to its resting value of –80 mV (Fig. 15.1), due to calcium-channel inactivation and the efflux of intracellular potassium ions through specific ion channels. In phase 4, the potential is maintained at a value of approximately –80 mV, since atrial and ventricular muscle fibres are effectively impermeable to sodium and calcium ions during diastole. During phase 4, the ionic movements across the myocardial membrane are reversed due to the activity

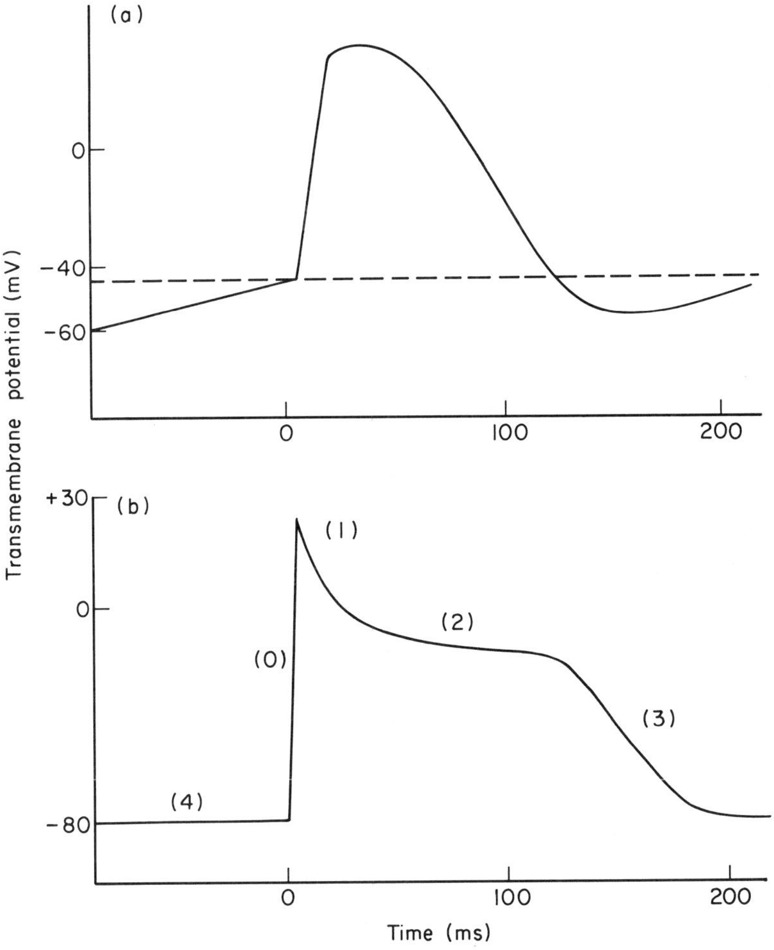

Fig. 15.1 Characteristic transmembrane potentials in (a) the sinoatrial (SA) node and (b) ventricular muscle. Figures in parentheses correspond to the five phases of the action potential in cardiac muscle fibres. The events shown in (a) and (b) are not intended to be simultaneous or synchronous.

of the ion pump (Na^+/K^+ ATPase), which exchanges three sodium ions for two potassium ions, resulting in a negative intracellular potential.

These electrophysiological differences between the SA node and ventricular muscle are reflected in other conducting tissues. Thus, the action potential of the AV node and the His–Purkinje system have characteristics that are intermediate between those of the SA node and normal ventricular muscle. The duration of the cardiac action potential (i.e. the beginning of phase 1 to the end of phase 3) is shorter in the bundle of His and ventricular muscle (150–200 ms) than in the terminal Purkinje fibres (250–300 ms). It is approximately equal in duration to the refractory period; this is the time after excitation during which cardiac muscle cells will not respond to a second stimulus. In myocardial cells, the refractory period is almost as long as the contractile response. In consequence, cardiac muscle (unlike skeletal muscle) cannot be tetanized (i.e. it will not rapidly respond to repeated electrical stimulation so that summation of the mechanical response occurs).

The origin and propagation of the cardiac impulse can be interpreted in terms of the electrophysiological differences between conducting tissues and contractile myocardial cells. The diastolic membrane potential reaches its threshold value in the SA node earlier than in other cardiac tissues (Fig. 15.1). Consequently, the SA node is depolarized sooner than other cells, and therefore initiates the cardiac impulse. Excitation is propagated over the right atrium by means of the internodal tracts, which are preferentially depolarized before atrial muscle cells. Similarly, the AV node and the His–Purkinje system are normally depolarized before ventricular muscle, since their threshold potential is closer to the resting value.

Physiology of cardiac arrhythmias

The occurrence of tachycardia and some tachyarrhythmias may be related to enhanced pacemaker activity or automaticity (i.e. to an increase in the rate of diastolic depolarization in the SA node). Alternatively, they may be due to the presence of an ectopic focus. When there is marked bradycardia or SA block, the cardiac impulse may be initiated by other junctional tissues (e.g. the AV node, the bundle or His or the His–Purkinje system). These cardiac impulses are known as escape beats; they may be induced by excessive vagal tone, and are responsible for the phenomenon of vagal escape. They are also commonly seen during halothane anaesthesia, which is frequently associated with sinus bradycardia and AV junctional escape rhythms (Chapter 8).

Cardiac arrhythmias that originate in ectopic foci may also be due to abnormal physiological mechanisms that are related to pathological changes in cardiac muscle. This type of arrhythmia may originate in the AV node, the His–Purkinje system or in atrial or ventricular muscle. In general, they are related to three different phenomena. These are:

1 Enhanced automaticity in conducting tissues or myocardial cells.
2 Re-entry or reciprocating mechanisms in abnormal cardiac cells.
3 The occurrence of pathological after-potentials.

These phenomena are believed to be concerned in the production of many tachyarrhythmias, e.g. atrial flutter, atrial fibrillation, ventricular extrasystoles, ventricular tachycardia and supraventricular tachycardias (including the Wolff–Parkinson–White syndrome).

Enhanced automaticity

Pathological damage to conducting tissues or myocardial cells may cause the development of an unstable membrane potential, resulting in spontaneous depolarization during diastole. Damaged myocardial cells may be slightly permeable to sodium ions during diastole (i.e. during phase 4 of the action potential). In consequence, their membrane potential may decrease (i.e. become less electronegative) during phase 4, and reach the threshold for depolarization before the cells of the SA node. Thus, ischaemia may produce pathological changes in myocardial muscle cells, and cause them to assume the electrical characteristics of pacemaker cells. Similar changes may be produced by hypokalaemia, which tends to cause an unstable resting membrane potential during phase 4. These conditions will favour the development of an ectopic focus in atrial or ventricular muscle (or in conducting tissues).

Re-entry and reciprocating mechanisms

Re-entry and reciprocating mechanisms usually arise in anatomical sites that possess the opportunity for differential rates of conduction along alternative pathways. These are particularly likely to occur when impulses can pass down alternative pathways with different conduction times and refractory periods, and when impulses can be blocked. These pathways may be present in the AV node and in terminal Purkinje fibres, as well as in damaged atrial and ventricular muscle. Terminal Purkinje fibres frequently branch as they approach the myocardium, so that a single cardiac muscle fibre can be innervated by more than one terminal (Fig. 15.2). If there is no delay in conduction, impulses can pass down both terminal arborizations and are extinguished in the muscle fibre. By contrast, if one of these terminals has a longer refractory period than the other (due to physiological or pathological causes),

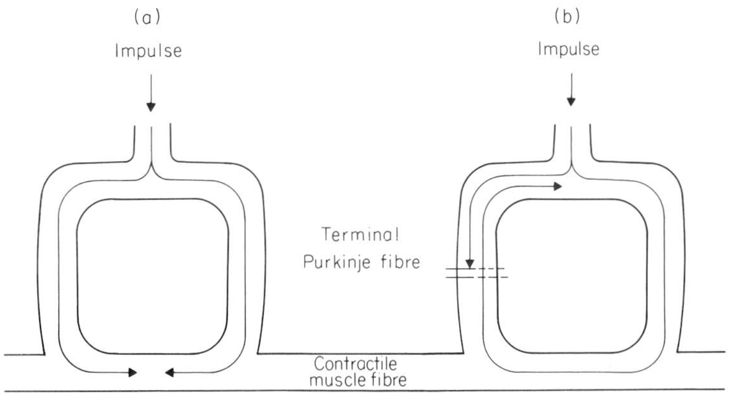

Fig. 15.2 The probable mechanism for the establishment of re-entrant arrythmias. (a) The impulse is conducted along two alternative pathways with normal conduction times in the terminal arborization of the Purkinje system. Normal conduction occurs down both pathways and the impulse is extinguished in the contractile muscle fibre. (b) One of the terminal branches has a prolonged conduction time and refractory period. If this branch is refractory on the arrival of the impulse, conduction only occurs down the opposite terminal. The impulse is not extinguished in the muscle fibre, and can approach the previously refractory arborization in a retrograde manner. If this branch has recovered, retrograde conduction of the impulse continues, followed by anterograde conduction in the opposite branch. In this manner, an ectopic focus is set up.

conduction may only occur down one branch, since the other may still be refractory. The impulse is not extinguished in the muscle fibre and can approach the previously refractory arborization in a retrograde manner. If this branch has recovered, retrograde conduction of the impulse occurs, followed by anterograde conduction in the contralateral limb (Fig. 15.2). A reciprocal rhythm is set up due to re-entry of the impulse; this phenomenon is probably responsible for many common atrial and ventricular arrhythmias.

Pathological after-potentials

Pathological changes in ischaemic myocardium may cause the generation of spontaneous after-potentials after the action potential. These changes may be related to entry of calcium or sodium ions along ion-specific channels.

Classification of antiarrhythmic drugs

In atrial flutter and atrial fibrillation, treatment is usually directed towards a reduction in the rate of ventricular response by the suppression of AV conduction. In most other arrhythmias, the aim of antiarrhythmic treatment is the restoration of sinus rhythm, either by decreasing the enhanced automaticity of ectopic foci, or by interruption (dissociation) of the process of re-entry. Drugs that produce these effects are usually divided into four groups, depending on their electrophysiological and ionic effects on cardiac muscle (Table 15.1). Consequently, antiarrhythmic drugs may act by:

Table 15.1 The antiarrhythmic activity of some common drugs.

	Antiarrhythmic activity			
Drug	Sodium-channel blockade (class 1)	β-Adrenoceptor antagonism (class 2)	Potassium-channel blockade (class 3)	Calcium-channel blockade (class 4)
Lignocaine	+			
Mexiletine	+			
Atenolol		+		
Propranolol	+	+		
Sotalol	+	+	+	
Verapamil				+
Adenosine				
Digoxin				
Disopyramide	+		+	
Flecainide	+			
Amiodarone			+	
Propafenone	+		+	

1. Sodium-channel blockade (class 1 antiarrhythmic activity).
2. β-Adrenoceptor blockade (class 2 antiarrhythmic activity).
3. Potassium-channel blockade (class 3 antiarrhythmic activity).
4. Calcium-channel blockade (class 4 antiarrhythmic activity).

Sodium-channel blockade (class 1 activity)

Some antiarrhythmic drugs reduce the entry of sodium ions into cardiac muscle fibres during depolarization, and thus decrease the maximum rate of rise of phase 0 of the action potential. Drugs that block sodium channels often affect other excitable tissues, and may have local anaesthetic and membrane-stabilizing activity.

They can be divided into three groups, depending on their effect on the refractory period of cardiac muscle. Class 1a drugs (e.g. quinidine, procainamide) increase the refractory period; class 1b drugs (e.g. lignocaine, mexilitine) reduce the refractory period; class 1c drugs (e.g. flecainide) do not affect the duration of the refractory period. The effects of class 1a and class 1b drugs on the duration of the refractory period are probably due to their action on the phase of repolarization (phase 3 of the cardiac action potential). Class 1a and 1b drugs also presumably modify calcium entry and/or potassium loss, affecting the duration of the action potential and the refractory period in opposite ways.

These drugs modify arrhythmias that are due to enhanced automaticity or to re-entry mechanisms. When cardiac arrhythmias are due to enhanced automaticity, class 1 drugs reduce the entry of sodium ions into cardiac cells, and reduce the rate of diastolic depolarization in abnormal ectopic foci. In these conditions, the diastolic potential in the ectopic focus reaches the threshold for depolarization less rapidly, and this may allow the SA node to reassume its normal role as a pacemaker. Some drugs with class 1 activity may also raise the threshold for depolarization. When cardiac arrhythmias are due to re-entry, drugs with class 1a activity may increase the refractory period of the pathway that is responsible for re-entry; this may prevent retrograde conduction of the impulse (Fig. 15.2) and produce bidirectional (rather than unidirectional) block in the pathway concerned. Conversely, drugs with class 1b activity may prevent the occurrence of unidirectional block and restore normal conduction, since they reduce the refractory period of cardiac muscle fibres.

β-Adrenoceptor blockade (class 2 activity)

Drugs that produce β-adrenoceptor blockade prevent the release or antagonize the effects of endogenous catecholamines on the heart. They may affect the terminal postganglionic sympathetic neurone and prevent the release of noradrenaline; alternatively, they may produce postsynaptic β-adrenoceptor blockade and protect the heart from circulating adrenaline, as well as the β-effects of locally released noradrenaline. β-Adrenoceptor agonists (e.g. adrenaline) increase the rate of diastolic depolarization (i.e. the slope of phase 4 of the action potential) in the SA node and conducting tissue, and increase the slow inward calcium current. Consequently, β-adrenoceptor antagonists slow the rate of diastolic depolarization and decrease inward movement of calcium ions. They produce their antiarrhythmic effects by slowing the sinus rate, inhibiting the automaticity of the conducting system during diastolic depolarization, and prolonging the effective refractory period of the AV node. β-Adrenoceptor antagonists are most useful in the management of arrhythmias produced by endogenous or administered catecholamines. Many β-adrenoceptor antagonists also produce sodium-channel blockade at high dose levels (sometimes known as local anaesthetic or membrane-stabilizing activity; Table 15.1).

Potassium-channel blockade (class 3 activity)

Some antiarrhythmic drugs prolong the duration of the action potential in both conducting tissues and in cardiac muscle fibres. Many of these drugs prolong the phase of repolarization (phase 3 of the cardiac action potential) by decreasing the rate of potassium loss through ion-specific channels (i.e. potassium-channel blockade) or by modifying the rate of calcium entry. This effect is most marked in the bundle of His, anomalous AV conduction pathways, and in atrial and ventricular muscle. Some drugs that prolong the action potential also antagonize the effects of catecholamines (e.g. sotalol) or modify the ionic changes responsible for the generation of the action potential (e.g. disopyramide). Nevertheless, these drugs primarily increase the duration of the action potential and consequently prolong the refractory period of the His–Purkinje system and cardiac muscle. Ectopic foci due to enhanced automaticity in atrial and ventricular muscle are suppressed; in addition, these drugs tend to interrupt reciprocal rhythms that are due to re-entry by preventing retrograde conduction in pathways with a prolonged refractory period. Antiarrhythmic agents that prolong the action potential may be of value in the management of patients with supraventricular tachyarrhythmias, or of arrhythmias associated with anomalous conduction pathways (e.g. the Wolff–Parkinson–White syndrome or the Lown–Ganong–Levine syndrome). In these conditions, high dosage may induce torsade de pointes (prolongation of the QT interval followed by episodes of ventricular tachycardia).

Calcium-channel blockade (class 4 activity)

Calcium antagonists prevent the voltage-dependent entry of calcium ions into cardiac muscle cells during depolarization. Certain cardiac cells (in particular, cells in the SA and the AV node) are almost entirely dependent on the slow inward calcium current for depolarization; calcium antagonists prevent this process and are particularly effective in preventing re-entrant arrhythmias in the AV node (including nodal tachycardia). Calcium ions also play an important part in the excitation of

Table 15.2 The site of action of some common antiarrhythmic drugs.

SA and AV node	Atrium	Ventricle
β-Adrenoceptor antagonists	Disopyramide	Lignocaine
Verapamil	Propafenone	Mexiletine
Adenosine	Amiodarone	Disopyramide
Digoxin		Flecainide
		Propafenone
		Amiodarone

SA, Sino-atrial; AV, atrioventricular.

vascular smooth muscle; consequently, calcium antagonists may decrease vascular tone and induce vasodilatation.

Although the classification of antiarrhythmic drugs by electrophysiological criteria emphasizes the differences between their mechanism of action, it does have certain disadvantages. For instance, it does not correspond to the clinical use of drugs in cardiac arrhythmias, and it does not include certain drugs with antiarrhythmic properties (e.g. digoxin, adenosine or drugs that modify vagal tone). In addition, many drugs possess more than one type of antiarrhythmic activity (Table 15.1). More than 40 drugs with antiarrhythmic properties are currently available in the UK; the site of action of the more commonly used antiarrhythmic drugs is shown in Table 15.2. For clinical purposes, antiarrhythmic drugs can be divided into three groups:

1 Drugs that are primarily used in ventricular arrhythmias (e.g. lignocaine, mexilitine).

2 Drugs that are primarily used in supraventricular arrhythmias (e.g. β-adrenoceptor antagonists, verapamil, adenosine, digoxin, anticholinergic drugs).

3 Drugs that are used in ventricular and supraventricular arrhythmias (e.g. disopyramide, flecainide, amiodarone, propafenone).

Drugs that are primarily used in ventricular arrhythmias

Lignocaine

The amide local anaesthetic lignocaine is widely used in the treatment of ventricular arrhythmias. It produces at least two distinct effects on the action potential in cardiac muscle, which probably account for its antiarrhythmic effects. In the first place, lignocaine prolongs the rise time of phase 0 of the action potential by slowing the entry of sodium ions into cardiac muscle fibres during depolarization. It may also increase the threshold for the depolarization of cardiac muscle cells. These effects reduce physiologically or pathologically enhanced automaticity in ventricular muscle fibres. In addition, lignocaine decreases the duration of the action potential and the refractory period of cardiac muscle, particularly in the preterminal Purkinje fibres. Consequently, lignocaine tends to suppress arrhythmias that are due to re-entry or established reciprocal rhythms. These effects are due to shortened repolarization (phase 3) of the cardiac action potential, and may reflect effects on calcium or potassium channels in the myocardial cell.

In general, therapeutic concentrations of lignocaine do not significantly affect AV conduction. Rarely, the drug may precipitate or exacerbate intraventricular conduction blockade. Moderate doses have little effect on heart rate, blood pressure or myocardial contractility.

Lignocaine is primarily used in the management of ventricular arrhythmias (particularly when induced by myocardial infarction or cardiac surgery). It is of little use in the treatment of atrial arrhythmias. It may produce toxic effects on the central nervous system (CNS) which are usually associated with high plasma concentrations of the drug (Chapter 9). Its safe and effective use in cardiac arrhythmias depends on accurate and controlled administration. The optimal antiarrhythmic effects are usually present at plasma concentrations of 2–4 $\mu g\ ml^{-1}$. These plasma concentrations can usually be produced by a bolus injection of 75–100 mg, followed by a constant infusion of 2–4 mg min^{-1}. After 2 h, a slower rate of infusion (e.g. 1 mg min^{-1}) is preferable. The terminal half-life of lignocaine in patients with normal hepatic and cardiac function usually ranges from 100 to 120 min. Thus, when the drug is infused at a constant rate, cumulation may occur for at least 7 h before a steady state is reached. In the presence of liver disease, cardiac failure or drugs that impair hepatic blood flow, this period may be prolonged.

Mexiletine

Mexiletine is chemically related to lignocaine, and has similar effects on ventricular arrhythmias. It slows the rise time of phase 0 of the cardiac action potential (i.e. it reduces the maximum rate of depolarization) without significantly affecting the resting membrane potential. The duration of the cardiac muscle action potential is slightly reduced, due to the shortening of repolarization (phase 3). Mexiletine (like lignocaine) is mainly used in the prevention and treatment of arrhythmias induced by coronary artery disease and myocardial infarction. It is effective when given orally or intravenously.

Mexiletine is used cautiously in patients with cardiac conduction defects. Its therapeutic ratio is low and the drug commonly causes side-effects. These may affect the CNS or the cardiovascular system. Mexiletine is mainly eliminated by hepatic metabolism; its terminal half-life is usually 10–15 h. Small amounts of the drug (approximately 10% of the dose) are excreted unchanged in urine.

Drugs that are primarily used in supraventricular arrhythmias

β-Adrenoceptor antagonists

β-Adrenoceptor antagonists prevent the diastolic depolarization induced in cardiac cells by catecholamines and produce bradycardia; in addition, they decrease cardiac excitability, prolong AV conduction and reduce myocardial contractility and cardiac output. Most β-adrenoceptor antagonists (with the exception of atenolol and nadolol) have a variable degree of local anaesthetic or membrane-stabilizing activity. In addition, sotalol prolongs repolarization and thus increases the duration of the action potential in cardiac muscle fibres (probably by blockade of potassium channels).

β-Adrenoceptor antagonists are primarily used in the treatment of certain atrial tachyarrhythmias (e.g. paroxysmal supraventricular tachycardia and sinus tachycardia prior to thyroidectomy), and when arrhythmias are due to increased sympathetic activity or increased concentrations of catecholamines. In atrial fibrillation, they may be used with digoxin to suppress a rapid ventricular response. They are also commonly used after myocardial infarction, in order to control arrhythmias and decrease the possibility of a recurrent attack. They should be avoided in patients with incipient or definitive heart block, since they increase the refractory period of the AV node and the bundle of His. They may also precipitate or exacerbate congestive cardiac failure. Their antiarrhythmic activity is mainly due to β-adrenoceptor blockade, since the suppression of ventricular arrhythmias usually occurs at plasma concentrations that are insufficient to produce membrane stabilization.

β-Adrenoceptor antagonists are considered in more detail in Chapter 12.

Verapamil

In the SA and AV nodes, depolarization is almost entirely dependent on the influx of calcium ions from extracellular fluid. Verapamil is a calcium antagonist that prevents calcium ion transport through voltage-sensitive slow channels (L channels) in SA and AV nodal cells; it has less marked effects on myocardial contractile tissue and vascular smooth muscle (Table 15.3). Consequently, the conduction velocity of the cardiac impulse in nodal cells is decreased (and their refractory period is increased). Verapamil can precipitate AV block in patients on other drugs that depress AV conduction (e.g. β-adrenoceptor antagonists, quinidine, procainamide). In addition, verapamil may cause bradycardia and precipitate or intensify cardiac failure. Although the drug has only limited effects on vascular smooth muscle, it may reduce the afterload on the heart and cause hypotension.

Verapamil can be given orally or intravenously; the usual oral dose ranges from 120–360 mg daily, given in divided doses. There may be considerable individual variability in the response to the drug. Although verapamil is well-absorbed after

Table 15.3 The effect of calcium-channel antagonists on the heart and the circulation.

	Heart rate	AV conduction	Myocardial contractility	Peripheral and coronary blood vessels
Phenylalkylamines e.g. verapamil (class 1 antagonists)	Decreased	Prolonged	Decreased	Slight dilatation
Dihydropyridines e.g. nifedipine (class 2 antagonists)	Increased*	Enhanced*	Increased*	Marked dilatation
Benzothiazepines e.g. diltiazem (class 3 antagonists)	Decreased	Prolonged	Slightly decreased	Moderate dilatation

* Mainly due to reflex effects induced by hypotension.
AV, Atrioventricular.

oral administration, it is subject to extensive presystemic metabolism, and its systemic bioavailability is only 20–30%. Verapamil is mainly metabolized by the liver to inactive metabolites, which are eliminated in urine. It is extensively (80–90%) bound to plasma protein, and its terminal half-life is usually 3–7 h.

Verapamil has been mainly used in the treatment of acute and chronic supraventricular tachycardias. In atrial fibrillation and flutter, it slows the ventricular rate and may restore sinus rhythm. Verapamil is not usually effective in ventricular arrhythmias. In addition to its use as an antiarrhythmic drug, verapamil has been used in the treatment of angina, hypertension and cardiomyopathy. Unfortunately, it may cause bradycardia, hypotension and congestive cardiac failure (particularly in patients on β-adrenoceptor antagonists and other drugs which depress AV conduction).

Adenosine

Adenosine is an endogenous nucleoside which consists of a purine base (adenine) linked to a pentose sugar (D-ribose). It is produced during normal metabolic activity by the action of various intracellular enzymes on high-energy phosphates (adenosine monophosphate (AMP), diphosphate (ADP) and triphosphate (ATP)), and is also formed by the conversion of *S*-adenosylhomocysteine to adenosine. Experimental studies indicate that extracellular levels of adenosine are significantly increased during hypoxic and ischaemic episodes. A number of cellular-protective effects are mediated by adenosine receptors; these include vasodilatation, inhibition of calcium flux and the release of excitatory neurotransmitters (e.g. glutamate), potassium-channel activation and an increase in energy production through glucose transport.

Adenosine has negative inotropic effects on the heart, and particularly affects SA automaticity, AV nodal conductivity and anomalous pathways. These effects are mediated by adenosine A_1 receptors (P_1 purinoceptors), which are coupled to G_i proteins; receptor activation produces a decrease in intracellular cAMP. Adenosine is used in the diagnosis and management of supraventricular arrhythmias (including those associated with anomalous pathways), and is given intravenously as a bolus dose (6–12 mg). Its effects are transient, as the plasma half-life of the drug is only 8–10 s. The drug has a number of side-effects (some of which may be mediated by other adenosine receptor subtypes); these include facial flushing, bronchospasm and chest pain. Adenosine, like digoxin, decreases the atrial refractory period and may induce atrial fibrillation or flutter. Severe bradycardia (which required temporary pacing) has also been reported. Concurrent administration of dipyridamole may considerably enhance the effects of adenosine.

ATP has been used during anaesthesia to attenuate the sympathetic responses to laryngoscopy and endotracheal intubation.

Digoxin

Digoxin is one of the most commonly used antiarrhythmic drugs. It is a glycoside derived from the dried leaves of the foxglove (*Digitalis lanata*); its parent glycoside (lanatoside C) is occasionally used as an alternative antiarrhythmic drug. Digoxin consists of a sugar (digitoxose) combined with an aglycone (digitoxigenin). The pharmacological and therapeutic effects of the drug are mainly dependent on the properties of digitoxigenin. Digoxin has little effect on the normal heart; its actions are most evident in patients with atrial flutter or atrial fibrillation.

The effects of digoxin can be divided into: (i) indirect effects, which are mediated by the vagus and antagonized by atropine; and (ii) direct effects, which are due to the inherent action of the drug on cardiac muscle and conducting tissue.

The indirect effects of digoxin cause bradycardia (by slowing the rate of phase 4 depolarization in the SA node), reduce the atrial refractory period and increases the refractory period of the AV node and the bundle of His; these actions are antagonized by atropine.

Digoxin also acts directly on the heart, and increases the refractory period of the AV node and the bundle of His, but decreases the ventricular refractory period. Ventricular excitability and the force of cardiac contraction are also increased (although digoxin does not affect the rate of contraction or the rate of relaxation). Some of the direct effects of digoxin are probably due to inhibition of sodium/potassium-activated adenosine triphosphatase (Na^+/K^+ ATPase), which plays a crucial role in governing the ionic balance in cardiac cells. Enzyme inhibition causes a rise in intracellular sodium; this is followed by sodium/calcium ion exchange (i.e. sodium efflux coupled to calcium influx), which increases the availability of calcium ions in myocardial cells, and increases the excitability and force of contraction.

Digoxin is widely used in the treatment of atrial flutter and fibrillation. In these conditions, numerous impulses impinge on the AV node; a proportion of them are conducted to the His–Purkinje system, resulting in a rapid and irregular ventricular rate. Digoxin (both indirectly and directly) increases the refractory period of the AV node and the bundle of His, and reduces their conductivity. The ventricular rate is decreased, allowing more time for ventricular filling to occur. Digoxin may increase the rate of the atrial arrhythmia, since it reduces the duration of the atrial refractory period.

Digoxin may also be used in the treatment of paroxysmal atrial tachycardia; it slows the heart by increasing vagal tone and may convert the arrhythmia to sinus rhythm. Digoxin should not be given to patients with ventricular extrasystoles or ventricular tachycardia, since it increases cardiac excitability and may precipitate fibrillation.

The use of digoxin in the treatment of chronic heart failure in patients in sinus rhythm has recently been challenged. Although it increases myocardial contractility and cardiac output in the short term, its positive inotropic effects may not be maintained during chronic treatment. In mild and moderate heart failure, diuretics and vasodilators may be more effective than digoxin.

Digoxin has a low therapeutic ratio (i.e. the relation between the therapeutic dose and the toxic dose is reasonably close). The initial effects of digoxin toxicity are often gastrointestinal (i.e. anorexia, nausea, vomiting, abdominal discomfort). Neurological side-effects (headache, fatigue, visual disturbances) occur frequently, and skin rashes and gynaecomastia are occasionally seen.

In addition, digoxin has serious toxic effects on the heart; almost any arrhythmia may be produced and can simulate cardiac disease. The commonest arrhythmias induced by digoxin are ventricular extrasystoles (including coupled beats), ventricular tachycardia and various types of AV block. Atrial arrhythmias are less frequent. Digoxin toxicity may be precipitated by electrolyte abnormalities (i.e. hypokalaemia or hypercalcaemia) or acid–base changes; it is particularly common in elderly subjects, and in patients with poor renal function. Digoxin therapy should be controlled (when possible) by the measurement of the serum concentration of the drug by radioimmunoassay. Serum concentrations of less than 1 ng ml^{-1} are usually ineffective; concentrations greater than 2.5 ng ml^{-1} are commonly associated with toxic effects.

Digoxin or digitoxin overdosage can be treated with digoxin-specific antibody fragments (Digibind). This preparation consists of the F(ab) fragments of immunoglobulin G (IgG) antibodies to digoxin, raised in sheep. The affinity of digoxin for the antibody fragments is more than 10 times greater than its affinity for Na^+/K^+ ATPase; consequently, digoxin is removed from the enzyme and other digoxin receptors and eliminated in urine as a protein-bound complex. Treatment with digoxin-specific antibody fragments is potentially hazardous, and should be restricted to severe and life-threatening cases of digoxin and digitoxin overdosage.

Digoxin is usually administered orally. Patients are commonly digitalized by the administration of 0.75–1.0 mg digoxin daily, until an optimum effect is obtained. Maintenance doses are usually 0.25–0.5 mg in 24 h. Digoxin is usually completely absorbed from the small intestine (as long as drug dissolution is complete). Maximum plasma concentrations are present within 30–60 min (although therapeutic effects are not observed for several hours). The plasma half-life of digoxin is approximately 36 h, and the drug is almost entirely eliminated by glomerular filtration. Consequently, cumulation may occur in elderly subjects or in patients with renal failure. Digoxin has a large volume of distribution (approximately $10\ l\ kg^{-1}$); the concentration of the drug in skeletal or cardiac muscle may be 20–30 times greater than the plasma level.

Anticholinergic agents

Anticholinergic drugs (e.g. atropine, glycopyrrolate) are widely used to prevent or antagonize bradycardia during general anaesthesia. They are considered in detail in Chapter 12.

Drugs that are used in ventricular and supraventricular arrhythmias

Disopyramide

Disopyramide produces blockade of sodium channels, and prolongs the rise time of phase 0 of the cardiac action potential; the threshold potential required to initiate phase 0 may also be increased. In addition, disopyramide increases the duration of the action potential in cardiac muscle fibres by delaying the repolarization of the cardiac action potential; consequently, it prolongs the effective refractory period of conducting tissue, as well as atrial and ventricular muscle. Disopyramide has considerable antimuscarinic (anticholinergic) activity, and may produce atropine-like effects in tissues innervated by the parasympathetic nervous system. Overdosage may cause depression of myocardial contractility, AV block, increased ventricular excitability and cardiac arrest.

Disopyramide is mainly used in the prevention and treatment of ventricular arrhythmias (particularly when they are induced by myocardial infarction, surgical procedures or digoxin overdosage). It is sometimes useful in arrhythmias that do not respond to lignocaine or mexiletine. Disopyramide is occasionally used in supraventricular tachycardia, atrial arrhythmias or in arrhythmias associated with anomalous conducting pathways.

Disopyramide is well-absorbed from the gastrointestinal tract, and can be given by oral or intravenous administration. After intravenous administration, the elimination half-life of disopyramide is 4–6 h; this is increased to 10–12 h in patients with cardiac failure. The drug is mainly eliminated unchanged by the kidney; in renal failure, the half-life of disopyramide is prolonged and the dosage of the drug should be modified.

Flecainide

Flecainide decreases sodium entry into myocardial cells, and prolongs the rise time of phase 0 of the action potential; however, it does not affect the duration of the cardiac action potential or the refractory period. It also affects conduction in all junctional tissues, and thus prolongs intra-atrial, nodal and intraventricular conduction times. In addition, it has negative inotropic effects, and may precipitate cardiac failure in susceptible patients.

Flecainide has been used in the treatment of atrial, junctional and ventricular arrhythmias. There is some evidence that its use is associated with an increased incidence of arrhythmias in patients with symptomless ventricular ectopic beats after myocardial infarction. In these circumstances, its use should probably be avoided. Flecainide may cause minor unwanted effects (e.g. nausea, dizziness, and tremor) in approximately 25% of patients. Its half-life is approximately 14 h, but may be prolonged in the elderly and in renal failure. Approximately 50% of the drug is metabolized by the liver; the remainder is eliminated unchanged in urine.

Amiodarone

Amiodarone produces blockade of potassium channels, and thus increases the duration of the action potential in the conducting system and the myocardium by approximately 20–30%. Repolarization is delayed and the maximum rate of repolarization is decreased. Consequently, the refractory period of the myocardium and the entire conducting system is increased.

Amiodarone is mainly used in arrhythmias associated with anomalous conducting pathways (particularly the Wolff–Parkinson–White syndrome); it is only used in other ventricular and supraventricular arrhythmias when standard drugs are ineffective. It commonly causes mild sinus bradycardia; when used with other drugs that slow the heart (e.g. digoxin, β-adrenoceptor antagonists, halothane), marked bradycardia and a reduction in cardiac output occurs. Amiodarone is an iodinated drug that affects thyroid function, and occasionally causes hypothyroidism. It commonly causes the formation of microdeposits of lipofuscin in the cornea; photosensitivity and pigmentation of the skin may also occur. Amiodarone is extensively bound to plasma protein, and has a relatively long elimination half-life (approximately 28 days). The drug is usually given orally, and may accumulate for some time after administration commences. An antiarrhythmic response usually occurs within 1 week, and may persist for 4–6 weeks after administration is stopped.

Metabolites of amiodarone have not been definitely identified, although the drug is deiodinated in the body.

Propafenone

Propafenone is a recently introduced antiarrhythmic agent which decreases the rate of depolarization of phase 0 of the action potential and slows conduction, particularly in the His–Purkinje system. The duration of the action potential and the effective refractory period is prolonged in atrial and ventricular muscle, as well as in anomalous pathways. Thus, propafenone may be of value in the management of both supraventricular and ventricular arrhythmias.

Propafenone is a chiral compound, and the s(+) enantiomer is a non-selective antagonist at β-adrenoceptors; it also has membrane-stabilizing activity. It has similar side-effects to procainamide, including minor gastrointestinal disorders, anticholinergic effects, drug rashes and occasional hypersensitivity responses; undesirable effects due to β_2-receptor antagonism (e.g. bronchospasm) have also been reported.

Propafenone is metabolized by an isoform of cytochrome P-450 which shows genetic polymorphism (CYP 2D6), and is more slowly metabolized (and may have enhanced effects) in patients with enzyme deficiency. It may also increase the bioavailability of other antiarrhythmic agents, particularly digoxin.

Other antiarrhythmic drugs

Quinidine

Quinidine is an isomer of quinine with more powerful antiarrhythmic effects. It has four main actions in cardiac arrhythmias. In the first place, it prevents sodium entry into myocardial cells, and slows the rise time of phase 0 of the action potential (i.e. it has local anaesthetic effects); second, it increases the threshold potential required for the electrical excitation of myocardial cells. Third, it directly prolongs the refractory period of conducting tissue and myocardial cells (without significantly affecting the duration of the action potential). Finally, it has antimuscarinic effects on the heart and antagonizes the effects of increased vagal tone.

At one time, quinidine was widely used in the management of certain arrhythmias (particularly supraventricular arrhythmias). In recent years, it has largely been replaced by other agents (or by cardioversion using direct current electric shock), since there are several disadvantages associated with its use.

In the first place, quinidine may cause tachycardia in patients with atrial flutter or fibrillation, and can precipitate ventricular arrhythmias. It is dangerous to use quinidine in patients with heart block or with digoxin-induced arrhythmias. Second, the therapeutic ratio of quinidine is relatively low, and the antiarrhythmic dose of the drug (1–3 g in 24 h) is close to the toxic dose. Quinidine may affect the central nervous system or produce various hypersensitivity responses; it may also potentiate the effects of non-depolarizing muscle relaxants.

Quinidine has a large apparent volume of distribution, and its concentration in cardiac and skeletal muscle is greater than the plasma level. It has a relatively short terminal half-life (4–5 h) which is decreased to 2–3 h by enzyme-inducing agents. Approximately 40% of the dose is eliminated unchanged in urine, and drug dosage does not require modification in renal and hepatic failure.

Procainamide

The actions of procainamide are similar to quinidine. Procainamide has four main effects:

1 It decreases the rise time of phase 0 of the action potential.

2 It increases the threshold for electrical activation of cardiac muscle.

3 It increases the refractory period of cardiac cells (with minimal effects on the duration of the action potential).

4 It has antimuscarinic (atropine-like) effects on the heart (although these are usually less marked than the effects of quinidine).

Procainamide is also said to have fewer myocardial depressant effects than quinidine.

Procainamide has been most commonly used in the management of ventricular arrhythmias. When the drug is injected intravenously, it may cause a dramatic fall in blood pressure. Oral administration is sometimes associated with minor gastrointestinal side-effects; occasionally drug rashes and central effects occur. A long-term hazard of chronic oral treatment is the development of antinuclear antibodies and a syndrome similar to systemic lupus erythematosus (SLE). The condition usually improves slowly when drug therapy is stopped.

Procainamide is partly metabolized and partly eliminated unchanged in urine (60%). The drug is slowly hydrolysed by amidases in the liver and in the plasma; it is also acetylated to an active metabolite with antiarrhythmic properties (*N*-acetylprocainamide). The acetylation of procainamide (like other drug acetylations) is controlled by genes that show polymorphism, so that patients can be divided into slow and fast acetylators. Slow acetylators may be more liable to develop signs of drug toxicity, including SLE. The plasma half-life of procainamide is relatively short (3–4 h), and the drug must be administered frequently in order to maintain a constant plasma concentration.

Due to the problems associated with its use, procainamide is not commonly used as an antiarrhythmic agent.

Phenytoin sodium

Phenytoin sodium depresses abnormal pacemaker activity and enhances conduction in the His–Purkinje system (particularly when conductivity is depressed by digitalis glycosides). Consequently, it depresses ectopic rhythms that are due to the escape of conducting tissue from the influence of the SA node. It has been used in the management of cardiac arrhythmias that are associated with digoxin toxicity. Approximately 200–300 mg of phenytoin is injected intravenously over 10 min. Although some of the antiarrhythmic effects of phenytoin are due to sodium-channel blockade, the drug has complex effects on excitable tissues that are dissimilar to other agents.

Magnesium salts

Magnesium is one of the commonest cations in the body (after sodium, potassium and calcium), and approximately 35–40% is found in cardiac and skeletal muscle. Decreased plasma magnesium concentrations have been associated with a variety of cardiac arrhythmias. The explanation for hypomagnesaemia is unclear, although the effects observed are similar to those induced by hypokalaemia. Alternatively, it has been suggested that magnesium deficiency may facilitate the influx of calcium ions.

Magnesium salts have been used in the treatment of supraventricular arrhythmias since the 1930s. Intravenous magnesium sulphate (8 mmol, given slowly over 15–20 min) has been used in the treatment of torsade de pointes induced by antiarrhythmic agents, or to reverse arrhythmias associated with digitalis toxicity. Magnesium salts have also been used after myocardial infarction; after a bolus dose, an infusion of 65–72 mmol in 24 h is recommended. Mortality appears to be reduced, and there may be a prophylactic effect on the development of arrhythmias. However, an improvement in coronary blood flow (due to the vasodilating properties of magnesium) and a reduction in platelet aggregation may also be contributory factors.

Antiarrhythmic drugs and general anaesthesia

General anaesthesia presents special hazards in patients on antiarrhythmic drug therapy. They may be related to the existence of cardiovascular disease or to its treatment with antiarrhythmic drugs. Verapamil and β-adrenoceptor antagonists reduce cardiac output, and the use of anaesthetic agents that produce similar effects may be hazardous. Similarly, many antiarrhythmic drugs increase the refractory period of junctional tissues and delay AV conduction. These effects may be potentiated by anaesthetic drugs that depress AV conduction (e.g. suxamethonium, neostigmine, inhalational anaesthetics, β-adrenoceptor antagonists), and partial or complete heart block may be precipitated.

Cardiac arrhythmias are not uncommon during general anaesthesia; they are often relatively benign and may require little or no intervention or treatment. Occasionally, they are dangerous or life-threatening and require the immediate administration of antiarrhythmic drugs. Although they may have no identifiable cause, they are often precipitated by physiological or pharmacological factors associated with general anaesthesia. Thus, arrhythmias may be due to electrolyte abnormalities (particularly in calcium or potassium levels), increased secretion of catecholamines (due to hypoxia or hypercarbia), surgical stimulation under light anaesthesia, or operative manipulations that reflexly alter vagal or sympathetic tone. Stimulation of the upper airways is associated with a reflex increase in sympathetic activity and increased catecholamine secretion; consequently, arrhythmias may occur during laryngoscopy, bronchoscopy, endotracheal intubation and extubation, and dental surgery. Traction or stimulation of the heart, the lungs and many intra-abdominal viscera may also cause reflex effects, including arrhythmias. Neurosurgical procedures in the posterior fossa, ocular surgery and stimulation of the carotid sinus may also cause bradycardia or arrhythmias. Alternatively, drugs used during anaesthesia (e.g. adrenaline, β-adrenoceptor antagonists, suxamethonium, atropine) may precipitate arrhythmias. Cyclopropane and halogenated hydrocarbons (e.g. trichlorethylene, halothane) sensitize the heart to the effects of administered or endogenous adrenaline, and may cause abnormalities in cardiac rhythm. Arrhythmias associated with catecholamines or increased catecholamine sensitivity are usually treated with propranolol (1.0 mg) injected over 1 min. The dose should be repeated at 2-min intervals until a response is observed, or a maximum dose of 5 mg has been given. In patients with obstructive airways disease, diabetes or peripheral vascular disease, a cardio-selective β-adrenoceptor antagonist (e.g. atenolol or metoprolol) should be used instead of propranolol. Arrhythmias produced by suxamethonium invariably respond to atropine (0.3–0.6 mg). Although atropine itself may produce arrhythmias, these are usually benign and of little importance.

Patients with pre-existing cardiovascular disease or with certain endocrine disorders (e.g. hyperaldosteronism, thyrotoxicosis, phaeochromocytoma) may develop arrhythmias during surgery. Arrhythmias associated with thyrotoxicosis, thyroid surgery or phaeochromocytomas usually respond to intravenous propranolol.

Drugs used in the treatment of angina

Anginal pain occurs when coronary blood flow cannot meet the metabolic demands of the myocardium (i.e. there is an imbalance between the oxygen supply and the oxygen requirement of the myocardium). Myocardial hypoxia leads to the accumulation of local metabolites, such as potassium ions, adenosine, prostaglandins, bradykinin or related mediators, resulting in precordial pain. Drugs are mainly useful in the prophylaxis rather than the treatment of anginal attacks (since the precordial pain usually rapidly responds to termination of the precipitating stimulus). Occasionally, anginal attacks are prolonged, and drug treatment is necessary.

Several different groups of drugs are commonly used to prevent attacks of anginal pain. These are:

1 Nitrates.

2 Calcium antagonists.

3 β-Adrenoceptor antagonists.

4 Potassium-channel activators.

These drugs have different modes and sites of action, and their use in combination may therefore be beneficial. Nitrates primarily dilate the venous system, and thus reduce the filling pressure (preload); calcium antagonists mainly affect the heart and dilate peripheral arterioles, decreasing arterial pressure (afterload); β-adrenoceptor antagonists reduce the work and the oxygen demand of the myocardium; while potassium channel activators increase K^+ loss from vascular smooth muscle, resulting in hyperpolarization and arteriolar vasodilatation.

Nitrates

Nitrates selectively dilate venules and small veins, resulting in the pooling of blood in capacitance vessels. Ventricular filling pressure (ventricular end-diastolic pressure) is reduced; this decreases both ventricular size and myocardial wall tension. Consequently, there is increased perfusion of subendocardial blood vessels (which are normally subjected to the greatest pressure during ventricular systole). Myocardial work and oxygen requirement are reduced, and blood is redistributed to ischaemic regions.

High concentrations of nitrates also act on the resistance vessels, some arteriolar dilatation occurs, and peripheral resistance is reduced. These effects reduce cardiac work (although compensatory tachycardia can cause a fall in coronary perfusion pressure). Finally, nitrates may directly dilate coronary arteries and coronary atherosclerotic stenoses; collateral flow is increased and the oxygenation of ischaemic myocardium is enhanced.

Since nitrates primarily affect capacitance vessels, they may produce postural hypotension. In supine patients, they have only minor effects on the blood pressure, although profound hypotension occurs on standing (particularly in younger subjects). The effects of nitrates on pulse rate is variable. Small doses may cause bradycardia; higher concentrations commonly produce tachycardia, due to a compensatory increase in sympathetic tone.

It is now generally accepted that the vasodilator effects of all nitrates (including sodium nitroprusside) is mainly due to their intracellular metabolism to nitric oxide (endothelium-derived relaxing factor). All organic nitroesters have the general formula R—C—O—NO_2, and are lipid-soluble compounds that readily penetrate many cells (including smooth-muscle and vascular endothelial cells). They are metabolized intracellularly (by glutathione-*S*-transferases and cytochrome P-450 enzymes) to nitrite ions and nitric oxide; this diffuses into vascular smooth muscle and reacts with sulphydryl groups to form reactive intermediates (*S*-nitrosothiols). Nitric oxide and/or nitrosothiols activate soluble guanylyl cyclase, increasing the conversion of guanosine triphosphate (GTP) to cyclic guanosine monophosphate (cGMP). This intermediate messenger subsequently activates protein kinases, resulting in the phosphorylation of membrane proteins and the relaxation of vascular smooth muscle (p. 87; Fig. 3.7).

All nitrates may rapidly induce the development of tolerance to their vasodilator effects. This phenomenon was first observed in munition workers, who were continually exposed to organic nitrates during the manufacture of nitroglycerine. It was also noticed that tolerance to nitrates was rapidly lost during the course of a drug-free weekend, resulting in 'Monday-morning headache'. Tolerance to the vascular effects of nitrates may develop within 24–48 h; it commonly occurs during continuous treatment with nitrates, unless there is a daily drug-free period of 6–8 h. Tolerance is associated with attenuation of the increase in guanylyl cyclase activity and the conversion of GTP to cGMP; it has been suggested that it is due to the depletion of sulphydryl (—SH) groups from vascular smooth muscle cells (which thus prevents the formation of *S*-nitrosothiols from nitric oxide). Nitrate tolerance is sometimes delayed or prevented by the infusion of drugs containing sulphydryl groups (e.g. acetylcysteine).

Glyceryl trinitrate tablets (0.3–1 mg) have been widely used in the management of anginal pain. They are mainly used to provide brief and rapid prophylaxis against anginal attacks, and to provide short-term extension of exercise tolerance, and should be taken sublingually approximately 1–2 min before any activity that is liable to provoke angina. After sublingual administration, the action of glyceryl trinitrate is almost immediate, and usually lasts for 20–30 min. Oral administration has little or no effect, due to the extensive presystemic metabolism of the drug by the gut wall and the liver. Glyceryl trinitrate tablets may deteriorate within 2–6 months of preparation.

In recent years, other preparations of glyceryl trinitrate have been extensively used to prevent or control anginal pain. Sustained-release sublingual or buccal tablets have an equally rapid onset but a longer duration of action than conventional preparations of glyceryl trinitrate. A metered aerosol spray may be used for buccal administration; this preparation is relatively stable, and may be useful in patients who require infrequent prophylaxis. Since glyceryl trinitrate is an extremely potent and lipid-soluble drug, it is also absorbed through the skin (although its permeability may affect the degree of absorption). A transdermal patch containing a slow-release formulation of glyceryl trinitrate produces acceptable bioavailability after application to any area of hairless skin in the body; the rate of drug delivery is controlled by a semipermeable membrane between the drug and the skin, and usually releases 5–10 mg of glyceryl trinitrate over a 24-h period. This preparation may be particularly useful in patients who suffer from nocturnal anginal attacks. An ointment containing glyceryl trinitrate is also used; after application, it should be covered by a dressing.

This preparation provides short-term prophylaxis for 2–3 h, but is inconvenient to apply and is unsuitable for long-term use. All of these preparations are associated with the rapid and sustained systemic absorption of glyceryl trinitrate, and avoid extensive presystemic metabolism by the liver. Although oral sustained-release tablets of glyceryl trinitrate are also available, they are generally of lesser value in the prophylaxis of anginal attacks.

Oral preparations of organic nitrates have also been widely used in the prophylaxis of angina. In general, these preparations decrease the frequency of anginal attacks and may extend exercises tolerance, but they are of no value in the immediate treatment of anginal pain. Pentaerythritol tetranitrate tablets have been widely used for many years; they slowly release nitrate ions and may provide sustained prophylaxis. More recently, oral preparations of isosorbide dinitrate and isosorbide mononitrate have been used. After oral administration, isosorbide dinitrate is variably absorbed from the small intestine; it is converted by the gut and the liver into two active metabolites (isosorbide-2-mononitrate and isosorbide-5-mononitrate). Most of the drug is present in the systemic circulation as isosorbide-5-mononitrate, which has a terminal half-life of approximately 5 h (i.e. about 10 times longer than the parent drug). Consequently, the prolonged prophylaxis produced by isosorbide dinitrate is mainly due to its active metabolite, isosorbide-5-mononitrate. This compound is also commonly used in its own right in the management of angina. Isosorbide mononitrate has a systemic bioavailability of 100%; it avoids the variable absorption and unpredictable presystemic metabolism of isosorbide dinitrate, and has a longer duration of action. It is probably preferable to isosorbide dinitrate in the management of angina. Isosorbide dinitrate may also be absorbed after sublingual administration (thus potentially avoiding any first-pass effects); however, its duration of action is usually no greater than sublingual glyceryl trinitrate.

Intravenous infusions of glyceryl trinitrate have also been used to provide controlled hypotension during surgical procedures.

Calcium antagonists

Calcium ions are intermediate mediators in many cellular processes, including glandular secretion, neuronal excitability, neurotransmitter release, excitation–contraction coupling and blood coagulation. In addition, they play an important role in the excitation and depolarization of cardiac muscle and vascular smooth muscle. During excitation, calcium ions pass from extracellular fluid into junctional and myocardial cells through specific voltage-sensitive ion channels, resulting in depolarization. Similar changes occur during excitation in vascular smooth muscle. Drugs that prevent calcium entry during depolarization are usually known as calcium antagonists or calcium-channel blockers; they may interfere with cardiac excitation or conduction, decrease the force of myocardial contraction or cause relaxation of vascular smooth muscle. Calcium antagonists selectively prevent ion entry through L-type calcium channels; they do not affect other types of ion channel.

The effects of calcium antagonists are extremely variable (possibly due to differences in their relative affinity for L-type channels in junctional tissues, cardiac muscle and vascular smooth muscle). In angina, they usually increase coronary and peripheral blood flow, reduce blood pressure, decrease the work of the heart and improve the efficiency of myocardial contraction; in these conditions, the imbalance between oxygen supply and demand may be corrected. In addition, calcium antagonists relax vascular spasm, and are usually effective in vasospastic angina (Prinzmetal's angina), as well as classical exertional angina. They are usually classified as:

1 Phenylalkylamines (class 1 antagonists), e.g. verapamil.
2 Dihydropyridines (class 2 antagonists), e.g. nifedipine, nicardipine, amlodipine.
3 Benzothiazepines (class 3 antagonists), e.g. diltiazem.

Other drugs may have non-selective effects on calcium channels (e.g. lidoflazine, prenylamine, perhexilene and possibly fluorinated anaesthetics).

Verapamil

In the SA and AV nodes, depolarization is almost entirely dependent on the influx of calcium ions from extracellular fluid. Verapamil prevents calcium ion transport through voltage-sensitive slow channels (L channels) in SA and AV nodal cells; it has less marked effects on myocardial contractile tissue and vascular smooth muscle. Consequently, verapamil is primarily used in the treatment of supraventricular arrhythmias (p. 515), although it may also be of value in the treatment of angina. It has significant negative inotropic effects and may cause bradycardia and congestive cardiac failure (particularly in patients on β-adrenoceptor antagonists and other drugs which depress AV conduction). Although verapamil has only limited effects on vascular smooth muscle, it may reduce peripheral resistance and cause hypotension. The usual oral dose ranges from 120 to 360 mg daily, given in divided doses.

Nifedipine

Nifedipine primarily affects the peripheral vasculature and the coronary circulation. It has little or no direct effect on myocardial contractility or AV conduction. It is unclear whether this is related to the preferential localization of the drug in vascular smooth muscle, or to its differential effects on calcium channels in the heart and the peripheral circulation. Current evidence suggests that nifedipine may reduce the duration of calcium-channel opening, and thus inhibit the entry of calcium ions into vascular smooth muscle during depolarization.

Nifedipine is a powerful vasodilator; it is approximately 30–50 times more potent than verapamil on vascular smooth muscle. It mainly affects calcium channels in arterioles, and has little or no effect on capacitance vessels. Consequently, nifedipine decreases systemic resistance and blood pressure, and increases peripheral and coronary blood flow (Table 15.3). In the isolated heart, nifedipine has direct depressant effects, and decreases myocardial contractility and AV conduction. In *in vivo* conditions, these effects are overshadowed by reflex tachycardia and increased stroke volume, resulting in a rise in cardiac output. Most of the side-effects of nifedipine are due to peripheral vasodilatation and the subsequent reduction in blood pressure (e.g. headache, flushing, dizziness, postural hypotension and palpitations). Occasionally, nifedipine (and other dihydropyridines) increase the frequency of anginal attacks and prolong ischaemic pain, due to decreased peripheral resistance and the associated reflex tachycardia.

Nifedipine may be given by oral, sublingual or intravenous administration (usual dose range = 20–80 mg day^{-1}). After oral administration, the drug is well-absorbed, although approximately 50% is eliminated by presystemic metabolism. The terminal half-life of nifedipine is approximately 5–6 h, and its clearance is 20–30% of liver blood flow. The drug is widely used in the treatment of angina and hypertension, but is of little or no value in the management of cardiac arrhythmias.

Nicardipine

Nicardipine is a dihydropyridine derivative closely related to nifedipine. It was originally introduced in Japan as a cerebral vasodilator, and was subsequently used in the treatment of essential hypertension. Nicardipine is a potent dilator of vascular smooth muscle; thus, it decreases systemic vascular resistance and diastolic blood pressure, and increases peripheral and coronary blood flow. It has less direct depressant effects on the heart than nifedipine; in *in vivo* conditions, it causes reflex tachycardia and an increase in cardiac output. After oral administration, nicardipine is rapidly absorbed and extensively metabolized by the liver. The systemic bioavailability is approximately 50%, due to extensive presystemic metabolism; little or none of the unchanged drug is eliminated in urine. The terminal half-life of nicardipine is 4–5 h, and its clearance is approximately 30–50% of liver blood flow.

Although nicardipine is used in the treatment of hypertension and angina, it is of no value in the management of cardiac arrhythmias.

Amlodipine

Amlodipine is a dihydropyridine calcium antagonist with similar effects to nicardipine. It produces selective effects on calcium channels in vascular smooth muscle; although it is used in angina, it is of no value in the treatment of cardiac arrhythmias.

Diltiazem

Diltiazem is a benzothiazepine derivative that affects calcium channels in the heart and in the peripheral circulation. Thus, it impairs cardiac conduction and contractility, and also causes vasodilatation in coronary and peripheral blood vessels (Table 15.3). Diltiazem reduces the automaticity of the SA node, and impairs conduction of the cardiac impulse in the AV node; the PR interval is usually prolonged, and heart rate is usually reduced. Diltiazem also affects calcium channels in vascular smooth muscle and the coronary circulation, and peripheral resistance is decreased. Systolic and diastolic blood pressure falls, due to the decrease in cardiac output and the reduction in peripheral resistance; reflex tachycardia does not usually occur. After oral administration, diltiazem is almost completely absorbed from the small intestine, but is subject to considerable presystemic metabolism. Consequently, the oral bioavailability of the drug is only 50–70%. Approximately 60% is metabolized by the liver (mainly to the active metabolite desacetyldiltiazem), while 40% is eliminated unchanged by the kidney. The terminal half-life of diltiazem is 4–6 h. Although diltiazem has antiarrhythmic effects, it is mainly used in the treatment of angina, hypertension and peripheral vascular disease (including Raynaud's disease).

β-Adrenoceptor antagonists

β-Adrenoceptor blockade reduces the work of the heart, decreases oxygen consumption and reduces systemic arterial pressure. In addition, the associated bradycardia improves coronary and myocardial perfusion. β-Adrenoceptor antagonists restore the balance between myocardial oxygen supply and demand, and decrease cardiac activity to a level that does not induce attacks of angina. They also modify sympathetic drive and the effects of circulating catecholamines, and thus reduce chronotropic and inotropic responses during exercise or stress. Consequently, β-adrenoceptor antagonists are widely used to decrease the frequency and severity of attacks of exertional angina. Unlike calcium antagonists, they are not usually of value in vasospastic (Prinzmetal) angina; occasionally they may exacerbate or provoke this condition by promoting α-adrenoceptor-mediated vasoconstriction of the coronary vasculature. They may also precipitate cardiac failure in patients with a poor cardiac reserve.

Non-selective β_1 and β_2-antagonists (e.g. nadolol, oxprenolol, pindolol, propranolol, sotalol) are widely used in angina; however, they may produce blockade at β_2-receptor sites, resulting in bronchospasm, decreased peripheral blood flow, hypoglycaemia and an increase in uterine tone. These effects are less common with the cardioselective β_1-antagonists (e.g. acebutolol, atenolol, metoprolol), and these drugs are often preferred in patients with obstructive airways disease, peripheral vascular disease and diabetes. The more polar agents (i.e. atenolol, nadolol and sotalol) are not significantly metabolized and have a relatively long half-life, so that once-daily oral administration may produce adequate β-blockade for up to 24 h. In addition, they do not readily cross the placenta or the blood–brain barrier. Both pindolol and oxprenolol may produce slight tachycardia, due to their partial agonist effects.

Potassium-channel activators

The normal resting potential in vascular smooth muscle is approximately –50 mV, and reflects the distribution of potassium ions across the cell membrane. Potassium ions diffuse from vascular smooth-muscle cells to extracellular fluid through potassium channels, which are divided into several subtypes. The basal tone and resting potential are mainly controlled by K_{IR}, BK_{Ca} and K_{ATP} channels; the voltage-sensitive, rapidly activating and inactivating K_A channel appears not to play an important role. In particular, the K_{ATP} channel may have an important influence on smooth-muscle tone during ischaemia and other pathophysiological states. Drugs that activate this channel (e.g. aprokalim, cromakalim, pinacidil, nicorandil) increase potassium loss from smooth-muscle cells, producing hyperpolarization and vasodilatation.

Nicorandil

Nicorandil (a nitrated derivative of nicotinamide) causes relaxation of vascular smooth muscle by two independent mechanisms. In the first place, it activates K_{ATP} channels, causing hyperpolarization and relaxation of vascular smooth muscle; patch-clamp studies with glibenclamide (a specific inhibitor of K_{ATP} potassium channels) suggest that nicorandil specifically activates potassium flux through K_{ATP} channels. Second, nicorandil releases nitrate ions, which indirectly stimulate guanylyl cyclase and increase the synthesis of cGMP. Subsequently protein kinases are activated, resulting in vasodilatation. Consequently, nicorandil has a dual mode of action on vascular smooth muscle; potassium-channel activation causes arteriolar vasodilatation in peripheral and coronary blood vessels, while the activation of guanylyl cyclase produces venous pooling in capacitance vessels. Nicorandil (and other drugs that activate K_{ATP} channels) accelerate recovery from myocardial contraction and may prolong the time for diastolic filling. In experimental studies, they have been shown to reduce infarct size, and they may have a cardioprotective effect in ischaemic conditions.

Nicorandil (20–60 mg day^{-1}) is used orally in the prophylaxis of angina. Many of its side-effects (e.g. headache, facial flushing, dizziness, postural hypotension and reflex tachycardia) appear to be related to nitric oxide production and activation of guanylyl cyclase.

Drug combinations in angina

Nitrates, calcium antagonists, β-adrenoceptor antagonists and potassium-channel activators have different modes and sites of action on the heart and the circulation, and their use in combination may therefore be beneficial. Nitrates primarily dilate the venous system, and thus reduce venous return and end-diastolic pressure; calcium antagonists mainly affect the heart and peripheral arterioles, decreasing arterial pressure, while β-adrenoceptor antagonists reduce the work and the oxygen demand of the myocardium. Combinations of nitrates and β-adrenoceptor antagonists are usually additive, and the drugs are often used together in the treatment of angina. Indeed, their disadvantages may be diminished by combined therapy, since β-receptor antagonists decrease tachycardia due to nitrates, while nitrates limit the alterations in ventricular size produced by β-adrenoceptor antagonists. Similarly, combinations of peripherally acting calcium antagonists (e.g. nicardipine, nifedipine and nisoldipine), β-adrenoceptor antagonists and nitrates are sometimes used in the control of anginal pain. Nicorandil can also be used with other drugs. However, combinations of verapamil with other antianginal drugs are potentially dangerous, due to its effects on cardiac conduction and myocardial contractility. This may precipitate heart failure in susceptible patients.

Angina and general anaesthesia

Classical angina is a sensitive and specific indication of the presence of coronary artery disease. Consequently, patients with angina usually have pre-existing cardiovascular pathology, and general anaesthesia may present special hazards. In general, the aim of anaesthetic management is to preserve a balance between myocardial supply and demand, and to maintain the circulation in a slightly hypodynamic state without prejudicing myocardial function. In particular, tachycardia and significant changes in blood pressure should be avoided. Preoperative drug therapy with nitrates, β-adrenoceptor antagonists, calcium antagonists and potassium-channel activators should be maintained until surgery, and resumed as soon as possible after surgery. Patients on low doses of β-adrenoceptor antagonists may require the dose to be slightly increased. Premedication should be sufficient to allay the undesirable haemodynamic effects of preoperative anxiety, and intravenous opioids may be useful in decreasing the requirements for intravenous agents and in suppressing the undesirable haemodynamic responses to laryngoscopy and intubation. Muscle relaxants that produce tachycardia should be avoided, while the choice of inhalational anaesthetics is controversial. Isoflurane may cause the redistribution of coronary blood flow away from ischaemic areas (Chapter 8). Intravenous anaesthetics, inhalational agents and other drugs may affect the cardiovascular response to antianginal drug therapy, and haemodynamic changes that are of little significance in healthy patients may result in serious morbidity or death.

Further reading

Abrams J. Glyceryl trinitrate (nitroglycerin) and the organic nitrates: choosing the method of administration. *Drugs* 1987; **34**: 391–403.

Abshagen U (ed.) Clinical pharmacology of antianginal drugs. In: *Handbook of Experimental Pharmacology* vol. 76, Berlin: Springer Verlag, 1985; 1–552.

Abshagen U, Betzie G, Endele R, Kaufmann B. Pharmacokinetics of intravenous and oral isosorbide-5-mononitrate. *European Journal of Clinical Pharmacology* 1981; **20**: 269–275.

Aggarwal A, Wartlier DC. Adenosine: present uses, future indications. *Current Opinion in Anaesthesiology* 1994; **7**: 109–123.

Amezcua JL, Dusting GJ, Palmer RMJ, Moncada S. Acetylcholine induces vasodilatation in the rabbit isolated heart through the release of nitric oxide the endogenous nitrovasodilator. *British Journal of Pharmacology* 1988; **95**: 830–834.

Antman EM, Stone PH, Muller JE, Braunwald E. Calcium channel blocking agents in the treatment of cardiovascular disorders. I. Basic and clinical electrophysiologic effects. *Annals of Internal Medicine* 1980; **93**: 875–885.

Aronow WS. Use of nitrates as antianginal agents. In: Neddleman PH (ed.) *Organic Nitrates. Handbook of Experimental Pharmacology*, vol. 40. Berlin: Springer Verlag, 1975; 163–174.

Barnett DB. Myocardial ischaemia: progress in drug therapy. *British Journal of Anaesthesia* 1988; **61**: 11–23.

Barnett DB. Myocardial β-receptor function and regulation in heart failure: implications for therapy. *British Journal of Clinical Pharmacology* 1989; **27**: 527–537.

Braunwald E. Mechanism of action of calcium-channel blocking agents. *New England Journal of Medicine* 1982; **307**: 1618–1627.

Brichard G, Zimmerman PE. Verapamil in cardiac dysrhythmias during anaesthesia. *British Journal of Anaesthesia* 1970; **42**: 1005–1072.

Britt BA. Diltiazem. *Canadian Anaesthetists Society Journal* 1985; **32**: 30–40.

Brogden RN, Todd PA. Disopyramide: a reappraisal of its pharmacodynamic and pharmacokinetic properties, and therapeutic use in cardiac arrhythmias. *Drugs* 1987; **34**: 151–187.

Campbell RWF. Mexiletine. *New England Journal of Medicine* 1987; **316**: 29–34.

Carson IW, Lyons SM, Shanks RG. Antiarrhythmic drugs. *British Journal of Anaesthesia* 1979; **51**: 659–670.

Dhalla NS, Pierce GN, Panagia V, Singal PK, Beamish RE. Calcium movements in relation to heart function. *Basic Research in Cardiology* 1982; **77**: 117–139.

DiCarlo FJ. Nitroglycerin revisited: chemistry, biochemistry, interactions. *Drug Metabolism Reviews* 1975; **4**: 1–38.

Fabiato A, Fabiato F. Calcium and cardiac excitation–contraction coupling. *Annual Review of Physiology* 1979; **41**: 473–484.

Fleckenstein A. History of calcium antagonists. *Circulation Research* 1983; **52** (suppl. 1): 3–16.

Foex P. The heart and autonomic nervous system. In: Nimmo WS, Smith G (eds) *Anaesthesia*. Oxford: Blackwell Scientific Publications, 1989; 115–161.

Funck-Brentano C, Kroemer HK, Lee JT, Roden DM. Propafenone. *New England Journal of Medicine* 1990; **322**: 518–525.

Gintant GA, Hoffman BF. The role of local anaesthetic effects in the actions of antiarrhythmic drugs. In: Strichartz GR (ed.) *Handbook of Experimental Pharmacology*, vol. 81. *Local Anaesthetics*. Berlin: Springer Verlag, 1987; 213–251.

Godfraind T, Govani S. Recent advances in the pharmacology of Ca^{2+} and K^{+} channels. *Trends in Pharmacological Sciences* 1995; **16**: 1–4.

Goldstein MM, Butterworth J. New roles for magnesium. *Current Opinion in Anaesthesiology* 1994; **7**: 98–108.

Hamilton TC, Weston AH. Cromokalim, nicorandil and pinacidil: novel drugs which open potassium channels in smooth muscle. *General Pharmacology* 1989; **20**: 1–9.

Henry PD. Comparative pharmacology of calcium antagonists: nifedipine, verapamil, and diltiazem. *American Journal of Cardiology* 1980; **46**: 1047–1058.

Hess P, Lansman JB, Tsien RW. Different modes of Ca channel gating behaviour favoured by dihydropyridine Ca agonists and antagonists. *Nature* 1984; **311**: 538–544.

Hoffman BF, Rosen MR. Cellular mechanisms for cardiac arrhythmias. *Circulation Research* 1981; **49**: 1–15.

Ijzerman AP, Soudijn W. The antiarrhythmic properties of β-adrenoceptor antagonists. *Trends in Pharmacological Sciences* 1989; **10**: 31–36.

Jones RM. Calcium antagonists. *Anaesthesia* 1984; **39**: 747–749.

Kaplinsky E. Management of angina pectoris. Modern concepts. *Drugs* 1992; **43** (suppl. 1): 9–14.

Krikler DM. A fresh look at cardiac arrhythmias. *Lancet* 1974; **i**: 851–854, 913–918, 974–976, 1034–1037.

Lablanche JM, Bauters C, McFadden EP, Quandalle P, Bertrand ME. Potassium channel activators in vasospastic angina. *European Heart Journal* 1993; **14**: (suppl. B): 22–24.

Mason JW. Amiodarone. *New England Journal of Medicine* 1987; **316**: 455–466.

Mikawa K, Maekawa N, Kaetsu H, Goto R, Yaku H, Obara H. Effects of adenosine triphosphate on the cardiovascular response to tracheal intubation. *British Journal of Anaesthesia* 1991; **67**: 410–415.

Morady F, Scheinman MM, Desai J. Disopyramide. *Annals of Internal Medicine* 1982; **96**: 337–343.

Nestico PF, Morganroth J, Horowitz LN. New antiarrhythmic drugs. *Drugs* 1988; **35**: 286–319.

Opie L. *The Heart. Physiology, Metabolism, Pharmacology and Therapy*. London: Grune & Stratton, 1986.

Palmer RMJ, Ashton DS, Moncada S. Vascular endothelial cells synthesize nitric oxide from L-arginine. *Nature* 1988; **333**: 664–666.

Platzer R, Reutemann G, Galleazzi RL. Pharmacokinetics of intravenous isosorbide dinitrate. *Journal of Pharmacokinetics and Biopharmaceutics* 1982; **10**: 575–585.

Prys-Roberts C. Anaesthetic considerations for the patient with coronary artery disease. *British Journal of Anaesthesia* 1988; **61**: 85–96.

Rasmussen H, Barrett PQ. Calcium messenger system: an integrated view. *Physiological Reviews* 1984; **64**: 938–984.

Reid JL, Prichard BNC, Bridgman KM. (eds) Calcium antagonists and their future clinical potential. *British Journal of Clinical Pharmacology* 1986; **21** (suppl. 2) 93S–204S.

Reiz S. Myocardial ischaemia associated with general anaesthesia. *British Journal of Anaesthesia* 1988; **61**: 68–84.

Roden DM. Risks and benefits of antiarrhythmic drug therapy. *New England Journal of Medicine* 1994; **331**: 785–791.

Rutherford JD. Pharmacologic management of angina and acute myocardial infarction. *American Journal of Cardiology* 1993; **72**: 16C–20C.

Smith TW. Digitalis: mechanisms of action and clinical use. *New England Journal of Medicine* 1988; **318**: 358–365.

Sorkin EM, Clissold SP. Nicardipine: a review of its pharmacodynamic and pharmacokinetic properties, and therapeutic efficacy, in the treatment of angina pectoris, hypertension, and related cardiovascular disorders. *Drugs* 1987; **33**: 296–345.

Taira N. Differences in cardiovascular profile among calcium antagonists. *American Journal of Cardiology* 1987; **59**: 24B–29B.

Taylor SH. α- and β-blockade in angina pectoris. *Drugs* 1984; **28** (suppl. 2): 69–87.

Thadani U. Role of nitrates in angina pectoris. *American Journal of Cardiology* 1992; **70**: 43B–53B.

Thompson RH. The clinical use of transdermal delivery-devices with nitroglycerin. *Angiology* 1983; **34**: 23–31.

Turner P, Feely J, Barrett P. (eds) Nicardipine: a new calcium antagonist. *British Journal of Clinical Pharmacology* 1986; **22** (suppl. 3): 191S–352S.

Vaughan Williams EM. Electrophysiological basis for a rational approach to antidysrhythmic drug therapy. *Advances in Drug Research* 1974; **9**: 69–102.

Vaughan Williams EM. Classifying antiarrhythmic actions: by facts or speculation. *Journal of Clinical Pharmacology* 1992; **32**: 964–977.

Weidmann S. Heart: electrophysiology. *Annual Review of Physiology* 1974; **36**: 155–169.

Why HJ, Richardson PJ. A potassium channel opener as monotherapy in chronic stable angina pectoris: comparison with placebo. *European Heart Journal* 1993; **14** (suppl. B): 25–29.

Wit AL, Rosen MR. Pathophysiological mechanisms of cardiac arrhythmias. *American Heart Journal* 1983; **106**: 798–811.

Woosley RL, Rumboldt TZ. Anti-arrhythmic drugs. In: Turner P, Shand DG (eds) *Recent Advances in Clinical Pharmacology*, vol. 1. Edinburgh: Churchill Livingstone, 1978; 93–122.

Zipes DP, Heger JJ, Prystowski EN. Pathophysiology of arrhythmias: clinical electrophysiology. *American Heart Journal* 1983; **106**: 812–827.

Chapter 16
Anticoagulants, Antiplatelet Drugs and Fibrinolytic Agents

Mechanisms of haemostasis and coagulation

Blood coagulation is a complex biological process which is intended to conserve blood volume in the event of vascular injury. Following tissue damage, arterioles contract immediately, and within a short time platelets become bound to collagen in the vessel wall and to each other. This process is activated by the release of adenosine diphosphate (ADP), and subsequently thromboxane, from the platelets themselves. Local stimulation of the coagulation process is initiated by a lipoprotein released from the vessel wall (tissue thromboplastin; factor III) and by phospholipids released from platelets. These interact with several components in the plasma (factors V, VII, X and calcium ions) to convert a glycoprotein, prothrombin, into the active proteolytic enzyme thrombin. Thrombin cleaves fibrinogen to release fibrinopeptides A and B and generate fibrin, which subsequently forms cross-links with adjacent monomers to produce an insoluble fibrin clot.

Thrombin also has important biological effects on platelets (leading to further aggregation and synthesis and secretion of thromboxane A), endothelial and smooth-muscle cells, leukocytes, the heart (influencing automaticity and repolarization) and neuronal activity. Thrombin appears to induce the proliferation of fibroblasts in pulmonary fibrosis associated with systemic sclerosis. Thrombin also activates certain coagulation factors (e.g. factor V, factor VIII) via specific thrombin receptors.

A different sequence of events occurs initially when blood is allowed to contact a foreign surface. More than a dozen proteins are involved in a cascading series of proteolytic reactions. Individual factors are considered as proenzymes; they are converted to active enzymes by each preceding action and then catalyse a subsequent reaction.

The two coagulation mechanisms described are usually distinguished as:

1 The intrinsic system, in which all the activating factors are present in the circulating plasma.

2 The extrinsic system, which is initiated by tissue injury.

This distinction has long been regarded as largely artificial as there is no clear demarcation between the systems in physiological events. Both systems lead to the formation of the prothrombin activating complex (factor Xa) and then proceed identically. Both pathways, which must be intact for adequate haemostasis, are further illustrated in Fig. 16.1.

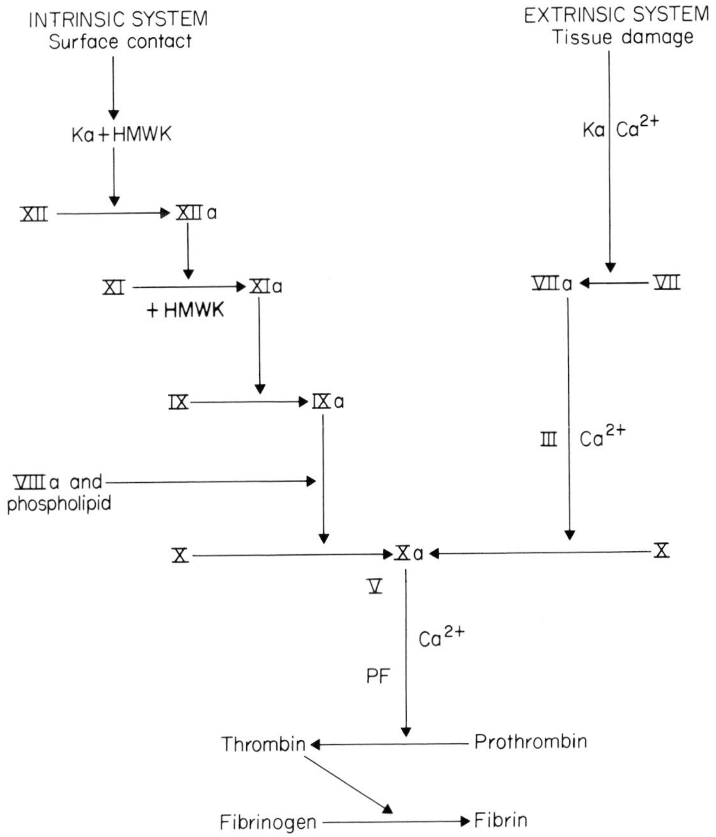

Fig. 16.1 Intrinsic and extrinsic systems of coagulation: the suffix a indicates the activated factor. PF, Platelet factor (phospholipid); Ka, kallikrein; HMWK, high molecular weight kininogen.

In clinical practice, two distinct laboratory investigations are normally performed to assess the efficacy of coagulation (or therapeutic anticoagulation). These are:

1 The activated partial thromboplastin time (aPTT). In this test, Ca^{2+}, negatively charged phospholipids and a particulate substance such as kaolin are added to blood which has previously been treated with citrate or a chelating agent to bind ionic calcium. In these circumstances the clotting time is normally 26–33 s, although this varies with the methods and reagents used.

2 The prothrombin time (PT). In this test, thromboplastin, which is a saline extract of brain containing tissue factor and phospholipids, is added to recalcified plasma. Clotting normally occurs in 12–14 s.

The international normalized ratio (INR), with a normal value of 1, is a ratio of the normal prothrombin time of a standard thromboplastin. It should only be used in the regulation of anticoagulant therapy, and permits the standardization of results between different laboratories throughout the world.

For all practical purposes, a patient with a prolonged aPTT and normal PT may be considered to have a defect in the intrinsic coagulation pathway. In contrast, an individual with a normal aPTT and a prolonged PT can be described as having a defect in the extrinsic pathway. When both values are prolonged, a defect in a common pathway is suggested.

Disorders of coagulation

Dietary factors

Vitamin K is a dietary constituent which is essential for the synthesis of certain coagulation factors in the liver. This was originally discovered during feeding experiments on chicks, when it was noted that deficiency of an ether-soluble substance caused a bleeding disease. It was subsequently elicited that there are at least two distinct natural forms of vitamin K: vitamin K_1 (phytomenadione), which is found in plants and is the only natural vitamin K available for therapeutic use, and vitamin K_2 (menaquinones), one or more compounds that are synthesized in the alimentary tract by Gram-negative bacteria. Both these types of vitamin K are fat-soluble, and intestinal absorption is dependent on the presence of bile salts in the duodenum.

Vitamin K deficiency may result from inadequacy of dietary intake or intestinal synthesis, failure of absorption or impaired utilization by the liver. The resultant effects will be a reduced availability of prothrombin and factors VII, IX and X, thus producing a bleeding tendency. Clinical situations in which this can occur include haemorrhagic disease of the newborn, various malabsorption syndromes, obstructive jaundice, biliary fistulae and cirrhosis of the liver. Phytomenadione (1 mg intramuscularly) is the treatment of choice in neonatal deficiency; larger doses (> 10 mg daily for 3 days preoperatively) should restore prothrombin levels to normal in the jaundiced patient, although if there is severe hepatocellular damage, infusion of fresh frozen plasma may be necessary. Vitamin K_3 (menadione) is a synthetic compound which can be converted into a water-soluble derivative (menadiol sodium phosphate); this may be administered orally in order to prevent vitamin K deficiency in malabsorption syndromes.

Hereditary disorders

Haemophilia is the classical example of a sex-linked coagulation defect. There are two types of haemophilia; haemophilia A (classical haemophilia), in which there is a deficiency of factor VIII (antihaemophilic globulin or AHG), and haemophilia B (Christmas disease) in which there is a deficiency of factor IX. Von Willebrand's disease is an autosomal dominant trait in which both males and females may be affected. In this condition, there is a deficiency of von Willebrand factor, which acts as a protective carrier for factor VIII in the circulation and is also involved in platelet adhesion to subendothelium. The haemostatic defect is therefore due to a lowering of factor VIII as well as a prolonged bleeding time. When such patients require surgery, concentrates of the appropriate factors will need to be administered in the perioperative period.

Thrombogenesis

Thrombogenesis is an altered state of haemostasis which results in the formation of an intravascular thrombus. The classical triad of Virchow implicates changes in the vessel wall, stasis and hypercoagulability as the main precipitating factors. Thrombi can form:

1 In arteries, leading to ischaemic changes in vital tissues or organs.

2 In veins, where there is a high risk of emboli becoming detached and occluding the pulmonary circulation.

3 As intramural deposits in the chambers of the heart, which can lead to embolic complications in systemic vessels.

Thromboembolic disease is a common cause of mortality and morbidity which may have special implications in the postoperative period. Undoubtedly, there are a number of preventable and treatable causes of vessel wall pathology (e.g. cigarette smoking, hypercholesterolaemia and other diseases such as essential hypertension) which produce the 'at-risk' patient. Furthermore, the venous stasis induced by prolonged surgery and postoperative immobilization may be remedied by a number of non-pharmacological measures (e.g. careful positioning during surgery, leg exercises, adequate hydration and the use of elasticated stockings).

A hypercoagulable state may be associated with changes which are conducive to thrombosis formation if additional factors, such as stasis, are present. Hypercoagulability can occur due to changes in coagulation factors, platelets, the fibrinolytic system or physiological inhibitors of haemostasis. Although increased levels of unactivated clotting factors do not increase the rate of fibrin formation, raised concentrations of factor VIII and fibrinogen are predictive of an increased risk of ischaemic heart disease. Diminished fibrinolysis constitutes a risk factor for venous thrombosis and results from insufficient availability or dysfunction of plasminogen activators, plasminogen (see Fig. 16.3) and fibrin cofactor activity.

Physiological inhibitors of the clotting mechanism include α_2-macroglobulin, α_1-antitrypsin, C1 esterase inhibitor, antithrombin III, protein C, protein S and heparin cofactor II. Congenital deficiencies of these endogenous substances are characterized by a predisposition to thrombotic disease (this group of conditions constitutes the thrombophilias). Activated protein C resistance is also associated with a mutation in the factor V gene (referred to as factor V Leiden). Paradoxically, a deficiency in the coagulation factor XII (which is also involved in the intrinsic pathway of fibrinolysis) may also predispose to thrombophilia.

In most cases of this type, the initial episode of venous thrombosis occurs between the ages of 20 and 30, and a precipitating factor can be determined in approximately 50% of these. If surgery is contemplated in such patients, the use of short-term anticoagulation should be considered (if long-term therapy is not already being used). Concentrates of antithrombin III or plasma administered on the day of surgery may also be useful.

There is also an increased risk of thromboembolism in the postoperative period in young women who are taking oral contraceptives; oestrogens have been shown to accelerate blood clotting and to raise the concentration of some coagulation factors. However, the role of factors influencing platelet aggregation may be of more significance. It has been shown that the abnormal coagulatory state may not revert to normal until about 3 months following cessation of oestrogen therapy. The problem is likely to be lessened when the oestrogen content of the oral contraceptive is low. However, the use of combined oral contraceptives containing third-generation progestogens (e.g. desogestrel, gestodene) has been associated with an increased risk of thromboembolism. It has been suggested that, when such patients present for major elective surgery or for all surgery on the lower limbs, the contraceptive drug should be discontinued for 4 weeks prior to operation and that in other types of surgery, the use of low-dose heparin regimes in the perioperative period should be considered. However, other authorities consider that there is insufficient evidence to support the cessation of such therapy, or the use of prophylactic anticoagulant regimes, unless other risk factors are also present.

In the remainder of this chapter, drugs which may be used in the prevention and treatment of thromboembolic disorders will be discussed. In general, they can be divided into three groups:

1 Drugs that interfere with the coagulation process (anticoagulant agents).

2 Drugs that inhibit platelet aggregation (antiplatelet or antithrombotic agents).

3 Drugs which promote the dissolution of thrombi (thrombolytic or fibrinolytic agents).

Anticoagulants

Two main types of anticoagulants are used in clinical practice. These are:

1 Heparin.

2 Oral anticoagulants.

Heparin

Heparin, as its name implies, is a naturally occurring substance which was originally found in the liver. It can also be obtained in large amounts from mast cells in the lung and intestinal mucosa. Heparin is a mucopolysaccharide containing many sulphate residues, and has a molecular weight of approximately 16 kDa. Heparin may be released in a macromolecular form from mast cells in the vascular endothelium in anaphylactic shock, and render the blood less coagulable.

The physiological role of heparin is not entirely clear, but a number of effects which are independent of its anticoagulant activity have been ascribed to heparin and associated endogenous heparinoids (e.g. heparan sulphate, chondroitin 4-sulphate). Heparin appears to have inhibitory effects on immune cell migration in inflammatory disorders and on tumour cell metastasis. Furthermore, heparin exhibits antiproliferative effects on smooth-muscle cells and fibroblasts; this may be relevant to anatomical changes in tissues which occur in diseases such as atherosclerosis or asthma. Many of these effects are undoubtedly due to the ability of heparin to bind (through electrostatic forces) to tissue proteins.

Heparin produces immediate anticoagulant effects, both *in vivo* and *in vitro*, but acts indirectly via a cofactor, an α_2-globulin which is present in plasma and known as antithrombin III.

1 In low concentrations, heparin binds to antithrombin III and accelerates its combination with thrombin to form an inactive complex. The activated Stuart factor (factor Xa), which promotes the conversion of prothrombin to thrombin, may be inhibited by a similar mechanism. These effects form the basis of action of low-dose heparin regimes.

2 When more elevated plasma levels of heparin are achieved, other activated clotting factors (IXa, XIa, XIIa) may also be neutralized. The synthesis of thrombin is thus further suppressed.

3 In high doses, heparin, in combination with antithrombin III, also inhibits the platelet aggregation which can be induced by thrombin.

Heparin also lowers plasma triglyceride levels, and thus reduces plasma turbidity, by activating a lipoprotein lipase in tissues. The resultant increase in free fatty acid levels which ensues can interfere with the plasma binding of certain drugs (e.g. propranolol, phenytoin) in blood sampled from cannulae which are intermittently flushed with heparin.

Heparin crosses membranes poorly because of its polarity and large molecular size. It is thus ineffective when administered orally or sublingually and does not readily traverse the placental and blood–brain barriers. When given as a single intravenous dose, the effect of heparin usually lasts for 4–6 h, although the half-life of the anticoagulant activity does appear to be dependent upon the amount administered. Heparin is metabolized in the liver by the enzyme heparinase, and the metabolites are excreted in the urine. The effects of the anticoagulant may thus be prolonged in renal failure or hepatic cirrhosis.

Heparin has a large number of anionic groups present at physiological pH which are essential for its anticoagulant action. Neutralizing these negatively charged groups with basic substances such as protamine or toluidine blue will rapidly abolish the pharmacological effects of heparin.

Commercial preparations of heparin are normally obtained from bovine and porcine lung tissue. Biological assay is necessary for standardization and the activity is measured in units. The concentration of preparations of heparin is normally expressed in terms of units per millilitre.

As heparin is derived from animal tissue, hypersensitivity responses may be anticipated and are occasionally observed, particularly in those patients with a history of an allergic disorder. Manifestations include fever, urticaria and anaphylactic shock. Thrombocytopenia may also occur. Hypersensitivity responses which occur immediately following the administration of heparin (and may include a mild form of thrombocytopenia) are thought to be anaphylactoid reactions and may involve the alternate complement pathway (Chapter 6). A more severe form of thrombocytopenia which presents at a later stage is considered to be a cytolytic (type II hypersensitivity) response. Patients who receive continuous or intermittent therapy with heparin will have a progressive reduction in antithrombin III activity and there is a possibility that a paradoxical increase in the thrombotic tendency may eventually occur. Alopecia and osteoporosis have also been reported after long-term use.

Clinical uses

Heparin is used in the prophylaxis and treatment of deep venous thrombosis, pulmonary embolism and myocardial infarction. Therapeutic doses of heparin are used to prevent thrombosis occurring during cardiac and major vascular surgery and during haemodialysis. Low-dose heparin is frequently advocated in the prophylaxis of thromboembolic complications in patients who undergo a wide variety of surgical procedures, particularly those who may be considered at special risk. Important factors include major surgery with prolonged immobilization, obesity, congestive cardiac failure, venous stasis in the lower limbs and previous thrombotic episodes. Heparin is contraindicated in haemorrhagic states, following recent ophthalmic or neurosurgery, in hypertensive patients with a diastolic pressure greater than 110 mmHg, peptic ulceration or oesophageal varices, and in cases of known hypersensitivity to heparin.

Dose regimes

Standard intravenous regime for the treatment of established thrombosis

Whenever possible, heparin should be administered intravenously and preferably by continuous infusion. A loading dose of 5000 units of heparin sodium is given, followed by 1000–2000 units h^{-1}. The dose is adjusted to maintain the aPTT between 1.5 and 2.5 times the normal value. In most instances where prolonged anticoagulation is required, oral anticoagulants (see below) are started at the same time and heparin can be withdrawn after these have achieved their therapeutic effect (this usually takes a minimum of 3 days).

Alternative regimes when intravenous administration is not feasible or oral anticoagulants are contraindicated (e.g. pregnancy)

In these instances heparin can be given by the subcutaneous route using a high-concentration preparation (25 000 units ml^{-1}). It is recommended that such injections are given into the anterolateral wall of the abdomen adjacent to the iliac crest or thigh. An initial dose of 10 000–20 000 units 12-hourly is administered and adjusted daily by laboratory monitoring. It is recommended that regular platelet counts should also be performed on patients receiving heparin for longer than 5 days.

Prophylactic regimes in 'high-risk' surgical patients

In these circumstances, heparin is usually administered subcutaneously. A dose of 5000 units is given 2 h before operation and repeated at 8–12-hourly intervals for 7 days, or until the patient is mobile. When subcutaneous routes are employed, calcium heparin preparations, which are thought to produce less haematomas at tissue injection sites, are often preferred. Laboratory monitoring of clotting activity is not necessary with low-dose regimes.

Low molecular weight heparins. The pharmacological effects and therapeutic regimes which have been described above relate to unfractionated heparin. In recent years low molecular weight heparins (LMWH) have been introduced into clinical practice. This group of compounds have been prepared by fractionating heparin to exclude the larger molecules (>10 kDa). LMWH molecules are unable to bind both thrombin and antithrombin III simultaneously. Thus they exert their effects by inhibiting activated factors IX–XII (via antithrombin III) but are devoid of any direct inhibitory actions on thrombin itself. LMWH have less effect on platelet function than unfractionated heparin and would be expected to produce fewer haemorrhagic complications in the perioperative period, although this has not been substantiated. However, there is evidence to suggest that LMWH are as safe and effective as unfractionated heparin in the prophylaxis of deep venous thrombosis and may induce a significant reduction in pulmonary embolism in patients undergoing general surgical or orthopaedic procedures. LMWH have greater bioavailability than unfractionated heparin; comparable dose requirements are less and the duration of action is longer.

Dalteparin, enoxaparin and tinzaparin are LMWH which are commercially available. They are usually administered once or twice daily in prophylactic regimes.

Dose requirements (usually expressed in milligrams) vary with individual drugs and with the degree of risk involved.

Danaparoid is a heparinoid which is also used for the prophylaxis of thromboembolism. These drugs are occasionally indicated when thrombocytopenia develops during the use of unfractionated heparin.

The publication of the National Confidential Enquiry into Perioperative Deaths (NCEPOD) implicated pulmonary embolism as an important cause of mortality (7% of all deaths) in postoperative surgical patients. There is little doubt that failure to administer prophylactic anticoagulant therapy to patients in whom it is considered appropriate may have important therapeutic and medicolegal consequences. However, a sense of balance must be achieved. There are many systemic and surgical contraindications to the use of heparin. Special care must be taken with patients who are concomitantly receiving non-steroidal anti-inflammatory drugs (NSAIDs). All drugs in this group may prolong the bleeding time; the concomitant use of ketorolac and low-dose heparin regimes in the perioperative period is specifically contraindicated, and dose-related effects can be anticipated when other NSAIDs are used. The timing of spinal and extradural blockade in the presence of anticoagulants must also be carefully considered. Present recommendations are that these blocks should be performed before heparin is administered, or at least 4–6 h after the last dose (a longer latent period should be observed when a LMWH is used).

Anticoagulation during surgical procedures

It is essential that anticoagulants are administered before cardiopulmonary bypass is commenced. The usual recommended dose is 300 units kg^{-1} given 4 min before the insertion of the cannulae. Further increments (50–100 units kg^{-1} for each hour of bypass) may be necessary; an *in vitro* test of coagulation, such as the activated clotting time (ACT), performed in theatre is helpful. A value approximately three times the control is desirable. Heparinization is also required prior to aortic clamping during peripheral vascular surgery. A dose of 150 units kg^{-1} is used initially and again measurement of the ACT in the operating theatre is of value in verifying control and the need for subsequent dosage.

Heparin has also been used in the treatment of disseminated intravascular coagulation (DIC). This condition is commonly associated with the introduction of thromboplastic material into the circulation and can occur following obstetric accidents, major trauma, severe infections, neoplastic disorders and liver failure. The widespread development of thrombi will consume clotting factors; fibrin degradation products are also liberated, the circulating blood becomes incoagulable and a haemorrhagic diathesis will ensue. Heparin may arrest the coagulation process by allowing the accumulation of clotting factors and lead to cessation of bleeding; however, the bleeding tendency may actually worsen. In these circumstances inhibitors of fibrinolysis (see below) may be of some value and reversal of the effects of heparin by protamine will be required. It is more important to replace platelets and fibrinogen (as cryoprecipitate) urgently, followed by other factors (such as fresh frozen plasma). Although the coagulation process in DIC can readily be controlled with heparin, patients often die from the adult respiratory distress syndrome (ARDS).

Protamine

Protamine is a highly basic compound which will rapidly neutralize the effects of heparin. Protamine is commercially available as a sulphate salt which is always administered by the intravenous route; slow rates of injection are employed in order to reduce the likelihood of anaphylactoid reactions. The dose required will depend on the time at which the heparin has been given previously but should not exceed 1 mg per 80–100 units of heparin (to a maximum dose of 50 mg). Overdosage may exacerbate any bleeding problems, as protamine is itself a weak anticoagulant which can inhibit the formation and activity of thromboplastin.

Oral anticoagulants

Oral anticoagulants were eventually introduced into clinical practice following the accidental discovery that cattle fed on a spoiled sweet-clover silage developed a haemorrhagic disorder. The cause was traced to a severe reduction in plasma prothrombin, and it was shown that the defect could be prevented by adding alfalfa, which is a rich source of vitamin K, to the diet. The haemorrhagic agents which was present in the silage was subsequently identified as dicoumarol. Dicoumarol was first used clinically as an anticoagulant in 1941. A racemic analogue, warfarin sodium, which was originally utilized as a rat poison and considered to be too toxic for use in humans, is now the drug of choice. A related group of compounds, the indanediones, are more likely to cause hypersensitivity responses than the coumarins.

Oral anticoagulants antagonize the action of vitamin K, which is involved in the synthesis of prothrombin and of factors VII, IX and X. The precursors of these clotting factors, which are produced in the liver and appear in the plasma, have antigenic properties but are biologically inactive. Their subsequent activation requires carboxylation of glutamic acid residues on the molecule; the resultant products can then chelate calcium (which allows them to bind to phospholipid membranes and produce their coagulant effects).

Carboxylation of the inactive precursors is coupled to the conversion of vitamin K from the reduced (hydroquinone) to the oxidized (epoxide) form. Subsequent regeneration (and thus further availability) of the hydroquinone requires the presence of a cofactor, NADH (the reduced form of nicotinamide adenine dinucleotide) and

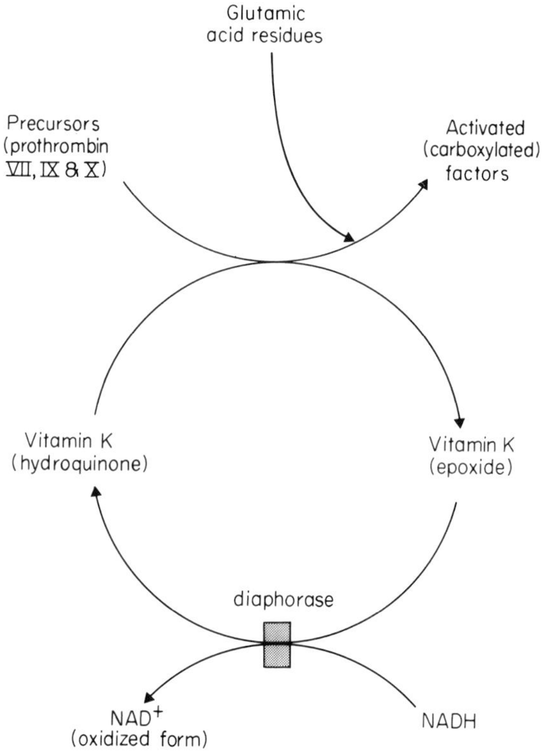

Fig. 16.2 The mode of action of vitamin K and its modification by oral anticoagulants. The principal site of action of warfarin and related compounds is denoted by the shaded box.

an enzyme, diaphorase (epoxide reductase). This latter reaction is considered to be inhibited by the oral anticoagulants (Fig. 16.2).

Oral anticoagulants will be without influence on previously activated clotting factors and thus be ineffective *in vitro*. Furthermore, their activity *in vivo* will be delayed whilst these circulating factors are removed from the plasma. The elimination half-lives of the various factors range from 5 to 60 h. The therapeutic effect of the initial dose will thus be delayed for up to 12 h, whilst the maximal required response may take 48–72 h to develop.

Warfarin is rapidly and completely absorbed from the gastrointestinal tract and peak plasma concentrations are achieved within 1 h. Warfarin is almost completely bound (95–98%) to plasma proteins. Diffusion across various membrane barriers (e.g. blood–brain barrier, glomerular membrane) is thus partly restricted and the volume of distribution (0.1 l kg^{-1}) reflects the volume of the vascular bed. However, the administration of warfarin during pregnancy may cause fetal bleeding and malformations, as it is relatively lipid-soluble and can readily cross the placental barrier. The elimination half-life of warfarin is normally about 35 h; the isomers undergo both oxidative and reductive metabolism and subsequently form glucuronide conjugates which are excreted in the urine.

Considerable variability may be observed in the response to oral anticoagulants, and three factors may be implicated:

1 The availability of vitamin K and the various clotting factors.
2 Pharmacogenetic differences.
3 The influence of other drugs administered concurrently.

Availability

Any condition which reduces the availability of vitamin K, (e.g. dietary deficiency, decreased synthesis or absorption in the gastrointestinal tract) will enhance the response to oral anticoagulants. Similarly, patients with liver disease will exhibit augmented effects, presumably due to impaired synthesis of the various clotting factors. Biotransformation of the vitamin K-dependent clotting factors is considerably influenced by the metabolic rate; thus the response to oral anticoagulants is decreased in myxoedema but enhanced in fever and hyperthyroidism.

Pharmacogenetic differences

Resistance to the effects of oral anticoagulants in some instances appears to be due to hereditary factors. The mechanism of action in these circumstances is unclear. Genetic variations in a suppressor substance which inhibits the synthesis of clotting factors, or the development of resistant forms of the enzyme diaphorase (epoxide reductase) which reduces vitamin K epoxide to its active form, have both been suggested. Congenital antithrombin III deficiency may give rise to severe reactions to warfarin.

The influence of other drugs

Oral anticoagulants may be involved in a number of drug interactions which can have serious clinical consequences. Aspirin and most NSAIDs will enhance the pharmacological effects of oral anticoagulants. Even a single dose of aspirin will reduce platelet aggregation, prolong bleeding time and impair haemostasis, whilst larger doses will inhibit prothrombin synthesis and decrease plasma levels. In addition to these mechanisms, phenylbutazone and related compounds will potentiate the anticoagulant effects by displacing warfarin from plasma-binding sites and by inhibiting the metabolism of the drug.

A number of other drugs can also prolong and enhance the response to oral anticoagulants and increase the likelihood of bleeding. In most instances competition for protein binding sites and metabolizing enzymes appears to be implicated. Drugs in this category include cimetidine, chloramphenicol, disulfiram, metronidazole and ketoconazole. Alcohol may prolong the clearance of warfarin.

Drugs with significant enzyme-inducing activity (e.g. barbiturates, dichloralphenazone, rifampicin, oral contraceptives) will stimulate the metabolism of oral anticoagulants and thus increase the dose requirement if these drugs are being used concomitantly. When the administration of the inducing agent is stopped the activity of the anticoagulant is increased, and dangerous or fatal haemorrhage may occur if the dosage is not adjusted accordingly.

Oral anticoagulants are used in the prophylaxis and treatment of deep venous thrombosis, pulmonary embolism, transient ischaemic attacks and in the management of poorly controlled atrial fibrillation. They are also used to prevent the deposition of thrombi on prosthetic heart valves and vascular grafts. When oral anticoagulant therapy is instituted, a baseline prothrombin time should be determined. The usual induction dose of warfarin is 10 mg daily for 3 days but this should be reduced in small or elderly subjects, in patients with liver disease or cardiac failure, or if the control prothrombin time is prolonged. The aim of treatment is to increase the prothrombin time so that the INR is maintained between 2 and 4.5. In the treatment of deep vein thrombosis, pulmonary embolism and transient ischaemic attacks, the ratio should be maintained between 2 and 3. However, in the management of recurrent deep vein thrombosis or pulmonary embolism, arterial grafts and cardiac prosthetic valves, a higher level (INR 3–4.5) is necessary. The maintenance dose will thus depend on the laboratory results desired and achieved; the INR should be determined on the second and third days of treatment and subsequently on alternate days until a stable level is attained. As previously mentioned, heparin must be administered simultaneously until the therapeutic effects of the oral anticoagulant have been achieved.

When surgery is contemplated on patients receiving oral anticoagulants, the INR should be measured. A level not greater than 2 is acceptable (and may even be desirable) as prophylaxis against further thrombotic episodes. However, the problems of perioperative control of warfarin levels due to surgical interference, and possible interactions with drugs which are administered during anaesthesia, suggest that in many cases a low-dose heparin regime should be substituted. When the INR is greater than 2, management will depend upon the urgency of the surgery and the need for anticoagulant control. An acceptable prothrombin level may be attained by withholding warfarin therapy for a day or two. If this cannot be achieved because of surgical necessity, the infusion of fresh frozen plasma (with appropriate haematological monitoring) is a rapidly effective and controllable method of correcting the coagulation defect. Vitamin K_1 should not be used as the reversal of its effects cannot be controlled easily.

Absolute or relative overdosage of oral anticoagulants can lead to frank haemorrhage. Bleeding may occur at various sites, including the gastrointestinal tract, lung, central nervous system and skin. In these circumstances, the administration of fresh frozen plasma or the various clotting factors is necessary and the cause must be investigated. In addition, phytomenadione may be given in a dose of 2.5–10 mg by slow intravenous injection.

Thrombin inhibitors

Inhibitors of thrombin (e.g. argatroban, hirudin) have been developed. They may act at various subsites on the molecule to produce reversible binding or the formation of slowly reversible complexes. They can directly inhibit clot-bound thrombin, are not affected by circulating inhibitors and function independently of antithrombin III. Some of these low molecular weight compounds may become available for oral administration.

Antiplatelet drugs

Drugs in this group will exert their effects by inhibiting platelet function. Platelets have long been known to play an important role in the production of arterial thrombi in patients with pre-existing vascular damage due to atheroma; there is some evidence to suggest that platelets may be involved in the process of atherogenesis itself. However, the role of platelets in the production of venous thrombi is less clear. Thus the principal indication for the use of antiplatelet agents is the prevention or management of thromboembolic episodes which originate on the arterial side of the circulation. These will include prophylaxis following cardiac or arterial surgery, the prevention and treatment of cerebral ischaemia or myocardial infarction, and the inhibition of thrombus formation in haemodialysis equipment or in pump oxygenators. Accelerated atherosclerosis in coronary arteries after heart transplantation and small-vessel occlusion in transplanted kidneys have been attributed to immune-mediated endothelial injury and may also be preventable by antiplatelet drugs.

Aspirin

Aspirin exerts an antiplatelet effect by acetylating and irreversibly inhibiting platelet cyclooxygenase. This enzyme promotes the synthesis of thromboxane A_2 (TXA_2), a potent vasoconstrictor (which also induces platelet aggregation by promoting the release of ADP). The production by vascular endothelium of prostacyclin (PGI_2), an autacoid whose biological effects are diametrically opposed to those of thromboxane, is similarly inhibited by aspirin. However, both clinical and experimental evidence suggests that the overall effect is a reduction in platelet aggregation. This may reflect an imbalance in the haemostatic mechanism due to a defect in the production of PGI_2 by damaged endothelium.

A large number of studies have been undertaken to assess the long-term effect of variable doses of aspirin (from 75 to 325 mg daily) in the prevention of primary and secondary myocardial infarction or cerebral ischaemia. Encouraging results have been obtained in reducing the frequency of transient ischaemic attacks and the incidence of strokes in male patients. Aspirin also appears to reduce the incidence of myocardial infarction in patients with unstable angina.

There is some evidence that the perioperative use of aspirin can reduce the incidence of thromboembolic phenomena following certain surgical procedures. In particular, a statistically significant reduction of these complications has been demonstrated after hip replacement surgery in male patients pretreated with aspirin. Other NSAIDs can produce the same effect, but are not normally used as antiplatelet drugs. However, the use of all NSAIDs during the perioperative period occasionally results in severe bleeding, during or after the surgical procedure, which can be difficult to control. The associated platelet deficiency and dysfunction suggest that hypersensitivity responses may be involved.

Dipyridamole

Dipyridamole is a drug which has many similar effects to those of papaverine, and was originally introduced into clinical practice for the treatment of angina. It is a potent coronary vasodilator, but apparently has little effect on vascular resistance and is therefore no longer used for this purpose. Dipyridamole appears to reduce platelet aggregation by two mechanisms.

1 Reversible inhibition of phosphodiesterase (isoenzyme V) activity in platelets occurs. The resultant increase in cyclic adenosine monophosphate levels may impair platelet aggregation by sequestrating calcium ions in the cytosol and inhibiting phospholipase activity.

2 Uptake of adenosine into erythrocytes is blocked by dipyridamole. The increased plasma concentration of adenosine may then reach a level at which adenosine diphosphate-induced platelet aggregation is inhibited.

Dipyridamole is used with oral anticoagulants to prevent thrombus formation on prosthetic heart valves, or independently as a prophylactic measure against transient ischaemic attacks. The drug is administered orally in three to four divided doses before food; the daily requirement is usually 300–600 mg. Side-effects include throbbing headache and postural hypotension. Dipyridamole can potentiate the effects of oral anticoagulants and special care must be taken in monitoring prothrombin activity when these drugs are used in combination.

Sulphinpyrazone

Sulphinpyrazone is a uricosuric agent which is used in the treatment of gout to prevent tubular reabsorption of urates. It has also been shown to be a reversible inhibitor of prostaglandin synthetase (cyclooxygenase) and to impair platelet aggregation. Initial studies suggested that long-term treatment with this drug significantly reduced the incidence of myocardial reinfarction, but these have not been substantiated. Sulphinpyrazone may potentiate the effects of oral anticoagulants, oral hypoglycaemic agents and phenytoin.

A number of other drugs have been in vogue at various times for their antiplatelet effect, and have been used either alone or in combination for the prophylaxis of deep venous thrombosis, particularly in the perioperative period. These include the antimalarial agent hydroxychloroquine, the lipid-lowering agent clofibrate, biguanide hypoglycaemic agents and certain anabolic steroids. In many cases the underlying mechanism of action is obscure and the likelihood of undesirable effects or drug interactions high. They can no longer be recommended in this context.

Dazoxiben is a drug which has been shown selectively to inhibit synthesis of TXA_2 *in vitro*. However, it does not appear to reduce platelet aggregation unless used in combination with low doses of aspirin, and has not as yet been introduced into clinical practice in the UK.

Ticlopidine appears to prevent platelet aggregation independently of any effect on prostaglandin synthesis. Ticlopinide inhibits the binding of fibrinogen to platelets by interacting with a specific glycoprotein receptor on the fibrinogen. The drug is available in the USA, and is currently used for prevention of thrombosis in cerebrovascular and coronary artery disease, and may be particularly recommended for patients unable to tolerate aspirin. Ticlopidine has also been used to prevent thrombus formation in heart–lung bypass machines.

Low molecular weight dextrans

Dextrans, which are sometimes used as plasma expanders, are polysaccharides which contain long chains of glucose units and are produced by fermentation of a sucrose medium with the bacterium *Leuconostoc mesenteroides*. These glucose polymers have molecular weights which range from 10 to 50 kDa and a number of preparations are commercially available.

Dextran 40 is prepared as a 10% solution in either 5% glucose or 0.9% saline. The resulting compound contains glucans with an average molecular weight of 40 kDa and has a slightly higher osmotic pressure than that due to plasma proteins.

Dextran 70 is produced as a 6% solution in either isotonic saline or dextrose; the average molecular weight of the contained glucans is of the order of 70 kDa and the osmotic pressure of the solution equates with that of plasma.

When added to blood *in vitro*, dextrans appear to have no effect on platelet function. However, following the infusion of these solutions, bleeding time may be prolonged, polymerization of fibrin impaired and platelet function reduced. Thus, in addition to their use as plasma substitutes to maintain blood volume in hypovolaemic shock, dextrans are sometimes administered in the prophylaxis of thromboembolic complications following surgical procedures. Furthermore, the infusion of dextran 40 can reduce the viscosity of plasma and the intravascular agglutination of erythrocytes, and may be indicated to enhance peripheral flow in small blood vessels.

The administration of dextrans is not without possible hazards. Overloading of the circulation may be especially dangerous in patients with pre-existing cardiac or renal disease. Anaphylactoid reactions, which may manifest as urticaria, bronchospasm or hypotension, can occur, and hypersensitivity responses observed in unconscious subjects are considered to be more extensive. Dextrans with higher molecular weights induce erythrocyte aggregation into rouleaux formation and increase the sedimentation rate; they may also interfere with blood grouping and cross-matching and certain biochemical tests.

Other colloidal volume expanders such as hydroxyethyl starch and urea-bridged gelatin (Haemaccel) may also diminish platelet aggregation to some extent.

Epoprostenol (PGI_2) is a naturally occurring prostaglandin which is produced by the intima of blood vessels. It is a potent vasodilator and produces dose-related inhibitory effects on platelet aggregation. Epoprostenol is now commercially available and is used as an alternative to heparin during renal dialysis. The plasma half-life of this agent is only about 3 min, so that it must be given by continuous intravenous infusion, usually at a rate of 5 ng kg^{-1} min^{-1}. Side-effects include flushing, headache and hypotension, whilst bradycardia, pallor and sweating may occur with higher doses.

Fibrinolytic agents

When the clotting mechanism is activated, an opposing process, the fibrinolytic system, is also initiated by tissue damage and results in the formation of a proteolytic enzyme (plasmin) which breaks down fibrin with subsequent dissolution of the clot. Plasmin itself is not normally present in the circulation but exists as an inactive precursor, plasminogen, contained in the α_2-globulin fraction of plasma protein. The conversion of plasminogen to plasmin results from the effects of tissue-bound plasminogen activators which are released from the endothelium of damaged blood vessels (e.g. the active form of the Hageman factor — factor XII) and from similar substances present in the circulation. The rate of fibrinolysis is normally controlled by antiplasmins which are also present in the plasma and may be released from the platelets. The principal steps involved in the fibrinolytic process are shown in Fig. 16.3.

Plasminogen activators are also produced at a number of other tissue sites and can be recovered from various secretions such as urine, milk, tears and sweat, where they may play a normal physiological role in preventing fibrin deposition in the ducts. One such substance, urokinase, was originally identified in human urine in 1885 and later prepared from cultures of human renal cells; a related compound, streptokinase, was obtained from group C haemolytic streptococci in 1945. Both of these agents have subsequently been introduced into clinical practice for the treatment of widespread venous thrombosis associated with pulmonary embolism, the management of myocardial infarction and for localized thrombolytic effects.

Urokinase

Urokinase is a globulin which directly converts plasminogen to plasmin in a two-stage reaction. It has been used in clinical trials for the treatment of pulmonary

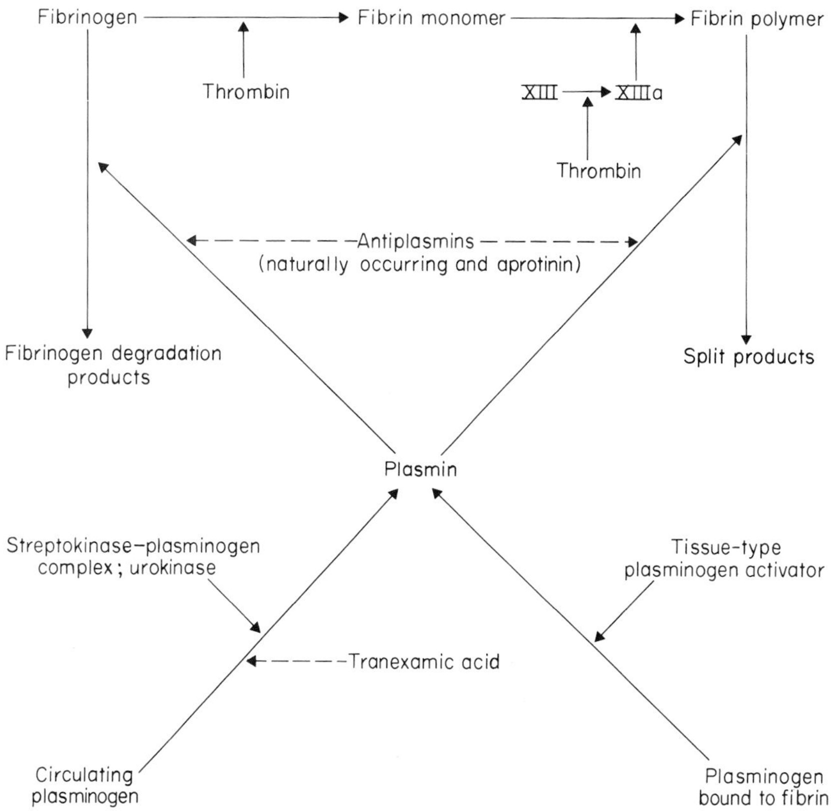

Fig. 16.3 The fibrinolytic system: stimulatory processes (solid arrows); inhibitory effects (broken arrows).

embolism, but the resultant systemic bleeding disorders have precluded its more generalized use. Urokinase is currently recommended for its local thrombolytic effects and may be instilled into an AV shunt to lyse a clot, or irrigated into the anterior or vitreous chambers of the eye in the treatment of refractory thrombi. In these circumstances a dose range of 5000–25 000 i.u. is used and haematological monitoring is not required. More recently, the use of genetic technology has led to the production of recombinant pro-urokinase or recombinant single-chain urokinase plasminogen activator; this has undergone trials in the treatment of acute myocardial infarction.

Streptokinase

Streptokinase forms a complex with plasminogen and this complex is rapidly converted to plasmin. Streptokinase has established a role in the treatment of various arterial and venous thromboembolic disorders. In many regimes, anticoagulant therapy is withdrawn, and a loading dose of 250 000 i.u. administered into a peripheral vein over 30 min; therapy is then maintained for up to 72 h, using a dose of 100 000 i.u. hourly. Haematological monitoring, including estimations of thrombin and prothrombin times, haematocrit and platelet levels is necessary before commencing treatment and during infusion. Following this regime, and when the thrombin time has returned to a value of less than twice the normal, heparin should be administered (preferably by continuous infusion) to prevent recurrent thrombosis. More commonly, streptokinase is used in the treatment of myocardial infarction in patients presenting within 6 h of the acute episode. In this context a dose of 1 500 000 i.u. is infused over 60 min.

Streptokinase is antigenic and may produce drug fever, allergic manifestations and overt anaphylaxis. The incidence of such side-effects is reduced by the use of slow infusion rates and the administration of prophylactic steroids. Treatment of major hypersensitivity responses may involve the use of adrenaline and both H_1- and H_2-receptor antagonists.

Streptokinase has also been administered locally in the treatment of myocardial infarction. Therapy is ideally given within 6 h of the onset of symptoms. Standard techniques for selective coronary angiography by either the brachial or femoral approach are used to identify the presence and location of the thrombus. In these circumstances a bolus dose of up to 250 000 i.u. is administered, followed by a continuous infusion of 4000 i.u. min^{-1} for up to 75 min until vessel patency is restored. Subsequent heparin therapy will again be necessary.

Intracoronary administration of streptokinase is a highly skilled and potentially hazardous procedure, which of necessity must be restricted to regional cardiology centres and other highly specialized units. Intravenous therapy with streptokinase involves a simpler and easily performed regime, although there is some evidence that recanalization of the occluded vessel is less likely with this method. Furthermore, there is theoretically an increased risk of bleeding complications due to a greater availability of plasmin in the systemic circulation. One attempt to circumvent this problem has been the use of improved drug-delivery systems for streptokinase.

Anisoylated plasminogen–streptokinase activator complex (APSAC) is a compound in which streptokinase forms a complex with an acylated (and thus a temporarily inactivated) form of plasminogen. Following intravenous injection of APSAC, deacylation to the activated form of plasminogen occurs by hydrolysis. The half-life of this deacylation process is approximately 40 min and it is considered that APSAC is relatively well-protected during its passage in the circulation to sites of recent thrombosis, where it acts preferentially on clot fibrin, whilst less systemic fibrinolysis occurs.

An alternative approach to more selective targeting of fibrinolytic therapy is in the development of tissue-type plasminogen activator (t-PA) for clinical use. t-PA has a much lower affinity for circulating plasminogen than for that which is bound to fibrin. Thus, very little plasmin is produced in the general circulation, even at high plasma concentrations of t-PA. This activator has been purified from cultured human melanoma cells and an identical material (rt-PA) reproduced using recombinant DNA techniques. However, it is as yet unclear whether APSAC or rt-PA produces a greater long-term benefit or a reduction in bleeding complications as compared with systemic streptokinase.

Stanozolol is an anabolic steroid with relatively low androgenic activity which can enhance endogenous fibrinolysis by increasing the synthesis and release of plasminogen activator in the vessel wall. Stanozolol is used in the treatment of Behçet's disease (Raynaud's syndrome associated with systemic sclerosis and lipodermatosclerosis), to control attacks of hereditary angioedema, and in the management of adhesive arachnoiditis associated with failed disc surgery.

Inhibitors of fibrinolysis

Drugs in this category can inhibit the conversion of plasminogen to plasmin, and in higher doses antagonize the effects of plasmin. They have been used as antidotes for the treatment of overdosage of a fibrinolytic agent. On occasions they have also been administered in the treatment of pathological states associated with hyperfibrinolytic activity, as may occur following obstetric accidents or prostatic surgery, and in the management of haemorrhage in haemophilic disorders.

Aminocaproic acid is a synthetic compound which is structurally related to lysine. It has been used as an oral preparation and also administered intravenously; in the latter case a slow rate of injection is important to avoid hypotension and arrhythmias. It is no longer commercially available in the UK.

Tranexamic acid, a cyclohexyl analogue of aminocaproic acid, is a more potent inhibitor of plasmin and has been used in similar circumstances. The occurrence of renal, hepatic and occasionally cardiac necrotic lesions has been reported following the use of these agents, and these have been attributed to failure of the fibrinolytic system to remove clots which have formed spontaneously. This undoubtedly accounts for the decline in their popularity and availability and they should only be administered, if at all, following expert haematological advice.

Miscellaneous agents

Ancrod

Ancrod is a proteolytic enzyme which has been isolated from the venom of the Malayan pit-viper. Ancrod reduces plasma fibrinogen by promoting the cleavage of fibrin. Microemboli are produced which are rapidly removed from the circulation; fibrinogen is depleted and the blood becomes less coagulable. The effect observed can be considered as a benign and controlled form of DIC. Ancrod has been used on occasions in the prevention and treatment of deep venous thrombosis. The drug can be given by intramuscular or intravenous routes; in the latter case a slow rate of infusion is necessary to avoid the rapid release of fibrin degradation products. Response can be monitored by observing clot size or by measuring plasma fibrinogen levels. The effects of overdosage can be reversed by a specific antivenom (which is itself antigenic) or by replacement of fibrinogen. In the UK, ancrod is now only available on a 'named-patient' basis.

Ethamsylate

Ethamsylate is sometimes used as a haemostatic agent in the treatment of menorrhagia and to control capillary bleeding during a variety of surgical procedures. Following systemic administration, the bleeding time is reduced, although platelet levels and clotting factors are unaffected. Ethamsylate is considered to act by improving capillary stability and by promoting the aggregation of platelets. The mechanism of action is unclear but may be related to an inhibitory effect on prostacyclins. The drug is marketed in the UK as Dicynene and is available both in tablet form and as a parenteral preparation. Side-effects are rare but may include headache, nausea and skin rashes; transient falls of blood pressure have been reported following intravenous administration.

Aprotinin

Aprotinin is a proteolytic enzyme inhibitor which exerts antiplasmin activity. It has been recommended for the treatment of severe haemorrhage in hyperfibrinolytic states, in particular those associated with malignant disease or ensuing from thrombolytic therapy. More recently, aprotinin has been used with success to reduce blood loss during open-heart surgery and other major surgical procedures. The drug is also a kallikrein (trypsin) inhibitor, and has been used in the treatment of acute pancreatitis. Aprotinin is always administered by slow intravenous infusion; localized thrombophlebitis has occasionally been associated with its use and severe hypersensitivity responses have occurred.

Desmopressin acetate

Desmopressin acetate (also known as DDAVP) is a synthetic analogue of vasopressin which lacks vasoconstrictor activity. It has been used to improve haemostasis in patients with mild haemophilia or von Willebrand's disease; in these conditions it apparently induces the release of the required coagulation factors. Desmopressin has also been employed to shorten the bleeding time in other conditions involving abnormal platelet function (e.g. uraemia, following ingestion of aspirin) and has been used successfully to reduce blood loss following cardiac surgery.

Further reading

Andersen JL, Marshall HW, Askings RW. A randomised trial of intravenous and intracoronary streptokinase in patients with acute myocardial infarction. *Circulation* 1984; **70**: 606–618.

Antiplatelet Trialists Collaboration. Secondary prevention of vascular disease by prolonged antiplatelet treatment. *British Medical Journal* 1988; **296**: 320–331.

Barnett DB. Myocardial ischaemia: progress in drug therapy. *British Journal of Anaesthesia* 1988; **61**: 11–23.

Bentley PG, Kakkar VV, Scully MF *et al.* An objective study of alternative methods of heparin administration. *Thrombosis Research* 1980; **18**: 1977–1987.

Beresford CH. Antithrombin III deficiency. *Blood Reviews* 1988; **2**: 239–250.

British Society for Haematology. Guidelines on the use and monitoring of heparin therapy: First Revision 1987: 1–12.

Brown JE, Kitchell BB, Bjornsson TD, Shand DG. The artifactural nature of heparin-induced drug protein-binding alterations. *Clinical Pharmacology and Therapeutics* 1981; **30**: 636–643.

Bull BS, Huse WM, Braven SS, Korpman RA. Heparin therapy during extracorporeal circulation. *Journal of Thoracic and Cardiovascular Surgery* 1975; **69**: 685–689.

Bullingham A, Strunin L. Prevention of postoperative thromboembolism. *British Journal of Anaesthesia* 1995; **75**: 622–630.

Campling E, Devlin H, Hoile R, Lunn J. *The Report of the National Confidential Enquiry into Perioperative Deaths 1991/2*. London: Eyre & Spottiswoode, 1993; 64–199.

Davie EW, Ratnoff OD. Waterfall sequence for intrinsic blood clotting. *Science* 1964; **145**: 1310–1312.

Evarts CM, Feil EJ. Prevention of thromboembolic disease after elective surgery of the hip. *Journal of Bone and Joint Surgery* 1971; **53A**: 1271–1280.

Gallus AS. Antiplatelet drugs: clinical pharmacology and therapeutic use. *Drugs* 1979; **18**: 439–477.

Gallus AS, Goodall KT, Tillet J *et al.* The relative contributions of antithrombin III during heparin treatment and of risk factors, to early recurrence of venous thromboembolism. *Thrombosis Research* 1987; **46**: 539–553.

GISSI. Effectiveness of intravenous thrombolytic therapy in acute myocardial infarction. *Lancet* 1986; **i**: 397–402.

Haagensen R, Steen PA. Perioperative myocardial infarction. *British Journal of Anaesthesia* 1988; **61**: 24–37.

Hambley H, Davidson JF, Walker ID, Menzies T. Prophylactic use of antithrombin concentrate following surgery in congenital antithrombin III deficiency. *Clinical and Laboratory Haematology* 1987; **9**: 27–31.

Hamilton PJ, Stalker AL, Douglas AS. Disseminated intravascular coagulation — a review. *Journal of Clinical Pathology* 1978; **31**: 609–619.

Hammond EC, Garfunkel L. Aspirin and coronary heart disease: findings of a prospective study. *British Medical Journal* 1975; **2**: 269–271.

Harris WH, Saltzman EW, Athanasoulis CA *et al.* Comparison of warfarin, low-molecular-weight dextran, aspirin and subcutaneous heparin in prevention of venous thrombo-embolism following total hip replacement. *Journal of Bone and Joint Surgery* 1974; **56A**: 1552–1562.

Harris WH, Saltzman EW, Athanasoulis CA *et al.* Aspirin prophylaxis of venous thrombo-embolism after total hip replacement. *New England Journal of Medicine* 1977; **297**: 1246–1249.

Hennekens CH, Peto R, Hutchinson GB, Doll R. An overview of the British and American aspirin studies. *New England Journal of Medicine* 1988; **318**: 923–924.

Hirsh J. Heparin. *New England Journal of Medicine* 1991; **324**: 1565–1574.

Hirsh J. Rationale for development of low molecular weight heparins and their clinical potential in the prevention of postoperative venous thrombosis. *American Journal of Surgery* 1991; **161**: 512–518.

Howell WH. Heparin, an anticoagulant. Preliminary communication. *American Journal of Physiology* 1922; **63**: 434–435.

Hull R, Hirsh J, Jay R *et al.* Different intensities of oral anticoagulant therapy in the treatment of proximal vein thrombosis. *New England Journal of Medicine* 1982; **307**: 1676–1681.

Ikram S, Lewis S, Bucknall C *et al.* Treatment of acute myocardial infarction with anisoylated plasminogen streptokinase activator complex. *British Medical Journal* 1986; **93**: 786–789.

Inman WH, Vessey MP, Westerholm B, Engleund A. Thromboembolism and the steroidal content of oral contraceptives: a report to the Committee of Safety of Drugs. *British Medical Journal* 1970; **2**: 203–209.

ISIS-2 Collaborative Group. Randomised trial of intravenous streptokinase, oral aspirin, both or neither among 17 187 cases of suspected acute myocardial infarction. *Lancet* 1988; **ii**: 349–360.

Kakkar VV, Scully MF. Thrombolytic therapy. *British Medical Bulletin* 1978; **34**: 191–199.

Kitchens CS. Concept of hypercoagulability: a review of its development, clinical application and recent progress. *Seminars in Thrombosis and Haemostasis* 1985; **11**: 293–315.

Kroll MH, Schafer AL. Biochemical mechanisms of platelet activation. *Blood* 1989; **74**: 1181–1195.

Lewis RJ, Trager WF. Warfarin. Stereochemical aspects of its metabolism and the interaction with phenylbutazone. *Journal of Clinical Investigation* 1974; **53**: 1607–1617.

Link KP. Discovery of dicumarol and its sequels. *Circulation* 1959; **19**: 97–107.

Ljungstrom K-G. Prophylaxis of postoperative thromboembolism with dextran 70: improvements of efficacy and safety. *Acta Chirurgica Scandinavica* 1983; **514** (suppl.): 1–39.

Loeliger EA. The optimal therapeutic range in oral anticoagulation. History and proposal. *Thrombosis and Haemostasis* 1979; **42**: 1141–1152.

Loscalzo J, Braunwald E. Drug therapy: tissue plasminogen activator. *New England Journal of Medicine* 1988; **319**: 925–931.

Lowe GDO, Greer IA, Cooke TG *et al*. Thromboembolic Risk Factors (THRIFT) Consensus Group. Risk of prophylaxis for venous thromboembolism in hospital patients. *British Medical Journal* 1992; **305**: 567–574.

McCann RL, Sabiston DC. Current management of venous thromboembolic disease. *British Journal of Surgery* 1989; **76**: 113–114.

Majerus PW, Broze GR Jr, Miletich JP, Tollefsen DM. Anticoagulant, thrombolytic, and antiplatelet drugs. In: Hardman JG, Limbird LE (eds) *Goodman & Gilman's The Pharmacological Basis of Therapeutics*, 9th edn. New York: McGraw-Hill, 1995.

Mannucci PM, Tripodi A. Laboratory screening of inherited thrombotic syndromes. *Thrombosis and Haemostasis* 1987; **57**: 247–251.

Macfarlane RG. An enzyme cascade in the blood clotting mechanism and its function as a biochemical amplifier. *Nature* 1964; **202**: 498–499.

Marciniak E, Gluckerman JP. Heparin-induced decrease in circulating antithrombin III. *Lancet* 1977; **ii**: 581–584.

Mishler JM. Synthetic plasma volume expanders — their pharmacological safety and clinical efficiency. *Clinics and Haematology* 1984; **13**: 75–92.

Morris GK, Mitchell JRA. Warfarin sodium in prevention of deep venous thrombosis and pulmonary embolism in patients with fractured neck of femur. *Lancet* 1976; **ii**: 869–872.

Morris GK, Mitchell JRA. The aetiology of pulmonary embolism and the identification of high risk groups. *British Journal of Hospital Medicine* 1977; **18**: 6–12.

Morris GK, Mitchell JRA. Preventing venous thromboembolism in elderly patients with hip fractures: studies of low dose heparin, dipyridamole, aspirin and flurbiprofen. *British Medical Journal* 1977; **1**: 535–537.

Morris GK, Mitchell JRA. Clinical management of venous thromboembolism. *British Medical Bulletin* 1978; **34**: 169–175.

O'Reilly RA. Vitamin K in hereditary resistance to anticoagulant drugs. *American Journal of Physiology* 1971; **221**: 1327–1330.

O'Reilly RA. Vitamin K and the oral anticoagulant drugs. *Annual Review of Medicine* 1976; **27**: 245–261.

Patrono C, Ciabattoni G, Bradrigani P *et al*. Clinical pharmacology of platelet cyclo-oxygenase inhibitors. *Circulation* 1985; **72**: 1177–1184.

Poller L, Taberner DA, Sandilands DG, Galasko CSB. An evaluation of APTT monitoring of low dose heparin dosage in hip surgery. *Thrombosis and Haemostasis* 1982; **47**: 50–53.

PRIMI Trial Study Group. Randomised double-blind trial of recombinant pro-urokinase against streptokinase in acute myocardial infarction. *Lancet* 1989; **ii**: 863–867.

Raskob GE, Carter CJ, Hull RD. Heparin therapy for venous thrombosis and pulmonary embolism. *Blood Reviews* 1989; **2**: 251–258.

Rees DC, Cox M, Clegg JB. World distribution of factor V Leiden. *Lancet* 1995; **346**: 1133–1134.

Rothermel JE, Wessnger JB, Stinchfield FE. Dextran 40 and thromboembolism in total hip replacement surgery. *Archives of Surgery* 1973; **106**: 135–137.

Salzman EW, Weinstein MJ, Weintrub RM *et al*. Treatment with desmopressin acetate to reduce blood loss after cardiac surgery. *New England Journal of Medicine* 1986; **314**: 1402–1406.

Schatt U, Bershus O, Jaremo J. Blood substitution and complement activation. *Acta Anaesthesiologica Scandinavica* 1987; **31**: 559–566.

Scheinberg P. Heparin anticoagulation. *Stroke* 1989; **20**: 173–174.

Sharnoff JG, DeBlasio G. Prevention of fatal postoperative thromboembolism by heparin prophylaxis. *Lancet* 1970; **i**: 1006–1007.

Taparelli C, Metternich R, Ehrhardt C, Cook NS. Synthetic low-molecular weight inhibitors: molecular design and pharmacological profile. *Trends in Pharmacological Sciences* 1993; **14**: 366–376.

Thomas DP. Current status of low molecular weight heparin. *Thrombosis and Haemostasis* 1986; **56**: 241–242.

Tyrrell DJ, Kilfeather S, Page CP. Therapeutic uses of heparin beyond its traditional role as an anticoagulant. *Trends in Pharmacological Sciences* 1995; **16**: 198–204.

Vessey MP, Doll R. Investigation of relation between use of oral contraceptives and thromboembolic disease: a further report. *British Medical Journal* 1969; **2**: 651–657.

Weiss HJ. Drug therapy. Antiplatelet therapy. *New England Journal of Medicine* 1978; **298**: 1344–1347, 1403–1406.

Weston-Smith S, Revell P, Savidge GF. Thrombophilia. *British Journal of Hospital Medicine* 1989; **41**: 368–371.

Chapter 17
Corticosteroids and Hypoglycaemic Agents

Corticosteroids

Corticosteroids (glucocorticoids) are drugs that are based on the steroid nucleus which have complex effects on carbohydrate, protein and fat metabolism. Naturally occurring glucocorticoids (e.g. hydrocortisone or cortisol) are secreted by the zona fasciculata of the adrenal cortex. In addition, a wide range of synthetic compounds with similar actions are used in medicine (e.g. prednisone, prednisolone, methylprednisolone, triamcinolone, betamethasone, dexamethasone). Both naturally occurring and synthetic compounds have similar biological effects.

Pharmacological effects

Protein and carbohydrate metabolism

Glucocorticoids stimulate and enhance gluconeogenesis (i.e. the deamination of proteins and amino acids, and their conversion to glucose and glycogen). Consequently, they cause an increase in protein breakdown and a reduction in protein synthesis; carbohydrate turnover is enhanced, and there is a rise in blood sugar and glycogen levels in liver and muscle. Although these actions are of little therapeutic importance, they are responsible for many of the side-effects of glucocorticoids. Increased protein breakdown causes retardation of growth, reduction in voluntary muscle mass, thinning and ulceration of the skin and mucosae, increased susceptibility to peptic ulceration, the appearance of striae, osteoporosis, vertebral collapse and a susceptibility to pathological fractures. Serum calcium is reduced, although its urinary elimination is enhanced; there is also a rise in the urinary elimination of nitrogen and phosphate. Increased carbohydrate turnover can cause hyperglycaemia, glycosuria and the precipitation of diabetes in predisposed individuals.

Lymphoid tissue and lymphocytes

Corticosteroids tend to cause the generalized atrophy of many lymphoid tissues. In particular, there is a marked decrease in the weight and cellular activity in the spleen, the thymus, the tonsils and lymph nodes. There is also a decrease in the number of circulating lymphocytes (particularly T cells); after intravenous hydrocortisone, the reduction in the lymphocyte count is maximal at 6–8 h. Glucocorticoids inhibit the synthesis and/or release of many lymphokines and interleukins; the reduction in lymphocyte proliferation is probably related to decreased synthesis of interleukin-2 (IL-2), which plays an important role in the division and multiplication of T cells after exposure to antigens. Consequently, glucocorticoids reduce the proliferation and immunological competence of T lymphocytes, and this may account for their effectiveness as immunosuppressant drugs after organ transplantation. They also reduce the concentration of complement, and may indirectly decrease the activity of B lymphocytes and the production of immunoglobulins.

Anti-inflammatory effects

Acute and chronic inflammatory responses are inhibited by corticosteroids, irrespective of their cause. In acute inflammation, corticosteroids decrease tissue transudation and oedema, reduce the diapedesis of polymorphs and macrophages, and prevent the access of immunoglobulins to inflamed tissues. Consequently, they decrease the accumulation of lymphocytes and neutrophil leukocytes at the site of the inflammation in tissues. Similar changes may occur in chronic inflammatory diseases. The activity of fibroblasts and osteoblasts is decreased, and bone density is reduced; in contrast, osteoclastic activity is increased.

The effects of corticosteroids on inflammatory responses may have undesirable effects. Thus, the reduction in the inflammatory response decreases the resistance to infection, and may lead to the reactivation of latent bacterial infections (e.g. tuberculosis). The symptoms and signs of infection may not be apparent until the condition is advanced. Corticosteroids may also lead to the reactivation of peptic ulceration, and gastrointestinal haemorrhage or perforation.

The anti-inflammatory potency of different glucocorticoids is extremely variable. Cortisone and hydrocortisone are the least potent steroids in current use. Prednisone and prednisolone are approximately four times more potent than hydrocortisone; methylprednisolone and triamcinolone are slightly more potent than prednisolone. Betamethasone and dexamethasone are the most potent steroids that are currently available; they are approximately 30 times more potent than hydrocortisone (Table 17.1). This range in potency is believed to reflect the differential affinity of glucocorticoids for intracellular steroid receptors.

Permissive effects

Glucocorticoids also have indirect or permissive actions, and their presence in the body in physiological concentrations is essential in order for certain hormones (e.g. insulin, adrenaline) to produce their effects. The synthesis of adrenaline by the

Table 17.1 The relative anti-inflammatory dose and potency of some common corticosteroids. The doses of each drug compared are equivalent to the daily physiological secretion rate of hydrocortisone.

	Equivalent anti-inflammatory dose (mg)	Equivalent anti-inflammatory potency
Cortisone	37.5	0.8
Hydrocortisone	30	1
Prednisone	7.5	4
Prednisolone	7.5	4
Methylprednisolone	6	5
Triamcinolone	6	5
Paramethasone	3	10
Betamethasone	1	30
Dexamethasone	1	30

adrenal medulla, and many of its metabolic effects, is indirectly dependent on corticosteroids in body fluids. In the presence of glucocorticoids, adrenaline causes lipolysis and increases free fatty acid levels in plasma; these effects are induced by the synthesis of cyclic adenosine monophosphate (cAMP) and a cAMP- and glucocorticoid-dependent protein kinase, which activates lipolytic enzymes in tissues. The general pattern of fat deposition is also affected by glucocorticoids; in continual dosage, they characteristically remove adipose tissue from the limbs, but increase its deposition in the neck, supraclavicular region, trunk, shoulders and face ('buffalo hump' and 'moon face'). Similarly, general anaesthesia in adrenocortical insufficiency may be associated with hypotension, vascular collapse, respiratory depression and delayed recovery; these effects are believed to reflect the resistance of vascular smooth muscle to adrenaline and other endogenous hormones in the absence of glucocorticoids.

Mineralocorticoid effects

Some glucocorticoids affect electrolyte balance and have actions that are similar to aldosterone (i.e. they also have mineralocorticoid effects). Thus, fludrocortisone (and, to a lesser extent, cortisone and hydrocortisone) act on the distal renal tubule, promoting the retention of sodium and chloride ions (and water) in exchange for the elimination of potassium and hydrogen ions. These mineralocorticoid effects are usually present in glucocorticoids whose anti-inflammatory potency is relatively weak; the more potent steroids (e.g. prednisone, prednisolone, triamcinolone, betamethasone, dexamethasone) only have minimal activity, and do not cause salt or water retention (except in very large doses). Corticosteroids with significant mineralocorticoid activity may cause oedema and precipitate hypertension or cardiac failure in susceptible patients.

Mode of action

Many of the pharmacological effects of glucocorticoids (particularly their anti-inflammatory actions) are dependent on their combination with intracellular steroid receptors in target cells, and their subsequent effects on DNA and ribosomal protein synthesis. Consequently, their onset of action is usually relatively slow (i.e. 1–6 h). Glucocorticoid receptors are discrete cytoplasmic proteins that are expressed in most cells, although their density is extremely variable; they are bound in a large-molecular-weight complex with other proteins (e.g. the heat shock protein, Hsp 90) which prevent their translocation to the nucleus. All glucocorticoids are highly lipid-soluble and readily diffuse across the cytoplasmic membrane in inflammatory and other cells, where they are reversibly bound by unoccupied receptors. After activation, the steroid–receptor complexes dissociate from other proteins, translocate to the nucleus and are bound by specific high-affinity binding sites on DNA (steroid regulatory/response elements). The transcription of 10–100 target genes in the immediate vicinity of the steroid-regulatory elements is modified, resulting in subsequent changes in messenger RNA and ribosomal protein synthesis. In addition, the activity of various transcriptional factors involved in inflammatory responses is modified. Thus, the expression of genes which are associated with the production of multiple inflammatory mediators is inhibited, and the synthesis of many of these factors (e.g. phospholipase A_2, cyclooxygenase-2, many cytokines and interleukins, vasocortin and inducible nitric oxide synthase) is decreased. In addition, glucocorticoids indirectly induce the synthesis and intracellular translocation of the lipocortins. This family of glycoproteins inhibit the enzyme phospholipase A_2, which mediates the conversion of membrane phospholipids to arachidonic acid in inflammatory cells (Fig. 17.1). In this manner, the formation of prostaglandins, leukotrienes and platelet-activating factor by target cells is reduced, producing anti-inflammatory effects.

Pharmacokinetics

All glucocorticoids are highly lipid-soluble compounds. Consequently, they are absorbed in the small intestine, highly bound to plasma proteins and extensively metabolized by the liver (usually with significant first-pass effects). Indeed, the effects of cortisone and prednisone are dependent on their initial metabolism in the liver (to hydrocortisone and prednisolone, respectively). After oral administration, the physiological steroids hydrocortisone and corticosterone are bound by a specific plasma globulin (corticosteroid-binding globulin), which is only present in small concentrations (35 mg l^{-1}); although it has a low capacity, it has an extremely high affinity for endogenous steroids. In addition, both naturally occurring and synthetic glucocorticoids (and their metabolites) are bound by albumin, which has a relatively low affinity for steroids.

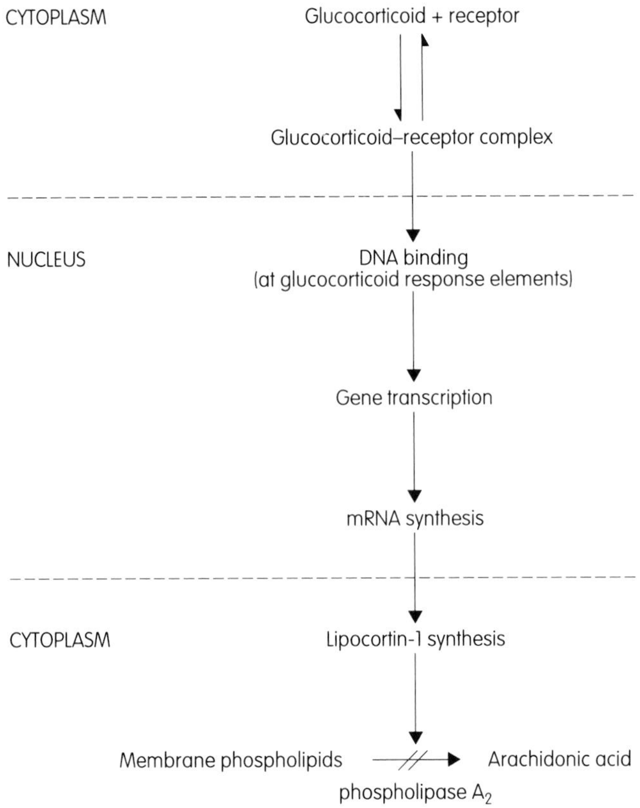

Fig. 17.1 The effects of glucocorticoids on gene transcription, the formation of lipocortin-1, and the synthesis of arachidonic acid by phospholipase A_2. —//→ represents enzyme inhibition by lipocortin-1.

After intravenous administration, most steroids (e.g. hydrocortisone and aldosterone) have a relatively short terminal half-life (90–120 min) due to their extensive hepatic metabolism. After reduction in the endoplasmic reticulum, they are usually eliminated in urine as glucuronide or sulphate conjugates.

Administration

Corticosteroids may be administered orally, parenterally or as local therapy to the skin, into joints or to the respiratory tract, ears or eyes.

Intravenous corticosteroids are most commonly used in emergency situations (e.g. shock, acute anaphylaxis and status asthmaticus). High doses can usually be given safely, as the risk of complications is negligible in patients on short-term therapy. Unfortunately, intravenous corticosteroids do not have an immediate action; although they often begin to act within 1 h, they may take up to 6 h to produce their maximum effects. Intravenous hydrocortisone (100–500 mg) is usually given as the sodium succinate salt, which requires reconstitution prior to injection.

Although the sodium phosphate salts of hydrocortisone or prednisolone can be given intravenously, they may cause unpleasant side-effects after rapid injection (e.g. generalized vasodilatation, pelvic and perineal discomfort), which may be related to their hydrolysis by phosphatase enzymes.

More commonly, corticosteroids are administered orally, and may be given as replacement therapy in Addison's disease, hypopituitarism or after hypophysectomy or adrenalectomy. In these conditions, hydrocortisone, usually supplemented with fludrocortisone, is used. Alternatively, they may be given non-specifically for their anti-inflammatory or antiallergic effects, in order to suppress the manifestations of various diseases. Some of the conditions in which corticosteroids are used are shown in Table 17.2.

Corticosteroids are also given by local application or administration in a wide variety of diseases. For instance, they are widely used in diseases of the skin (e.g. in eczema, lichen planus, discoid lupus erythematosus, neurodermatoses); in diseases of the mouth (oral and perioral ulceration); in ear, nose and throat diseases (allergic rhinitis and eczematous otitis externa); in ophthalmological conditions (e.g. allergic conjunctivitis, keratitis, uveitis); in respiratory diseases (e.g. bronchial asthma, bronchospasm); and intestinal conditions (e.g. ulcerative colitis, proctitis). Local preparations of corticosteroids are used whenever possible in order to limit their systemic side-effects. When oral or parenteral preparations are used in the management of rheumatic, inflammatory or autoimmune diseases, the doses required to control or suppress pathological processes are usually associated with the presence

Table 17.2 Conditions in which corticosteroids are used systemically in order to suppress pharmacological or pathological processes.

Active chronic hepatitis
Acute anaphylaxis
Bronchial asthma
Bronchospasm
Cerebral oedema
Crohn's disease
Gout
Haemolytic anaemia (acquired)
Malignant conditions (acute leukaemia; non-Hodgkin's lymphoma)
Nephrotic syndrome
Polyarteritis nodosa
Polymyalgia rheumatica
Polymyositis
Rheumatoid arthritis
Rheumatic carditis
Systemic lupus erythematosus
Systemic sclerosis
Temporal arteritis
Thrombocytopenic purpura
Transplantation reactions
Ulcerative colitis

of serious and unavoidable side-effects. Indeed, some of these effects may be observed after the use of potent local preparations (particularly when used in the treatment of diseases of the skin). Adverse reactions to systemic corticosteroids are often a limiting factor in their use; although some of these reactions are due to the exaggerated pharmacological effects of steroids, others are obscure in origin (Table 17.3).

Table 17.3 Adverse reactions to systemic corticosteroids.

Causal effects	Reaction
Increased tissue and protein breakdown	Retardation of growth Muscle wasting Myopathy Osteoporosis Vertebral collapse Fractures Thinning of skin, mucosae and hair Cutaneous striae Ecchymoses and bruising Subcutaneous and petechial haemorrhages Gastrointestinal bleeding Impaired wound healing
Increased carbohydrate turnover	Hyperglycaemia Glycosuria Diminished carbohydrate tolerance Diabetes mellitus
Anti-inflammatory effects	Suppression of normal immunological responses Suppression of manifestations of infection Diminished resistance to infection Reactivation of latent infection Peptic ulceration
Salt and water retention	Oedema Cardiac failure Hypertension Hypokalaemia
Abnormal fat deposition	Facial roundness Buffalo hump Supraclavicular fat deposition Truncal obesity
Of uncertain origin	Habituation and dependence Euphoria Psychoses Mental depression Acne Leukocytosis Cataract Amenorrhoea Peripheral neuropathy

Suppression of pituitary–adrenal function

Undoubtedly the most serious long-term complication of corticosteroid therapy is suppression of the hypothalamic–pituitary–adrenal axis. Corticosteroid administration increases the plasma concentration of hydrocortisone or similar glucocorticoids, which suppresses the secretion of both corticotrophin-releasing factor by the hypothalamus and adrenocorticotrophic hormone (ACTH) by the anterior pituitary (Fig. 17.2). The decreased secretion of ACTH reduces the physiological release of hydrocortisone and corticosterone by the adrenal gland to negligible levels (although the secretion of aldosterone by the zona glomerulosa is little affected). Functional suppression of the hypothalamic–pituitary–adrenal axis may be followed by atrophy (particularly of adrenal cortical cells), which persists for a variable time (possibly as long as 3–12 months) after treatment is stopped. In consequence, when patients are stabilized on corticosteroids in doses greater than the normal physiological secretion rate (30–90 μmol, i.e. 11–33 mg hydrocortisone in 24 h), the sudden withdrawal of steroids is dangerous, since pituitary–adrenal function is suppressed and the adrenocortical response to stress may be impaired or defective. It is therefore important slowly to decrease corticosteroid dosage after chronic therapy, so that functional recovery of the hypothalamic–pituitary–adrenal axis can occur. The

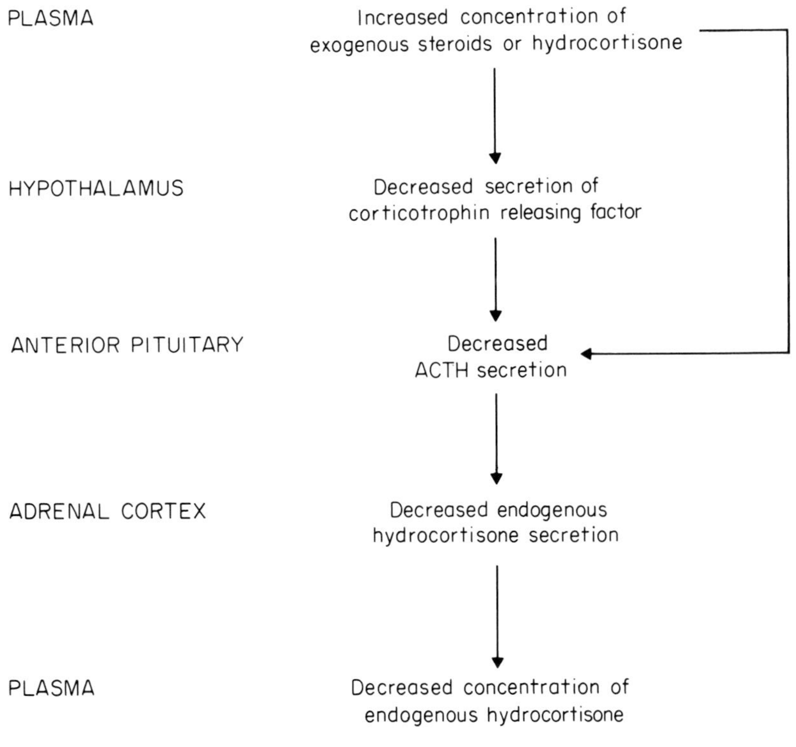

Fig. 17.2 The control of hydrocortisone secretion by the hypothalamic–pituitary–adrenal axis.

physiological integrity of the axis can be tested by the morning plasma hydrocortisone concentration or the response to insulin-induced hypoglycaemia, which normally causes a prompt increase in the physiological secretion of hydrocortisone.

Suppression of the hypothalamic–pituitary–adrenal axis by systemic corticosteroid therapy can be limited by various methods. These include:

1 The use of as low a steroid dose as possible for as short a period as possible.

2 Intermittent corticosteroid therapy.

3 The use of a single daily dose, given in the morning (in order to mimic the normal circadian rhythm of hydrocortisone secretion).

4 The use of a double dose on alternate mornings.

5 The use of ACTH or tetracosactrin.

ACTH is a polypeptide containing 39 amino acids; only part of the molecule (the first 24 amino acids) is identical in all mammalian species and is responsible for the biological effects of the hormone. The remaining amino acid sequence is not identical in all mammals (e.g. it is different in humans, pigs and cattle), and is responsible for the immunological specificity of ACTH. The hormone used in humans sometimes causes allergic and hypersensitivity reactions. Tetracosactrin only contains the biologically active part of the molecule (i.e. the first 24 amino acids), and hypersensitivity reactions are less likely, although they can occur. Both ACTH and tetracosactrin are available as depot preparations that are complexed with gelatin or zinc, and their action may last for 16–48 h.

Although they increase the secretion of hydrocortisone from the adrenal cortex, they suppress the production of corticotrophin-releasing factor and endogenous ACTH. These effects are only occasionally of clinical significance. ACTH and tetracosactrin increase the secretion of endogenous anabolic steroids from the adrenal cortex, and may be less likely to induce muscle atrophy, osteoporosis and retardation of growth during childhood than corticosteroids. Unfortunately, the adrenocortical response is variable, and the effectiveness of ACTH and tetracosactrin is also variable, since they can only increase the basal secretion of hydrocortisone 5–10 times (i.e. from 20 to 100–200 mg day^{-1}).

Normal hypothalamic, pituitary and adrenal function also plays an important role in the metabolic response to surgery. In a normal subject, the response to stress (including surgical operations and dental extraction) is complex; it may be influenced by the extent and nature of the surgical procedure, by drugs used during anaesthesia, and by other factors. One of the important metabolic responses to general anaesthesia and major surgery is an increase in the endogenous secretion of ACTH and hydrocortisone. The secretion rate of hydrocortisone may rise from 20–30 mg daily to 100–300 mg daily in response to operative stress, and remain elevated for a variable period after surgery. Aldosterone secretion is also increased. These responses are dependent on the integrity of the hypothalamic–pituitary–adrenal axis. In patients taking the equivalent of 30 mg hydrocortisone (or more) daily, the axis is partially or completely suppressed. Some adrenal suppression may persist for at least 2 months (and possibly longer) after corticosteroid therapy has been slowly reduced and stopped.

The degree of adrenal suppression and its duration depend on the dose and the duration of previous steroid therapy. In these conditions, the physiological increase in hydrocortisone secretion normally associated with surgical stress is partially obtunded or absent, and its absence may cause severe hypotension and cardiovascular collapse during surgery. In patients undergoing major surgical procedures, these complications can be prevented by the administration of hydrocortisone (100 mg 8-hourly, by intramuscular injection) on the day of surgery. This dose should be given to all patients on corticosteroids (or who have been on corticosteroids during the previous 3 months) on the day of major surgical procedures. Hydrocortisone sodium succinate must also be available during surgery. During the postoperative period, the dosage of steroids can be slowly reduced, and progressively replaced by the normal oral steroid therapy (if any). This process is usually complete by the third to fifth postoperative day. During and after adrenalectomy, a similar regime may be followed, and oral therapy (usually hydrocortisone and fludrocortisone) progressively introduced following surgery.

The use of corticosteroids during minor surgical procedures (or in patients whose steroid therapy has been stopped 3–12 months earlier) is less clearly defined. There is considerable evidence that the use of hydrocortisone on the day of surgery alone (either in three divided doses, or possibly as a single injection) provides ample protection against peripheral vascular collapse. Nevertheless, intravenous steroids should be available during surgery.

Hypoglycaemic agents

In diabetes mellitus, there is a relative or absolute deficiency of insulin. The disease may be due to the degeneration, destruction or exhaustion of the β cells of the islets of Langerhans, to the failure of tissues to respond to circulating insulin, or to the presence or excessive secretion of insulin antagonists (e.g. antibodies, ACTH, hydrocortisone and other corticosteroids, and possibly glucagon and somatostatin). The relative or absolute deficiency of insulin results in defective carbohydrate metabolism, hyperglycaemia and glycosuria; secondary effects on fat metabolism occur, resulting in the formation of ketones (aceto-acetate and β-hydroxybutyrate). Gluconeogenesis, i.e. the deamination of proteins and amino acids and their conversion to glucose, is also affected.

The aim of the treatment of diabetes mellitus is the correction of the immediate metabolic abnormalities and the prevention of long-term complications (e.g. retinopathy, nephropathy, neuropathy, hypercholesterolaemia, peripheral vascular damage) by the use of hypoglycaemic drugs. Current evidence suggests that most or all of these long-term complications can be prevented or avoided by the close control of blood glucose within physiological limits, using individualized treatment regimes.

Hypoglycaemic drugs can be divided into four groups:

1 Insulin and its derivatives.
2 Sulphonylureas and related drugs.
3 Biguanides.
4 α-Glucosidase inhibitors.

Insulin and its derivatives

Insulin is a polypeptide with a molecular weight of approximately 5800. It contains 51 amino acid residues, in two peptide chains (A and B), which are linked by two disulphide bridges (Fig. 17.3). The hormone is synthesized in the Golgi complex of β cells from a larger polypeptide (proinsulin), in which the A and B chains are linked by a larger fragment (the connector peptide or C-peptide). When insulin is released into the circulation in response to hyperglycaemia, the C-peptide is also released and can be measured separately. Although the C-peptide has no known function, it can be used to monitor insulin secretion.

Until the introduction of human insulins, all of the hormone used in the treatment of diabetes was extracted from the pancreas of pigs (porcine insulin) or cattle (bovine insulin), and purified by crystallization. There are minor differences in the amino acid sequences of these insulins and human insulin; thus, human insulin differs

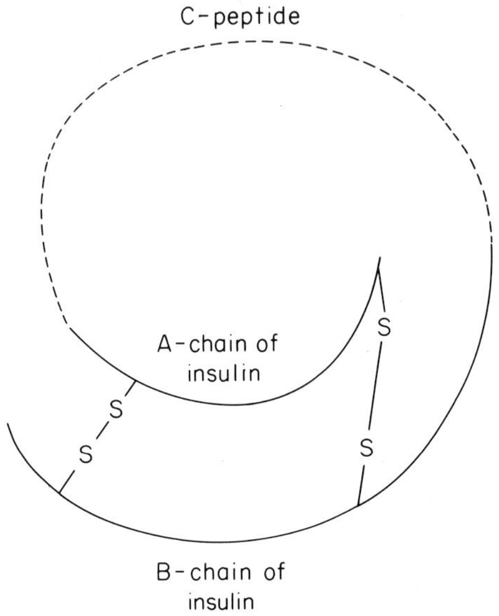

Fig. 17.3 Diagrammatic representation of the structure of pro-insulin. The A-chain and the B-chain of insulin (solid lines) are connected by disulphide bridges; C-peptide (broken line) is released from pro-insulin when it is converted to insulin.

from porcine insulin by one amino acid, and from bovine insulin by three amino acids. In impure preparations of porcine or bovine insulin, both proinsulin and the C-peptide may be present; in the past, subcutaneous injection of these impure crystallized insulins frequently gave rise to localized or generalized insulin allergy, insulin resistance or fat atrophy (lipodystrophy), which was often distressing and disfiguring. These are believed to be immunological reactions, which were mainly dependent on the species differences between proinsulins (particularly the C-peptide fragment). In recent years, their occurrence has been minimized by the use of highly purified preparations of porcine or bovine insulin, in which almost all the proinsulin and C-peptide impurities have been removed by gel filtration and ion-exchange chromatography. In the UK, all insulin preparations of animal origin are now highly purified, and immunological reactions are now relatively uncommon.

During the past 15 years, human insulins have been synthesized and used in the treatment of diabetes; approximately 80–90% of patients are now stabilized on the natural endogenous hormone. Human preparations of insulin are prepared semisynthetically, by the enzymic modification of porcine insulin (enzyme-modified porcine or emp insulin); alternatively they are made biosynthetically by *Escherichia coli* (prb insulin) or yeast organisms (pyr insulin), using recombinant DNA technology. The insulin requirement of diabetic patients is usually reduced by 10–15% when bovine insulin is replaced by human insulin; the requirement of patients stabilized on porcine insulin is usually unchanged. Hypoglycaemia may be commoner in patients stabilized on human insulin, since the hormone is commonly used in diabetic regimes that depend on the tight control of blood glucose concentrations.

Insulin lowers blood sugar by activating specific insulin receptors, which are widely present in many tissues, and are subject to up-regulation and down-regulation by the plasma concentration of the hormone. Insulin receptors are tetrameric glycoproteins, consisting of two α subunits linked by disulphide bonds to two β subunits; the two β subunits have inherent tyrosine kinase activity. When the extracellular α units are bound by insulin, the transmembrane β subunits are activated and their tyrosine residues are phosphorylated, enhancing their tyrosine kinase activity. Subsequent phosphorylation of several different intracellular proteins results in increased glucose uptake, which is mediated by specific glucose transport proteins. Glucose enters cells by facilitated diffusion (Chapter 1), where it is immediately phosphorylated by hexokinase to glucose-6-phosphate; insulin also has secondary effects on enzymes concerned with glycogen synthesis. Consequently, the storage of glucose as glycogen in liver and muscle is increased, and glycogenolysis is reduced. Insulin also stimulates the synthesis of fat; lipogenesis is increased, the concentration of most plasma lipids is decreased, and lipolysis is reduced. Similarly, protein synthesis from amino acids is enhanced, protein catabolism is diminished, and gluconeogenesis is reduced.

Endogenous insulin secretion is mainly dependent on the concentration of glucose in blood. In pancreatic islet β cells, glucose reduces potassium diffusion through adenosine triphosphate (ATP)-sensitive potassium channels (K_{ATP} channels); depolarization is prolonged and calcium entry through voltage-sensitive L-type channels is increased. In these conditions, insulin secretion is enhanced. It is also modified by amino acids, and by drugs that affect α- and β-adrenoceptors (Chapter 12). In the circulation, insulin has a short half-life (4–6 min); it is rapidly taken up by tissues and broken down by insulin-degrading enzymes (insulinases) in the liver, kidney and other organs.

Since insulin is a polypeptide, it is broken down in the gut and must be given by injection (subcutaneously, except in the treatment of hyperglycaemic coma). Insulin is injected into the arms, thighs or abdomen, and its absorption may be affected by the site of injection and local blood flow; consequently, absorption is increased by massage, local heat and physical exercise. It is usually given by disposable plastic syringes with prefixed or unfixed needles, although reusable glass syringes with disposable needles are sometimes used. Portable injection devices (pen injectors) which deliver a metered dose are also widely employed. Alternatively, soluble insulin can be given by continuous subcutaneous infusion, using a battery-operated portable pump. This technique provides a continuous basal infusion of soluble neutral insulin (with the option of differential infusion rates during the day and the night), and the use of supplementary bolus injections before the main meals. In spite of its disadvantages, diabetic control and the quality of life may be improved.

Neutral insulin is a buffered solution of soluble insulin (pH 7.0). It may be prepared from human insulin or highly purified animal insulins. After subcutaneous injection, it normally acts within 30–60 min; its maximum activity is from 2 to 4 h, and its action lasts for up to 8 h. Human neutral insulin preparations may have a more rapid onset of action, and a shorter duration of action (due to their enhanced aqueous solubility). Neutral insulin may be given intramuscularly and intravenously, as well as subcutaneously, and is the most suitable preparation for diabetic emergencies, and during the perioperative period. It is commonly mixed with longer-acting preparations of insulin, and is widely used in multiple injection regimes.

The duration of action of soluble neutral insulin can be prolonged by decreasing the solubility of insulin, and delaying its absorption after subcutaneous injection. This can be achieved by complexing the hormone with various proteins (e.g. protamine), or with zinc alone in specialized conditions (e.g. in insulin zinc suspensions). After subcutaneous injection, the insulin present in these preparations is released and absorbed at different rates, resulting in preparations with either an intermediate onset and long duration of action (maximum activity between 4 and 12 h); or a slower onset and long duration of action (maximum activity between 6 and 24 h).

The preparations that are commonly used in the UK are shown in Table 17.4. Preparations with an intermediate duration of action are usually given twice daily; those with a longer duration of action are given once daily. In general, they may be mixed with neutral insulin before injection. Protamine zinc insulin should not be

Table 17.4 Preparations of human and animal insulin in current use.

Type of preparation	Name of preparation		Subcutaneous injection: Onset of action (h)	Maximum activity (h)	Duration of action (h)
Short-acting	Neutral insulin (soluble insulin)	Human Actrapid (H) Human Velosulin (H) Humulin S (H) Pork Velosulin (P) Hypurin Neutral (B)	0.5	2–4	6–8
Intermediate-acting	Isophane insulin (NPH)*	Human Insulatard (H) Humulin I (H) Pork Insulatard (P) Hypurin Isophane (B)	2	4–12	18–24
	Biphasic insulin†	Human Mixtard 10, 20, 30, 40, 50 (H) Humulin M1, M2, M3, M4, M5 (H) Pork Mixtard 30/70 (P) Rapitard MC (P and B)	0.5	2–12	18–24
	Insulin zinc suspension (amorphous)	Semitard MC (P)	2	6–12	15–18
Long-acting	Insulin zinc suspension‡ (mixed)	Human Monotard (H) Humulin Lente (H) Lentard MC (P and B) Hypurin Lente (B)	3	6–15	18–24
	Insulin zinc suspension (crystalline)	Human Ultratard (H) Humulin Zn (H)	6	12–24	24–36
	Protamine zinc insulin	Hypurin protamine zinc (B)	6	12–24	24–36

* Neutral protamine Hagedorn (NPH) insulin.
† Biphasic insulin consists of a mixture of soluble and isophane insulin.
‡ A mixture of 30% amorphous and 70% crystalline insulin zinc suspension.
H, Human sequence insulin; P, porcine highly purified insulin; B, bovine highly purified insulin.

mixed with neutral soluble insulin before injection; however, this preparation is only rarely used.

Sulphonylureas and related drugs

The sulphonylureas initially lower blood glucose by increasing the secretion of insulin by functioning β cells in the islets of Langerhans. In experimental conditions, they cause degranulation of β cells; they also increase the number and cause hyperplasia of functioning β cells. Some sulphonylureas may also reduce the secretion of glucagon and decrease the activity of hepatic insulinase. During chronic administration, plasma insulin tends to decrease to pretreatment levels, although the hypoglycaemic effect is maintained; the explanation for this phenomenon is obscure.

The cellular effects of sulphonylureas are probably due to their actions on ATP-sensitive potassium channels in the cytoplasmic membrane of islet β cells. Sulphonylureas produce blockade of K_{ATP} channels, decreasing potassium permeability, resulting in membrane depolarization and delayed repolarization. In these conditions, Ca^{2+} entry is enhanced, resulting in increased insulin secretion.

Since sulphonylureas mainly act by enhancing the physiological secretion of insulin, their effects are dependent on the presence of functioning islet cells. Consequently, they are mainly used in patients with type II diabetes (i.e. maturity-onset, non-insulin-dependent diabetes) who are not controlled by diet alone. Sulphonylureas are of little value in insulin-dependent diabetes, in patients with ketosis or in subjects with an insulin requirement of more than 30 units per day.

The sulphonylureas are almost completely absorbed after oral administration. They are usually extensively metabolized in the liver (with the exception of chlorpropamide); some of their metabolites possess hypoglycaemic activity, but this is not usually of clinical significance. Most sulphonylureas are extensively bound to plasma proteins, and have a relatively short half-life (3–11 h) and a volume of distribution similar to extracellular fluid volume (200 ml kg^{-1}). Chlorpropamide, unlike other sulphonylureas, is partly eliminated unchanged in urine, and has a longer half-life (24–48 h). It may produce prolonged hypoglycaemia, particularly in elderly subjects and in patients with renal or hepatic disease.

The sulphonylureas may produce gastrointestinal side-effects (e.g. nausea, heartburn, anorexia, diarrhoea); hypersensitivity reactions (skin reactions, cholestatic jaundice, blood dyscrasias) occasionally occur. The chronic administration of some sulphonylureas (particularly tolbutamide and chlorpropamide) is associated with alcohol intolerance; genetically susceptible patients on these drugs may develop intense facial flushing due to vasodilatation on drinking alcohol. The hypoglycaemic effects of most sulphonylureas may be enhanced by some other drugs (phenylbutazone, salicylates, sulphonamides, probenecid, monoamine oxidase inhibitors, anticoagulants, clofibrate, β-adrenoceptor antagonists), and antagonized by others (thiazide diuretics and corticosteroids). Some sulphonylureas (e.g. glibenclamide) produce slight diuresis; others (e.g. chlorpropamide) can have slight antidiuretic effects, and have been used in the treatment of diabetes insipidus.

The sulphonylureas that are currently available in the UK are shown in Table 17.5.

Biguanides

Metformin is the only biguanide that is currently used in the treatment of diabetes.

Table 17.5 Sulphonylureas in current use as hypoglycaemic agents.

Drug	Proprietary name	Dose range (mg day^{-1})	Plasma half-life (h)	Elimination
Chlorpropamide	Diabinese	100–500	24–48	25% excreted unchanged; remainder metabolized
Glibenclamide	Daonil Euglucon	5–15	4–8	Mainly metabolized; some metabolites are active*
Gliclazide	Diamicron	40–320	9–13	Extensively metabolized; no active metabolites
Glipizide	Glibenese Minodiab	5–40	2–5	Extensively metabolized; no active metabolites
Gliquidone	Glurenorm	30–180	3–7	Extensively metabolized; no active metabolites
Tolazamide	Tolanase	100–1000	5–9	Extensively metabolized
Tolbutamide	Rastinon	1000–1500	3–7	Mainly metabolized to carboxytolbutamide (inactive)

* Active metabolites are not usually of clinical significance.

It has little or no effect on blood glucose in normal subjects, although it decreases insulin requirements in diabetes. Its mode of action is controversial. Although metformin decreases carbohydrate absorption from the small intestine and reduces hepatic gluconeogenesis, it may mainly act by increasing the peripheral uptake and metabolism of glucose by voluntary muscle. It also affects fat metabolism and lowers the plasma concentration of cholesterol, triglycerides and low-density lipoproteins.

Metformin is extensively absorbed from the small intestine and is eliminated unchanged in urine. Although it frequently produces gastrointestinal side-effects, the most serious complication is the occasional occurrence of lactic acidosis, which often has an insidious onset. Metformin may predispose to this condition by increasing lactate levels in blood, and its use in the elderly, in patients with renal or hepatic impairment or in alcoholic subjects may be particularly dangerous.

Nevertheless, metformin is occasionally used in patients with type II (non-insulin-dependent) diabetes who are not adequately controlled by diet and sulphonylurea drugs alone.

α-Glucosidase inhibitors

α-Glucosidase inhibitors reduce the intestinal absorption of polysaccharides and disaccharides by preventing their hydrolysis to monosaccharides by the enzyme α-glucosidase, which is present in the brush border of the small intestine. Inhibition of the enzyme slows the absorption of carbohydrates as monosaccharides and attenuates the normal postprandial increase in plasma glucose concentration by retarding the absorption of glucose from the small intestine.

Acarbose is the only α-glucosidase inhibitor that is currently used in the treatment of diabetes. In addition to inhibition of α-glucosidase, it also affects the activity of other enzyme systems concerned with the hydrolysis and absorption of carbohydrates. Acarbose may be combined with sulphonylureas in the treatment of type II (non-insulin-dependent) diabetes; in these conditions, hypoglycaemia should be prevented or treated with the monosaccharide dextrose (grape sugar) rather than the disaccharide sucrose (cane or beet sugar). Although acarbose is not significantly absorbed from the gut, it may cause an increase in the fermentation of unabsorbed carbohydrates. Consequently, abdominal distension, eructation and flatulence are not uncommon.

Hypoglycaemic drugs and general anaesthesia

Surgical procedures in diabetic patients are associated with an increased morbidity and mortality. Diabetic subjects are a high-risk group of surgical patients who are more likely to develop several postoperative problems, including metabolic and electrolyte abnormalities, cardiovascular sequelae, infection and delayed wound healing. Management of the disease in the perioperative period is complicated by several factors (e.g. altered calorie intake, the metabolic response to stress and the effects of procedures and agents that are used during anaesthesia). The metabolic response to stress is particularly difficult to assess and varies considerably in different patients. Unfortunately, some diabetic patients may not be recognized or detected prior to surgery; the presence of glycosuria should always be excluded (or a fasting blood glucose determined) in all patients before any operative procedure.

In normal circumstances, surgical stress causes a rise in the metabolic rate, changes in carbohydrate, fat and protein metabolism and the increased urinary elimination of nitrogen, phosphorus, potassium and calcium. The secretion of many pituitary hormones (e.g. antidiuretic hormone, ACTH, growth hormone, prolactin) and adrenal hormones (adrenaline, aldosterone, hydrocortisone) is increased. Surgical stress also affects the secretion of pancreatic hormones; glucagon levels are increased, and may be raised for several days. By contrast, insulin secretion is normal or decreased during surgery, despite the presence of hyperglycaemia. It is generally accepted that the normal or reduced insulin levels are due to changes in the plasma concentration of endogenous catecholamines (mainly adrenaline). In the postoperative period insulin secretion rises, although hyperglycaemia is sustained (possibly due to enhanced gluconeogenesis). These metabolic changes are related to the extent and duration of surgery. They are slight and unimportant during minor procedures, but are enhanced during major surgery, particularly when complicated by shock or infection.

The management of diabetic patients during anaesthesia and surgery is aimed at the prevention of intraoperative or postoperative hypoglycaemia, and the avoidance of excessive metabolic responses or decompensation. Many regimes have been proposed and used for this purpose, and the management of diabetes during surgery has been a matter of some controversy. Ideally, the use of insulin should reflect the physiological changes in secretion that occur during surgical procedures in non-diabetic subjects.

It is generally accepted that patients who are controlled by diet alone, or who are stabilized on low doses of short-acting sulphonylureas do not require additional therapy during minor surgical procedures. The morning dose of the sulphonylurea should be omitted on the day of surgery. Small amounts of intravenous glucose may be required preoperatively, depending on the blood glucose concentration. Patients stabilized on chlorpropamide should probably be admitted to hospital several days prior to surgery and stabilized on insulin, given twice or three times daily (particularly if diabetic control is poor or major surgery is contemplated). Similarly, metformin may be stopped and changed to insulin before surgery, in order to prevent the possibility of intraoperative hypoglycaemia and lactic acidosis. The aim of these procedures is to ensure that diabetic patients are well-controlled, normoglycaemic, non-ketotic and have adequate glycogen reserves prior to surgery.

In the past, several different regimes have been used for the administration of insulin and the control of blood glucose levels during surgery and the perioperative period. One common method involved the administration of half the daily insulin requirement subcutaneously on the morning of surgery, followed by the infusion of sufficient dextrose to maintain normoglycaemia (or slight hyperglycaemia). It is now recognized, particularly when patients are undergoing major surgical procedures, that these regimes are less satisfactory than methods that depend on the intravenous infusion of insulin, and the monitoring of its effects on blood glucose. In diabetic patients stabilized on insulin who are undergoing major surgical procedures, mixed intravenous infusions of glucose, insulin and potassium salts are now widely used during the perioperative period. One common regime is based on the addition of neutral insulin (usually 16–20 units) and potassium chloride (10 mmol) to each unit of dextrose (10%), which is then infused at the rate of 100 ml h^{-1}. This regime can be modified if hyperglycaemia is marked, or if fluid restriction is necessary. Although there is no danger of patients receiving insulin alone, some may be absorbed by glass or by plastic. Alternatively, insulin and dextrose (with potassium chloride) can be separately infused; the rate of insulin infusion (usually 1–3 units h^{-1}) is controlled by frequent blood glucose determinations. Sufficient potassium is added to maintain its plasma concentration within normal limits (3.5–5.0 mmol l^{-1}).

In the postoperative period, there is commonly an increased insulin requirement (particularly if infection or other complications occur), and a moderate degree of hyperglycaemia is not unusual; frequent monitoring of blood glucose may be needed to prevent the development of decompensation or ketosis. Infusion of intravenous fluids containing glucose, insulin and potassium salts may be continued for several days, while normal feeding is gradually established. As soon as the patient can take food or fluids orally, normal antidiabetic drug therapy can be resumed. Emergency surgery (particularly in the uncontrolled or ketotic diabetic patient) presents particular problems; it is generally accepted that ketosis and abnormal fluid balance must be controlled before anaesthesia is induced.

It should be emphasized that the optimum control of diabetic patients during surgery depends on the frequent measurement of blood glucose (and potassium) concentrations. Blood glucose can be rapidly determined on the ward or in theatre by semiquantitative methods (i.e. glucose testing strips with a glucose meter) which provide a reasonably accurate assessment of the metabolic state. Most authorities consider that the determination of glucose in urine during the perioperative period is an extremely misleading guide, since the blood glucose may be changing rapidly. Although certain anaesthetics (e.g. ether, cyclopropane) can cause hyperglycaemia, most agents in current use (including nitrous oxide, fluorinated agents, intravenous barbiturates, opioid analgesics and all muscle relaxants) have little or no effect on blood glucose. Nevertheless, other drugs that may be used before, during or after surgery (e.g. ketamine, diazoxide, adrenaline, trimetaphan, β-adrenoceptor antagonists, corticosteroids) may significantly modify blood glucose levels. β-Adrenoceptor antagonists are particularly hazardous, since they may induce hypoglycaemia and obscure all its peripheral clinical signs.

Increased secretion of endogenous adrenaline may cause marked hyperglycaemia in the unpremedicated, nervous and excitable patient. Similarly, hypoxia and hypercarbia increase adrenaline secretion, and may cause a considerable rise in blood glucose concentration.

Further reading

Adams R, Siderius N. Postoperative acute adrenal cortical insufficiency. *Journal of the American Medical Association* 1957; **165**: 41–44.

Alberti KGMM. Diabetic emergencies. *British Medical Bulletin* 1989; **45**: 242–263.

Alberti KGMM, Thomas DJB. The management of diabetes during surgery. *British Journal of Anaesthesia* 1979; **51**: 693–710.

Allison SP. Changes in insulin secretion during open-heart surgery. *British Journal of Anaesthesia* 1971; **43**: 138–143.

Bailey CJ. Biguanides and NIDDM. *Diabetes Care* 1992; **15**: 755–772.

Bayliss RIS. Surgical collapse during and after corticosteroid therapy. *British Medical Journal* 1958; **2**: 935–936.

Bowen DJ, Daykin AP, Nanciekievill ML, Norman J. Insulin-dependent diabetic patients during surgery and labour. *Anaesthesia* 1984; **39**: 407–411.

Bressler R, Johnson D. New pharmacological approaches to therapy of NIDDM. *Diabetes Care* 1992; **15**: 792–805.

Burke CW. Adrenocortical insufficiency. *Clinics in Endocrinology and Metabolism* 1985; **14**: 947–976.

Byyny RL. Management of diabetes during surgery. *Postgraduate Medicine* 1980; **68**: 191–202.

Cheatham B, Kahn CR. Insulin action and the insulin signaling network. *Endocrinological Reviews* 1995; **16**: 117–142.

Chou CK, Dull TJ, Russell DS *et al*. Human insulin receptors mutated at the ATP-binding site lack protein tyrosine kinase activity and fail to mediate postreceptor effects of insulin. *Journal of Biological Chemistry* 1987; **262**: 1842–1847.

Christiansen CL, Schurizek BA, Malling B, Knudsen L, Alberti KGMM, Hermansen K. Insulin treatment of the insulin-dependent diabetic patient undergoing minor surgery — continuous intravenous infusion compared with subcutaneous administration. *Anaesthesia* 1988; **43**: 533–537.

Chrousos GP. The hypothalamic–pituitary–adrenal axis and immune-mediated inflammation. *New England Journal of Medicine* 1995; **332**: 1351–1362.

Clarke RSJ. Anaesthesia and carbohydrate metabolism. *British Journal of Anaesthesia* 1973; **45**: 237–243.

Davis SN, Thompson C, Brown MD, Home PD, Alberti KGMM. A comparison of the pharmacokinetics and metabolic effects of human regular and NPH insulin mixtures. *Diabetes Research and Clinical Practice* 1991; **13**: 107–117.

Diethelm AG. Surgical management of complications of steroid therapy. *Annals of Surgery* 1977; **185**: 251–263.

Diltoer M, Camu F. Glucose homeostasis and insulin secretion during isoflurane anesthesia in humans. *Anesthesiology* 1988; **68**: 880–886.

Dunnet JM, Holman RR, Turner RC, Sear JW. Diabetes mellitus and anaesthesia — a survey of the perioperative management of the patient with diabetes mellitus. *Anaesthesia* 1988; **43**: 538–542.

Dunnett SR. Insulin infusion pump. *British Medical Journal* 1985; **291**: 1808–1809.

Feiwel M, James VHT, Barnett ES. Effect of potent topical steroids on plasma cortisol levels of infants and children with eczema. *Lancet* 1969; **i**: 485–487.

Ferner RE, Neil HAW. Sulfonylureas and hypoglycaemia. *British Medical Journal* 1988; **296**: 949–950.

Fletcher J, Langman MJS, Kellock TD. Effect of surgery on blood sugar levels in diabetes mellitus. *Lancet* 1965; **ii**: 52–54.

Flower RJ. Lipocortin and the mechanism of action of the glucocorticoids. *British Journal of Pharmacology* 1988; **94**: 987–1015.

Fraser CG, Preuss FS, Bigford WD. Adrenal atrophy and irreversible shock associated with cortisone therapy. *Journal of the American Medical Association* 1952; **149**: 1542–1543.

Galloway JA, Shuman CR. Diabetes and surgery. A study of 667 cases. *American Journal of Medicine* 1963; **34**: 177–191.

Gill GV, Alberti KGMM. Surgery and diabetes. *Hospital Update* 1989; **5**: 327–336.

Hall GM. Diabetes and anaesthesia — a promise unfulfilled? *Anaesthesia* 1984; **39**: 627–628.

Hall GM. The anaesthetic modification of the endocrine and metabolic response to surgery. *Annals of the Royal College of Surgeons* 1985; **67**: 25–29.

Hall GM, Desborough JP. Diabetes and anaesthesia — slow progress. *Anaesthesia* 1988; **43**: 531–532.

Halter JB, Pflug AE. Effects of anaesthesia and surgical stress on insulin secretion in man. *Metabolism* 1980; **29**: 1124–1127.

Hermann LS, Schersten B, Bitzen PO, Kjellstrom T, Lindgarde F, Melander A. Therapeutic comparison of metformin and sulfonylurea, alone and in various combinations. *Diabetes Care* 1994; **17**: 1100–1109.

Hertzberg LB, Shulman MS. Acute adrenal insufficiency in a patient with appendicitis during anesthesia. *Anesthesiology* 1985; **62**: 517–519.

James ML. Endocrine disease and anaesthesia: a review of anaesthetic management in pituitary, adrenal and pituitary diseases. *Anaesthesia* 1970; **25**: 232–252.

Jarrett RJ, Keen H. Oral hypoglycaemic drugs. *British Journal of Hospital Medicine* 1974; **11**: 265–267.

Kahn CR. Banting lecture. Insulin action, diabetogenes, and the cause of type II diabetes. *Diabetes* 1994; **43**: 1066–1084.

Kahn CR, White MF. The insulin receptor and the molecular mechanism of insulin action. *Journal of Clinical Investigation* 1988; **82**: 1151–1156.

Keen H, Jarrett J. Modern management of diabetes. *Medicine* 1978; **11**: 530–536.

Kehlet H. A rational approach to dosage and preparation of parenteral glucocorticoid substitution therapy during surgical procedures. *Acta Anaesthesiologica Scandinavica* 1975; **19**: 260–264.

Kehlet H, Binder C. Adrenocortical function and clinical course during and after surgery in unsupplemented glucocorticoid-treated patients. *British Journal of Anaesthesia* 1973; **45**: 1043–1048.

Lacoumenta S, Yeo TH, Burrin JM, Paterson JL, Hall GM. The effects of cortisol supplementation on the metabolic and hormonal response to surgery. *Clinical Physiology* 1987; **7**: 455–464.

Leslie RDG, Mackay JD. Intravenous insulin infusion in diabetic emergencies. *British Medical Journal* 1978; **2**: 1343–1344.

MacKenzie CR, Charlson ME. Assessment of perioperative risk in the patient with diabetes mellitus. *Surgery, Gynecology and Obstetrics* 1988; **167**: 293–299.

Munck A, Guyre PM, Holbrook NJ. Physiological functions of glucocorticoids in stress and their relation to pharmacological actions. *Endocrinological Reviews* 1984; **5**: 25–44.

Nordenstrom J, Sonnenfeld T, Arner P. Characterization of insulin release after surgery. *Surgery* 1989; **105**: 28–35.

Oyama T. Endocrine responses to anaesthetic agents. *British Journal of Anaesthesia* 1973; **45**: 276–281.

Oyama T, Takiguchi M. Prediction of adrenal hypofunction in anaesthesia. *Canadian Anaesthetists Society Journal* 1972; **19**: 239–249.

Page MMcB, Watkins PJ. Cardiorespiratory arrest and diabetic autonomic neuropathy. *Lancet* 1978; **i**: 14–16.

Philipson LH, Steiner DF. Pas de deux or more: the sulfonylurea receptor and K^+ channels. *Science* 1995; **268**: 372–373.

Pilkis SJ, Granner DK. Molecular physiology of the regulation of hepatic gluconeogenesis and glycolysis. *Annual Review of Physiology* 1992; **54**: 885–909.

Plumpton FS, Besser GM, Cole PV. Corticosteroid treatment and surgery. *Anaesthesia* 1969; **24**: 3–18.

Rees GAD, Hayes TM, Pearson JF. Diabetes, pregnancy and anaesthesia. *Clinics in Obstetrics and Gynaecology* 1982; **9**: 311–331.

Ringold GM. Steroid hormone regulation of gene expression. *Annual Review of Pharmacology and Toxicology* 1985; **25**: 529–566.

Salam AA, Davies DM. Acute adrenal insufficiency during surgery. *British Journal of Anaesthesia* 1974; **46**: 619–622.

Salassa RM, Bennett WA, Keating FR, Sprague RG. Postoperative adrenal cortical insufficiency: occurrence in patients previously treated with cortisone. *Journal of the American Medical Association* 1953; **152**: 1509–1515.

Sampson PA, Brooke BN, Winstone NE. Biochemical confirmation of collapse due to adrenal failure. *Lancet* 1961; **i**: 1377.

Sampson PA, Winstone NE, Brooke BN. Adrenal function in surgical patients after steroid failure. *Lancet* 1962; **ii**: 322–325.

Schleimer RP. The mechanisms of anti-inflammatory steroid action in allergic diseases. *Annual Review of Pharmacology and Toxicology* 1985; **25**: 381–412.

Simpson IA, Cushman SW. Hormonal regulation of mammalian glucose transport. *Annual Reviews of Biochemistry* 1986; **55**: 1059–1089.

Slaney G, Brooke BN. Postoperative collapse due to adrenal insufficiency following cortisone therapy. *Lancet* 1957; **i**: 1167–1170.

Symreng T, Karlberg BE, Kagedal B, Schildt B. Physiological cortisol substitution of long-term steroid-treated patients undergoing major surgery. *British Journal of Anaesthesia* 1981; **53**: 949–959.

Thomas DJB, Platt HS, Alberti KGMM. Insulin-dependent diabetes during the peri-operative period. An assessment of continuous glucose–insulin–potassium infusion, and traditional treatment. *Anaesthesia* 1984; **39**: 629–637.

Uchida I, Asoh T, Shirasaka C, Tsuji H. Effect of epidural analgesia on postoperative insulin resistance as evaluated by insulin clamp technique. *British Journal of Surgery* 1988; **75**: 557–562.

White MF, Kahn CR. The insulin signaling system. *Journal of Biological Chemistry* 1994; **269**: 1–4.

Wright PD, Henderson K, Johnston IDA. Glucose utilisation and insulin secretion during surgery in man. *British Journal of Surgery* 1974; **61**: 5–8.

Glossary

The glossary contains most of the common abbreviations used in the book. The mathematical symbols used in Chapters 2 and 3 are defined separately. Common chemical symbols (e.g. H^+, K^+, Na^+ and Ca^{2+}) have not been included.

Units of length, mass, volume and time

m	metre
mm	millimetre
μm	micrometre (micron)
nm	nanometre
g	gram
kg	kilogram
μg	microgram
mg	milligram
l	litre
ml	millilitre
h	hour
ms	millisecond
min	minute
s	second

Other abbreviations

AChE	acetylcholinesterase
ACTH	adrenocorticotrophic hormone
ADH	antidiuretic hormone
AMP	adenosine monophosphate
ATP	adenosine triphosphate
AV	atrioventricular
B.P.	British Pharmacopoeia
BP	blood pressure
b.p.m.	beats per minute
CCK	cholecystokinin
CGRP	calcitonin-gene–related peptide
ChE	cholinesterase
CNS	central nervous system
COMT	catechol-*O*-methyltransferase
COX	cyclooxygenase
CSF	cerebrospinal fluid
CTZ	chemoreceptor trigger zone
δ-ALA	delta-aminolaevulinic acid
Da	Dalton
EC	excitation–contraction
ECG	electrocardiogram
ED_{50}	median effective dose
EEG	electroencephalogram
ENT	ear, nose and throat
GABA	γ-aminobutyric acid
GH	growth hormone
GMP	guanosine monophosphate
GTP	guanosine triphosphate
G6PD	glucose-6-phosphate dehydrogenase
^3H	tritium labelled
5-HT	5-hydroxytryptamine
Hz	Hertz (a frequency of 1 stimulus per second)
ICP	Intracranial pressure
IgE	immunoglobulin E
IgG	immunoglobulin G
i.m.	intramuscular
iu	international unit
i.v.	intravenous
IVRA	intravenous regional analgesia
kPa	kilopascals (1 kilopascal = 7.5 mmHg)
LD_{50}	median lethal dose
MAC	minimum alveolar concentration
MAOI	monoamine oxidase inhibitors
MHPG	3-methoxy-4-hydroxy-phenylethylene-glycol
MSH	melanocyte stimulating hormone

mV	millivolt
NADPH	reduced nicotinamide adenine dinucleotide phosphate
NGF	nerve growth factor
NSAID	non-steroidal anti-inflammatory drug
$P\text{co}_2$	carbon dioxide tension
$P\text{aco}_2$	carbon dioxide tension in arterial blood
$P\text{ao}_2$	oxygen tension in arterial blood
pH	$-\log_{10}[H^+]$
$\text{p}K_a$	dissociation constant, negative logarithm of
PAG	periaqueductal grey matter
PG	prostaglandin
p.p.m.	parts per million
PRA	plasma renin activity
RNA	ribonucleic acid
SA	sino-atrial
s.c.	subcutaneous
sp. gr.	specific gravity
$t_{1/2}$	half-life
t.d.s.	thrice daily
TX	thromboxane
u	unit
UDP	uridine diphosphate
V	volume
v/v	volume for volume
VMA	3-methoxy-4-hydroxy-mandelic acid (vanillylmandelic acid)

Greek letters

α	alpha
β	beta
γ	gamma
δ	delta
ε	epsilon
κ	kappa
λ	lambda
μ	mu
π	pi
ρ	rho
σ	sigma

Symbols

≈	approximately equals
∝	is proportional to
≡	is congruent to

Index